THE AMERICAN ACADEMY OF ORTHOPAEDIC SURGEONS

Instructional
Course
Lectures

Volume XXXV 1986

THE AMERICAN ACADEMY OF ORTHOPAEDIC SURGEONS

Instructional Course Lectures

Volume XXXV 1986

Edited by

Lewis D. Anderson, M.D.

Professor and Chairman,
Department of Orthopaedic Surgery,
College of Medicine,
University of South Alabama,
Mobile, Alabama

With 565 illustrations

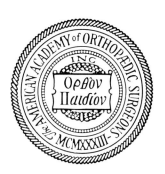

The C. V. Mosby Company

ST. LOUIS • WASHINGTON, D.C. • TORONTO   1986

MOSBY

A TRADITION OF PUBLISHING EXCELLENCE

Editor: Eugenia A. Klein
Developmental editor: Kathryn H. Falk
Project editor: Sylvia B. Kluth
Manuscript editor: John A. Rogers
Book design: Staff
Production: Florence Fansher

Volume XXXV

Printed in the United States of America

International Standard Book Number 0-8016-0104-5
Library of Congress Catalog Card Number 43-17054

The C.V. Mosby Company
11830 Westline Industrial Drive, St. Louis, Missouri 63146

T/MV/MV   9 8 7 6 5 4 3 2 1   11/A/136

Contributors

James Aronson, M.D.

Assistant Professor,
Children's Trauma and Reconstructive Surgery,
Department of Orthopaedic Surgery,
University of Arkansas for Medical Sciences,
Little Rock, Arkansas

Yoram Ben-Menachem, M.D.

Professor of Radiology,
Baylor University College of Medicine,
Attending Radiologist, Ben Taub General
Hospital and Staff Radiologist,
V.A.M.C. Hospital,
Houston, Texas

James B. Bennett, M.D.

Associate Professor of Orthopaedic Surgery,
Baylor University College of Medicine,
Houston, Texas

J. Dennis Bobyn, Ph.D.

Research Director,
Anderson Orthopaedic Research Institute,
Arlington, Virginia

Robert E. Booth, Jr., M.D.

Associate Professor of Orthopaedic Surgery,
University of Pennsylvania,
Philadelphia, Pennsylvania

Barry D. Brause, M.D.

Clinical Associate Professor of Medicine,
Cornell University Medical College,
Infectious Disease Consultant,
The Hospital for Special Surgery,
The New York Hospital,
New York, New York

Bruce D. Browner, M.D.

Associate Professor of Orthopaedic Surgery,
University of Texas Health Science Center,
Houston, Texas

Richard S. Bryan, M.D.

Professor of Orthopaedic Surgery,
Mayo Medical School,
Rochester, Minnesota

John J. Callaghan, M.D.

Former Fellow in Hip Surgery,
Former Instructor of Orthopaedic Surgery,
The Hospital for Special Surgery,
Cornell University Medical College,
New York, New York;
Attending in Orthopaedic Surgery,
Walter Reed Army Medical Center,
Washington, D.C.

William N. Capello, M.D.

Associate Professor of Orthopaedic Surgery,
Indiana University School of Medicine,
Indianapolis, Indiana

Guy L. Clifton, M.D.

Associate Professor,
Division of Neurological Surgery,
Medical College of Virginia,
Virginia Commonwealth University,
Richmond, Virginia

Dennis K. Collis, M.D.

Assistant Clinical Professor of
Orthopaedic Surgery,
University of Oregon,
Eugene, Oregon

Ralph W. Coonrad, M.D.

Associate Clinical Professor of
Orthopaedic Surgery,
Duke University School of Medicine,
Durham, North Carolina

Roy D. Crowninshield, Ph.D.

Vice President, Research
Orthopaedic Implant Division,
Zimmer, Inc., Warsaw, Indiana

Eugene J. Dabezies, M.D.

Professor of Orthopaedic Surgery,
Louisiana State University School of Medicine,
New Orleans, Louisiana

Robert D'Ambrosia, M.D.

Professor and Chairman,
Department of Orthopaedic Surgery,
Louisiana State University
School of Medicine,
New Orleans, Louisiana

Charles A. Engh, M.D.

Assistant Professor of Orthopaedic Surgery,
Georgetown University,
Washington, D.C.;
National Hospital for
Orthopedics and Rehabilitation,
Arlington, Virginia

Frederick C. Ewald, M.D.

Associate Clinical Professor of
Orthopaedic Surgery,
Harvard Medical School,
Boston, Massachusetts

Victor H. Frankel, M.D.

Chairman of Orthopaedic Surgery,
Hospital of Joint Diseases,
Orthopaedic Institute,
New York, New York

Gerard Gabel, M.D.

Resident, Former Research Fellow,
Division of Orthopaedic Surgery,
Baylor College of Medicine,
Houston, Texas

Ramon B. Gustilo, M.D.

Chief, Department of Orthopaedics,
Hennepin County Medical Center,
Professor of Orthopaedic Surgery,
University of Minnesota,
Minneapolis, Minnesota

Warren G. Harding III, M.D.

Clinical Instructor,
College of Medicine,
University of Cincinnati Medical Center,
Cincinnati, Ohio

Kevin D. Harrington, M.D.

Clinical Associate Professor of
Orthopaedic Surgery,
University of California,
San Francisco, California

William H. Harris, M.D.

Clinical Professor of Orthopaedic Surgery;
Chief, Hip and Implant Surgery,
Department of Orthopaedic Surgery,
Harvard Medical School,
Massachusetts General Hospital,
Boston, Massachusetts

David A. Heck, M.D.

Assistant Professor,
Department of Orthopaedic Surgery,
Indiana University Medical Center,
Indianapolis, Indiana

Robert S. Heidt, Jr., M.D.

Clinical Instructor,
University of Cincinnati Medical Center,
Cincinnati, Ohio

Robert S. Heidt, M.D.

Assistant Clinical Professor,
University of Cincinnati Medical Center,
Cincinnati, Ohio

Duane M. Ilstrup, M.S.

Statistician,
Section of Medical Research Statistics,
Mayo Clinic,
Rochester, Minnesota

John N. Insall, M.D.

Attending Orthopaedic Surgeon,
The Hospital for Special Surgery, and
The New York Hospital;
Professor of Orthopaedic Surgery,
Cornell University Medical College; and
Director of the Knee Service,
The Hospital for Special Surgery,
New York, New York

Richard C. Johnston, M.D.

Professor of Orthopaedic Surgery,
University of Iowa,
Des Moines, Iowa

Herbert Kaufer, M.D.

Professor of Orthopaedic Surgery,
University of Michigan,
Ann Arbor, Michigan

Donald B. Kettlekamp, M.D.

Associate Dean,
Texas Tech University Health Sciences,
Regional Academic Health Center at El Paso,
School of Medicine, El Paso, Texas

Andrew King, M.D.

Associate Professor of Orthopaedic Surgery,
Louisiana State University School of Medicine,
New Orleans, Louisiana

Kenneth A. Krackow, M.D.

Associate Professor,
The Johns Hopkins University,
School of Medicine,
Department of Orthopaedic Surgery,
Baltimore, Maryland

S. Michael Lawhon, M.D.

Clinical Instructor,
University of Cincinnati Medical Center,
Cincinnati, Ohio

Jack E. Lemons, Ph.D.

Professor,
Departments of Biomaterials, Biomedical
and Materials Engineering, Surgery and
Public Health,
The University of Alabama Schools of Medicine
and Dentistry, and the University of Alabama
at Birmingham, Birmingham, Alabama

Emile LeTournel, M.D.

Professor of Orthopaedic Surgery,
Centre Chirurgicaldelo Porte De Choisy,
Paris, France

L.C. Lucas, Ph.D.

Associate Professor,
Departments of Biomedical Engineering,
Biomaterials and Materials Engineering,
The University of Alabama at Birmingham,
Birmingham, Alabama

Roger A. Mann, M.D.

Associate Clinical Professor of Orthopaedic
Surgery,
University of California,
San Francisco, California

Joel M. Matta, M.D.

Assistant Professor,
Department of Orthopaedics,
University of Southern California,
School of Medicine, Los Angeles, California

Larry S. Matthews, M.D.

Professor of Orthopaedic Surgery,
University of Michigan, Ann Arbor, Michigan

Paul R. Meyer, Jr., M.D.

Professor of Orthopaedic Surgery,
Northwestern University Medical School;
Director, Acute Spine Injury Center,
Northwestern Memorial Hospital,
Chicago, Illinois

Edward H. Miller, M.D.

Clinical Professor of Orthopaedic Surgery,
University of Cincinnati;
Associate Director,
The Bone and Joint Institute,
The Christ Hospital, Cincinnati, Ohio

Bernard F. Morrey, M.D.

Associate Professor of Orthopaedic Surgery,
Mayo Medical School, Rochester, Minnesota

William R. Murray, M.D.

Professor and Chairman,
Department of Orthopaedic Surgery,
University of California, School of Medicine,
San Francisco, California

Carl L. Nelson, M.D.

Professor and Chairman;
Head, Section of Reconstructive Surgery,
University of Arkansas for Medical Sciences,
Little Rock, Arkansas

P.C. Noble, M.S.

Research Assistant Professor,
Baylor College of Medicine,
Houston, Texas

Paul M. Pellicci, M.D.

Assistant Attending Surgeon,
The Hospital for Special Surgery,
Cornell University Medical College,
New York, New York

Lowell F.A. Peterson, M.D.

Professor of Orthopaedic Surgery,
Mayo Medical School, Rochester, Minnesota

Robert Poss, M.D.

Associate Professor of Orthopaedic Surgery,
Harvard Medical School,
Brigham and Women's Hospital,
Boston, Massachusetts

James A. Rand, M.D.

Assistant Professor of Orthopaedic Surgery,
Mayo Medical School, Rochester, Minnesota

Eduardo A. Salvati, M.D.

Chief of Hip Clinic,
The Hospital for Special Surgery,
Clinical Professor of Orthopaedic Surgery,
Cornell University Medical College;
Attending Orthopaedic Surgeon,
The Hospital for Special Surgery,
The New York Hospital,
New York, New York

Douglas Shepard, M.D.

Former Fellow,
Division of Orthopaedic Surgery,
Baylor College of Medicine,
Houston, Texas;
Attending Orthopaedic Surgeon,
Memorial Medical Center, and
Driscoll Hospital,
Corpus Christi, Texas

Mack A. Thomas, M.D.

Chief, Anesthesiology VA Medical Center,
New Orleans, Louisiana;
Clinical Associate Professor,
Department of Anesthesiology and Surgery,
Louisiana School of Medicine,
New Orleans, Louisiana

Donald D. Trunkey, M.D.

Chairman and Professor,
Department of Surgery,
Oregon Health Sciences University,
Portland, Oregon

Hugh S. Tullos, M.D.

Head, Division of Orthopaedic Surgery,
Baylor College of Medicine,
Houston, Texas

Michael C. Welch, M.D.

Assistant Clinical Professor of
Orthopaedic Surgery,
University of Cincinnati,
Cincinnati, Ohio;
Attending Surgeon,
Joint Replacement Center,
The Christ Hospital Bone and Joint Institute,
Cincinnati, Ohio

Kaye E. Wilkins, M.D.

Associate Professor of Pediatrics,
Orthopaedics and Pediatrics,
University of Health Science Center
of San Antonio,
San Antonio, Texas

Philip D. Wilson, Jr., M.D.

Surgeon-in-Chief,
The Hospital for Special Surgery,
Professor of Surgery (Orthopaedics),
Cornell University Medical College,
New York, New York

Karl Zweymüller, M.D.

Assistant Professor,
Department of Orthopaedic Surgery,
Orthopaedic University,
Clinic of Vienna,
A-1090-Vienna, Austria

Preface

The first Instructional Course Lectures Series was organized by James E.M. Thompson, M.D. and presented at the 10th Annual Meeting of the American Academy of Orthopaedic Surgeons in 1942. From its inception, The Instructional Course Lectures have been recognized as one of the most important and authoritative instruments that we have for orthopaedic education, both at the level of the resident and at that of the practicing orthopaedist.

Volume 35 of the American Academy of Orthopaedic Surgeons Instructional Course Lectures was prepared during 1985 from selected courses presented at the 52nd Annual Meeting of the American Academy of Orthopaedic Surgeons in Las Vegas in January of 1985. Each of the chapters in this volume was among the 119 Instructional Courses presented in 1985 and was selected for inclusion because of its timeliness and importance to current orthopaedic knowledge.

There are a variety of topics covered in Volume 35, but the emphasis of the volume is on total hip and total knee replacement. The committee thinks the emphasis is timely and important, especially as it relates to planning the operation, new techniques and materials, and complications.

Each of the authors in the volume has a proven track record in his special field. Of course, not all authors agree, but this is to be expected. Also, in selecting chapters we attempt to achieve a balance between what is established and well proven and what is new, fresh, and appealing. We hope that this balance has been realized in Volume 35.

I would like to thank the essayists for their contribution of excellent chapters to this volume. I would also like to thank the members of the Committee on Instructional Courses for their many hours of hard work, without which the Instructional Course Lectures of the American Academy of Orthopaedic Surgeons 1985 and this Volume 35 would not be possible.

Lewis D. Anderson, M.D.

1985 Chairman
Committee on Instructional Courses

Committee Members:

Frank H. Bassett III, M.D.
Paul P. Griffin, M.D.
John A. Murray, M.D.
E. Shannon Stauffer, M.S.

Contents

BIOMECHANICS AND HIP JOINT TRAUMA

Chapter 1

Biomechanics of the hip joint

VICTOR H. FRANKEL

The normal hip joint allows for the wide range of motion required for such diverse activities as walking, sitting, bending, and squatting. To accomplish such activities without difficulty requires, however, that the acetabulum remain precisely aligned with the femoral head.

The hip joint bears large forces; a derangement of the ball-and-socket configuration can produce abnormal stresses throughout the joint cartilage and bone. Stresses and strains in the hip joint also can lead to degenerative arthritis, which, when coupled with the already large forces borne by the joint, may produce further damage to the hip.[2]

Hip joint motion occurs in all three planes, but it is greatest in the sagittal plane where flexion ranges up to 140 degrees and extension up to 15 degrees.[19] In the frontal plane abduction ranges up to 30 degrees, whereas adduction is slightly less, up to 25 degrees. In the transverse plane external rotation ranges up to 90 degrees, whereas internal rotation ranges up to 70 degrees, when the hip joint is flexed. Less rotation occurs during extension, however, as a result of the restrictive function of the soft tissues.

Johnson and Smidt,[16] using an electrogoniometer, studied hip joint motion in the frontal and transverse planes during the gait cycle (Fig. 1-1). It was found that in the frontal plane abduction occurs during the swing phase and reaches a peak just after toe off. The hip joint then reverses into adduction at heel strike and continues until late stance phase.

As age increases, the gait pattern changes considerably, demonstrating a diminished range of motion in the joints of the lower limb. One particular study[20] examined the walking patterns of 67 normal men of similar height and weight, ranging in age from 20 to 87 years. When the gait patterns of the younger and older men were compared, the differences in the sagittal position at heel strike of the two groups were dramatic (Fig. 1-2). The older men displayed shorter leg lengths, limited range of hip flexion and extension, decreased plantar flexion of the ankle, and a decreased heel-floor angle of elevation of the toe of the forward limb.

SURFACE JOINT MOTION

Surface motion in the hip joint may be viewed as the sliding of the femoral head on the acetabulum. This sliding of the joint surfaces is produced by the pivoting action of the ball-and-socket configuration in three planes around the center of rotation of the femoral head.[3] If incongruity occurs in the femoral head, with a displaced center of rotation, sliding may not be parallel or tangential to the surface, and the joint cartilage may be abnormally compressed or distracted, creating a plowlike action. An instant center analysis that would detect derangements in a joint such as the knee is not possible in the hip since motion occurs in all three planes simultaneously.

KINETICS

Large forces are imposed on the hip during simple, everyday activities. The balanced distribution of these forces depends on a rational neutralization of the forces of gravity by physiologic counterforces. The diverse factors and circumstances that produce these considerable forces must first be determined fully, if a rational and effective rehabilitation program is to be de-

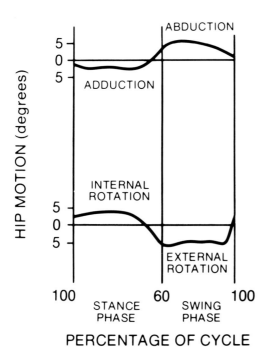

Fig. 1-1. Typical pattern for range of motion in the frontal *(top)* and transverse *(bottom)* planes during level walking for one gait cycle. (Modified from Johnston, R.C., and Smidt, G.L.: J. Bone Joint Surg. **51A:**1083, 1969.)

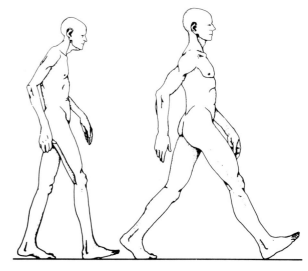

Fig. 1-2. Significant differences in the sagittal body position of older and younger men at the moment of heel strike. Older men exhibit shorter leg lengths, restricted range of hip flexion and extension, decreased plantar flexion of the ankle, and decreased heel-floor angle of the tracking limb. Older men also show decreased dorsiflexion of the ankle and elevation of the toe of the forward limb. (Modified from Murray, M.P., Kory, R.C., and Clarkson, B.H.: J. Gerontol. **24:**169, 1969.)

veloped for pathologic conditions of the hip.

Statics, the study of forces that act on a body in equilibrium, and dynamics, the study of forces that act on a body and do not sum to zero, are the two chief analytic methods of kinetics. Kinetic analysis allows the surgeon to determine the magnitude and direction of the forces imposed on the hip joint, which are produced by the muscles, body weight, connective tissues, and externally applied loads. More important, kinetic analysis can help to identify those loading situations that may produce excessively high, damaging forces.

The two main methods for determining the joint reaction force imposed on the head of the femur are the free body technique for coplanar forces and the moment method with the use of equilibrium equations.[17]

Dynamics

Several investigators have studied the forces imposed on the femoral head during dynamic activities.[21,22,23,25] Using a force plate system and kinematic data for the normal hip, Paul[21] studied the joint reaction force on the femoral head during gait in normal men and women and correlated the peak magnitudes with specific muscle activities that were recorded electromyographically. In the group of men two peak forces were generated during the stance phase when the abductor muscles contracted to stabilize the pelvis. A peak of approximately four times body weight occurred just after heel strike and another, greater magnitude of about seven times body weight was attained just before toe off (Fig. 1-3, *A*). When the foot was flat, the joint reaction force decreased to less than body weight because of the rapid lowering of the body's center of gravity. In the swing phase the joint reaction force was produced by contraction of the extensor muscles, which were engaged in decelerating the thigh mass; the magnitude here was low, about equal to body weight.

In the group of women studied the force pattern was similar, but the magnitudes were significantly lower, attaining a maximum of only four times body weight in the late stance phase (Fig. 1-3, *B*). This lower magnitude of joint force

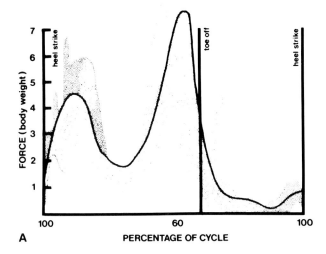

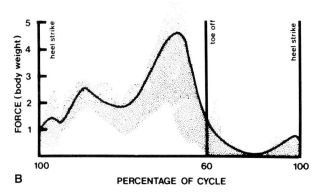

Fig. 1-3. Hip joint reaction force measured in multiples of body weight during walking for one gait cycle. Shaded portions indicate variations among subjects. **A,** Joint force pattern for men. **B,** Joint force pattern for women. (Modified from Paul, J.P.: master's thesis, Chicago, 1967, University of Chicago.)

may be attributed to several factors: a wider pelvis in females, a difference in the inclination of the neck-shaft angle, a difference in footwear, and general differences in the gait pattern.

In an earlier study by Rydell,[23] intravital measurements recorded through an instrumented prosthesis also demonstrated that a large joint reaction force acts on the femoral head during the late stance phase of a gait cycle. More important, the study indicated that at a faster pace the forces imposed on the prosthesis were greatly increased because of a proportional increase in muscle activity. The forces recorded in the swing phase were about half the magnitude of the forces during the last stance phase.

In another study an instrumented nail plate was used to measure the forces acting on a radiotelemeterized internal fixation device during common everyday activities following osteotomy or fracture of the femoral neck (Fig. 1-4).[10,17] The instrumented device measured forces on the nail plate but not on the hip joint itself. Through static analysis, however, it was possible to calculate the proportion of the load imposed on the implant and also to determine the total load imposed on the hip joint. Such diverse activities as raising onto a bedpan, transferring to a wheelchair, and walking imposed very large forces on the appliance.

The instrumented nail plate study demonstrated that for a bedridden patient with a fractured femoral neck or an osteotomy, the forces acting on the femoral head during common daily activities were similar in magnitude to the forces acting on the implanted device during walking with external supports.

THE MECHANICAL PROPERTIES OF BONE

Strength and stiffness, measured as a function of stress and strain, are the key mechanical properties of bone. Stress-strain curves are used to determine the relative loading behavior of cancellous and cortical bone and of other different materials, such as steel, used in prosthesis design. Stress can be described as the load per unit area on a plane surface, as a result of an externally imposed load. Strain is the percentage of deformation, a measurement of the lengthening or shortening of a material at a point under active loading.

Cortical bone, which is stiffer than cancellous bone, can withstand greater stresses but only comparable strains before failure. When the strain in vivo exceeds 2% of the original length, cortical bone fractures. Cancellous bone can withstand somewhat greater strains before fracturing because of its greater porosity—30% to 90%. The porosity of cortical bone is only 5% to 30% in comparison.[5]

Muscle contraction also plays a vital role in the supportive functions of the hip joint. During propulsion, bending moments are applied at the femoral neck, and tensile stress and strain are produced on the superior cortex. The contraction of the gluteus medius, however, generates a compressive stress and strain that, acting as a counterbalance, neutralize the tensile stress and strain.

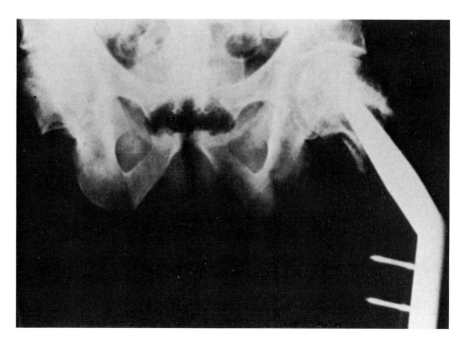

Fig. 1-4. An instrumented nail plate in the upper end of the femur, used to determine the forces imposed on the implant during common everyday activities following fracture of the femoral neck. In this case the nail plate was found to transmit one fourth of the total load on the hip joint. (Modified from Frankel, V.H., and Nordin, M.: Basic biomechanics of the skeletal system, ed. 2, Philadelphia, 1986, Lea & Febiger.)

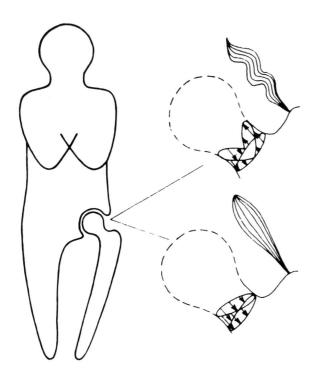

Fig. 1-5. Distribution of tensile and compressive stresses in a femoral neck subjected to bending. *Top,* When the gluteus medius muscle is relaxed the femoral neck is loaded in a nonphysiologic, more vertical, manner such as in the case of severe muscle fatigue. Large tensile stresses are found in the superior cortex while higher compressive stresses act on the inferior cortex. *Bottom,* Contraction of the gluteus medius neutralizes the tensile stresses in the superior cortex, while increasing compressive stresses act on the inferior cortex, thus loading the shaft in a physiologic manner.

The overall result is that neither the compressive nor the tensile stress and strain act significantly on the superior cortex, which enables the femoral neck to sustain higher loads than otherwise would be possible (Fig. 1-5).

The testing of bone in vitro demonstrates that bone fatigues rapidly when the load or deformation approximates the yield strength of the bone, and the number of repetitions needed to produce a fracture decreases.[4] In repetitive loading the frequency of loading, as well as the magnitude of the load and the number of repetitions, affects the fatiguing process. Fatigue fractures are usually sustained as a result of continuous, strenuous physical activity that causes the muscles to gradually fatigue. When the fatigue point is reached, the muscles' ability to contract and thus store energy and neutralize the stress on the bone is seriously diminished. The energy storage capacity of bone also varies directly according to the speed with which it is loaded.

Failure may occur on the tensile side, the compressive side, or on both sides of the bone. In the case of a backpacker who continues to hike strenuously with a heavy pack on the back, abductor muscle fatigue may produce the loading configuration shown in Fig. 1-5. The high tensile strains on the superior surface may lead to an overload fracture of the femoral neck; or as pointed out by Chamay,[5] fatigue fracture results at the site of compression in a bending bone caused by a "slip line" formation in the collagen fibers of the bone.

THE MECHANICAL PROPERTIES OF TISSUE

The collagenous tissues—the ligaments, including the joint capsule, and tendons—are very different from common engineering materials. The most important mechanical properties of collagenous tissues are strength and stiffness.[8]

Several theories and techniques of measuring tissue behavior have been reported.[6,12,14,24] Adequate testing describes the strain or load rate since the ultimate stress, strain, and energy absorption depend directly on the strain rate.

In bone the relation of the orientation of collagen fibers to the mechanical properties of the bony tissue is all-important.[7,8] A rough approximation of the relative elasticity of stainless steel to cortical bone to cancellous bone to articular cartilage under compressive loading is 1000:100:10:1.

The direction of the joint reaction force imposed on the head of the femur may be correlated with the anatomy of the upper end of the femur.[15,21] The interior of the femoral neck is composed of cancellous bone, which is divided into the medial and lateral trabecular systems. The joint reaction force on the femoral head parallels the trabeculae of the medial trabecular system (Frankel[9]), indicating that this system is important in supporting the joint reaction force. The lateral trabecular system probably resists the compressive force produced by the contraction of the abductor muscles. The epiphyseal plate is at right angles to the trabeculae of the medial trabecular system and is considered to be perpendicular to the joint reaction force on the femoral head.[15] The thin shell of cortical bone around the superior femoral neck gradually thickens in the inferior region. With the aging process the femoral neck gradually undergoes degenerative modifications wherein the cortical bone is thinned and cancellated and the trabeculae are gradually resorbed. These degenerative modifications may predispose the femoral neck to fracture.

FRACTURE MECHANISMS

Experimental studies also have indicated that fracture characteristics depend on the resultant direction of the joint reaction force on the femoral neck, not on the total exerted force.[19] Typical subcapital fractures resulted from high axial-to-bending load ratios. Intermediate ratios produced subcapital fractures with a "spike of neck." McLaughlin and Frankel[18] also analyzed the data from the earlier experimental study by classifying the bones according to degree of osteoporosis.[26] It was found that the strength of the bone steadily decreased with age; older bones absorbed about 25% less energy to failure than did younger bones.

An investigation into the biomechanical energetics of fractures of the femoral neck showed that two distinct mechanisms of fracture were operable.[11] In one type, where a person slips but does not fall, sufficient muscle force must be exerted to fracture the femoral neck. If the average femoral neck of an elderly female requires 600 kg_f to produce a fracture, then the amount of muscle tissue that must contract simultaneously to produce sufficient fracture is available in the muscle that spans the hip joint (120 to 300 cm^2 at a ratio of 2 to 5 kg of force per cm^2). Indeed, weakness of the neck and osteoporosis are not necessarily contributing factors because fractures have been known to occur as a result of muscle forces during electric shock, in the "stiff-man syndrome,"[27] and during seizures. Instead of deficient bone strength, such fractures may be caused by aging of the neuromuscular appa-ratus—for example, the overloading of the bone that may occur because of a lack of inhibitory impulses to the muscles during a slip.

Similarly, femoral neck fractures sustained dur-ing actual falls may not be primarily caused by weak bone tissue. The mechanism that dissipates the potential energy stored by an elderly female who falls is depicted in Fig. 1-6. In the illustrated example 3700 kg$_f$ cm must be dissipated. Since the femoral neck can absorb only 60 kg$_f$ cm of energy before failure, other absorption and dis-sipation systems are active. Most of the energy in a fall is absorbed by active muscle contractions; the quadriceps alone can absorb 10 times more energy than can the femur during a fall. In this situation, however, about 40 times the energy necessary to fracture the femoral neck is avail-able, and this energy cannot be dissipated quickly enough through muscle contractions or through the conversion of strain to kinetic energy. Conse-quently, when the level of stored energy in the neck of the femur rises above its threshold level, a fracture will occur.

Similar relationships between stored energy and the ability of the musculoskeletal system to absorb that energy also exist for a younger per-son. A typical subcapital fracture was observed in a healthy, vigorous skier who attempted to negoti-ate a 360-degree turn on an icy slope. Although the skier was accustomed to falling in snow, the event occurred so suddenly that the neuromuscu-lar mechanisms for energy dissipation could not respond in time.

Energy absorption-dissipation studies for con-ditions such as femoral neck fractures, disloca-tions of the hip joint, intertrochanteric fractures,

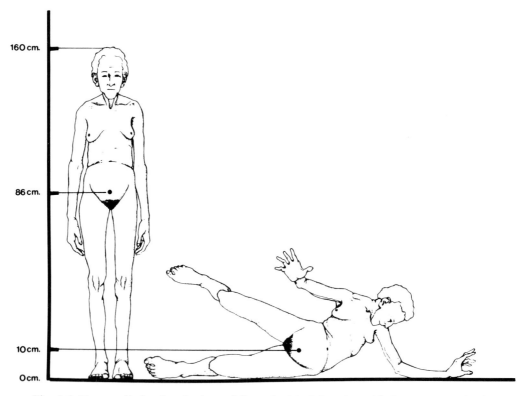

Fig. 1-6. Energy dissipation during a fall on the hip joint. A rapid change occurs in the vertical alignment of the center of gravity of an elderly woman weighing 50 kg—from 86 cm to 10 cm. Potential energy equals weight × height (50 kg × 76 cm), equaling 3700 kg/cm of energy to be dissipated during the fall. (Modified from Frankel and Burstein.)

and acetabular fractures should account for the role played by muscle forces, as well as ground reaction forces and externally applied loads. Neuromuscular control data and the effect of aging on the neuromuscular system should also be taken into account. One study[1] found that patients with diabetes, hemiplegia, and rheumatoid arthritis—all conditions associated with possible neuromuscular pathologies—sustained a greater incidence of fracture of the femoral neck than normal.

SUMMARY

A great deal of biomechanical research remains to be done in the area of hip joint trauma so that bioengineers and other medical scientists can work with accurate bone failure data, which are essential to the design of sports equipment, vehicles, workplace situations, and prostheses.

The application of biomechanical data, in addition to being essential in prosthesis design and ergonomics, also can be useful in such diverse problems as pathogenesis of degenerative joint disease, management of the postfracture patient, bracing in Perthes' disease, and in many other pathologic conditions.

REFERENCES

1. Alffram, P.A.: An epidemiologic study of cervical and trochanteric fractures of the femur in an urban projection, Acta Orthop. Scand. Suppl. **65,** 1964.
2. Backman, S.: The proximal end of the femur, Acta Radiol. Suppl. **146,** 1957.
3. Bartel, D.L., and Johnston, R.C.: Mechanical analysis and optimization of a cup arthroplasty, J. Biomech. **2:**97, 1969.
4. Carter, D.R., and Hayes, W.C.: The compressive behavior of bone as a two-phase porous structure, J. Bone Joint Surg. **59A:**954, 1977.
5. Chamay, A.: Mechanical and morphological aspects of experimental overloads and fatigue in bone, vol. 3, London, 1970, Pergamon Press Ltd.
6. Currey, J.D.: The mechanical properties of bone, Clin. Orthop. **24:**72, 1970.
7. Evans, F.G.: Stress and strain in bones, Springfield, Ill., 1957, Charles C Thomas, Publisher.
8. Evans, F.G., and Vincentelli, R.: Relation of collagen fiber orientation to some mechanical properties of human cortical bone, J. Biomech. **2:**63, 1969.
9. Frankel, V.H.: The femoral neck: function, fracture mechanisms, internal fixation, Springfield, Ill., 1960, Charles C Thomas, Publisher.
10. Frankel, V.H.: Mechanical fixation of unstable fractures about the proximal end of the femur, Bull. Hosp. Joint Dis. **24:**1, 1963.
11. Frankel, V.H., and Burstein, A.H.: Force and energetics of femoral neck fractures, Proceedings Dixieme Congress International de Chirurgie Orthopaedique et de Traumatologie, Paris, 1966.
12. Frankel, V.H., and Burstein, A.H.: Orthopaedic biomechanics, Philadelphia, 1970, Lea & Febiger.
13. Frankel, V.H., and Nordin, M.: Basic biomechanics of the skeletal system, ed. 2, Philadelphia, 1986, Lea & Febiger.
14. Frisen, M., Magi, M., Sonnerup, L., and Vidik, A.: Rheological analysis of soft collagenous tissues, J. Biomech. **2:**13, 1969.
15. Inman, V.T.: Functional aspects of the abductor muscles of the hip, J. Bone Joint Surg. **29:**607, 1947.
16. Johnston, R.C., and Smidt, G.L.: Measurement of hip joint motion during walking: Evaluation of an electrogoniometric method, J. Bone Joint Surg. **51A:**1083, 1969.
17. Lygre, L.: The loads produced on the hip joint by nursing procedures: a telemeterization study, M.S. master's thesis (nursing), Cleveland, 1970, Case Western Reserve University.
18. McLaughlin, T., and Frankel, V.H.: A parametric study of the strength of the upper end of the femur, Unpublished data, 1970.
19. Murray, M.P.: Gait as a total pattern of movement, Am. J. Phys. Med. **46:**290, 1967.
20. Murray, M.P., Kory, R.C., and Clarkson, B.H.: Walking patterns in healthy old men, J. Gerontol. **24:**169, 1969.
21. Paul, J.P.: Forces at the human hip joint, master's thesis, Chicago, 1967, University of Chicago.
22. Rydell, N.W.: Forces in the hip joint. In Kenedi, R.M., Biomechanics and related bioengineering topics, London, 1965, Pergamon Press Ltd.
23. Rydell, N.W.: Forces acting on the femoral head prosthesis, Acta Orthop. Scand. Suppl. **88,** 1966.
24. Sedlin, E.D.: A rheological model for cortical bone, Acta Orthop. Scand. Suppl. **83,** 1965.
25. Seirig, A., and Arvikar, R.J.: The prediction of muscular load sharing and joint forces in the lower extremities during walking, J. Biomech. **8:**89, 1975.
26. Singh, M., Nagrath, A.R., and Naini, P.S.: Changes in trabecular pattern of the upper end of the femur as an index of osteoporosis, J. Bone Joint Surg. **52A:**457, 1970.
27. Smith, L.D.: Hip fractures: A role of muscle contraction or intrinsic forces in the causation of fractures in the femoral neck, J. Bone Joint Surg. **35A:**367, 1953.

THE MULTIPLY INJURED PATIENT

Chapter 2

Fracture treatment for the multiply injured patient

EUGENE J. DABEZIES

ROBERT D'AMBROSIA

Epidemiologic studies have shown that trauma, now redefined as a disease, has serious effects on our society in terms of deaths, lost wage earners, and disability.[1,40,43] The treatment of civilian trauma continues to evolve, and surgical treatment is advocated because of beneficial effects.[2,25,36,37] The appropriate specialists working cooperatively can salvage traumatized persons with combined system injuries and restore most to their vocational and recreational activities. This multidiscipline approach to treatment requires an understanding of the physiology of injury combined with established treatment priorities and goals. In this section our consultants provide us with current concepts of treatment in their areas and relate these concepts to the whole patient.

Although the problem of treating the multiply injured patient was appreciated by our predecessors, recent research has better defined the concept. In the past, after careful examination, physicians would prescribe nasal oxygen; we now recognize incipient lung failure (ARDS) as evidenced by decreasing arterial oxygen pressure (PaO_2) when arterial blood gases (ABG) are obtained. Orr[31] in 1941 stressed "the importance of primary reduction and immobilization in compound fractures." Bone healing without chronic infection was the primary goal, and frequently joint mobility had to be sacrificed. In 1901 Rudolph Matas,[27] a New Orleans surgeon, reported the use of "ambulating splints and orthopedic appliances" and stressed the value was in "abbreviating the period of convalescence after the fracture and in shortening the stay in bed." He cited an example of a man with an infected, ununited fracture of the proximal femur. This patient was described as "reduced to a marasmic condition." The wound was drained, and necrotic bone fragments were removed. The man was placed in a long-leg brace with a thigh and calf lacer and an ischial support. He remained in New Orleans for 1 month and returned to his own country, where he resumed his military duties and the fracture healed "without appreciable lameness." The concept of cast bracing, mobilization, and nutrition was understood in 1901.

In the United States, with shifting emphasis in various disciplines within surgery, it is the orthopaedic surgeon's responsibility to care for fractures. The challenge is to establish priorities of treatment of multiple-system injury and dysfunction and provide fracture care.

In the emergency room, diagnostic evaluation and resuscitation, whether hemodynamic, pulmonary, neurologic or abdominal, take precedence. Life-saving procedures are to be done first and then are to be followed by limb-saving procedures. After life-threatening injuries to the head, chest, or abdomen are treated, the orthopaedic surgeon can proceed with fracture treatment. Because monitoring such an injured patient is extremely important, the anesthesiologist assumes a most important role in the operating room. We are dependent on this monitoring to continue appropriate treatment, to maintain blood volume, pulmonary and renal function, and to recognize and treat clotting defects.

The double-antibiotic regimen (Table 2-1)[7] has the most to offer in preventing infection; treatment should be started in the emergency room and continued in the operating room.[13,32] Studies have advocated the use of antibiotics in open fractures.[13,32] Our data have shown a decrease in infection in Class III open fractures from 34% to 10.7%, with an overall infection rate in open fractures of 4% with this double coverage (Dabezies, E.J., Marier, R., and Hernandez, A., unpublished L.S.U. data).

During the acute phase of injury, protein is mobilized to meet the caloric requirements for life and the glucose-dependent metabolism of the CNS and leukocytes. This protein is mobilized from the somatic protein of skeletal muscle and visceral protein of blood components. Fat is mobilized later, during the adaptive and chronic phase. Recent work by Border[2], Laduca and others[25] suggests that there is an obligatory catabolism of isoleucine and leucine of skeletal muscle as a source of organ energy. Nutritional support is required to prevent protein exhaustion.

In general, a normal, 70 kg man requires 3500 kcal/day (50 kcal/kg/day) to maintain positive nitrogen balance after trauma. For more accuracy, nitrogen balance studies can be obtained easily with cooperation from the clinical dietitian. Positive nitrogen balance of 2 to 4 g/day should be the goal for these patients for maintaining immune competence to resist infection and for preventing the emaciation that precipitates multiple organ failure syndrome. (See box.[20])

Table 2-1. Clinical use of antibiotics

Setting*	Drug regimen
Emergency room	Cephapirin (Cefadyl) 2 g IV stat Tobramycin (Nebcin) 1.5 mg/kg IV stat Cephapirin 1 g IV every 6 hours Tobramycin 1.5 mg/kg IV every 8 hours
Postoperatively	Adjust tobramycin according to renal function and serum peak (4 to 8 μg) and trough (<2 μg) levels Continue antibiotics for 5 days after the last surgical procedure, then stop and assess the wound

*Also use penicillin for heavily contaminated wounds: in emergency room give 4 million units IV; postoperatively give 4 million units IV every 4 hours.

NITROGEN BALANCE DETERMINATION

$$\frac{\text{Protein intake (grams/24 hr)}}{6.25} - (\text{UUN} + 3) =$$
$$> \text{2-4 g N/day for injured}$$

Protein intake is determined from diet by dietitian: 1 g N = 6.25 g protein; UUN = 24 hours urinary urea nitrogen; 3 = non-urea nitrogen loss.

Table 2-2. Classification of open fractures

	I	II	III
Energy	Low (ski)	Moderate (fall, football)	High (car bumper)
Bone comminution	None	Minimal	Segments (butterfly)
Contamination	None	Minimal	Moderate to major

Soft tissue	Laceration	Contused
		(no loss)
			Extensive damage
			Prognosis worsened
			  Skin or muscle loss
			  Vascular injury
			  Dirt, water
			  Short-range shotgun
			  High velocity gunshot wound
			  More than 6 hours old

WOUND AND FRACTURE CARE

A classification that combines the soft tissue and bone injury in open fractures was popularized by the AO/ASIF and has been modified to assist in treatment and prognostication (Table 2-2). The Class III fractures have the worst outlook. Treatment of Class III fractures is easier when the soft tissue envelope has survived. When loss of skin or muscle is extensive, particularly in tibial fractures, early muscle rotation flaps[12] or free vascularized flaps[10,29,42] to cover the exposed bone should be considered before infection becomes an overwhelming problem.

Soft tissue care

Assessment and care of soft tissue is critical to the outcome, particularly with tibial fractures. Contused and degloved skin has the propensity to slough, even in closed fractures. Therefore exposures for internal fixation have to respect damage to skin and muscle. Incisions are planned carefully to avoid jeopardizing the tenuous blood supply. All open fractures need adequate exposure for irrigation and debridement. Nothing is to be gained by closing the compound wound, but the extending incisions may be closed if there is no tension. Debrided wounds usually will not become infected if hematoma and tissue exudates are allowed to drain.

Severe resting pain, pain with passive motion, and dyesthesia are signals of a compartment syndrome. Decompression of the compartment and stabilization of the fracture are the requisite treatment. Residual flexion contracture of toes does not mean that the tendon is "caught in the fracture site" but rather that an ischemic compartment syndrome was not recognized.

Fracture treatment

We cannot discuss all fractures, but we should consider treatment of those fractures that threaten survival, whether they occur as a single event or in combinations.

Modes of fixation of fractures remain a challenge. Modern metallurgy has produced implants that are sufficiently strong and corrosion-resistant to be used for the treatment of various fractures. Clinical experience has shown that certain devices are suited better for certain bones, and innovations in technology—such as the image-intensified mobile C-arm fluoroscopic unit—have allowed development of intramedullary rodding techniques for the femur, tibia, and humerus.

To the AO/ASIF surgeons go the credit for combining the engineering and medical disciplines. These surgeons have developed an ever-evolving system of implants for fractures. Bone is now treated as a material, as well as a living tissue. The physiologic studies in the laboratory and clinical studies of the patients have demonstrated that advantages of rigid fixation of fractures in multiply injured patients in terms of decreased mortality and morbidity.[30,38]

Femur. The classic treatment of fractured femurs has evolved from traction to cast bracing to intramedullary rodding. Closed treatment is associated with problems of fracture healing (28%), refracture (9%), and long convalescence.[5,17] G. Kuntscher[23,24] demonstrated the value of intramedullary rodding of fractured femurs. In fact he even developed a system of locking the nail with transfixion screws. The closed rodding technique has reduced a difficult problem to a relatively standard treatment plan.[15,16] We prefer the supine position because of ease in setup and more standard anatomic frame of reference (Fig. 2-1).

Compound fractures of the shaft of the femur are debrided, dressed open, and placed in traction. At about 48 to 72 hours, the wounds are closed, and within 1 week closed intramedullary rodding is done. Occasionally the rodding will be done without closure of the wound. For certain severe Class III open fractures, a Wagner external fixator may be the device of choice.[8] For many comminuted fractures the locked nail (Fig. 2-2) allows superb stabilization. We have used this nail in 40 cases without loss of position and all have gone on to union.

In a series of 130 fractures of the femur we have had a 1% infection incidence, no failure of union, and an average range of motion of 110 degrees of the knee.

Proximal femoral fractures are stabilized best with a sliding screw plate device. Supracondylar fractures require restoration of joint congruity; stabilization can be achieved with a 90-degree screw-side plate, or with the 95-degree supracondylar plate. This latter device is demanding technically. Postoperative mobilization of supracondylar fractures must be done very cautiously. Bone grafting of subtrochanteric and supracondylar fractures is indicated when there is a loss of cortical integrity.

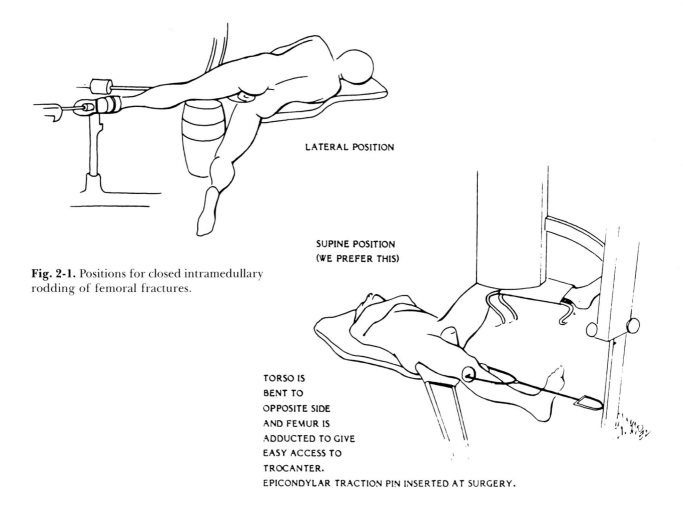

LATERAL POSITION

SUPINE POSITION
(WE PREFER THIS)

Fig. 2-1. Positions for closed intramedullary rodding of femoral fractures.

TORSO IS
BENT TO
OPPOSITE SIDE
AND FEMUR IS
ADDUCTED TO GIVE
EASY ACCESS TO
TROCANTER.
EPICONDYLAR TRACTION PIN INSERTED AT SURGERY.

Stabilization of femoral fractures does seem to help prevent major lung failure. We have experienced no occurrence of the fat embolism syndrome and 8% incidence of adult respiratory distress syndrome (ARDS), defined by PaO_2 less than 50 mm Hg and $PaCO_2$ greater than 50 mm Hg on room air. There have been no serious respiratory problems after ORIF of pelvis and acetabular fractures. Riska and associates reported a 4% incidence of ARDS in operative treatment, whereas in nonoperatively treated cases ARDS occurred in 22% of patients.[36,37]

Tibia. Open fractures of the tibia continue to be a serious problem. Treatment with a walking cast produces reliable results with minimal complications.[9]

Surgical stabilization has much to offer a patient with several long-bone fractures. For open fractures, stabilization has increased limb salvage, improved the functional end result, decreased infection, and improved mobility. Moreover, it has not decreased the rate of bone union. If a patient has a stable tibial fracture, the surgeon can concentrate on soft tissue problems and skin coverage.

The choices for fracture treatment are plates, external fixators, and intramedullary rods.[14] The AO/ASIF makes a strong case for plates in a 13-year review showing delayed healing in 6.8% and infection in 9.5% of open tibial fractures.[30]

An equivalent method is to use external fixation frames until soft tissue coverage is achieved and then to apply an ambulatory cast. This has been our preferred method. It has produced consistently good results, particularly in highly contaminated wounds from motorcycles and ditch water (Fig. 2-3).[21,22]

Intramedullary rodding of tibial fractures is being reassessed and offers a third alternative.[41] We have used intramedullary rods for closed tibial fractures in patients with multiple extremity fractures and for some selected Class III open

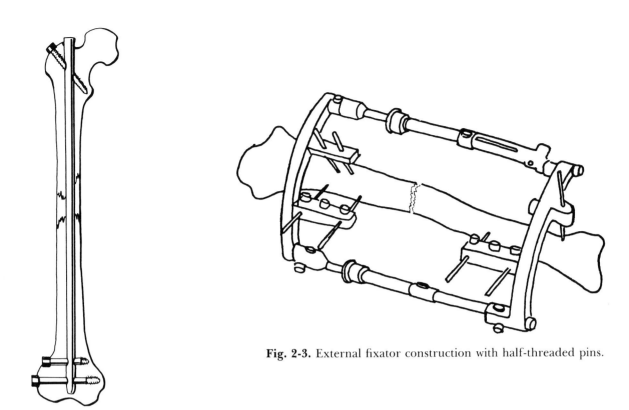

Fig. 2-3. External fixator construction with half-threaded pins.

Fig. 2-2. Gross-Kempf interlocking femoral rod.

tibial fractures with soft tissue coverage. The surgery for the Class III fractures is done on a delayed basis to get the patient out of a cast, when there are problems maintaining fracture position, or for delayed unions. Early results have been pleasing, but no recommendations can be made at this point because some infections have recurred.

The trend for treating open tibial fractures is toward surgical stabilization to facilitate soft tissue coverage and closure. If there is soft tissue loss, then early coverage with gastrocnemius muscle rotation flap for the proximal tibia should be considered.[12] The soleus rotation flap can be used in the middle third but is more demanding surgically.[11] For the middle and distal third, free vascularized flaps can provide the needed soft tissue coverage.

Pelvis. Mortality is decreasing to the range of 5% to 20% because we are becoming aware of associated vascular and urologic injuries and have developed methods of stabilization, urinary drainage, and arterial embolism that do not jeopardize the patient. The classification of Pennal and Tile (Fig. 2-4) is valuable because it provides insight into the mechanics of injury.

Lateral compression alerts us to the possibility of urethral injury by disruption of the urogenital diaphragm. This occurs because the anteroposterior diameter of the pelvis is lengthened with lateral compression.[33,34,39]

The *vertical shear* injury may damage the superior gluteal or other hypogastric pelvic vessels and the sciatic nerve. Disruption of the symphysis pubis is best treated via a Pfannenstiel incision and two-plate fixation. The diastasis of the symphysis should be fixed first. Then the patient is rolled onto the abdomen and the SI joint or fractured sacrum stabilized by two threaded Harrington sacral bars with washers and nuts going from one posterior iliac crest to the other but superficial to the sacrum (Fig. 2-5). This posterior fixation system provides very rigid stability and is much easier than placing screws into the sacrum. We have been unable to reduce an SI joint dislocation with an external fixator, so we prefer this method of stabilization. If the anterior fracture extends through the obturator foramen, then it is probably easier to achieve the anterior reduction, stabilization, and closure of the pelvis using the external fixator combined with pos-

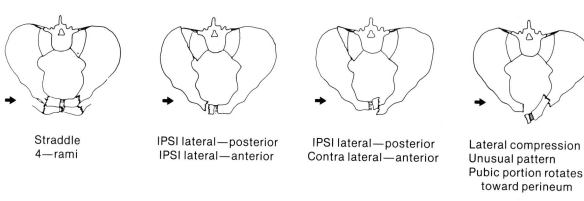

Straddle
4—rami

IPSI lateral—posterior
IPSI lateral—anterior

IPSI lateral—posterior
Contra lateral—anterior

Lateral compression
Unusual pattern
Pubic portion rotates
toward perineum

Lateral compression

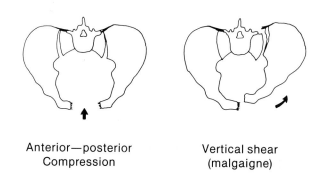

Anterior—posterior
Compression

Vertical shear
(malgaigne)

Patterns of pelvic disruption

Fig. 2-4. Pennal-Tile classification of pelvic fracture. (Modified from Rowe, C.R., and Lowell, J.D.: J. Bone Joint Surg. **43A:**30-59, 1961.)

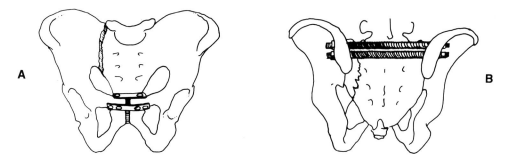

Fig. 2-5. Unstable pelvic fracture. Open reduction and fixation of anterior and posterior lesion. **A,** Symphysis diastasis fixed with two plates via Pfannenstiel incision. **B,** SI joint and sacrum stabilized by two threaded Harrington sacral bars via parallel incisions over posterior ilium.

terior double rods (Fig. 2-6). The alternative is to plate the superior pubic ramus, but this is technically demanding.

Restoration of the anatomy and stabilization of the pelvis usually will stop the persisting hemorrhage; however, selected embolization (discussed in another section) should not be overlooked.[26]

For urethral injuries (discussed later), suprapubic drainage is appropriate. If the general or urologic surgeon is going to do an abdominal procedure, the symphysis diastasis should be plated at that time, and the posterior SI joint fracture-dislocation then should be stabilized if there is a posterior injury. An option is to use a simple configuration external fixator to treat the anterior lesion.

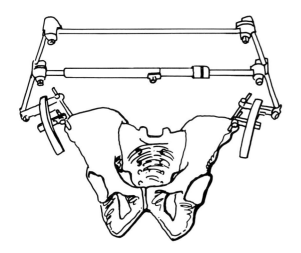

Fig. 2-6. External fixation frame for pelvic fracture.

Acetabulum. A fracture classification[28] that recognizes instability of the acetabulum is important because these unstable fractures produce unacceptable results.[4,5,38] Our choice for surgical exposure is through a transtrochanteric approach as described by Reudi.[35] Since this is a formidable undertaking, one should have special experience before accepting the surgeon's responsibility. Satisfying results can be achieved with restoration of the joint in these unstable fractures. Even if the joint fails, later reconstruction procedures such as total joint arthroplasty are easier because the anatomic pillars have been reconstructed.

Humerus. Treating a humerus with the plaster immobilization of a hanging arm cast presents a major problem in the multiply injured patient. We have been satisfied using plates for the humerus when surgery is indicated in multiple trauma. Such stabilization frees this injured extremity, allows venous access, and provides the patient with increased mobility. In our experience no fractures have failed to unite in this situation. We have found external fixation to be fraught with problems.

Restoration of elbow fractures is accomplished best through a posterior approach with the patient prone. Reconstruction of the elbow joint offers the best hope or a stable, nonpainful, and mobile elbow joint (Fig. 2-7).[18,19]

Forearm. Fractures of the radius and ulna are treated best with the compression plate technique. Comminuted distal radius fractures can be treated with distraction pinning whether a short-arm cast or an external fixator frame is used.[6]

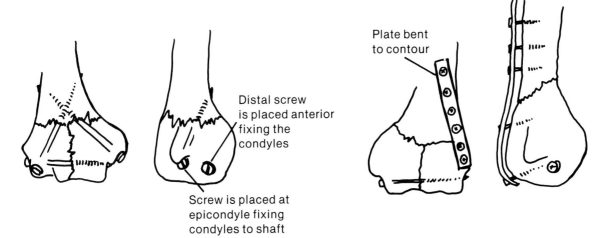

Distal screw is placed anterior fixing the condyles

Screw is placed at epicondyle fixing condyles to shaft

Plate bent to contour

Fig. 2-7. Techniques for stabilizing distal humerus fractures.

SUMMARY

Multiply injured patients are benefited by an intradisciplinary approach to treatment. Consultants provide expertise in the treatment of particular injured systems. Resuscitation and diagnostic evaluation are life-saving priorities of treatment in the emergency room. Definitive surgical treatment of body cavity injury is combined with careful monitoring while the patient is under anesthesia. The orthopaedic surgeon's responsibility then is to stabilize the fractures, thus minimizing the risk of infection, lung failure, and debilitation so that the patient may be gotten out of bed and rehabilitation started. Prolonged recumbency is probably the worst thing that can happen to a traumatized patient. The goal of fracture treatment is bone union without infection and with stable soft tissue coverage and normal motion of associated joints. It is important to realize that in these multiply injured people, fractures of the femoral or tibial shafts and unstable pelvic fractures threaten survival and should be surgically treated as soon as feasible. The operative treatment of fractures of the humerus, forearm, knee, and ankle can be addressed on an emergent basis. The condition of the skin around the ankle and knee influences the timing of surgery; a 24-hour delay may preclude surgery for weeks because of swelling and blisters.

Orthopaedic surgeons now are beginning to understand the concepts of spine instability and have devices to stabilize the fractures. We think that unstable fractures should be given the same priority that fractures of major long bones receive.

Free vascularized tissue provides excellent coverage when skin loss occurs over the distal two-thirds of tibial fractures. Skin loss over the proximal tibia can be covered quite nicely with gastrocnemius rotation muscle flaps and split-thickness skin grafting. Rotation flaps raised with the deep fascia are not as sure a method of obtaining coverage. The trend is early coverage of soft tissue defects with muscle flaps or vascularized free tissue transfer.

Nutrition must be maintained, because, unless the massive caloric requirements are met, there is an impairment of immune competence, which sets the stage for infection and a prolonged convalescence or, at worst, multiple organ failure syndrome. During the acute phase, there is obligatory catabolism of skeletal muscle to meet the demands for amino acids and glucose. Nitrogen balance studies should be done for the multiply injured patient targeting 3500 kcal (50 kcal/kg/day) as the minimum.

A two-drug antibiotic regimen (cephalosporin and aminoglycoside) is therapeutic against both gram-negative and gram-positive organisms and helps to reduce the incidence of infection. Proper soft tissue and bone wound care cannot be replaced by any chemotherapeutic regimen.

Plans should be made within a community so that hospitals that receive multiply traumatized patients have facilities and consultants dedicated to their care.

REFERENCES

1. Baker, C.C.: Epidemiology of trauma deaths, Am. J. Surg. **140:**144-150, 1980.
2. Border, J.: Trauma and sepsis. In Worth, M.H.: Principles and practice of trauma, Baltimore, 1982, Williams & Wilkins.
3. Caldwell, J.A.: Treatment of fractures of the shaft of the humerus by hanging cast, Surg. Gynecol. Obstet. **70:**421-425, 1940.
4. Carnesale, P.G., Stewart, M.J., and Barnes, S.: Acetabular disruption and central fracture dislocation of the hip, J. Bone Joint Surg. **57A:**1054-1059, 1975.
5. Carr, C.R., and Wingo, C.H.: Fractures of the femoral diaphysis, a retrospective study of the results and costs of treatment by intramedullary nailing and by traction in a spica cast, J. Bone Joint Surg. **55A:**690-700, 1973.
6. Dabezies, E., Chuinard, R., and Kitziger, R.: Distraction pinning for radical metaphysis fractures, Orthopedics **1:**294-298, 1978.
7. Dabezies, E.J., and D'Ambrosia, R.D.: Treatment of the multiply injured patient: Plans for treatment and problems of major trauma. In The American Academy of Orthopaedic Surgeons: Instructional course lectures, vol. 33, St. Louis, 1984, The C.V. Mosby Co.
8. Dabezies, E.J., D'Ambrosia, R.D., Shoji, H., Norris, R., and Murphy, E.: Fracture of femoral shaft treated by external fixation with the Wagner device, J. Bone Surg. **66A:**360-364, 1984.
9. Dehne, E., Metz, C.W., and Deffer, P.A.: Nonoperative treatment of the fractured tibia by immediate weight-bearing, J. Trauma **1:**514-533, 1961.
10. Faust, D.C.: Advanced techniques of soft tissue cover in the extremities, Paper presented at the Louisiana Orthopedic Association meeting, New Orleans, Oct. 1984.
11. Fitzgerald, R.H., Jr., Ruttle, P.E., Arnold, P.G., Kelly, P.J., and Irons, G.B.: Local muscle flaps in the treatment of chronic osteomyelitis, J. Bone Joint Surg. **67A:**175-185, 1985.
12. Ger, R.: The management of pretibial skin loss, Surgery **63:**757-763, 1968.
13. Gustillo, R.B., and Anderson J.T.: Prevention of infection in the treatment of 1025 open fractures of long bones, J. Bone Joint Surg. **58A:**453-458, 1976.

14. Gustilo, R.B., Simpson, L., Nixon, R., Ruiz, A., and Indeck, W.: An analysis of 511 open fractures, Clin. Orthop. **66**:148-154, 1969.

15. Hanson, S.T., and Winquist, R.A.: Closed intramedullary nailing of fractures of the femoral shaft, Part 2, technical considerations. In The American Academy of Orthopaedic Surgeons: Instructional course lectures, vol. 27, St. Louis, 1978, The C.V. Mosby Co.

16. Hanson, S., and Winquist, R.: Closed intramedullary nailing of the femur: Kuntsche technique with reaming, Clin. Orthop. **138**:56-61, 1979.

17. Hartmann, E.R., and Brav, E.A.: The problem of refracturing fractures of the femoral shaft, J. Bone Joint Surg. **36A**:1071-1079, 1954.

18. Helfet, D.: Bicondylar intraarticuular fractures of the distal humerus in adults: Their assessment, classification, and operative management, Adv. Orthop. Surg. **8**:223-235, 1985.

19. Jupiter, J., Ursneff, M., Holzach, P., and Allgower, M.: Intercondylar fractures of the humerus: An operative approach, J. Bone Surg. **67A**:226-239, 1985.

20. Kaminski, M.V., Jr., and Ruggiero, R.P.: Nutritional assessment and support: Why, when, how? Resident Staff Physician **26**:94-108, 1980.

21. Karlstrom, E., and Olerud, S.: Fractures of the tibial shaft, a critical evaluation of treatment alternatives, Clin. Orthop. **105**:82-115, 1974.

22. Karlstrom, E., and Olerud, S.: Percutaneous pin fixation of open tibial fractures: Double framed anchorage using Vidal-Adrey method, J. Bone Joint Surg. **57A**:915-924, 1975.

23. Kuntscher, G.: The intramedullary nailing of fractures, Arch. F. Clin. Chir. **200**:5-12, 1940.

24. Kuntscher, G.: Intramedullary surgical technique and its place in orthopedic surgery, J. Bone Joint Surg. **47A**:809-818, 1965.

25. Laduca, J.N., Bone L.L., Seibel, R.W., and Border, J.R.: Primary open reduction and internal fixation of open fractures, J. Trauma **20**:580-586, 1980.

26. Matalon, T., Athanasoulis, C., Margolies, M., Waltman, A., Novelline, R., Greenfield, A., and Miller, S.: Hemorrhage with pelvic fractures: efficacy of transcatheter embolization, Am. J. Roentgenol. **133**:859-864, 1979.

27. Matas, R.: The relative prevalence and fatality of fractures in the white and colored races, Transactions of the Louisiana State Medical Society, New Orleans, April 18-20, 1901.

28. Muller, M.E., Allgower, M., Schneider, R., and Willengger, H.: Manual of internal fixation: Techniques recommended by the AO-group, ed. 2, New York, 1979, Springer-Verlag.

29. Nunley, J.A.: Electric microsurgery for orthopedic reconstruction. In The American Academy of Orthopaedic Surgeons: Instructional course lectures, vol. 33, St. Louis, 1984, The C.V. Mosby Co.

30. Oertlid, Matter, P., Scharplatz, D., and Zehnderr: Evaluation of surgically treated shaft fractures: Analysis of the Swiss AO/ASIF documentation, 1967-1980, AO Bull. June 1984.

31. Orr, H.W.: Wounds and fractures, Springfield, Ill, 1941, Charles C Thomas, Publisher.

32. Patzakis, M.J., Harvey, J.D., and Irler, D.: The role of antibiotics in the management of open fractures, J. Bone Joint Surg. **56A**:532-540, 1974.

33. Peltier, L.F.: Complications associated with fractures of the pelvis, J. Bone Joint Surg. **47A**:1060-1069, 1965.

34. Pennal, G.F., Tile, M., Waddelm, J.P., and Garside, H.: Pelvic disruption: Assessment and classification, Clin. Orthop. **151**:12-21, 1980.

35. Reudi, T.: Surgical approach for internal fixation, New York, 1984, Springer-Verlag.

36. Riska, E.B., Von Bonsdorff, H., Hakkinen, S., Jaroma, H., Kiviluoto, O., and Paavilainen, T.: Prevention of fat embolism by early internal fixation of fractures in patients with multiple injuries, Injury **8**:110-116, 1976.

37. Riska, E.B., Von Bonsdorff, H., Hakkinen, S., Jaroma, H., Kiviluoto, O., and Paavilainen, T.: Primary operative fixation of long bone fractures in patients with multiple injuries, J. Trauma **17**:111-120, 1977.

38. Rowe, C.R., and Lowell, J.D.: Prognosis of fractures of the acetabulum, J. Bone Joint Surg. **43A**:30-59, 1961.

39. Tile, M.: Fractures of the pelvis and acetabulum, Baltimore, 1984, Williams & Wilkins.

40. Trunkey, D.D.: The value of trauma centers, Bull. Am. Coll. Surg. **67**:5-7, 1982.

41. Velazco, A., Whitesides, Jr., T.E., and Fleming, L.L.: Open fractures of the tibia treated with the Lottes nail, J. Bone Joint Surg. **65A**879-885, 1983.

42. Weiland, A.J.: Current concepts review: Vascularized free bone transplants, J. Bone Surg. **63A**:166-169, 1981.

43. West J., Trunkey, D.D., and Lim, R.C.: Systems of trauma care, a study of two counties, Arch. Surg. **114**:455-460, 1979.

Chapter 3

Initial resuscitation of trauma victims

DONALD D. TRUNKEY

RAPID EVALUATION

Resuscitation of the trauma patient can be chaotic. It is usually unplanned yet involves life-and-death decisions; information is limited, and speed is of the utmost importance. Order can come out of chaos, however, if the primary resuscitator remains calm and maintains leadership. Panic kills.

Resuscitation is a series of decision trees rooted in priorities that must be established quickly (box); thus rapid, accurate assessment is mandatory. One of the first decisions to be made concerns the patient's relative stability. I base my decisions on what is called the "one-second optical scan test," used to describe which of three categories—apparently dead or dying, unstable, or stable—is most appropriate. This "one-second"

PRIORITIES IN EVALUATION AND RESUSCITATION OF THE TRAUMA VICTIM

FIRST PRIORITIES

Establish airway
Control of rapid external hemorrhage
Cardiovascular resuscitation
  Pump problems must first be assessed and then corrected
  Restore blood volume

SECOND PRIORITIES

The second examination
Neurologic examination performed
Fracture management
Diagnosis and treatment of occult hemorrhage
Radiographic procedures: definitive diagnosis and care

---

preliminary evaluation actually should take no longer than a few seconds, and it does require the "sixth sense" that comes only with experience. Sometimes it is clear even as the patient is wheeled into the resuscitation room that the appropriate category is apparently dead or dying. When it is not so obvious, the physician must quickly assess airway, pulse, level of consciousness, neck veins, and peripheral perfusion.

INITIAL RESUSCITATION
Airway

If the patient is apparently dead or dying, decisions on resuscitative steps must be taken immediately. Let us examine the most urgent: extensive airway problems. If these problems are not treated promptly, the patient will die within a few minutes. Sometimes airway obstruction and ventilatory insufficiency are not completely obvious but certain signs are clear—stridor, cyanosis, anxiety, intercostal retraction, use of accessory muscles of respiration, and tachypnea with a ventilatory rate of more than 25 breaths per minute. Sometimes the signs are subtle to begin with and, as the patient weakens or begins to die, diminish further.

The oropharynx should be cleared with a tonsil sucker or the examiner's fingers. The back of the tongue should be brought forward, away from the oropharynx, by displacing the angles of the jaw anteriorly (insertion of an oral or nasal airway sometimes helps keep the tongue forward), or if the patient has massive maxillofacial injuries, the tongue can be pulled forward with either a towel clip or the examiner's fingers.

When practicable, the patient should be given several breaths of 100% oxygen with an Ambutype bag and a face mask and then intubated through the mouth or nose. However, bag placement is not always possible, as when all bony structures have been destroyed. High-flow nasal or face oxygen should be started for such patients as the resuscitator prepares for intubation.

If oral or nasal intubation fails to secure an airway within 60 seconds and if the patient cannot be ventilated with a mask, the physician should gain access to the trachea through the cricothyroid membrane. This is done by cutting down on the membrane with a no. 11 blade, inserting the handle of the scalpel into the trachea, twisting it to enlarge the tracheal opening, and inserting a no. 5 or no. 6 cuffed endotracheal tube. The single contraindication for cricothyrotomy is complete tracheal-laryngeal separation.

In less extreme cases tracheostomy or emergency intubation is not subject to the same time constraints. If there is no sign of head or neck injury, the patient's head can be turned to the side and the oropharynx cleared with a sucker. If the airway is still obstructed, the tongue should be brought forward by displacing the angles of the jaw forward or by inserting a pharyngeal airway. These maneuvers are usually sufficient to secure the airway in the conscious patient. If they are not, the patient should be intubated. Conscious patients frequently assume the position that gives them the best airway and should not be forced into a recumbent position. For example, the patient with a fractured mandible may sit up and hang his or her head forward to let the mandible and its attached tongue fall away from the back of the throat.

Since conscious patients tend to struggle as attempts are made to establish an airway, the physician must show fine judgment in this situation. On the one hand, many struggling patients are more than strong enough and awake enough to maintain their airways and oxygenate and ventilate themselves, and too vigorous attempts at suctioning and passage of endotracheal tubes may only lead to vomiting and aspiration. On the other hand, some conscious patients begin to struggle when they become hypoxemic, and in this situation the physician must be aggressive in securing the airway.

To distinguish between the two situations, the physician should note whether struggling is associated specifically with ventilatory insufficiency—stridor, intercostal retraction, use of accessory muscles, and tachypnea—indicating a need to proceed aggressively. If the patient's struggles are nonspecific, the physician can be more deliberate.

Ventilation

Once the airway is established, ventilation must be ensured. Open pneumothoraxes are closed with occlusive dressings. Flail segments of the chest wall are stabilized by placing sandbags next to the flail or by turning the patient so that the flail segment is against the mattress. Chest tubes are inserted to evacuate pneumothoraxes and massive hemothoraxes. If the patient requires intubation, positive pressure ventilation is provided mechanically.

Bleeding

External bleeding usually has been controlled by paramedics on the way to the emergency room. If this has not been done, it should be controlled simultaneously with establishment of airway and ventilation. Simple pressure applied directly to the bleeding site almost always will achieve control until definitive treatment can be given; tourniquets rarely are indicated except for traumatic amputations. Wounds should not be probed, and blind clamping is contraindicated because it jeopardizes the chances for primary vascular repair and can lead to permanent nerve injury.

Shock

The next priority in the treatment of apparently dead, dying or unstable patients, after establishing an airway and controlling bleeding, is cardiovascular assessment. One of the first things I do in the trauma room is feel the patient's extremities. Then, as I turn to assess and treat the airway, I look at the neck veins. If the patient is cool and pale or capillary filling is delayed, shock is assumed present until proved otherwise. If neck veins are flat, shock is assumed to be hypovolemic until proved otherwise. If, on the other hand, neck veins are distended, five conditions must be ruled out immediately: tension pneumothorax, pericardial tamponade, air embolism, myocardial contusion, and myocardial infarction (Fig. 3-1).

Cardiovascular status

A tension pneumothorax impedes venous return by increasing thoracic pressures and by

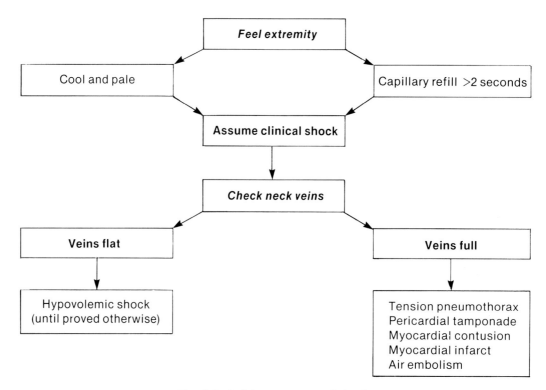

Fig. 3-1. Quick assessment of shock.

shifting the mediastinum and kinking the great veins as they enter the chest. Ventilatory function is compromised because one lung is collapsed and the other is compressed. Patients with a full-blown tension pneumothorax will be in shock and may have distended neck veins, respiratory distress, a trachea deviated from the involved hemithorax, hyperresonance, and diminished breath sounds on the involved side. A chest radiograph may confirm a collapsed lung with a shifted mediastinum.[8,9]

However, tension pneumothorax may not produce these signs in some patients. If the patient is hypovolemic, the neck veins may be flat, or fat around the neck may obscure the veins. The patient may not be lying in a perfectly symmetric manner, making evaluation of a deviated trachea difficult. Ambient noise may make percussion and auscultation difficult. In addition, most patients with a tension pneumothorax will be unstable, and chest radiographs are not readily obtained. Thus, because a tension pneumothorax can be fatal quickly and because the diagnosis can be difficult to make, physicians often must—and should—treat presumptively by inserting a 16-gauge needle in the second intercostal space in

the midclavicular line of the involved side. Tube thoracostomy is the definitive treatment.

Pericardial tamponade also is often a life-threatening emergency. It may be suspected when a patient is in shock and has distended neck veins but displays no evidence of tension pneumothorax. If pericardial tamponade is diagnosed early, pericardiocentesis may be a helpful temporary treatment. This is done by inserting an 18-gauge spinal needle in the subxiphoid area (Larrey's point) at a 45-degree angle, advancing slowly while aiming at the left shoulder. Monitoring the V lead of the ECG can pinpoint the tip of the needle; when the needle touches the epicardium, the noisy QRS complex inverts. Removal of as little as 10 ml of blood sometimes dramatically reverses hypotension.

If pericardiocentesis is unsuccessful in removing clotted blood, which is usually the case, or if tamponade induces cardiac arrest, immediate emergency thoracotomy should be done on the left side unless tamponade results from penetrating trauma, when it should be done on the side of injury. The incision is started in the intercostal space just below the nipple and carried medially to the sternum where, to facilitate exposure, the costochondral cartilage can be incised above and below the incision. The incision is carried laterally as far as possible, and the pericardium is opened along its anterior surface in a caudal-to-cephalad direction, avoiding the phrenic nerve that runs along the posterior lateral aspect of the pericardium.[2,3]

Clots are quickly evacuated, and any holes in the heart are occluded with the physician's finger. If there is no spontaneous cardiac activity, open heart massage with the fingers and palm should be begun. Arterial pH should be corrected, and 5 to 10 ml of 1:10,000 solution of epinephrine should be administered to try to establish coarse fibrillation. Electrical defibrillation then should be attempted, with internal paddles set at 20 to 40 watt-seconds or with external paddles set at 400 watt-seconds. If resuscitation is successful, the heart can be repaired in the emergency room, keeping in mind that it is done more ideally in the operating room.

Air embolization is usually a consequence of injury to the lung parenchyma from either blunt or penetrating trauma. This condition usually is seen in patients with major lung lacerations caused by rib fractures or by stab or gunshot wounds. Instituting positive pressure ventilation in such patients can force air from the tracheobronchial tree into the pulmonary venous circulation. Although embolization of air to most organs causes few recognizable acute changes, air embolization to the brain can cause hemiparesis or other severe neurologic deficits, and air embolization to the coronary arteries can cause cardiogenic shock. If this condition is recognized in the ER, the treatment is emergency thoracotomy on the involved side and occlusion of the lung hilum.[2,3] Definitive therapy, such as repair of the laceration, lobectomy, or pneumonectomy, can be done later.

Myocardial contusion usually is the result of blunt chest trauma and can cause serious arrhythmias, often within the first hour. This injury should be suspected if any patient has been struck in the anterior chest, particularly if sternal fractures are noted. If the patient is a child, the physician must be especially suspicious, because the high compliance of a child's bony thorax may permit the injury without the usual fracture. The ECG may show an injury pattern, and these patients should be continuously monitored for arrhythmias. Lidocaine or other antiarrhythmics

should be given if needed, and inotropic support should be provided.

Myocardial infarction also must be considered if the trauma patient is in cardiogenic shock. The infarction may have preceded the injuries or may have resulted from blood loss, hypoxemia, or stimulation from circulating catecholamines. Therapy is the same as for myocardial contusion.

Fluid replacement

If hypovolemia is the cause of the patient's unstable status, resuscitation consists of gaining access to the circulation and giving fluids. The first priority is vascular access. If the patient is in mild shock, a 16-gauge or larger catheter is placed percutaneously in an upper-extremity vein. If the patient is in moderate or severe shock, access is gained by one or more cutdowns, the number depending on the clinical severity of the shock. The safest and quickest cutdown is on the long saphenous vein, over the medial malleolus. An additional cutdown on the basilic vein in the antecubital space, passing the catheter centrally, allows monitoring of the central venous pressure. Catheters inserted by cutdown should be as large as possible to maximize flow rates of the fluids administered; in the average adult they should be 14 gauge or larger. The catheters inserted in the saphenous vein at the ankle should be short, again to maximize flow, but a long catheter is used for the antecubital cutdown to produce the benefit of central venous monitoring. I prefer a no. 5 or no. 8 French pediatric feeding tube as the central venous monitoring line. Catheters should not be inserted in injured extremities. As fluid resuscitation proceeds, catheters may be placed percutaneously in upper-extremity veins as they begin to distend. In some circumstances, as when a single physician is guiding the resuscitation or if a physician is uncomfortable with the surgical technique of a cutdown, percutaneous femoral vein punctures may allow rapid access to the circulation without major complications.

I discourage central percutaneous subclavian or internal jugular punctures if the patient is hypovolemic. Although such punctures may be easy and safe when the patient is quiet or hypervolemic, they can be difficult and dangerous if the patient is restless, combative, or hypovolemic. A severely hypovolemic patient has empty central veins, and such attempts at cannulation carry at least a 15% complication rate.

```
┌─────────────────────────────────────┐
│        INDEXES OF SUCCESSFUL         │
│            RESUSCITATION             │
│ Atrial filling pressures            │
│     Keep at or near normal          │
│ Urine output 0.5 ml/kg/hr           │
│ Level of consciousness              │
│ Peripheral perfusion                │
│ Cardiac output                      │
└─────────────────────────────────────┘
```

As soon as the first intravenous line is established, blood should be drawn for type and cross-match, hematocrit, and white blood count. Part of the specimen should be reserved to determine electrolytes, BUN, creatinine, amylase, blood sugar, and toxicology if indicated by history or subsequent course.

In general, 2 liters of balanced salt solution can be infused with impunity in the hypovolemic patient. The amount of blood administered should be governed by the clinical situation and by the amount and kind of other intravenous fluid replacement.

If severe shock has occurred, I prefer to initiate resuscitation with a balanced salt solution, because it helps alleviate metabolic acidosis and decreased blood viscosity. It also enhances perfusion of the microvasculature and replenishes interstitial fluid losses. If the patient remains in shock after 3 liters of balanced salt solution have been given, control of hemorrhage becomes part of the resuscitation and the patient should be taken to the operating room immediately.[10] If the patient's response to the initial infusion of balanced salt solution reflects improved mental status and improved skin perfusion, increased urine output, and restoration of normal vital signs, I proceed with a deliberate diagnostic workup. (See box.)

Type-specific whole blood offers several advantages in the emergency situation: it can be administered rapidly through intravenous lines, in contrast to packed red cells that tend to sludge; it is quicker to obtain than cross-matched blood; and it is tolerated well by most patients. The risk of transfusion reaction with type-specific blood is small. Low-titer O-negative blood may be used if type-specific blood is not available, but it occasionally causes difficulties with typing and cross-matching for subsequent transfusions.[5,6]

Autotransfusion also provides compatible blood with minimal delay.[4] In the most favorable situation, blood can be drained from hemothoraxes into containers with a citrate anticoagulant. Blood from the abdominal cavity can also be used, but the physician must be certain it is free from contamination by bowel contents, an assurance that is rare at the beginning of the operation when blood is needed most. Only small amounts of autologous blood should be transfused since large amounts will cause coagulopathies. Ideally, the severely traumatized patient's hematocrit should be kept at or near 30%, which is a compromise between desired levels of viscosity and oxygen-carrying capacity.

Defective hemostasis occurs with massive transfusion. The exact cause of transfusion coagulopathy is incompletely defined. The labile factors (factors V and VIII) are the only hemostatic factors that decay significantly during liquid preservation of blood. Moreover, if the patient has been hemodynamically resuscitated, factor VIII levels actually will be higher than normal because of the accelerated manufacture of factor VIII by the liver. Therefore factor V is the only clotting factor that is lowered significantly in massive blood transfusion. Fresh frozen plasma provides the necessary clotting components, but its effectiveness in transfusion-related bleeding is not firmly established.

More important, all blood routinely dispensed from the blood bank should be assumed to lack functioning platelets. Platelets lose their ability to aggregate in cold storage, and preservatives do not maintain platelet viability beyond 72 hours. In addition, most blood banks with component programs routinely remove the platelets from the donated unit. For these reasons it should be assumed that blood received by routine order contains no platelets. During massive blood transfusions, the quantity and function of platelets in the recipient are roughly proportional to the number of units of blood administered. In general it is advisable to administer platelet concentrates or "packs" whenever 10 units of blood have been administered in less than 1 hour.

Neurologic evaluation

This initial neurologic examination should take no more than 20 seconds; it is done only to establish baselines against which later examinations can be compared. It is not the purpose of this examination to make a definitive neurologic diagnosis. The patient's state of consciousness is categorized as alert, responsive to vocal stimuli, responsive only to pain, or unresponsive. The pupils are assessed for size and reactivity. The extremities are checked for movement—either spontaneous or in response to command or to pain. Trauma to the brain can cause any of a number of alterations in mental status, including coma, obtundation, confusion, agitation, combativeness, "paranoid" delusions, or even euphoria. All these altered states of consciousness also can be produced by hypoxemia or hypovolemic shock or, indeed, by inebriation.

The primary priority when treating the trauma patient who has an altered state of consciousness is to recognize and treat hypoxemia and shock.[7] The second priority is to recognize and treat brain damage. The physician should never ascribe an altered state of consciousness to brain damage or inebriation until hypoxemia and shock either have been ruled out or dealt with.

Once resuscitation has been initiated and tentatively assessed, a second evaluation can be performed. Since the need for speed here conflicts with the need for thoroughness, the resolution of this conflict depends on the patient's condition. If the patient remains unstable or deteriorates, operation becomes part of the resuscitation. If the patient stabilizes, a complete examination is done, and definitive surgery proceeds as indicated by the examination and special diagnostic studies.

SECOND PRIORITIES
The second examination

Once the airway is controlled, rapid external bleeding is stopped, the heart is able to maintain adequate arterial pressure, intravenous lines are established with the appropriate fluids administered, and blood is sent for initial laboratory analysis (hematocrit, toxicology, type and crossmatch), it is then time to begin the next series of evaluations.

A rapid but thorough examination from head to toe, including all systems, such as neurologic, cardiovascular, gastrointestinal-abdominal, urologic, and musculoskeletal, must be done. The physician must be thorough, because an injury that is missed at this time may go unrecognized for many more hours.

Table 3-1. Correlation between clinical signs and levels of brain function

Brain function	Clinical signs
Cerebral hemispheres	Verbal responses
	Purposive movements
Brainstem	Reflex motor movements: decortication, decerebration
Reticular activating system	Eye opening
Midbrain CN III	Reactive pupils
Pons CN V + VII, CN VIII, VI, III + MLF	Corneal reflex
	Doll's eyes and icewater responses
Medulla	Breathing, blood pressure
Spinal cord	Deep tendon reflexes

The neurologic examination

Ideally, a neurologic examination should be performed in the field or during transportation to the emergency department. However, it definitely should be performed as soon as possible after arrival in the emergency department. This clinical examination is the most important assessment of neurologic injury and may be all that is required to establish the need for exploratory burr holes and decompressive craniotomy.

The essentials include: assessment of hemispheric function (such as the Glasgow Coma Score), brain stem function (by cranial nerve activity, motor activity, and respirations), spinal cord function by motor activity, sensation, and bulbocavernous reflex (Table 3-1). Obvious or suspected cervical spine fractures should be treated by maintaining axial orientation using Gardner-Wells tongs.

If the patient stabilizes as a result of resuscitation, further diagnostic tests such as CT scanning and arteriography may be warranted. This decision should be governed by both the clinical course and repeated neurologic examinations.

Fracture management

Ideally, patients with major fracture injuries should arrive in the emergency room with splints in place. Unsplinted fractures should be splinted as soon as possible after initial resuscitation to prevent further blood loss and neurovascular damage, reduce pain, and prevent continued microembolization. Open fractures should be cultured and Gram's stain performed on the smear. They should be wrapped temporarily in clean dressings in preparation for irrigation and debridement in the operating room. If the patient stabilizes during the resuscitation, x-ray films should be obtained of all areas where fracture is suspected.

If a displaced fracture has caused vascular compromise to an extremity, the fracture should be manipulated as early as possible into a better alignment to reestablish distal blood flow. Arteriograms should be taken of all fractures and dislocations associated with diminished pulses if the patient is hemidynamically stable.

Diagnosis and treatment of occult hemorrhage

The clinician must be aware of the likely locations of occult blood loss. Since each hemithorax may contain up to 2 liters of blood, a chest x-ray film is essential before proceeding to the operating room. The film can be extremely helpful to the surgeon in determining the surgical approach. Another highly suspect area of hidden blood is the abdomen. Distention is a late and very unreliable sign. If a patient is in shock, if the chest x-ray film is normal, and if there is no other external signs of bleeding, it must be assumed that there is intraabdominal hemorrhage. The pelvis is considered part of the abdomen and can conceal large amounts of blood. Also, the thigh may contain 4 to 6 units of whole blood after a major fracture or crush injury.

In some circumstances the pneumatic antishock trouser may be used to temporarily control hemorrhage. If the patient arrives in the emergency room with an antishock suit already in place, it is imperative not to remove it until there is access to the circulation and the surgeon is ready to treat the specific injury. In general the antishock suit is best removed in the operating room with the patient prepared for or already under anesthesia.

The most extreme example of hemorrhage occurs in the patient who has a cardiac arrest from hypovolemia. In this instance the only chance for salvage is immediate emergency thoracotomy and open chest cardiac massage, because it is impossible to resuscitate an empty heart with closed chest massage. Emergency thoracotomy also allows access to the descending aorta, which can be controlled with a vascular clamp or the clinician's hand. What little blood volume that remains may then be preserved for the two

critical organs: the heart and the brain. As resuscitation progresses and the patient's blood volume is restored, it is important not to let the left ventricle distend.

Radiographic procedures: definitive diagnosis and care

If the patient remains unstable, the only mandatory diagnostic test is a chest x-ray film. If the patient stabilizes or arrives in a stable condition, definitive diagnostic tests may be necessary to determine the extent of injury.

In the more stable patient the cervical spine is the most critical area to examine if there is any question of spinal injury. A cross-table lateral cervical spine film, with all seven cervical vertebrae carefully demonstrated, usually is obtained at the same time as the chest x-ray film. Until the cervical spine is cleared of fracture, continuous care must be taken to avoid flexion, lateral rotation, or hyperextension. The neck should be maintained in a neutral position with a cervical collar or sandbags.

A well-equipped emergency room should have x-ray equipment in the same room that is used for resuscitation, and initial films of the chest and cervical spine should be obtained without moving the patient. If fixed overhead x-ray equipment is not available in the emergency room, portable films should be obtained. Patients should not be transported to the x-ray suite for better films until they have stabilized and have been examined, as discussed. During the initial examination, seriously injured patients must be observed at all times by a physician or skilled nursing personnel. Patients are taken too often to x-ray suites unattended; fortunately, serious consequences are infrequent.

Additional x-ray films are ordered depending on the specific injuries encountered. Plain skull films are obtained if a patient has experienced head trauma and has a history of unconsciousness but no focal neurologic deficits. This procedure allows rapid identification of skull fractures. When focal neurologic deficits exist, CT is the examination of choice. Only in exceptional circumstances must an unstable patient with a focal neurologic deficit be taken to the operating room without a preoperative CT of the head. CT generally has replaced arteriography in the evaluation of head injuries.

The question of thoracic aorta injury often is

raised after blunt chest trauma. The most common sites of aortic tear associated with deceleration injuries are just distal to the aortic valve and the descending aorta beyond the subclavian artery, where fixation occurs at the ligamentum arteriosum. Findings derived from x-ray films that suggest aortic injury include widening of the superior mediastinum adjacent to the aortic knob, obliteration of the aortic shadow, left pleural apical cap, downward displacement of the left mainstem bronchus, displacement of the trachea or esophagus to the right, left hemothorax, or fracture of the first or second ribs. First-rib fractures have special significance because they usually are caused by severe trauma. These fractures often are associated with aortic and major bronchial tears and a high mortality. Sternal fractures also are caused by serious trauma and are associated frequently with cardiovascular injury, particularly myocardial contusion. Physical findings suggesting traumatic aortic rupture include a systolic murmur over the precordium or medial to the left scapula, hypertension in the upper extremities, weak pulses in lower extremities, or hoarseness or voice change resulting from the pressure of the hematoma on the left recurrent laryngeal nerve. Aortic arch angiography must be done promptly if aortic injury is suspected.

In lower chest or abdominal penetrating injuries where violation of the peritoneum is uncertain, peritoneal lavage may be a useful diagnostic technique. This technique has become the principal method of determining potential intraabdominal injury since as little as 10 milliliters of blood in the peritoneal cavity can cause a lavage to be positive. In addition, falling serial hematocrits may suggest peritoneal irritation. An elevated serum amylase level may suggest pancreatic or small-bowel injury. Plain films of the abdomen generally demonstrate nonspecific changes when there is only a small amount of blood present in the peritoneal cavity. Peritoneal lavage is also useful in examining some patients with blunt abdominal trauma, particularly those who are uncooperative or unconscious or who may be lost to clinical follow-up for some time. This last group of patients includes those requiring CT scans, arteriography, or operative procedures such as craniotomy or fixation of fractures.

Selective visceral angiography is occasionally helpful with the stable patient if the diagnosis of

abdominal injury is in doubt and the indications for surgery are equivocal. Angiography is not useful in patients with clinical indications for laparotomy. Angiography has generally been used after the acute injury phase. Aortography and selective studies are used for suspected injury to the liver, spleen, kidney, or pancreas.

The patient with a suspected but unproved visceral abdominal injury should benefit from both ultrasound and CT in the clinical setting. CT, in particular, is valuable in examining upper abdominal and retroperitoneal organs. Ultrasound is useful in identifying pelvic and lateral abdominal gutter fluid; unfortunately, its value is negated by the fact that peritoneal lavage has usually been performed first. The problem with radionuclide studies of the liver and spleen is that it is difficult to distinguish the margins of organs, and it is precisely this accurate definition that is required.

An intravenous pyelogram (IVP) should be performed promptly using a "high-dose" drip infusion technique for hematuria or a suspected renal injury. Tomography should be used whenever possible. The IVP should not be relied on to determine the presence or absence of bladder injuries; for these, a retrograde cystogram should be performed. Theoretically, bladder extravasation from a retrograde cystogram may obscure later ureteral extravasation during an IVP. For this reason the IVP should be obtained first whenever possible. If there is gross penile bleeding, a retrograde urethrogram should be performed before Foley catheter insertion.

As indicated in the box, neck injuries below the sternal notch (level I) require femoral angiography to visualize the great vessels and determine the appropriate operative approach. Neck in-

---

**INDICATIONS FOR
ARTERIOGRAPHY AFTER TRAUMA**

Neck injuries—zones I and III
Chest injuries: mediastinal widening, first rib fracture, deviation of trachea to the right
Abdominal injuries: nonvisualization of a kidney by intravenous pyelogram, selected pelvic fractures
All penetrating wounds of extremities in proximity to major vessels
Dislocation of the knee
All fractures associated with abnormal pulses

juries above the angle of the jaw (level III) require angiography to determine the status of the internal carotid artery and assess the quality of intracranial collaterals.

All neck wounds penetrating the platysma should have formal surgical exploration. Since this exploration cannot be done safely in the emergency room, active bleeding should be controlled with pressure rather than injudicious probing. Only 10% of penetrating neck wounds can be watched, even by the most experienced surgeons, rather than explored. There is no question that injuries to a significant structure can be missed by plain films, angiography, or esophageal swallows. Since missing a significant injury can have disastrous consequences and since the morbidity of a negative neck exploration is essentially zero, all wounds should be explored. If a patient has a gunshot wound near the spinal column, the head and neck must be maintained continuously in a neutral position until cervical spine films are obtained.

Additional indications for angiography after trauma are presented in the box on p. 29.

REFERENCES

1. Alexander, R.H., et al.: The effect of advanced life support and sophisticated hospital systems on motor vehicle mortality, J. Trauma **24:**486, 1984.
2. Burns, C.M.: Surgery in the resuscitation of critically injured patients, Can. J. Surg. **27:**461, 1984.
3. Callaham, M.: Pericardiocentesis in traumatic and non-traumatic cardiac tamponade, Ann. Emerg. Med. **13:**924, 1984.
4. Demling, R.H., Duy, N., Manohar, M., et al.: Comparison between lung fluid filtration rate and measured Starling forces after hemorrhagic and endotoxic shock, J. Trauma **20:**856, 1980.
5. Demling, R.H., Manohar, M., and Will, J.A.: Response of the pulmonary microcirculation to fluid loading after hemorrhagic shock and resuscitation, Surgery **87:**552, 1980.
6. Demling, R.H., Niehaus, G., and Will, J.A.: Pulmonary microvascular response to hemorrhagic shock, resuscitation, and recovery, J. Appl. Physiol. **46:**498, 1979.
7. Lucas, C.E., Ledgerwood, A.M., and Higgins, R.F.: Impaired salt and water excretion after albumin resuscitation for hypovolemic shock, Surgery **86:**544, 1979.
8. Smith, B.P., et al.: Prehospital stabilization of critically injured patients: A failed concept, J. Trauma **25:**65, 1985.
9. Stoutenbeck, C.P., et al.: The prevention of superinfection in multiple trauma patients, J. Antimicrob. Chemother. **14:**203, 1984.
10. Trunkey, D.D.: Trauma, Sci. Am. **249:**28, 1983.

Chapter 4

Massive blunt trauma: radiologic diagnosis and intervention

YORAM BEN-MENACHEM

Hemorrhage is the common denominator in the majority of deaths in massive non-CNS trauma. The relationship between death and hemodynamic instability on admission is direct, as it is between the severity of posttraumatic hemorrhage and multiple organ failure.[11,15,21] Therefore in victims of wide-impact trauma, rapid and precise identification and control of all sources of hemorrhage—both active and imminent—must be given first priority. Yet despite major advances in the diagnosis and management of trauma, uncontrolled hemorrhage continues to account for a sizable percentage of deaths of patients with potentially survivable injuries.[23] Indeed, a missed or delayed diagnosis is twice as common in eventual nonsurvivors than it is in survivors (33% vs. 17%, respectively).[10] The fact that these ratios have remained constant for 20 years[10] is indicative of an elusive deficiency in the initial investigation of trauma victims.

In my experience the missing element is almost always the etiologic assessment. Knowledge of the etiology is vital to the understanding of its resultant wounding pattern, and the judicial application of this knowledge is a key to a rapid, logical diagnosis of critical injuries.[1-6] Its exclusion from consideration reduces the reliability of the clinical, laboratory, and radiologic assessment of trauma and is therefore a premier source of missed, delayed, or erroneous diagnoses.[2-7]

ETIOLOGIC ASSESSMENT OF MASSIVE TRAUMA

The etiology has two components. The first is a mechanism of injury: the intensity, direction, and type of force causing the injury such as intervehicular collisions, pedestrian accidents, crushing industrial accidents, and falls from height. The second is an accident environment: the location of the victim at the moment of impact. The interior of a car can be described as an accident environment, but that is nonspecific and therefore of little use. Each position in the car the victim may occupy—front or rear, left or right—is a distinctly different accident environment, and every one of these has two major variants: with seatbelts or without them. These are important to recognize, because the performance of the same mechanism of injury differs in relation to specific accident environments. Thus it results in different wounding patterns, that is, the nature, number, distribution, and severity of injuries.

A wounding pattern is a list of injuries characteristic of its causative etiology. However, the same or very similar injuries may be caused by several etiologies. For example, a ruptured thoracic aorta is part of the wounding pattern of an unrestrained frontal car collision at freeway speed;[1,5] it is also part of the wounding pattern of a broadside impact.[4] However, even though the aortic lacerations in both events may look alike, they differ in character, extent, location, and even in the respective underlying mechanics and dynamics of rupture.[1,4,5] Also, the abdominal component of a frontal-collision wounding pattern includes midline and bilateral injuries, but the most serious injuries that result from the broadside impact involve the side of the victim nearest the impact.[1,4] A wounding pattern tends to repeat itself in all victims of the causative etiology, al-

31

though it does not always appear in its entirety. Still, despite its lack of specificity, the concept of wounding patterns is very important: Those who become familiar with the various etiologies can use their respective wounding patterns as mental checklists, each including one or more imminently lethal injuries. The wounding pattern creates instant suspicion that leads to early diagnosis of those injuries.[1,3-6]

Etiologic assessment is an analysis of the etiology and its wounding pattern. With the delineation of a wounding pattern all potentially lethal injuries are identified. It is then the duty of the attending surgeon and radiologist to make the presumption that these injuries indeed have occurred and proceed to prove or to refute the presumption, irrespective of the initial clinical and roentgenographic presentation of the patient.[3-6] This approach is recommended highly in view of some serious shortcomings of the clinical and roentgenographic assessment of trauma patients.

COMMON CLINICAL AND ROENTGENOLOGIC PITFALLS

The postulation that an injury has occurred just because a patient was exposed to the etiology that can cause it is sometimes the only logical clue to the presence of such injury. In massive trauma, clinical and laboratory examinations, tests, and parameters lose reliability because often they fall outside the context of the etiology. Prominent among them are the patient's external appearance,[4,17] physical examination,[5,10,20] urinalysis,[2,4,5] and especially peritoneal lavage.* In fact, the diagnostic specificity of lavage is low enough to make it inferior to CT in diagnosis of abdominal and extraperitoneal injuries in stable patients.[12] For the same reason, exploratory angiography should be preferred over lavage and exploratory laparotomy for diagnosis and control of hemorrhage in many unstable multitrauma patients, especially those with pelvic fractures.†

The inadequacies of the clinical investigation are compounded by those of the roentgenographic assessment. Most emergency-room roentgenograms are relatively inferior in quality, and their informatory value is inherently limited. Even "old faithful," the chest film, is downright

unreliable in the diagnosis of aortic wounding.[4,13,18] It "shows you a lot, but still hides the essentials" faithfully describes the chest film or a bikini.[9]

The most ominous roentgenologic pitfall in trauma is the indiscriminate requisitioning of numerous x-ray films, of which the great majority are unnecessary for the initial, that is, life-saving, investigation and treatment. Such practice is aimed at obvious lesions, thereby diverting attention from critical injuries in favor of superficial wounds. It interferes with the diagnosis and control of hemorrhage and is therefore a direct cause of death by exsanguination.[14]

The practice of diversionary radiology by taking multiple unnecessary films comes with a variety of unacceptable excuses. A most prevalent error is the biblical-sequence approach to radiology: in the beginning God created the KUB and the IVP, and they forever must be done as a prelude to CT. The fact that they have become obsolete must interfere in no way with tradition. Other emergency room films as well offer poor or partial information; taking 10 times as many of the same films will still fail to enrich it. The production of a multitude of unnecessary plain films and minimum-contrast examinations may be driven by a sincere, although misguided, desire to avoid necessary but invasive or expensive radiologic studies, to fend off possible future litigation, or simply "to cover all contingencies" (whatever that means). Regardless of the excuse, whole-body radiography can cost more than a financial fortune: it may cost the patient's life.[14] Finally, when members of five surgical subspecialties simultaneously declare "their" respective injuries irrevocably the most important and deserving of priority attention and then proceed to "order" films, redundancy becomes aggravated by confusion, and damage to the patient may be extreme. If there is any duty at all for the radiologist in the trauma room, it is to prevent such practice.

SELECTION OF ROENTGENOLOGIC PROCEDURES

The initial roentgenologic assessment of multitrauma patients must be governed by a few elementary but logical rules:

1. On admission, the most severely injured patient needs only three films: chest, pelvis, and a lateral C-spine.[3] If tube-thoracostomy was per-

---

*References 5-8, 11, 12, 15, 16, 19, 21.
†References 3, 4, 6, 7, 22, 24.

formed, a second chest film is needed. At this point, based on physical examination, lavage, and the three admission films, the surgeon already has a working diagnosis that usually mandates emergency laparotomy or craniotomy. All radiologic work must stop because there is no time for it.

The number of x-ray films permitted in the emergency room must be inversely proportional to the severity of the injuries.

2. In a small number of cases—in my estimate no more than 15% of severely injured patients—further radiologic study of the torso and limbs is required to assess need, direction, and priority of surgical intervention or to obtain help in stabilizing the patient. These patients come in with a very complex or confusing clinical presentation, and one may be misled easily by multiple obvious injuries.

Obvious wounds are superficial. Superficial wounds are irrelevant.

3. The same principle applies to laboratory examinations: positive peritoneal lavage in a patient with pelvic fractures is not an indication for laparotomy. Indeed, pelvic ring disruption is a contraindication to lavage,[4,21,22] and a negative lavage must be discounted in patients after violent impact to the abdomen. The same applies to negative urinalysis:[2-5] hematuria is the rule in trauma, but some patients with the most serious renal-pedicle injuries have normal urine. Therefore it follows that *hematuria is irrelevant:* when present, we must find its source; when absent we must find out why.

Do not accept any finding at face value if that finding is etiologically out of context.

4. In the small group of patients who require further investigation the study must be designed to identify all possible life-threatening injuries that could be caused by the etiology to which the patient was exposed, and it must be able to cover the whole body quickly, in fine detail, using only one x-ray table.

Select the minimum number of radiologic studies (one, preferably) with the maximum informatory yield.

Only two methods in radiology meet these specifications: CT and angiography. Since all the rest are limited in scope or detail, I have discarded them. The choice between angiography and CT depends on the etiology, the patient's clinical status, and the information one is looking for. Information is most reliable when derived from direct evidence; the modality that provides it on that basis should be preferred over one that offers only indirect evidence. In vascular wounding, extravasation is direct evidence and a hematoma is indirect; the preferred method is therefore angiography. In parenchymal trauma (i.e., hematoma) the third dimension offered by CT makes it the better diagnostic method as long as the patient is hemodynamically stable. To assist in control of hemorrhage in unstable patients, the radiologist needs an intraarterial catheter, and angiography becomes the only viable method of study.

The summary selection of method is thus very clearly defined: *If your patient is stable, and you are looking mainly for parenchymal wounding, refer to CT.* This indication includes patients who were exposed to violent trauma but, in your opinion probably did not suffer any injury. *If you are looking for vascular injuries or if your patient is hemodynamically unstable with any type of injury, refer the patient for exploratory angiography.* Again, this indication includes patients who may appear relatively unhurt but have come in after violent trauma.

ANGIOGRAPHIC CONTROL OF HEMORRHAGE

Transcatheter control of hemorrhage often is safer and more effective than hemostasis by surgical intervention and is preferred especially when surgery is either undesirable or impossible.[6,7] Control of pelvic arterial hemorrhage, which almost invariably is from branches of the internal iliac arteries, is no longer a surgical matter. Surgical ligation of the internal iliac arteries via laparotomy is ineffective and lethal. Since the effectiveness of exploratory angiography and transcatheter embolization of bleeding arteries has been proved, leading traumatologists now advocate angiographic hemostasis in pelvic ring disruptions.[21,22]

Outside the pelvis, either transcatheter embolization or balloon occlusion has been used extensively in control of hemorrhage from almost every artery in the body, including the brachiocephalics. In most instances hemostasis by angiography is easier and more selective than with any surgical technique. It usually is accomplished with little if any loss of functioning tissue and has a negligible complication rate.

Given that death by hemorrhage in a hospital is almost always preventable[6,14] and having established the superiority of angiography as a means of exploration and hemostasis, one must also urge its liberal use. The lethal potential of uncontrolled hemorrhage is so high that, when surgery is not the best immediate option, it is much safer to perform a few "unnecessary" angiograms (an unnecessary angiogram is a necessary one that came out negative) than to risk not doing one at all. After violent trauma, a very early decision for angiography is recommended, sometimes even when the patient is not in hemorrhagic shock. It is an error to assume that a 70-year-old pedestrian who has just absorbed a 20-ton impact will remain stable indefinitely.[4,6,7] At this juncture one might also recommend the slaughter of a sacred cow: "never move an unstable patient" must be declared illegitimate. Neither surgery nor angiography is a trauma-room procedure. Patients must be transferred without delay to one of the two units, unstable as they may be, if they are to be prevented from bleeding to death.

THE HIGH PRICE OF COST CONTAINMENT

Angiography and CT are attractive targets for cost cutters because of their apparently high cost. However, given the diagnostic accuracy and specificity of both modalities, either is a worthwhile investment. The importance of making that investment becomes manifest if one considers the price of not making it. I am unable to attach a price tag to preventable death, but I will try to describe one for a preventable amputation.

Apart from the permanent psychologic scarring that will affect the victim for life, what is the total cost to the national medical economy of an above-knee amputation in a 17-year-old, an amputation that could have been prevented with a timely $800.00 arteriogram? An impromptu survey of a small group of orthopaedic surgeons yielded an average estimate of total cost to completion of rehabilitation at $300,000.00

For that amount we can use CT with 1000 patients or pay for 375 angiograms.

Countless millions of dollars are spent annually to screen the population for cancer, diabetes, hypertension, and a colorful variety of venereal diseases, to name a select few. These screenings are of perfectly healthy people. Still we hope that

we just may find something in perhaps one of the 15,000 and "cure" whatever it is we found. Having done that, we are then called to the emergency room to see a kid who has just rear-ended a semitrailer, and with him we decide to play Ring Around the Dollar? We have not the right.

REFERENCES

1. Ben-Menachem, Y.: The mechanism of injury. In Ben-Menachem, Y.: Angiography in trauma: a work atlas, Philadelphia, 1981, W.B. Saunders Co.
2. Ben-Menachem, Y.: Pitfalls in the clinical and laboratory investigation of trauma. In Ben-Menachem, Y.: Angiography in trauma: a work atlas, Philadelphia, 1981, W.B. Saunders Co.
3. Ben-Menachem, Y.: Logic and logistics of radiography, angiography, and angiographic intervention in massive blunt trauma, Radiol. Clin. North Am. **19**:9-15, 1981.
4. Ben-Menachem, Y.: Radiological evaluation of torso vascular trauma, Paper presented at the Proceedings of the 6th Annual National Trauma Symposium, Baltimore, Nov. 17-19, 1983, Philadelphia, 1984, Centrum.
5. Ben-Menachem, Y., Fisher, R.G., and Ward, R.E.: Are "occult" intra-abdominal and extraperitoneal injuries really occult? Radiol. Clin. North Am. **19**:125-140, 1981.
6. Ben-Menachem, Y., Handel, S.F., Ray, R.D., and Childs, T.L., III: Embolization procedures in trauma: A matter of urgency, Semin. Interv. Radiol. **2**:107-117, 1985.
7. Ben-Menachem, Y., Handel, S.F., Ray, R.D., and Childs, T.L., III: Embolization procedures in trauma: The pelvis, Semin. Interv. Radiol. **2**:158-181, 1985.
8. Cetro, T.F., Rogers, F.B., and Pilcher, D.B.: Review of care of fatally injured patients in a rural state: 5-year followup, J. Trauma **23**:559-565, 1983.
9. Dontigny, L.: Comments to the annual session of the AAST, Colorado Springs, Sept. 11, 1982, J. Trauma **23**:298, 1983.
10. Dove, D.B., Stahl, W.M., and DelGuerico, L.R.M.: A five-year review of deaths following urban trauma, J. Trauma **20**:760-766, 1980.
11. Faist, E., Baue, A.E., Dittmer, H., et al.: Multiple organ failure in polytrauma patients, J. Trauma **23**:775-787, 1983.
12. Federle, M.P., Crass, R.A., Jeffrey, R.B., et al.: Computed tomography in blunt abdominal trauma, Arch. Surg. **116**:645-650, 1982.
13. Fisher, R.G., Hadlock, F., and Ben-Menachem, Y.: Laceration of the thoracic aorta and brachiocephalic arteries by blunt trauma, Radiol. Clin. North Am. **19**:91-100, 1981.
14. Foley, R.W., Harris, L.S., and Pilcher, D.B.: Abdominal injuries in automobile accidents: review of care of fatally injured patients, J. Trauma **17**:611-615, 1977.
15. Gilliland, M.D., Ward, R.E., Barton, R.M., et al.: Factors affecting mortality in pelvic fractures, J. Trauma **22**:691-693, 1982.
16. Gilliland, M.D., Ward, R.E., Flynn, T.C., Miller, P.W., Ben-Menachem, Y., and Duke, J.H., Jr.: Peritoneal lavage and angiography in the management of patients with pelvic fractures, Am. J. Surg. **144**:744-747, 1982.
17. Greendyke, R.M.: Traumatic rupture of the aorta: Special reference to automobile accidents, JAMA **195**:119-122, 1966.

18. Gundry, S.R., Burney, R.E., Mackenzie, J.R., et al.: Assessment of mediastinal widening associated with traumatic rupture of the aorta, J. Trauma **23:**293-299, 1983.

19. Hubbard, S.G., Bivins, B.A., Sachatello, C.R., et al.: Diagnostic errors with peritoneal lavage in patients with pelvic fractures, Arch. Surg. **114:**844-846, 1979.

20. Laasonen, E.M., Penttila, A., and Sumuvuori, H.: Acute lethal trauma of the trunk: Clinical, radiologic, and pathologic findings, J. Trauma **20:**657-662, 1980.

21. Mucha, P., and Farnell, M.B.: Analysis of pelvic fracture management, J. Trauma **24:**379-386, 1984.

22. Peltier, L.F.: Comments to the forty-third annual session of the American Association for the Surgery of Trauma, Chicago, Sept. 21-Oct. 1, 1983, J. Trauma **24:**385, 1984.

23. Ramenofsky, M.L., Luterman, A., Quindlen, E. et al.: Maximum survival in pediatric trauma: the ideal system, J. Trauma **24:**818-823, 1984.

24. Shah, R., Max, M.H., and Flint, L.M., Jr.: Negative laparotomy: Mortality and morbidity among 100 patients, Am. Surg. **44:**150-154, 1978.

Chapter 5

Acute head injuries

GUY L. CLIFTON

DEFINITION OF A HEAD INJURY

A head injury may be diagnosed in a patient who, as a result of trauma, has sustained a loss of consciousness, has sustained a skull fracture, or has an altered level of consciousness.

1. In the neurologically normal patient without a skull fracture, a head injury may be diagnosed historically. The patient who has had a loss of consciousness will have a period of posttraumatic amnesia extending for the period of unconsciousness and perhaps longer.

2. A skull fracture may be detected radiographically or on physical examination. Palpation of a depressed skull fracture through an open laceration, bilateral periorbital ecchymoses, or a retromastoid ecchymosis (the battle sign) are physical signs of a skull fracture.

3. An altered level of consciousness or a focal motor deficit is indicative of significant brain injury. Level of consciousness is quantified by the Glasgow Coma Score, an essential clinical tool in diagnosis and triage.

NEUROLOGIC EXAMINATION OF THE PATIENT WITH SIGNIFICANT BRAIN INJURY
Glasgow Coma Score

The Glasgow Coma Score (GCS) (Table 5-1), described by Brian Jennett and Graham Teasdale in 1974, is used worldwide to assess neurologically the patient with an altered level of consciousness after trauma. A standard definition of coma is absence of eye opening, unintelligible speech, and an inability to follow commands. This corresponds to a Glasgow Coma Score of 7 or less. GCS 3 describes a patient with no motor response, no eye opening, and no speech, whereas a

Coma score of 15 is that of a neurologically normal patient.

Pupils and strength

Two other elements of the neurologic examination of the patient who has a head injury are assessment of pupillary reactivity and extraocular motility and examination for loss of motor function, specifically hemiparesis. Extraocular motility can be evaluated by rapid turning of the head from side to side or injection of iced saline into the external auditory canal. After evaluation of the cervical spine, the head may be safely turned. The eyes tonically deviate to the side opposite to which the head is turned. Slight flexion of the neck produces maximal deviation of the eyes. Iced saline also may be injected into the external auditory canal if the canal is first examined with an otoscope. Hemotympanum, laceration of the external auditory canal, or CSF leakage are contraindications to caloric testing. The eyes tonically deviate toward the side of the injection with the iced saline. The neurologic finding that is sought in this examination is presence of an isolated third nerve palsy, which is characterized by inability to adduct the affected eye. This, in the presence of an unreactive pupil of the same eye, is indicative of a herniation syndrome.

TRIAGE OF HEAD INJURIES

No consensus for triage of head injury has been reached by neurosurgical organizations; however, some generally accepted guidelines for triage can be discussed. The patient with a skull fracture, whether basilar, linear or depressed, is admitted routinely to the hospital. Surgical management is required for a depressed skull fracture; however,

36

Table 5-1. Glasgow Coma Score*

Best motor response	Obeys	M6
	Localizes	5
	Withdraws	4
	Abnormal flexion	3
	Extensor response	2
	Nil	1
Verbal response	Oriented	V5
	Confused conversation	4
	Inappropriate words	3
	Incomprehensible sounds	2
	Nil	1
Eye opening	Spontaneous	E4
	To speech	3
	To pain	2
	Nil	1

*M, motor; V, verbal; E, eye.

observation is the only treatment generally undertaken for the patient with basilar or linear skull fractures. The incidence of late intracranial hematoma is higher in patients with skull fractures than in those without; therefore these patients are not generally discharged from the emergency room but are admitted for observation.

Patients who are neurologically normal without skull fractures but with posttraumatic amnesia or clear historical evidence of loss of consciousness of less than 5 minutes are admitted to the hospital for observation by many neurosurgeons. If conditions at home are consistent with dependable observation for a period of 24 hours, it is becoming increasingly common for those patients to be discharged for observation by the family. Late complications for neurologically normal patients who have had a brief loss of consciousness (concussion) and no skull fracture are very rare.

The patient with an altered level of consciousness as defined by the Glasgow Coma Score is, of course, always admitted under the care or observation of a neurosurgeon. The etiology of the altered level of consciousness may not be always clear. For example, alcohol ingestion frequently complicates motor vehicle accidents and head injuries, so it is safest to assume that a patient who has an altered level of consciousness after trauma, and who is also inebriated, has sustained a head injury. The etiology can only be sorted out by CT scanning and observation of the patient during the first 24 hours after injury. Some general guidelines are that the patient who has a GCS 13-14 may be observed carefully, usually in the

intensive care unit or emergency room. Evaluation with an initial CT scan is not necessary in the absence of a skull fracture or focal neurologic signs. Patients who are not in coma but who have significantly altered levels of consciousness consistent with a GCS <13 or who do not follow commands undergo either careful observation or, more common, CT scanning initially to rule out intracranial hematoma or to detect significant cortical contusions.

The management of the patient in coma from trauma is substantially different from that of the patient who is not comatose. The mortality rate from traumatic coma is 30%, whereas the mortality rate of the patient with an altered level of consciousness from trauma and not in coma is approximately 5%.[2] Management of the noncomatose patient with a head injury (GCS 8-14) hinges on diagnosis, early surgery for hematomas, and careful observation. Patients with altered levels of consciousness who are not in coma infrequently develop intracranial hypertension from cerebral edema and so do not commonly require maximal physiologic support. The comatose patient, however, has a much more severe brain injury, with a 40% incidence of the development of cerebral edema after surgery and resuscitation and a 40% chance of harboring a significant hematoma on admission.[1,4] These patients require maximal physiologic support, very early surgery, and sophisticated early management. Because of the extensive care requirements of the patient who does not follow commands, I believe that in urban areas these patients should be directly taken from the roadside to a level I trauma facility (by the American College of Surgeons criteria). In rural areas, after stabilization at a nearby hospital, evacuation to the nearest level I facility is advised. Patients with lesser degrees of injury who are able to follow commands require less urgent and less extensive management. In urban areas, they may be appropriately cared for at the nearest hospital served by a neurosurgeon. It is important to emphasize that a consensus by organized neurosurgery has not been reached on these issues of triage.

EARLY MANAGEMENT OF THE COMATOSE PATIENT
From the roadside to the emergency room

The test of any system of management of major trauma is the rapidity and effectiveness with which the ABCs of trauma management are delivered: airway, breathing, and circulation. A mounting volume of data suggests that two factors in early care are critical to outcome: prevention of secondary hypoxic insults to the brain and early evacuation of mass lesions. Hypoxia has been found to be associated with a significantly worse neurologic outcome than that found in normoxic, comatose patients.[5] Hypoxia may result from airway obstruction but also may result from chest injury, pulmonary shunting, or systemic hypotension. The importance of rapid neurosurgical management has been corroborated recently by a study of patients with acute subdural hematoma in which the most influential factor in outcome was the time from injury to hematoma evacuation. A tenfold increase in mortality resulted from a delay of over 4 hours in surgical evacuation.[6]

To deliver early intubation, early support of circulation, and early evacuation of mass lesions, an extensively organized system of trauma care is required. Trained paramedics may control bleeding from an open wound by applying pressure, also, they may administer intravenous fluid and medications, protect the fractured spine, and perform tracheal intubation under a physician's order.

Following roadside management, it is essential that the patient be transferred quickly to a facility organized for the care of the critically ill trauma patient. In urban areas stops at hospitals not equipped for neurosurgical management will often delay definitive treatment of the patient. If neurosurgical facilities are far from the accident site, an initial stop at a nearby hospital for resuscitation may be life-saving.

Emergency room management

Whether the patient is admitted to the facility of primary treatment or arrives for stabilization before transfer, the same series of physical assessments and treatment should be administered. The first priorities of management are the ABCs of trauma. Comatose patients are unable to control their airway. Two thirds of nonintubated, comatose patients have been found to be hypoxic.[3] Early intubation and volume ventilation with supplemental oxygen will prevent hypercapnia and hypoxia. Beginning hyperventilation immediately is an effective treatment for intra-

cranial hypertension and is advisable until an intracranial diagnosis is made.

Systemic hypotension may be caused by hypoxia and, if so, is corrected by intubation and ventilation. Hypotension from hypovolemia is treated by volume expansion with blood and crystalloid solutions. Hypotension in comatose patients always should be attributed to systemic injury. Hypotension is the result of brain injury itself only in patients who are moribund with advanced brainstem compression (GCS 3).

After resuscitation, a rapid neurologic assessment should consist of the Glasgow Coma Score, assessment of strength of the right and left extremities, and examination of extraocular motility and pupillary reactivity. A rapid physical assessment will determine the extent of other injuries. Peritoneal lavage should be performed as part of the physical assessment even if systemic hypotension is not present, because significant intraabdominal bleeding may not be detectable on physical examination in the comatose patient. Any available history at this point is valuable. The history of a lucid interval or a neurologic deterioration after injury should alert the physician to the probability of an expanding intracranial hematoma.

Emergency room radiographic evaluation should include cervical spine, pelvic, and skull radiographs. Spine films should be done as soon as possible after admission. During intubation and movement of the patient, the possibility of a cervical fracture should be kept in mind if cervical radiographs have not yet been obtained. After evaluation and stabilization, the patient then may be removed from the emergency room for CT scan and operative management. Measures to control elevated intracranial pressure, such as hyperventilation, head elevation, and mannitol (0.25 to 1 g/kg), should be begun in the emergency room before definitive intracranial diagnosis by CT scan and intracranial pressure monitoring. For the patient who is posturing or spontaneously moving, paralysis with pancuronium bromide (Pavulon) and sedation with morphine will facilitate medical treatment of increased intracranial pressure and provide a diagnostic-quality CT scan.

At this point in management, craniotomy for hematoma or placement of devices for intracranial pressure monitoring is the next step.

REFERENCES

1. Becker, D.P., Miller, J.D., Ward, J.D., Greenberg, R.P., Young, H.F., and Sakalas, R.: The outcome from severe head injury with early diagnosis and intensive management, J. Neurosurg. **47:**491-502, 1977.
2. Clifton, G.L.: Traumatic lesions. In Rosenberg, R.N., and Grossman, R.G., editors, The clinical neurosciences, New York, 1983, Churchill Livingstone.
3. Frost, E.A.M., Arancibia, C.U., and Shulman, K.: Pulmonary shunt as a prognostic indicator in head injury, J. Neurosurg. **50:**768, 1979.
4. Miller, J.D., Becker, D.P., Ward, J.D., Sullivan, H.G., Adams, W.E., and Rosner, M.J.: Significance of intracranial hypertension in severe head injury, J. Neurosurg. **47:**503-516, 1977.
5. Miller, J.D., Sweet, R.C., Narayan, R., and Becker, D.P.: Early insults to the injured brain, JAMA **240**(5):439-442, 1978.
6. Seelig, J., Becker, D.P., Miller, J.D., Greenberg, R.P., Ward, J.D., and Choi, S.C.: Acute traumatic subdural hematoma: Major mortality reduction in comatose patients treated under four hours, N. Engl. J. Med. **304:**1511-1518, 1981.

Chapter 6

Spinal column trauma

ANDREW G. KING

Probably the two most important assessments facing the physician treating spinal column injuries concern the stability of the fracture and the need for operative or conservative treatment. These assessments are made easier if they are based on a clear understanding of the pathologic anatomy involved. The pathologic lesion frequently involves a combination of bony and ligamentous disruption. The bony disruption will be shown by appropriate radiologic imaging. The ligamentous disruption, however, may be more difficult to determine and may have to be surmised, often based on an innate knowledge of the fracture born from years of experience. Alternatively, the ligamentous component can be assessed more precisely by recognizing where the fracture as a whole fits into a known mechanistic classification. Over the past 10 years mechanistic classifications have been published for a number of specific fractures and regions of the spine, such as Jefferson's fractures, odontoid fractures, and hangman's fractures. These classifications often are tedious to memorize and give an added degree of complexity to the management of these injuries. However, I believe that this added complexity is necessary since it gives a clearer understanding of the pathoanatomy and forms the basis for a more rational choice of treatment.

CRANIOCERVICAL REGION

The craniocervical region consists of the base of the skull, the atlas, the odontoid, and the body of the axis. It is clinically and biomechanically a distinct area, separate from the remainder of the cervical spine (Fig. 6-1).[42,44] High stress areas are found at the junction between the skull and atlas and between the axis and C3. This area has

particular importance in the assessment of the severe road trauma case. Studies involving postmortem radiographic examinations after fatal traffic accidents[1,12] show a marked preponderance of fractures and dislocations in this area (Table 6-1).

BURSTING ATLANTAL FRACTURE (JEFFERSON'S FRACTURE)

The mechanism of injury with a bursting atlantal fracture is an axial-loading force that is applied to the vertex of the skull, and transmitted through the occipital condyles. It meets an opposing force transmitted by the spine to the lateral atlantoaxial joints. These joints have a sloping articular surface, and a disrupting tension is produced in the ring of the atlas.[2] The classic Jefferson's fracture is a four-part bursting fracture of C1. Interestingly, these fractures, rarely encountered in high-energy road traffic trauma patients, appear to be caused by lesser degrees of force. It is not uncommon, however, for there to be an association with fractures elsewhere in the cervical spine. In contrast, isolated fractures of the posterior arch of C1 should not be called Jefferson's fractures. They do not affect the stability of the C1 to C2 complex and usually heal uneventfully. These fractures can be treated in a Philadelphia collar for comfort.[28]

It is important to differentiate between the stable Jefferson's fracture, in which the transverse ligament is intact, and the unstable fracture, in which it is ruptured. The key to determining the stability of these fractures is the open-mouthed odontoid x-ray film. Lateral subluxation of the lateral masses to a point where the combined overhang measures greater than 7 mm indicates

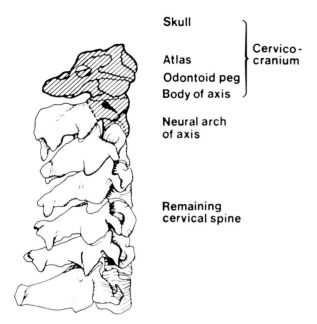

Skull

Atlas ⎫
       ⎪ Cervico-
Odontoid peg ⎬ cranium
              ⎪
Body of axis ⎭

Neural arch
of axis

Remaining
cervical spine

Fig. 6-1. The cervico cranium: clinically and biomechanically an area to be considered separate from the remainder of the cervical spine. (From Williams, T.G.: J. Bone Joint Surg. **57B**:82, 1975.)

Table 6-1. Distribution of neck injuries

Level	Number of cases
A0	19
C1	21
C2	30
C3	7
C4	3
C5	5
C6	5
C7	8

(From Alker, G.J., Oh, Y.S., and Leslie, E.V.: Othop. Clin. North Am. **9**:1005, 1978. Reprinted with permission from W.B. Saunders Co.)

that the transverse ligament must be either plastically deformed or ruptured. Theoretically, this instability should persist even after bony union, since it is doubtful that the transverse ligament will heal sufficiently. Therefore some authors advocate primary occiput to C2 fusion[39]; however, most authors have found that immobilization in a halo vest for 3 months will result in spontaneous stabilization.[37] In the rare case in which persistent instability is found, the fusion can then be confined to a C1 to C2 arthrodesis, since the posterior arch of C1 will have healed. A Jefferson's fracture in which the transverse liga-

ment is intact may be treated in an intermediate orthosis such as an S.O.M.I. brace.[28]

ODONTOID REGION

The mechanism of injury in the odontoid fractures probably is a shearing force in either a forward or backward direction transmitted through the skull. The force therefore is transmitted to the dens either by the anterior arch of the atlas or the strong transverse ligament. Minimally displaced odontoid fractures often are missed in the emergency room, particularly if they are seen in association with a more obvious fracture in the lower cervical spine. It is therefore important to keep a high index of suspicion, particularly when the patient has persistent occipital pain. The standard AP and lateral x-ray films should be supplemented, if necessary, with AP and lateral tomograms. The high-resolution CT scan often will miss the fracture because the transaxial slices are in the same plane as the fracture. The CT scan, however, remains ideal in delineating the Jefferson's fracture and atlantoaxial rotatory subluxations.

The treatment of an odontoid fracture will be dictated by the fracture classification of Anderson and D'Alonzo (Fig. 6-2).[4] Type I, which is extremely rare and stable, is an avulsion of the attachment of the alar ligament. The Type III fracture, which is the more common injury in the younger patient, is through cancellous bone of the C2 body. Because of its large contact area, the fracture usually will heal if the patient is immobilized in a halo body jacket for 12 weeks.

The treatment of Type II injuries, in which the fracture line is through the cortical bone at the base of the odontoid just distal to the articular surface in contact with the anterior arch of the atlas, is controversial. Even with prolonged immobilization in a halo body jacket, the failure of fusion has been reported at a rate of between 30% and 60%.[4,33,35,36]

When the multiply injured patient has numerous long-bone fractures, an unstable odontoid fracture causes considerable concern with regard to transfers and anesthesia for stabilization of the long bones. At our institution, the first procedure that is carried out with such patients is a primary C1 to C2 fusion on all Type II odontoid fractures. The surgical construct selected, however, must be one that confers immediate stability to the atlantoaxial joint.[42] The choice therefore

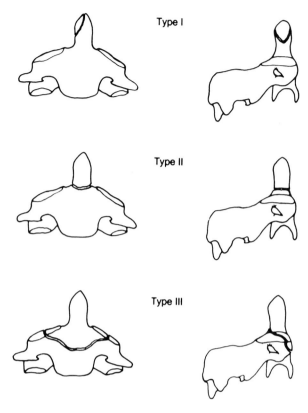

Fig. 6-2. Fracture classification of D'Alonzo and Anderson. (From Anderson, L.D.: Fractures of the odontoid process of the axis: The cervical spine. Philadelphia, 1983, J.B. Lippincott Co.)

should be a wedge compression type arthrodesis, as was first described by Brooks.[11,23,42] Type II odontoid fractures may be associated with a fracture of the posterior arch of C1, which should always be looked for before deciding to carry out a Brooks fusion, because in that case alternative methods of stabilization would have to be used.

We also advocate primary altantoaxial fusion for displaced Type II odontoid fractures for elderly patients and for those with anterior or posterior translational displacement greater than 4 mm.

TRAUMATIC SPONDYLOLISTHESIS OF THE AXIS (HANGMAN'S FRACTURE)

The popular name for traumatic spondylolisthesis comes from its similarity to the lesion produced in judicial hanging. Francis and Fielding[20] pointed out, however, that the mechanism of injury in judicial hanging is that of distraction and extension, whereas in the civilian form of this injury the force is usually hyperextension combined with axial loading. The point of application of the major force vector therefore will be to the face or the forehead, where there is often a concomitant injury. Francis and Fielding proposed grades of severity of this injury.[20] With progressive force, the fracture propagated first through the pars interarticularis, then through the anterior and posterior longitudinal ligaments, thus totally separating the cervicocranium from the remainder of the cervical spine.

Levine and Edwards[29] divided these fractures into three types, each caused by different forces and requiring important differences in the mode of treatment. Type I fractures, isolated fractures through the pars interarticularis, were stable and were treated with collar protection. Type II injuries resulted from initial hyperextension and axial loading followed by severe flexion. They showed fracture through the neural arch with significant anterior rotation or displacement of the body of C2. Care must be taken with IIA injuries in the acute situation because they may show increased angulation with traction. Type II fractures may show dangerous distraction in traction. Clearly, in the emergency situation traction must be applied with care to any Type II fracture. Weight must be applied in small increments with frequent lateral x-ray films taken.

The Type III fracture consists of the neural arch fracture with bilateral dislocated facet joints at C2 to C3. It is difficult to understand how this fracture could be caused by compression and extension alone. An element of distractive flexion must predominate. These fractures are grossly unstable and require surgical stabilization.

Thus there is a spectrum of stability in hangman's fractures. An unstable fracture should be suspected if there is marked anterior displacement or angulation of the body of C2 or C2 to C3 dislocation. Evidence of C2 to C3 disk disruption may be hinted at by an avulsion fracture from the anterior and superior aspect of C3 or, less commonly, from the anterior and inferior aspect of C2. Large retropharyngeal hematomas also will be present where the anterior longitudinal ligament has been disrupted.

THE CRANIOCERVICAL REGION IN CHILDREN

Although cervical fractures and dislocations are uncommon in children, when they do occur the craniocervical region predominates. The fulcrum of normal cervical spine motion in children under 8 years old is C2 to C3, compared with C5 to C6 in the adult. This area is hard to evaluate on x-ray films of children. A lateral x-ray film frequently will show C2 misaligned relative to C3 by as much as 4.5 mm, and such misalignment may be a normal variant.[13] The anterior atlantoaxial distance in children may be as much as 4.5 mm without injury. Odontoid fractures are rare in children younger than 7 years old. The fracture is more commonly a Type III fracture, which normally heals; surgical fusion is rarely necessary. Strong evidence indicates, however, that the late presentation of an "os odontoideum" probably means that the patient had had an unrecognized Type II odontoid fracture in the past.[13,19]

The emergency room physician also should be aware of two other factors in the radiologic evaluation of the cervical spine in children. First, the dens is separated from the body of C2 by a region of growth cartilage. This cartilage begins to disappear between the ages of 5 and 7, but a ghost of that structure may remain for several years, often causing it to be confused with a fracture. Second, the soft tissue swelling seen on the lateral x-ray study in the retropharyngeal area is not as reliable an indication of occult cervical spine trauma as it is in adults. A crying infant may balloon this area considerably.[6]

LOWER CERVICAL SPINE REGION

Radiology. The most important factor in the assessment of trauma to the midcervical spine is adequate x-ray films. It is a rule of our institution that, in all cases of a suspected unstable spinal column injury, a physician must be present while the x-ray films are being taken. The physician should supervise and assist the radiographer in positioning the patient and also evaluate the adequacy of the x-ray studies as they are being taken. By far the most information is gained from the lateral x-ray film of the cervical spine. This view must show at least the seventh cervical vertebra, and in most cases of cervical spine trauma, it will require a physician to don a lead apron and pull down on the patient's arms while the x-ray film is being taken.

Oblique views are necessary to demonstrate facet fracture or dislocation. In addition, the pillar or neural arch view also is important. The neural arch is the most vulnerable area of the cervical spine to fracture, accounting for up to

Table 6-2. Checklist and point value system to determine spinal stability

Element	Point value
Anterior elements destroyed or unable to function	2
Posterior elements destroyed or unable to function	2
Relative sagittal plane translation >3.5 mm	2
Relative sagittal plane rotation >11 degrees	2
Positive stretch test	2
Medullary (cord) damage	2
Root damage	1
Abnormal disk narrowing	1
Dangerous loading anticipated	1

From White, A.A., Southwick, W.O., and Panjabi, M.M.: Spine **1**:22, 1976.
*Total of 5 or more, unstable.

20% of cervical fractures. Without the pillar view, many of these fractures are dismissed as sprains. The view is taken by angling the x-rays 30 degrees to the vertical and aiming toward the suprasternal notch with the neck rotated to either side.[22]

In my experience stress x-ray films are rarely required; however, the traction stress x-ray film will confirm suspicion of a total disruption of the anterior column through the disk in association with a posterior fracture.[43]

Questions most commonly asked about cervical spine fractures in the acute situation are: Is this fracture stable or unstable? What is the mechanism of injury? Does it require surgery or would a halo body jacket suffice? If surgery is required, is decompression of the neural elements necessary?

Stability. Stability has been defined as "the ability of the spine under physiological loads, to maintain the relationship between vertebrae in such a way that there is neither damage nor subsequent irritation of the spinal cord or nerve roots, and in addition, no development of deformity with excessive pain."[43]

White and associates,[43] the authors of this definition, proposed a checklist and point value system to determine stability (Table 6-2). For points to be given accurately according to this checklist, detailed radiographic evaluation is a necessity. Bony integrity will be obvious on the x-ray film; however, the ligamentous integrity often must be surmised. The ligamentous integrity and thus the stability of the fracture can be assessed better by linking the fracture to a valid classification. The Galveston classification is the first to categorize comprehensively all indirect lower cervical spine injuries by mechanism of injury.[2] Although this classification adds complexity to the study of cervical spine fractures, it is a necessary addition. As the authors stated, "There is an awesome state of vagueness in the cervical spine literature. Previous papers have grouped fractures according to descriptive terms such as 'teardrop fracture,' 'burst fracture,' and 'wedge fracture.' Within such groupings, fractures with totally different mechanisms have been displayed."

An analogy can be drawn between this classification and the Lauge-Hansen classification for ankle fractures. As in ankle fractures, a specific history of an injury mechanism rarely can be elicited in cervical spine fractures. The authors indicated five categories (phylogenies) and identify four or five stages within each classification as

increasing force is put through the motion segment (Fig. 6-3). In correlating the classification with clinical material, they found increasing incidence of incomplete and complete neurologic deficit with each stage within the phylogeny. (Previous authors had noted a lack of correlation between the degree of vertebral displacement and the severity of the spinal cord lesion.[5,15]) We have found this classification useful in clinical management of cervical spine fractures. Compressive extension stage IV lesions, for example, may closely resemble, at least on the lateral x-ray film, the unilateral jumped facet, which comes under the diametrically opposite mechanism of distractive flexion. They clearly must be managed both acutely and definitively by different modes. In a recent study 139 unstable cervical spine fractures managed nonoperatively in halo vest immobilization were grouped according to the Galveston classification.[32] The halo vest was applied for 14 weeks. At the end of this time, 96 had achieved

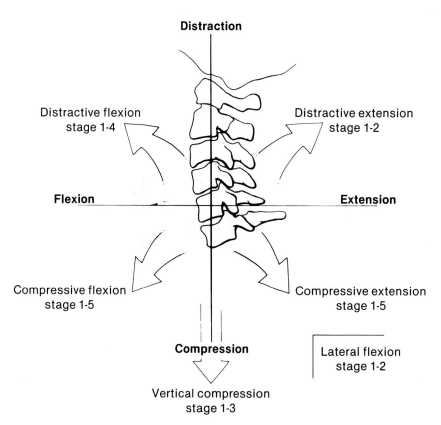

Fig. 6-3. Soaphic representation of the Salvestor mechanistic classification of lower cervical spine injuries, indicating the graphic representation of the Galveston Mechanistic Classification, six phylogenies or groupings and the stages within each phylogeny.

bony union, 22 required surgery as a result of pin tract infection, and a further 21 required surgery because of residual instability. Fractures with distractive and compressive flexion predominated. This finding could be expected, because in these injuries the damage is largely ligamentous. The spontaneous fusions that occur in up to 50% of unstable cervical spine fractures treated in a halo brace could not be expected to occur. Thus a case could be made for early surgical treatment of these particular fractures, avoiding unnecessary time in a halo brace.

Fusion of the cervical spine. The commonly cited reasons for surgical fusion of the cervical spine are that surgical fusions (1) reduce pain, (2) improve stability, (3) improve overall prognosis, (4) facilitate nursing care, and (5) reduce hospitalization time. We agree with White and associates, who stated, "There is no convincing evidence in the literature to support or condemn these indications."[43] Operative treatment is not essential. Most cervical fractures will undergo spontaneous fusion if treated conservatively by traction or halo body jacket for 8 weeks and intermediate control orthosis for 8 weeks.

Fusion should be performed in the following situations:

1. Where surgery has been required for open reduction or for decompression
2. Sometimes to aid in the overall aggressive management of the multiply injured patient
3. When stability after conservative treatment is going to depend primarily on ligamentous healing. The question is unanswered as to whether ligamentous healing in any given case of spinal trauma is of satisfactory strength to withstand physiologic loads[43]

Injuries that occur mainly through bone, such as are seen in grade I hangman's fracture and in the compressive extension phylogeny, will heal through bone and can be expected to be stable once healing has occurred. Ligamentous disruption gives unpredictable healing as is seen in a unilateral facet dislocation. The common treatment of traction to reduce these fractures may not be successful because of the resistance of the intact disk and capsule on the undislocated side. Manual reduction probably is indicated in most cases as long as it is carried out within 48 hours of the injury. Many of these injuries may be reduced, but they redislocate when transferred into an orthosis, because of the torn capsular and

interspinous ligaments, and ligamentum flavum. We believe that if a unilateral facet dislocation is over 48 hours old or if it has redislocated, open reduction and wire fixation accompanied by local fusion should be carried out.[16]

Decompression. The indication for decompression is the demonstration of disk or bone material in the medullary canal in a patient with a partial neurologic lesion.[43] The spine should be decompressed on the same side as the defect's location. If this is impossible to determine, then it should be on the side where the major damage to bone or ligamentous structures has occurred. Most complete neurologic injuries occur instantaneously with the impact of the disk or bone against the cord, and decompression hours later is usually of little value. Decompression, however, has been advocated in complete lesions to allow for root sparing and may be of great value in the treatment of quadriplegics who are injured at C5 or C6.[8]

If fusion is chosen, should it be done anteriorly or posteriorly? If, as in most distractive flexion and compression flexion injuries, the major disruption is of the posterior ligamentous structures with sparing of the anterior longitudinal ligament, then posterior wiring and fusion are indicated. Anterior interbody fusion in this instance may be harmful. Loss of the anterior longitudinal ligament, the sole remaining stabilizing structure, may lead to a recurrent instability that is difficult to treat.[7,40]

Laminectomy rarely is indicated. It is the most common cause of increased neural deficit in the treatment of lower cervical fractures. In addition, it causes increased instability and allows further subluxation or dislocation.[7,31]

The routine use of methyl methacrylate in spine trauma other than that caused by pathologic fractures is not recommended. Wire and acrylic is strongest at insertion and progressively becomes weaker with secondary loosening and metal fatigue. Bone graft is weakest at insertion but progressively becomes stronger with time. Reports on the use of methyl methacrylate show a high instance of deep infection and lost reduction.[17]

Cervical orthoses. The effectiveness of an orthosis in controlling cervical spine motion will depend on its inherent rigidity and its length. In practice, there are three groups. The most secure is the halo body jacket; the least secure is a soft cervical collar, and other orthoses are of intermediate range.[25]

The soft collar restricts motion by only 25%. Its main function therefore is to remind the patient that activities should be curtailed. The Philadelphia collar improves fixation by molded mandibular and occipital caps. It is reasonably effective in restricting flexion and extension, although weakest in controlling rotation. Intermediate orthoses gain control of the occiput and mandible with a more rigid superstructure and with a more extended thoracic support.

Although the classic four-poster brace is still used, we prefer the Guilford orthosis, which has a rigid neck ring and a thoracic strap. The S.O.M.I. is an intermediate orthosis that is particularly effective in controlling flexion of the atlantoaxial and C2 to C3 segments. This fact makes it a good orthosis for a hangman's fracture or in the later stages of treatment for a fractured odontoid. All intermediate braces, however, still allow up to 50% of lateral bending, 20% of rotation, and 20% of flexion. Thus they are clearly unsuitable for the initial conservative treatment of an unstable cervical spine fracture. The halo with a plastic body vest allows only a few degrees of movement in all planes. Control is best when a halo is attached to a well-fitting plaster body jacket as opposed to the plastic jacket. The jacket, however, should not be molded around the iliac crest as is seen in a Risser cast applied for scoliosis. The fixation thus is too rigid and the torque is applied to the pins, causing more rapid loosening.[35] In the large majority of cases the plastic jacket suffices, and it has the advantage of comfort. A halo that has four posts, which allows lateral x-ray films to be taken is preferred.

The Minerva cast can achieve a similar degree of immobilization as the halo, but to do so the jaw must be enclosed to the point where the patient finds it difficult to eat. The cast is difficult to apply, it is poorly tolerated in warm climates, and it has up to a 20% chance of incidence of occipital and mandibular pressure sores. We no longer use it.

IMMOBILIZATION OF THE CERVICAL SPINE IN THE ACUTE PHASE

Crutchfield tongs. Crutchfield tongs are difficult to apply because their use requires shaving the head, incising the scalp, and making small holes in the outer table of the skull with a drill. Because insertion is not at the maximum diameter of the skull, the tongs occasionally loosen.

Gardner-Wells tongs. Gardner-Wells tongs can be applied simply and quickly in the emergency room. The tongs are applied at the maximum diameter of the head just behind the external auditory meatus. They can be applied at any early stage in the emergency room to give some stability during transfers and during radiologic procedures.

Halo. It has been argued that the halo should be fitted in the emergency room. Such fitting will allow traction to be applied through the initial phase and later will allow fitting to a halo body jacket for prolonged immobilization. However, recent reports have shown a high rate of loosening in patients treated conservatively with halo body jacket fixation. If the halo is expected to last 6 weeks to 3 months or even longer, it must be applied with precision and due regard to biomechanical principles. Halo size, pin length, and halo angulation all have been shown to be important. Fitting a halo can be done best by using a halo jig, of which several models are available commercially. Too often these choices are not found in the hectic world of a busy emergency room. In addition, protruding pins in the posterior aspect of the halo may catch on a bed, dangerously jerking the head and inhibiting traction.

For this reason we recommend that Gardner-Wells tongs be used as the initial form of traction. If a halo body jacket is required at a later date, it is applied as an elective procedure by a skilled practitioner. If these conditions are met, we believe the despondency created by the longevity of halo body jacket fixation is largely unwarranted.

Beds. A standard orthopaedic bed with divided mattresses is adequate for the large majority of spinal column–injured patients with or without neurologic deficit. An egg crate should be applied and a log-rolling schedule involving at least two nurses instituted.

The Stryker frame. The Stryker frame has been a mainstay in the treatment of patients with these injuries. We have discontinued using it because of reports of loss of reduction on turning, decrease in vital capacity of quadriplegic patients in the prone position, a definite incidence of decubitus ulcer in the occipital areas, and the marked apprehension of the patient during turning.[38]

Rotorest bed. The Rotorest bed, with its constant motion, from side to side and up and down, is excellent for the high-quadriplegic patient, particularly the patient with pulmonary atelectasis or pneumonia. Patient acceptance is usually good, although some report "seasickness" and anxiety.

Anesthesia in acute unstable cervical spine fractures. It is the duty of the orthopaedic surgeon to ensure that the anesthesiologist is aware of the stability of a cervical spine fracture before inducing anesthesia. If the cervical spine is unstable, the orthopaedic surgeon must be present at the time of induction to stabilize the head and prevent excessive movement of the cervical spine. The safest form of intubation is an awake-blind nasal intubation. In small communities and non-trauma centers, however, anesthesiologists may not be facile with this procedure and will prefer to carry out a standard endotracheal intubation. This procedure indeed may be less traumatic in the easy cases, but in other more difficult cases it may require excessive and dangerous extension of the neck.

If awake-blind nasal intubation is unsuccessful, it is important that a fiberoptic endoscope be available. Even more important is the availability of an anesthesiologist or surgeon who knows how to use it.

LESIONS OF THE UPPER THORACIC SPINE, T2 TO T10

Lesions of the upper thoracic spine require special mention. They differ from cervical or thoracolumbar spine fractures in evaluation and treatment guidelines. There is a high degree of associated injuries of the chest, head, and cervical spine, and, often, associated life-threatening emergencies in the cardiovascular or pulmonary systems or severe head trauma. The care of these emergencies usually takes precedence over the spine and spinal cord injury.[9]

The spinal canal here is narrowed between the first and tenth vertebrae. There is an area of critical blood supply to the spinal cord between the fourth and eighth vertebrae. Thus spinal cord injury with small amounts of displacement of the spine is not uncommon. Bohlman's review of fractures in this region showed that five sixths of the patients sustained a complete cord lesion with resulting complete paraplegia. One sixth had some sort of incomplete cord syndrome, often a

Brown-Sequard syndrome, from stab wounds into the spinal canal.

These fractures often are reasonably stable because of the strong ligamentous attachment of the ribs to the vertebral bodies.[9] Displaced fractures always will be accompanied by painful rib fractures and often underlying lung contusion. The uncommon fracture that is displaced the length of the vertebral body or greater may fall into increasing kyphosis and therefore require reduction and internal fixation. Most of the remainder of fractures in this region can be treated conservatively with spontaneous ankylosis anticipated. Patients with complete cord injuries lasting more than 48 hours should not be considered for a decompressive procedure. Patients with an incomplete cord injury with demonstrable anterior cord compression by bone or disk fragments should have anterior decompression and fusion, which should be carried out as soon as the medical status of the patient permits.[9]

THORACOLUMBAR FRACTURES AND DISLOCATIONS

Classifications. Holdsworth divided the fractures into two categories: stable and unstable.[24] In the stable category are wedge compression fractures and burst compression fractures. Unstable fractures include dislocations, extension fracture dislocations, and rotational fracture dislocations.[24] This classification still is useful, although many burst compression fractures will be classified as unstable according to current definitions of stability.

Kelly and Whitesides introduced the two-column concept of the spine.[26] With only one column destroyed, collapse is incomplete. Destruction of both columns permits pronounced collapse. With one column destroyed by trauma and one by laminectomy, the spine is again rendered unstable.

Denis more recently introduced the middle column concept, an osteoligamentous column consisting of the posterior wall of the vertebral body, the posterior longitudinal ligament, and the posterior annulus fibrosis (Fig. 6-4).[14]

Careful assessment of the integrity of the middle column is crucial in determining stability of a fracture and selecting the appropriate treatment. In wedge compression fractures, the middle column remains intact. In burst fractures, compression failure of the middle column allows frag-

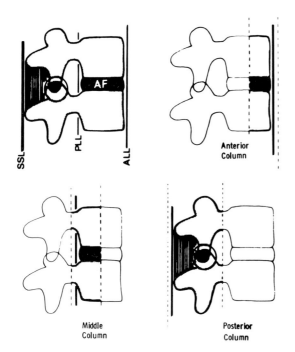

Fig. 6-4. Anatomic boundaries of the three spinal columns. (From Denis, F.: The three column spine and its significance in the classification of acute thoracolumbar spinal injuries, Spine **8:**817-831, 1983.)

ments to be retropulsed into the spinal canal. In fracture dislocations, the middle column fails under tension, rotation, or shear. In seatbelt-type fractures, the failure mode is tension.

Radiology. The integrity of the middle column is difficult to ascertain by the standard AP and lateral x-ray film. The height of the middle column on the lateral x-ray film can be compared with that of the adjacent unaffected vertebrae. Widening of the pedicles as seen on the AP plain film in a burst compression fracture has, in our experience, always been associated with retropulsed fragments in the canal. The CT scan gives much more information on the middle column and should be mandatory in all major thoracolumbar spinal column injuries.[27]

Treatment. There are no universally accepted guidelines for the treatment of thoracolumbar fractures. The major decisions are whether to reduce spinal deformity or to allow healing in situ, whether reduction should be achieved by operative or nonoperative means, and whether decompression of the spinal canal is required. No one criterion should be used exclusively in making these decisions. Rather, decisions should be based on a composite knowledge of the fracture, which is gained from adequate radiologic evaluation and classification of the fracture, use of a stability checklist, the neurologic status of the patient, and, equally important, the experience and skill of the physician.

Classification alone should not be used as the criterion. Wedge compression fractures are generally described as stable, yet if the degree of vertebral body collapse is greater than 50% anteriorly, they may leave an unacceptable late, painful deformity. Holdsworth classified burst fractures as stable, not meaning they could be mobilized immediately without fear of collapse or neurologic deficit but that with an adequate period of conservative rest and subsequent bony healing, they would then resist further deformity.[24]

McAfee and colleagues described the stable burst compression fracture, that is, one with an intact posterior arch but with failed anterior and middle columns.[30] We continue to mobilize stable burst compression fractures in a body jacket after a short period of bed rest to relieve initial pain symptoms and ileus. This procedure may be done even in the presence of a mild degree of retropulsed fragments if a patient is neurologically intact and without major canal compromise. These fractures were managed effectively this way for years before the CT scan showed us that many fractures previously considered benign indeed had some degree of fragment retropulsion.

Through-bone chance fractures will heal predictably with a cast applied with the patient in extension.

Surgical treatment. The indications for the surgical treatment of thoracolumbar spine fractures in the neurologically intact patient have not been well defined. The ideal treatment would realign the disrupted spine to an anatomic configuration, while at the same time causing little or no compromise of the motion segment. In some cases residual bony deformity after conservative care in a cast or brace causes less morbidity than a reduction done with Harrington rods, particularly if the lower end point of the fusion is required to be L4, L5, or the sacrum. For this reason many burst compression fractures of L4 and L5 are better treated conservatively with bed rest and a plaster cast.[21]

Surgical realignment generally is performed in the following situations: (1) a wedge compression fracture where the anterior vertebral height has been reduced more than 50%; (2) a burst compression fracture either with pedicle widening (indicating disruption of the posterior elements in at least two levels) or with retropulsed fragments occupying greater than one third of the canal; (3) most torsional and translational injuries (as these often have extensive ligamentous disruption with a propensity for both acute and chronic deformity)[18]; (4) chance fractures through soft tissue, and (5) injuries causing complete neurologic deficit. We believe that most patients who have complete neurologic deficit require stabilization to allow more rapid mobilization and rehabilitation.

Decompression. The indications for decompression are similar to those outlined for the cervical spine: the presence of a significant partial neurologic deficit with evidence of canal compromise by bone or disk material. In thoracolumbar fractures, the side for decompression almost always will be anterior. In injuries below L3, where cauda equina is involved, decompression can be more adequately carried out posteriorly.

Instrumentation. In recent years many new forms of instrumentation for spine fractures have become available. Each new device or technique does not necessarily supercede the one preceding it. What is emerging is that, with a clearer classification of the fracture and knowledge of its basic anatomic features, a more appropriate instrumentation can be assigned to each individual fracture. A surgeon adept only in the placement of dual Harrington distraction rods no longer is able to treat adequately all spine fractures.

Our current philosophy is shown in the accompanying algorithm (Fig. 6-5). The column on the left of the figure shows that in the uncomplicated, unstable fracture, we still rely on bilateral Harrington distraction rods and spinal fusion. In most cases lordosis should be contoured into the rods, necessitating the use of square-ended lower hooks. Harrington compression rods are dangerous if there is middle column disruption; compression may extrude disk or bone fragments into the canal and cause or exacerbate a neurologic deficit. If the anterior longitudinal ligament is disrupted, distraction rods may cause dangerous overdistraction of the spine or fail to stabilize the fracture, and later loosening may result.[30] In this situation, we use segmental spinal instrumentation, either sublaminar or through the spinous process.

The point of application of the corrective force of Harrington rods is the posterior element at the apex of the kyphosis, which is usually the fractured vertebra. If there is a comminuted fracture here or if the patient has had a wide laminectomy, the rod must be applied at points above and below the apex. In these cases we would advocate using Edward's sleeves or sublaminal wires attached to the Harrington rod to aid in application of the corrective force.

I do not advocate the use of sublaminal wires with Harrington distraction rods in uncomplicated, neurologically intact cases. The risk of neurologic damage by passing sublaminal wires in an area that may be swollen with edema fluid and with a possible swollen spinal cord is dangerously high. It has not been of much practical value because properly placed Harrington distraction rods without added wires can be confidently immobilized in a Jewett brace without fear of loss of fixation.

In cases of complete loss of neurologic function, however, the concern for neurologic damage does not apply and the advantage of more secure fixation and less need for external fixation on insensate skin is important.[3,41]

Decompression is carried out only on the patient whose neurologic deficit is significantly incomplete, with bone or disk present in the canal. In our opinion, a single nerve root lesion on one side is not an indication for anterior decompression, because this problem usually improves spontaneously. After decompression, we have been using the Dunn device for anterior stabilization, along with autogenous fibular strut grafts. Although this device is bulky and has mechanical disadvantages, we believe it is the best available at this stage.

In addition, in the rarer instance of an unstable fracture of L3 or L4, we believe anterior fixation *may* be preferable in an effort to save intact motion segments below the instrumentation.

We do not advocate anterior decompression and fixation in the neurologically intact patient regardless of the apparent degree of compromise of the canal by bone or disk. Some, but not all, of the canal compromise will be reduced with distraction. It is unknown whether unreduced canal fragments will lead to symptomatic spinal stenosis in the future, despite adequate stabilization and fusion of the fracture area. There is an equal possibility that these fragments, if they regain an

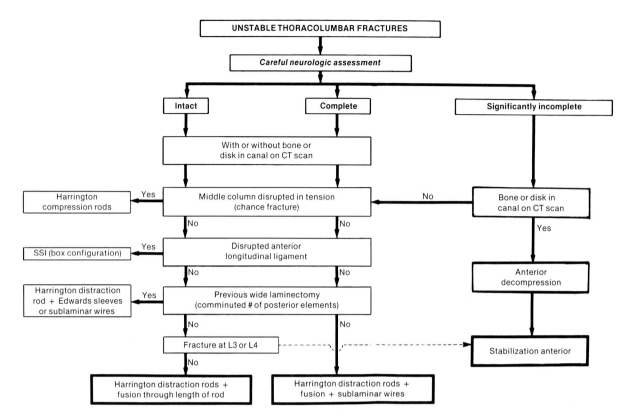

Fig. 6-5. Current LSU algorithm for instrumentation of thoracolumbar spine fractures.

adequate blood supply, will resolve spontaneously in the same way that posterior vertebral body osteophytes in the cervical spine have been shown to resolve after solid fusion.[34]

Finally, a word of caution. Complications in spine fracture surgery, hindering recovery of the patients, increasingly are being reported. When looked at carefully, these complications have been shown to have a high correlation with errors in technique.[10] The spinal surgery should be carried out by surgeons who have adequate training and a full knowledge of available options. Facilities and backup must be adequate. Spinal cord monitoring now should be accepted as standard practice. If not, the surgeon and anesthesia staff should be well-versed in the wake-up test technique.

REFERENCES

1. Alker, G.J., Jr., Young, S.O., and Leslie, E.V.: High cervical spine and craniocervical junction injuries in fatal traffic accidents: A radiological study, Orthop. Clin. North Am. **9**(4):1003-1010, 1978.
2. Allen, B.L., Ferguson, R.L., Lehmann, T.R., and O'Brian, R.P.: A mechanistic classification of closed, indirect fractures and dislocations of the lower cervical spine, Spine **7**:1-27, 1982.
3. Akbarnia, B.A., Fogarty, J.P., and Smith, K.R.: New trends in surgical stabilization of thoracolumbar spinal fractures with emphasis for sublaminar wiring, Paraplegia **23**:27-33, 1985.
4. Anderson, L.D., and D'Alonzo, R.T.: Fractures of the odontoid process of the axis, J. Bone Joint Surg. **56A**:1663-1678, 1974.
5. Barnes, R.: Paraplegia in cervical spine injuries, J. Bone Joint Surg. **30B**:234-244, 1948.
6. Boger, D.C.: Cervical prevertebral soft tissues in children: An indicator of cervical spine trauma, Contemp. Orthop. **5**:31-34, 1982.
7. Bohlman, H.H.: Acute fractures and dislocations of the cervical spine: An analysis of 300 hospitalized patients and review of the literature, J. Bone Joint Surg. **61A**:1119-1142, 1979.
8. Bohlman, H.H.: Late anterior decompression for spinal cord injury: A review of 100 cases with long-term results, Orthop. Trans. **4**:42-43, 1980.
9. Bohlman, H.H., Freehafer, A., and Dejak, J.: The results of treatment of acute injuries of the upper thoracic spine with paralysis, J. Bone Joint Surg. **67A**:360-369, 1985.
10. Bradley, G.W., King, H.A., and Dunn, H.K.: Surgical stabilization of spine fractures: A community experience, Orthopedics **3**:38-43, 1980.
11. Brooks, A.L., and Jenkins, E.B.: Atlantoaxial arthrodesis by the wedge compression method, J. Bone Joint Surg. **60A**:279-284, 1978.

12. Bucholz, R.W., and Burkhead, W.Z.: The pathological anatomy of fatal atlanto-occipital dislocations, J. Bone Joint Surg. **61A:**248-250, 1979.

13. Cattel, H.S., and Filtzer, D.L.: Pseudosubluxation and other normal variations in the cervical spine in children, J. Bone Joint Surg. **47A:**1295-1309, 1965.

14. Denis, F.: The three column spine and its significance in the classification of acute thoracolumbar spinal injuries, Spine **8:**817-831, 1983.

15. Durbin, F.C.: Fracture dislocations of the cervical spine, J. Bone Joint Surg. **39B:**23-38, 1957.

16. Edwards, C.C., Matz, S.O., and Levine, A.M.: Oblique wiring technique for rotational injuries of the cervical spine, Paper presented to the twelfth annual meeting of the Cervical Spine Research Society, New Orleans, Dec. 5-8, 1984.

17. Eismont, F.J., Bohlman, H.H.: Posterior methyl methacrylate fixation for cervical trauma, Spine **6:**347-353, 1981.

18. Ferguson, R.L., and Allen, B.L.: A mechanistic classification of thoracolumbar spine fractures, Clin. Orthop. **189:**77-87, 1984.

19. Fielding, W.J., Hensinger, R.N., and Hawkins, R.J.: Os odontoideum, J. Bone Joint Surg. **62A:**376-383, 1980.

20. Francis, W.R., and Fielding, W.J.: Traumatic spondylolisthesis of the axis, Orthop. Clin. North Am. **9**(4):1011-1027, 1978.

21. Fredrickson, B.E., Yuan, H.A., and Miller, H.: Burst fractures of the fifth lumbar vertebra: A report of four cases, J. Bone Joint Surg. **64A:**1088-1094, 1982.

22. Gehweiler, J.A., Osborne, R.L., Jr., and Becker, R.F.: The radiology of vertebral trauma, Philadelphia, 1980, W.B. Saunders Co.

23. Griswald, D.M., Southwick, W.O., Albright, J.A., Schiffman, E., and Johnson, R.: Atlantoaxial fusion for instability, J. Bone Joint Surg. **60A:**285-292, 1978.

24. Holdsworth, F.: Fractures, dislocations, and fracture dislocations of the spine, J. Bone Joint Surg. **52A:**1531-1551, 1970.

25. Johnson, R.M., Hart, D.L., Simmons, E.F., Ramsby, G.R., and Southwick, W.O.: Cervical orthoses: A study comparing the effectiveness in restricting cervical motion in normal subjects, J. Bone Joint Surg. **59A:**332-339, 1977.

26. Kelly, R.P., and Whitesides, T.E.: Treatment of lumbodorsal fracture dislocations, Ann. Surg. **167**(5):705-715, 1968.

27. King, A.G.: High resolution CAT scanning of burst compression and wedge compression thoracolumbar fractures, Paper presented to the eighteenth annual meeting of the Scoliosis Research Society, New Orleans, Sept. 28-Oct. 1, 1983.

28. Levine, A.M.: Fractures of the atlas, Paper presented to the American Academy of Orthopaedic Surgeons, Las Vegas, Jan. 1985.

29. Levine, A.M., and Edwards, C.C.: The management of traumatic spondylolisthesis of the axis, J. Bone Joint Surg. **67A:**217-225, 1985.

30. McAfee, P.C., Yuan, H.A., Fredrickson, B.E., and Lubicky, J.P.: The value of computed tomography in thoracolumbar fractures: An analysis of 100 consecutive cases and a new classification, J. Bone Joint Surg. **65A:**461-473, 1983.

31. Morgan, T.H., Wharton, G.W., and Austin, G.N.: The results of laminectomy in patients with incomplete spinal cord injuries, Paraplegia **9:**14-23, 1971.

32. Nelson, R., Capen, D.A., Waters, R.L., Garland, D.E., Passoff, T.L., and Zigler, J.: Non-operative stabilization of cervical spine fractures and dislocations—A series review and long-term follow-up, Paper presented at the American Academy of Orthopaedic Surgeons Annual Meeting, Atlanta, Feb. 1984.

33. Roberts, A., and Wickstrom, J.: Prognosis of odontoid fractures, J. Bone Joint Surg. **54A:**1353, 1972.

34. Robinson, R.A.: The results of anterior interbody fusion of the cervical spine, J. Bone Joint Surg. **44A:**1569-1586, 1962.

35. Ryan, M.D., and Taylor, T.K.: Odontoid fractures: a rational approach to treatment, J. Bone Joint Surg. **64B:**416-421, 1982.

36. Schatzker, J., Rorabeck, C.H., and Waddell, J.P.: Fractures of the dens (odontoid process), an analysis of 37 cases, J. Bone Joint Surg. **53B:**392-405, 1971.

37. Sherk, H.H.: Fractures of the atlas and odontoid process, Orthop. Clin. North Am. **9:**973-984, 1978.

38. Slabaugh, P.B., and Nickel, V.L.: Complications with use of the stryker frame, J. Bone Joint Surg. **60A:**1111-1112, 1978.

39. Spence, K.F., Decker, S., and Sell, K.W.: Bursting atlantal fracture associated with rupture of the transverse ligament, J. Bone Joint Surg. **52A:**543-549, 1970.

40. Stauffer, E.S., and Kelly, E.J.: Fracture-dislocations of cervical spine: Instability and recurrent deformities following treatment by anterior interbody fusion, J. Bone Joint Surg. **59A:**45-48, 1977.

41. Sullivan, J.A.: Sublaminar wiring of harrington distraction rods for unstable thoracolumbar spine fractures, Clin. Orthop. **189:**178-185, 1984.

42. White, A.A., and Panjabi, M.M.: The clinical biomechanics of the occipito-atlantoaxial complex, Orthop. Clin. North Am. **9**(4):867-878, 1978.

43. White, A.A., Southwick, W.O., and Panjabi, M.M.: Clinical instability in the lower cervical spine: A review of past and current concepts, Spine **1**(1):15-27, 1976.

44. Williams, T.G.: Hangman's fracture, J. Bone Joint Surg. **57B:**82-88, 1975.

Chapter 7

Anesthesia and the trauma patient

MACK A. THOMAS

Physicians involved in the care of the trauma patient are presented with one of the most challenging circumstances in medical practice. Assessing the trauma patient demands accurate and rapid decision making from both diagnostic and therapeutic viewpoints. The condition of the injured patient varies from the previously healthy person to the individual with preexisting medical problems. The following is a brief overview of the problems confronted and the alternatives available from the anesthetist's viewpoint.

Problems presented to the anesthetist can be divided into those related to induction, maintenance, emergence, and postanesthetic recovery.

An initial evaluation of airway competence, breathing, and circulatory status (the ABCs) is accomplished quickly. Indications for an artificial airway (most commonly an endotracheal tube) can be listed as follows:

1. Upper airway obstruction
2. Tracheobronchial hygiene
3. Airway protection
4. Mechanical ventilation (prolonged)

Instability of the cervical spine dictates the use of various techniques to gain airway control and maintain traction. Each circumstance must be evaluated independently for the most appropriate intubation technique. Insertion of the airway may be accomplished by blind nasal intubation, fiberoptic or retrograde techniques, or crycothyroidotomy.

Aspiration of gastric contents is a major concern in the treatment of the emergency patient. The vast majority of traumatized patients have full stomachs, and if general anesthesia is used, aspiration becomes the leading cause of anesthetic morbidity and mortality. Although regional anesthesia may allow the patient to maintain airway control, loss of protective airway reflexes may occur due to high levels of spinal or epidural anesthesia or rapid vascular absorption of local anesthetics leading to seizure activity. Supplemental sedation must be used cautiously, if at all, if the patient has a full stomach.

Aspiration of gastric contents is associated with emergency surgery. In fact, when aspiration occurs, 92% are emergency procedures; 30% occur with upper abdominal procedures, and 25% occur in the prone position. If the volume of the aspirate is 20 cc or greater and the aspirate has a pH of 2.5 or less, the *mortality* rate is 60% to 70%.[5] Intubation of the airway when general anesthesia is needed may be accomplished acceptably by either of the following techniques:

1. Awake intubation with or without topical anesthesia to the pharyngeal structures
2. Rapid sequence induction with cricoid pressure (Sellick's maneuver) maintained during intubation

Once the airway has been secured, maintenance of anesthesia is accomplished by inhalation or intravenous agents usually combined with muscle relaxants. Frequently a combination of both agents may be used. Ventilation is accomplished by using positive pressure in a controlled mode.

Most anesthesia techniques produce vasodilation with resultant venous pooling. The use of positive pressure breathing (PPB) may cause hypotension. Most anesthetic agents also reduce myocardial contractility. This reduction varies from essentially no depression with fentanyl to significant depression with halothane. Because of these effects, it is of the utmost importance that vascular volume be replenished as quickly as possible. Without adequate venous return, cardiac output will be decreased and tissue oxygenation will suffer. Adequate fluid resuscitation can be gauged by the usual signs of pulse, blood pressure, and urine output. In many cases central monitoring may be necessary to assess accurately the vascular space to vascular volume relationship.

It is imperative to appreciate that venous volume is critical to ensure adequate return to the right ventricle. A pressure gradient must be maintained between the peripheral venous system and the right atrium so that venous return can be maintained. In many instances a greater volume than might be expected is necessary to accomplish atrial filling. During the period of stress, sympathetic discharge is usually at its maximum output. It can be seen by referring to Fig. 7-1 that the goal of sympathetic outflow is restoration of vascular volume and increasing venous return.

Because patients who are under anesthesia tend to become poikilothermic, hypothermia is a common occurrence during surgery and anesthesia. Factors that may bring about hypothermia include:

1. Immobility and depression of the thermostat with absence of normal regulatory mechanisms
2. Autonomic and motor blockade with impairment of heat generation
3. Vasodilation
4. Wet skin surfaces
5. Exposure to low ambient temperature
6. Unheated, dry anesthetic gases
7. Unwarmed fluids and blood products

All of these factors are present to a greater or lesser degree during anesthesia and surgery.[3]

Elderly patients and those undergoing long operations are at high risk for the development of hypothermia. One group of investigators found that most temperature change occurred during exposure and preparation before surgical incision.[6]

Consequences of hypothermia include an increase in O_2 consumption and a shift to the left of the oxyhemoglobin dissociation curve because of cold and hypocapnia associated with decreased CO_2 production.[3] Lowered CO_2 results in decreases in cerebral perfusion with peripheral vasoconstriction. The attendant vasoconstriction may result in a central shift of blood volume with misleading central pressure measurements

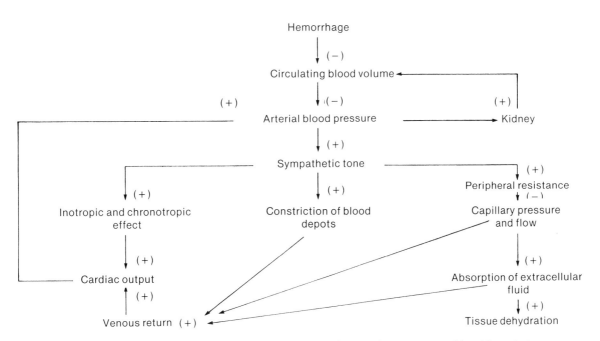

Fig. 7-1. Diagram of the vascular and autonomic changes in response to blood loss. **(+)**, increase; **(−)**, decrease.

leading to inadequate volume replacement. Peripheral vasoconstriction may cause further decrease in perfusion, endangering the trauma patient's extremities, which already have marginal circulation.

In the postoperative patient shivering may create 300% to 800% increases in oxygen demand. During this period, patients unable to meet this additional stress can sustain such serious sequalcae as myocardial damage.

Pulmonary volumes during general anesthesia may decrease because of the following factors: (1) position, (2) a paralyzed diaphragm caused by muscle relaxants, (3) lack of airway defense, (4) decreased surfactant production, and (5) incision site—abdominal or thoracic.[2] If a patient breathes spontaneously at the termination of the operation and is extubated, the effects of the anesthetic do not persist beyond 4 to 6 hours. It is a common myth among surgical practitioners that spinal anesthesia is less risky than general anesthesia. The preponderance of evidence reveals no difference in morbidity or mortality and specifically no difference in respiratory morbidity and mortality however measured.[1] At the termination of the procedure, patient status must be elevated as to the ability to maintain spontaneous ventilation and airway protection.

Lung function may be impaired in the trauma patient because of direct injury, such as pulmonary contusion, pneumothorax, and flail chest, as well as abdominal injury with restriction of abdominal and diaphragmatic motion. These effects lead to restrictive lung dysfunction in the surgical patient, which is always accompanied by a decrease in lung volume. Additional lung injury may be caused by multiple blood transfusions, large volumes of fluid, and vasoconstriction resulting from sympathetic discharge.

The hypoperfused lung is unable to metabolize many of the substances released during the period of stress. The inability of the lung to meet these metabolic demands effectively may lead to lung injury that can result in the development of acute postoperative respiratory problems. Adult respiratory distress syndrome (ARDS) is the term associated with this type of postoperative dysfunction. ARDS usually is diagnosed when a patient with previously normal lungs develops the clinical findings of stiff lungs (decreased compliance and high airway pressure), arterial hypoxemia, and

bilateral lung infiltrates on chest x-ray films. The frequent development of sepsis in the postoperative period is in all likelihood responsible for the most severe cases of ARDS. If reconstructive surgery has successfully stabilized the effects of trauma and if sepsis is effectively treated, the outcome is good. When sepsis cannot be controlled, the outcome from the pulmonary point of view is an unresponsive hypoxemia resulting in a hypoxic death.

The goals of postoperative pulmonary management include:

1. Adequate oxygenation
2. Clearance of secretions
3. Maintenance of respiratory acid-base balance (pH 7.35 to 7.45; P_{CO_2} 35 to 45)
4. Resumption of spontaneous ventilation as soon as possible

In order to accomplish these goals, use of airway pressure (PEEP), oxygen therapy, respiratory therapy maneuvers (chest physiotherapy, drainage, incentive spirometry), and appropriate antibiotic therapy usually are necessary. Most surgical intensivists believe that the use of 5 to 10 cm of PEEP in the immediate postoperative period is useful in maintaining adequate lung volumes in the trauma patient. Several clinical studies have suggested that the use of PEEP is the only effective means of maintaining lung volumes in the postoperative period.[2]

The brain is of course at high risk during periods of hypoperfusion. Some degree of protection is offered to the central nervous system in that all anesthesia techniques decrease cerebral metabolic oxygen requirements. Additionally, barbiturates are thought to be scavengers of free radicals that are associated with brain injury, and they have been used in brain resuscitation in the form of bolus doses or barbiturate coma.

Based on extensive studies of patients in shock who survived, Shoemaker[7] concluded the following optimal therapeutic values:

1. Cardiac output 30% above normal
2. Pulmonary vascular resistance normal to slight increase
3. Systemic vascular resistance normal to slight increase
4. Blood volume 500 ml above normal
5. Normal or slightly alkaline pH (7.4 to 7.45)
6. O_2 consumption 10% to 15% above normal

REFERENCES

1. Boutros, A.K., and Weisel, N.: Comparison of effects of three anesthetic techniques on patients with severe pulmonary obstructive disease, Can. Anaesth. Soc. J. **18:**286-292, 1971.
2. Dueck, R.: Gas exchange. Effects of anesthesia and surgery on pulmonary mechanisms and gas exchange. In Jones, J.G., editor: Int. Anesthesiol. Clin. vol. 22, no. 4, Boston, 1984, Little, Brown & Co.
3. Flacke, J.W., and Flacke, W.E.: Inadvertent hypothermia: Frequent, insidious, and often serious, Semin. Anesth. vol. II no. 3, 1983.
4. Godfrey, P.J., Greenan, J., Ranesinghe, D.D., et al.: Ventilatory capacity after three methods of anesthesia for inguinal hernia repair: A randomized controlled trial, Br. J. Surg. **68:**587-589, 1981.
5. Modell, J.H.: Aspiration pneumonitis. In Hershey, S.G., editor: ASA refresher courses in anesthesiology, vol. 10, Philadelphia, 1982, J.B. Lippincott Co.
6. Roizen, M.F., Sohn, Y.J., L'Hommedieu C.S., et al.: Operating room temperature prior to surgical draping: Effect on patient temperature in recovery room, Anesth. Analg. **59:**852-855, 1980.
7. Waxman, K., and Shoemaker, W.C.: Physiologic responses to massive intraoperative hemorrhage, Arch. Surg. **117:**470-475, 1982.

THE ELBOW

Chapter 8

Applied anatomy and biomechanics of the elbow joint

BERNARD F. MORREY

A detailed understanding of the specific anatomy of the elbow joint, as well as the practical aspects of the mechanics of this joint, is important knowledge for the clinician to have to treat the joint properly when it becomes diseased or injured. As with any other joint, elbow joint function is described clinically by noting motion, stability, and strength. These aspects of a joint are defined by its specific anatomy. The applied anatomy of the elbow joint therefore will be described as it relates to the three biomechanical considerations that detail its function: kinematics, joint constraints, and force transmission.

KINEMATICS: JOINT MOTION

The motion of any joint is based on the unique features of its articular surface and orientation. For this reason an understanding of the humeral ulnar and radial contributions to the elbow joint is required.

The humeral articulation

The distal humerus is comprised of the capitellar and trochlear cartilaginous surfaces that make an angle of approximately 6 degrees of valgus when viewed in the anteroposterior plane. It is rotated anteriorly about 30 degrees as viewed in the lateral projection and demonstrates a slight but definite 3- to 5-degree internal rotation with respect to the epicondylar line (Fig. 8-1).[11] The articular surface of the trochlea is covered by hyaline cartilage in an arc of approximately 330 degrees. The capitellum comprises an almost perfect hemisphere with an arc of 180 degrees.

The ulnar articulation

The articular surface of the proximal ulna consists of a greater sigmoid fossa that makes an approximate 4-degree valgus angulation with the shaft of the ulna; it is rotated posteriorly approximately 30 degrees with respect to the long axis as viewed in the lateral projection (Fig. 8-2). The angular relationship of the distal humerus and proximal ulna defines the carrying angle of the extremity.[2] The posterior rotation of the articular surface of the ulna matches the 30-degree anterior rotation of the distal humerus, thus providing stability in full extension. The articular surface of the greater sigmoid notch comprises an arc of at least 180 degrees, but it is not continuous with hyaline cartilage in the midsection.

In over 90% of individuals the midportion is comprised of a fatty, fibrous tissue.[16] This anatomic feature explains the propensity of fractures to occur in this area, since this portion of the greater sigmoid fossa is not supported by the stronger subchondral bone. This anatomic aspect also justifies the use of a transolecranon osteotomy to expose the elbow in certain conditions. The articular surface of the proximal ulna matches that of the trochlea in a way that results in the elbow joint as one of the most congruent and constrained joints in the body.

Radius

Approximately four fifths of the 360-degree circular margin of the radial head consists of articular cartilage with strong subchondral bone. This arc articulates with the lesser sigmoid fossa

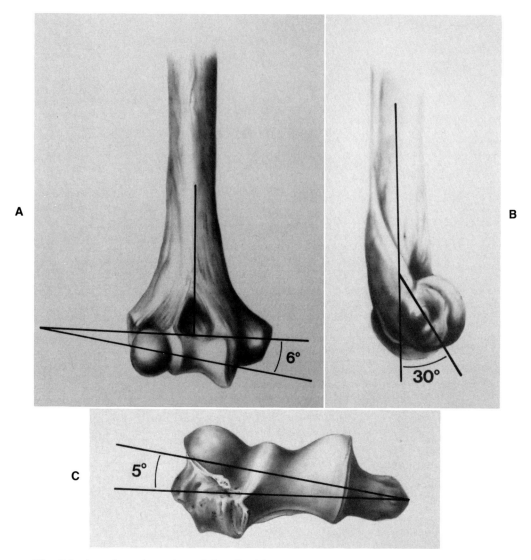

Fig. 8-1. Angular orientation of the distal humerus in the anteroposterior **(A)**, lateral **(B)**, and axial projections **(C)**. (From Morrey, B.F., editor: The elbow and its disorders, Philadelphia, 1985, W.B. Saunders Co.)

of the proximal ulna. The anterolateral aspect of the radial head lacks the stronger subchondral bone associated with hyaline cartilage. This explains the propensity for the marginal or slice radial head fracture to occur with falls on the outstretched hand when the elbow is flexed and slightly pronated. The radial neck makes an angle of approximately 15 degrees away from the radial tuberosity (Fig. 8-3). This degree of angulation, coupled with the bowing of the radius, allows forearm rotation to occur about an arc of almost 180 degrees, while the radial head maintains precise axial alignment with the capitellum.

Elbow motion: axis of rotation

The unique articular orientations previously described allow elbow motion up to approximately 150 degrees of flexion. The mean pronation is approximately 75 degrees, and the mean supination is approximately 85 degrees for an arc of forearm rotation averaging 160 to 170 degrees.[4] The axis of elbow flexion and extension is approximated by a locus that resides in the center of the trochlea and capitellum as viewed on the lateral projection (Fig. 8-4).[10,14] This fact has important connotations with respect to elbow ligaments and the rationale of such reconstructive

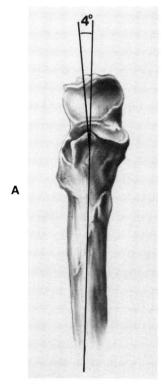

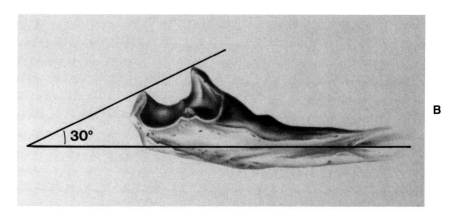

Fig. 8-2. Angular orientation of the proximal ulna in the anteroposterior **(A)** and lateral projection **(B)**. (From Morrey, B.F., editor: The elbow and its disorders, Philadelphia, 1985, W.B. Saunders Co.)

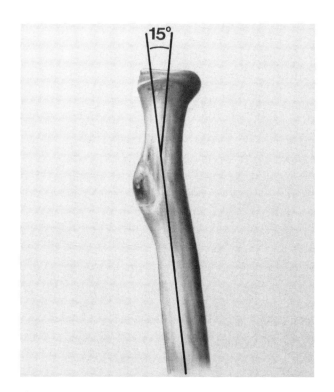

Fig. 8-3. Angular orientation of the radial head and neck with respect to the shaft of the radius. (From Morrey, B.F., editor: The elbow and its disorders, Philadelphia, 1985, W.B. Saunders Co.)

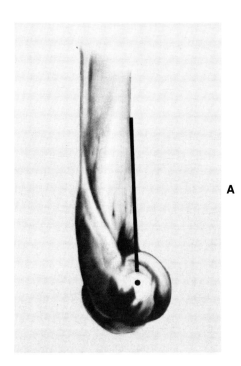

Fig. 8-4. Axis of rotation of the elbow in flexion and extension is through the center of the trochlea, colinear with the distal anterior cortex of the humerus **(A)**.

Continued.

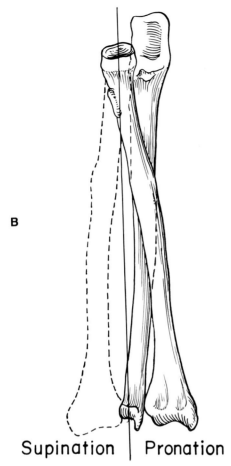

B

Supination | Pronation

Fig. 8-4, cont'd. Forearm rotation occurs about an axis through the center of the medial head and base of the ulnar styloid **(B)**. (From Morrey, B.F., editor: The elbow and its disorders, Philadelphia, 1985, W.B. Saunders Co.)

procedures as distraction arthroplasty.

The axis of the forearm rotation is through the center of the radial head and the capitellum and along a line extending through the base of the ulna styloid (Fig. 8-4).

JOINT CONSTRAINTS: STABILITY

The stability of any joint is caused by certain static and dynamic elements. The static stability is contributed by the articular surface and the ligamentous and capsular structures. At the elbow, the medial and lateral collateral ligaments, as well as the anterior capsule, are the major static soft tissue stabilizing elements.

The collateral ligaments

The medial collateral ligament complex demonstrates a constant pattern of anterior and posterior bundles with a transverse ligament that consists of a thickening of the capsule and expands the greater sigmoid notch (Fig. 8-5).

Unlike the medial collateral ligament, which demonstrates a very consistent pattern, the lateral ligamentous complex, which is not so well understood, demonstrates more individual variation. In addition to the classical radial collateral ligament, which originates from the lateral epicondyle and inserts on the annular ligament, a posterior bundle of fibers also has been identified; it originates from the posterior aspect of the lateral epicondyle that transveres the annular ligament and

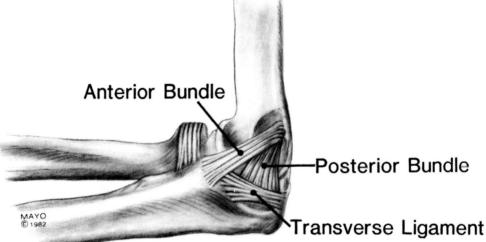

Anterior Bundle

Posterior Bundle

Transverse Ligament

MAYO © 1982

Fig. 8-5. Classical representation of the medial collateral ligament complex consisting of an anterior and posterior oblique bundle as well as a transverse component. (From Morrey, B.F., editor: The elbow and its disorders, Philadelphia, 1985, W.B. Saunders Co.)

attaches to the christa supinatoris.[13] This structure appears to be present in about 90% of individuals (Fig. 8-6). This portion of the lateral collateral ligament complex might be termed justifiably the lateral ulnar collateral ligament. Observations in the laboratory support the idea that the function of this portion of the lateral complex is to stabilize the elbow against varus stress. It is this portion of the lateral collateral ligament that accounts for the stability of the elbow after the radial head has been excised.

Variable laxity of the anterior and posterior portions of the medial and collateral ligament has been observed.[13] The anterior bundle becomes taut after about 20 to 30 degrees of flexion, but the posterior portion is lax until about 60 degrees of flexion. We have correlated the variable length of these ligament segments as the function of elbow flexion and, with their origin, referable to the axis of rotation (Fig. 8-7). It was shown that the origins of these two ligament segments do not lie on the axis of elbow flexion. Thus the so-called cam effect occurs. On the lateral aspect of the joint the origin of the lateral collateral ligament is coincident with the axis of rotation. Thus a more uniform length-flexion relationship of this ligament is noted (Fig. 8-8).

Functional implications

Clinical experience and biomechanical testing have established the anterior portion of the medial collateral ligament as the prime stabilizer of the elbow joint.[12,15] The limitation of elbow extension is provided primarily by the anterior capsule. However, a taut anterior bundle in the medial collateral ligament also may play a role. In addition, excision of the fat pad from the olecranon fossa allows some additional extension, usually about 5 degrees, thus suggesting this mechanism also provides some constraint to elbow extension.

Articular contribution—elbow stability

The articular contribution of the ulnohumeral joint is important clinically, since excision of the proximal ulna sometimes is recommended and indicated for comminuted fractures of the olecranon. Analysis of the composite stability of the varus/valgus, internal/external rotation, and anterior and posterior displacement of the ulna on

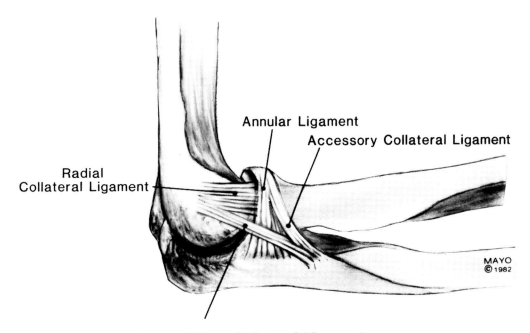

Fig. 8-6. A typical pattern of the more variable radial collateral ligament complex consists of a contribution from the humerus to the ulna that may be termed the lateral ulnar collateral ligament. (From Morrey, B.F., editor: The elbow and its disorders, Philadelphia, 1985, W.B. Saunders Co.)

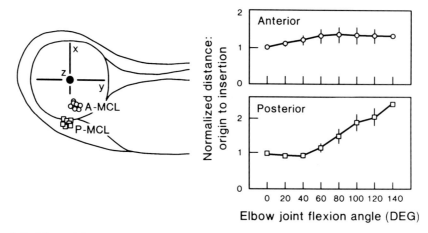

Fig. 8-7. The origins of the medial collateral ligament do not coincide with the axis of rotation of elbow flexion and extension, thus accounting for the laxity observed in these portions of the ligament complex associated with elbow flexion.

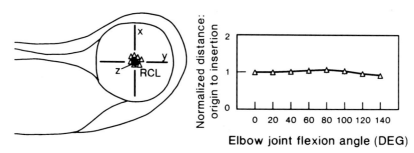

Fig. 8-8. The origin of the radial collateral ligament does originate from the axis of rotation, thus little change is observed in the length of the segment during elbow flexion.

the humerus in full extension and at 90 degrees of flexion has been investigated. Serial removal of 25%, 50%, 75%, and 100% of the olecranon results in a near linear decrease in the stability provided by the ulnohumeral joint (Fig. 8-9).[11] There is some increased loss of stability with removal of the last 25%, because this portion of the olecranon is also associated with release of the anterior portion of the ulnar collateral ligament.

Finally, the stabilizing contribution of the radial head is currently under investigation. Experiments in our laboratory and those of others have demonstrated[12] that the radial head does provide some resistance to valgus stress varying from 15% to 30% depending on the loading configurations and orientation of the elbow joint. Additional information is required, however, before a complete understanding of the role of the radial head

in transmitting forces and stabilizing the elbow is understood fully.

In general, elbow stability may be considered to be approximately 50% a function of the joint articulation, primarily from the ulnohumeral joint, and 50% a function of the collateral ligaments and anterior capsule.[12]

FORCES

A final consideration of the functional anatomy of the elbow joint relates to the generation of strength and the transmitted forces across this joint. Force transmission is dependent primarily on the muscles that cross the joint.

The variation and the participation of force transmission of a given muscle are dependent on three characteristics of that muscle: (1) its physiological cross-sectional area, (2) the

Fig. 8-9. Serial removal of 25%, 50%, 75%, or 100% of the proximal ulna **(A)** results in a near linear decrease of the constraint contribution provided by that segment **(B).** (From Morrey, B.F., editor: The elbow and its disorders, Philadelphia, 1985, W.B. Saunders Co.)

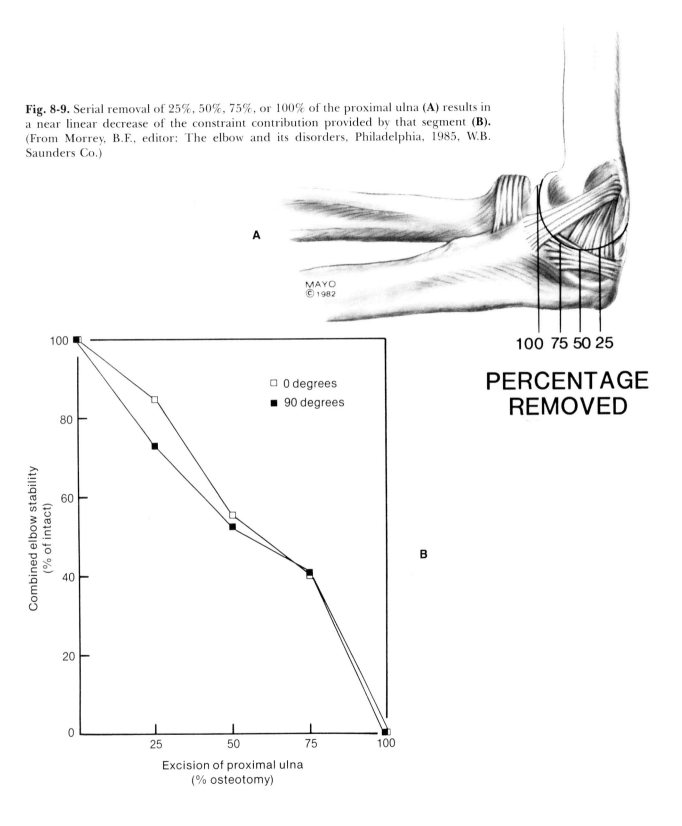

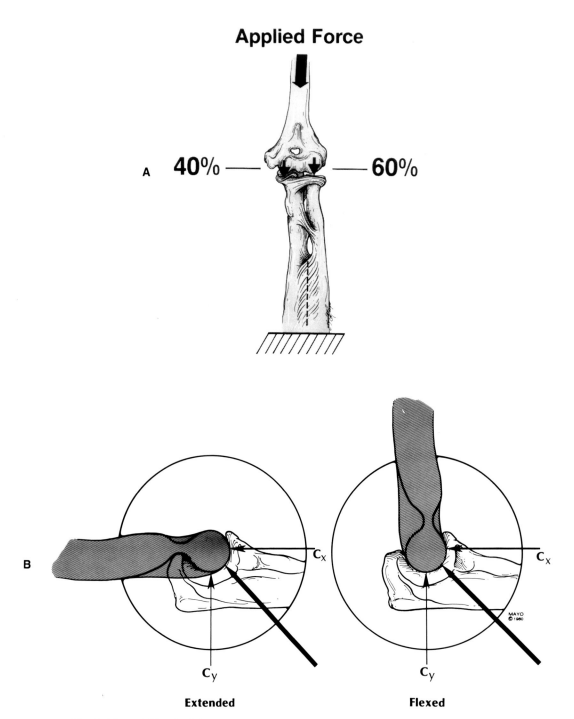

Fig. 8-10. Axial load of the upper extremity results in transmission of about 60% of the force across the radiohumeral joint **(A),** with flexion and extension the resultant vector results in a cyclic load being imparted to the distal humerus **(B).**

mechanical advantage, and (3) the EMG activity with a given function. Although numerous muscles do cross the elbow joint, the major flexors of this joint consist of the brachialis, biceps, and brachioradialis; the primary extensors are the triceps and the anconeus muscles.[1,6]

Although the amount of force transmitted across the joint does depend on the loading configurations and the angular orientation of the joint, a magnitude of up to three times body weight has been predicted in certain functions.[1,8] Activities of daily living are carried out with approximately one half body weight transmitted across the joint with the maximum force transmission occurring in about 90 degrees of flexion.[5,9] Experiments have indicated further that approximately 60% of the axial load transmitted across the joint occurs at the radiohumeral joint and 40% at the ulnohumeral joint.[7,16] The dynamic distribution of these forces during activities of daily living has not yet been defined. It has been

shown, however, that with use the resultant vector of the transmitted force changes its orientation, depending on the position of the elbow joint (Fig. 8-10). It is the cyclic loading pattern of the distal humerus that has been implicated in the early problem of loosening of the humeral component of constrained elbow prostheses.

Strength measurement in the clinical setting usually is estimated by the maximum isometric strength generated with the elbow at 90 degrees of flexion. A study of over 100 normal individuals has demonstrated the following clinically pertinent information regarding normal elbow strength: extension strength is approximately 70% that of flexion strength.[3] The difference between the dominant and nondominant side is 3% to 8%, but this difference is statistically significant. The strength of males averages twice that of females in all functions tested: flexion and extension, pronation and supination, and grip strength (Fig. 8-11).

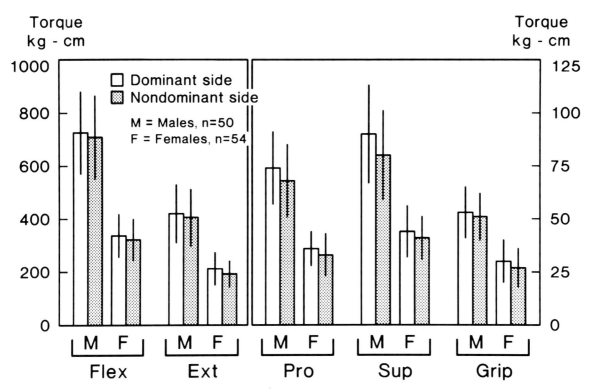

Fig. 8-11. Normal strength variation with different functions, between male and female, and between dominant and nondominant extremities. (From Morrey, B.F., editor: The elbow and its disorders, Philadelphia, 1985, W.B. Saunders Co.)

SUMMARY

A clear understanding of the unique anatomic features of the elbow joint aids in a more full appreciation of the biomechanical aspects of this joint. This knowledge may, it is hoped, be translated into a broader understanding of the scientific basis of the management of elbow problems.

REFERENCES

1. An, K.N., Hui, F.C., Morrey, B.F., Linscheid, R.L., and Chao, E.Y.: Muscles across the elbow joint: A biomechanical analysis, J. Biomech. **14:**659-669, 1981.
2. An, K.N., Morrey, B.F., and Chao, E.Y.: Carrying angle of human elbow joint, J. Orthop. Res. **1:**369-378, 1984.
3. Askew, L.J., An, K.N., Morrey, B.F., and Chao, E.Y.: Functional evaluation of the elbow: Normal motion requirements and strength determinations. Transactions of the twenty-seventh annual meeting of the Orthopaedic Research Society. **6:**183, 1981.
4. Boone, D.C., and Azen, S.P.: Normal range of motion of joints in male subjects, J. Bone Joint Surg. **61A:**756-759, 1979.
5. Elkins, E.C., Leden, U.M., and Wakim, K.G.: Objective recording of the strength of normal muscles, Arch. Phys. Med. **32:**639-647, 1951.
6. Funk, D.: An EMG analysis of muscles controlling elbow motion, Master's thesis, Minneapolis, 1984, Mayo Clinic.
7. Halls, A.A., and Travill, R.: Transmission of pressures across the elbow joint, Anat. Rec. **150:**243, 1964.
8. Hui, F.C., Chao, E.Y., and An, K.N.: Muscle and joint forces at the elbow during isometric lifting, (abstract) Orthop. Trans. **2:**169, 1978.
9. Larson, R.F.: Forearm positioning on maximal elbow-flexor force, Phys. Ther. **49:**748-756, 1969.
10. London, J.T.: Kinematics of the elbow, J. Bone Joint Surg. **63A:**529-535, 1981.
11. Morrey, B.F., editor: The elbow and its disorders, Philadelphia, 1985, W.B. Saunders Co.
12. Morrey, B.F., and An, K.N.: Articular and ligamentous contributions to the stability of the elbow joint, Am. J. Sports Med. **11:**315, 1983.
13. Morrey, B.F., and An, K.N.: Functional anatomy of the collateral ligaments of the elbow joint, accepted for publication, CORR: **201:**84-90, 1986.
14. Morrey, B.F., and Chao, E.Y.S.: Passive motion of the elbow joint, J. Bone Joint Surg. **58A:**501-508, 1976.
15. Travill, A.A.: Electromyographic study of the extensor apparatus of the forearm, Anat. Rec. **144:**373-376, 1962.
16. Walker, P.S.: Human joints and their artificial replacement, Springfield, Ill., 1977, Charles C Thomas, Publisher.

Chapter 9

Adult elbow dislocations: mechanism of instability

H.S. TULLOS

JAMES BENNETT

DOUGLAS SHEPARD

P.C. NOBLE

GERARD GABEL

The function of the human elbow is complex, and this complexity is manifested by the movements of the ulnotrochlear joint, the radio-capitellar joint, and the proximal radioulnar joint. Although the elbow functions in flexion and extension, as well as supination and pronation, its primary purpose is not motion per se but positioning the hand in space to facilitate activity.

When the elbow is analyzed in terms of forces that occur within the activities of daily living, work, and sports, the dominant ligamentous force is valgus stress (Fig. 9-1).[1] This valgus stress is reflected in the ligament anatomy of the elbow joint.[9,14] On the lateral side of the elbow there appears to be no true lateral collateral ligament per se. Recent studies by Morrey have identified a rudimentary lateral collateral ligament;[7] however, there is no functional ligament spanning the lateral aspect of the joint.

The lateral support ligament is not a true collateral ligament. Because it arises from the lateral epicondyle and inserts into the annular ligament (Fig. 9-2), it does not perform the function of a true ligament with bone to bone attachment of the collateral ligament. The only major structure that does conform to a true lateral collateral ligament is the anconeus muscle, which originates from the lateral epicondyle and inserts on the proximal ulna. It may be hypothesized that the primary function of the anconeus muscle is to aid in elbow stabilization resulting from varus stress (Fig. 9-3), but this is not yet proved.

In contrast, on the medial side of the elbow, the medial collateral ligament is well defined; it originates from medial epicondyle and inserts into the coronoid process at the medial olecranon. It is composed of two primary bundles: the anterior oblique and posterior oblique ligament group.[7] The characteristics of the posterior oblique are well understood. This ligament, which is absent in many primates, is taut only in flexion and lax in extension (Fig. 9-4). In addition, in anatomic specimens, sectioning of the posterior oblique ligament does not influence the stability of the elbow to valgus stress (Fig. 9-5) if the anterior oblique ligament is left intact.

The anterior oblique ligament is taut both in flexion and extension. This is a result of the anatomic characteristic of the ligament itself. Because it is rectangular, the ligament uses the anterior fibers to hold the joint taut in extension and the posterior fibers to hold the joint taut in flexion (Fig. 9-6). In addition, if the anterior oblique ligament is sectioned while the posterior oblique ligament is left intact, the cadaveric elbow

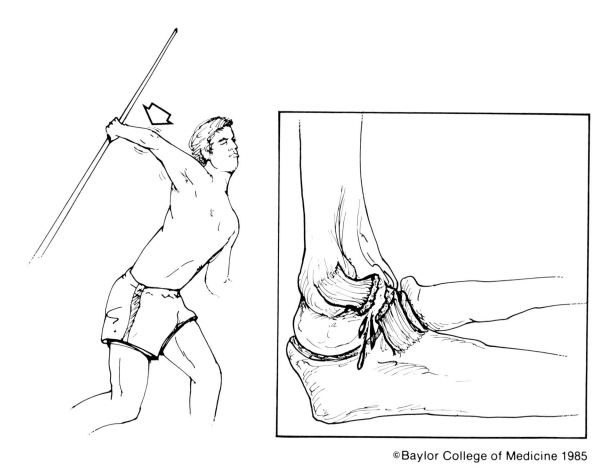

©Baylor College of Medicine 1985

Fig. 9-1. Javelin thrower with elbow at valgus stress. Insert shows rupture of medial collateral ligament.

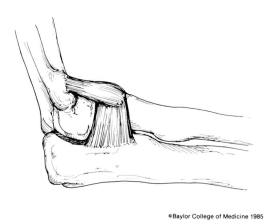

©Baylor College of Medicine 1985

Fig. 9-2. Lateral collateral ligament insertion into the annular ligament.

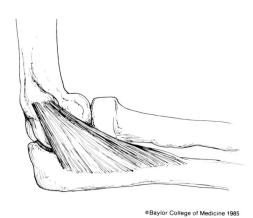

©Baylor College of Medicine 1985

Fig. 9-3. Anconeus muscle as the lateral collateral ligament.

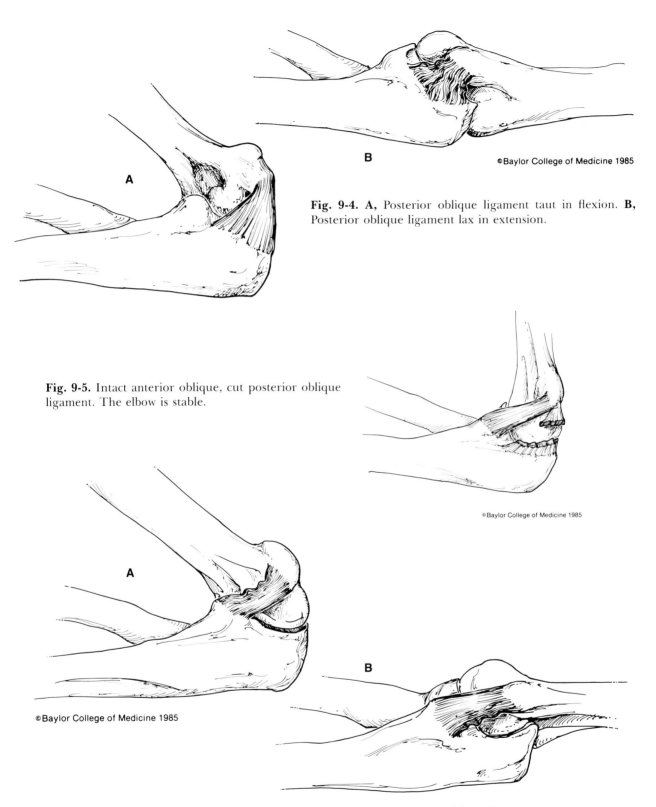

©Baylor College of Medicine 1985

Fig. 9-4. A, Posterior oblique ligament taut in flexion. **B,** Posterior oblique ligament lax in extension.

Fig. 9-5. Intact anterior oblique, cut posterior oblique ligament. The elbow is stable.

©Baylor College of Medicine 1985

©Baylor College of Medicine 1985

Fig. 9-6. A, Anterior oblique ligament taut in flexion. **B,** Anterior oblique ligament taut in extension.

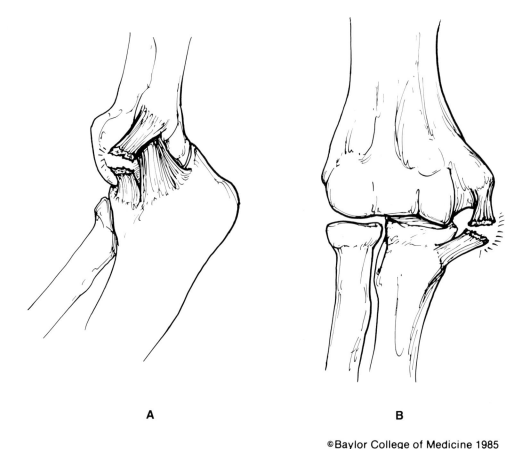

A   B

©Baylor College of Medicine 1985

Fig. 9-7. A, Lateral view: posterior oblique intact, anterior oblique ligament cut. The elbow is unstable. **B,** Anteroposterior view: posterior oblique intact, anterior oblique ligament cut.

becomes grossly unstable and dislocation may occur (Fig. 9-7).[2,14]

ELBOW DISLOCATIONS

Traumatic dislocation of the elbow joint is not a common occurrence.[3,6] Many other joints are far more prone to dislocate, particularly the patellofemoral articulation and the glenohumeral joint. Nonetheless, traumatic dislocations of the elbow do occur, and virtually every orthopaedist will encounter this injury at some time.

An axiom of orthopaedic treatment is that relocation for this injury, with or without general anesthesia, is all that is necessary. The elbow will be stable following a closed reduction, and the end results will be satisfactory. Although this statement is generally true, it is not always so. After relocation elbows are periodically unstable

Table 9-1. Redislocation rate (simple)

Conn and Wade (1961)	0%
Roberts (1969)	0%
Linscheid and Wheeler (1965)	3%

and either will redislocate in plaster (Fig. 9-8) or will be very difficult to maintain unless the elbow is held in extremes of flexion.[12,15,19]

Examples of persistent instability following redislocation can be extrapolated from the literature of previous series on simple elbow dislocations. In the reported series (Table 9-1) the redislocation rate following a simple closed reduction was very low.[13,20] This is consistent with many other reviews of this injury that have appeared in the literature. Indeed, the only re-

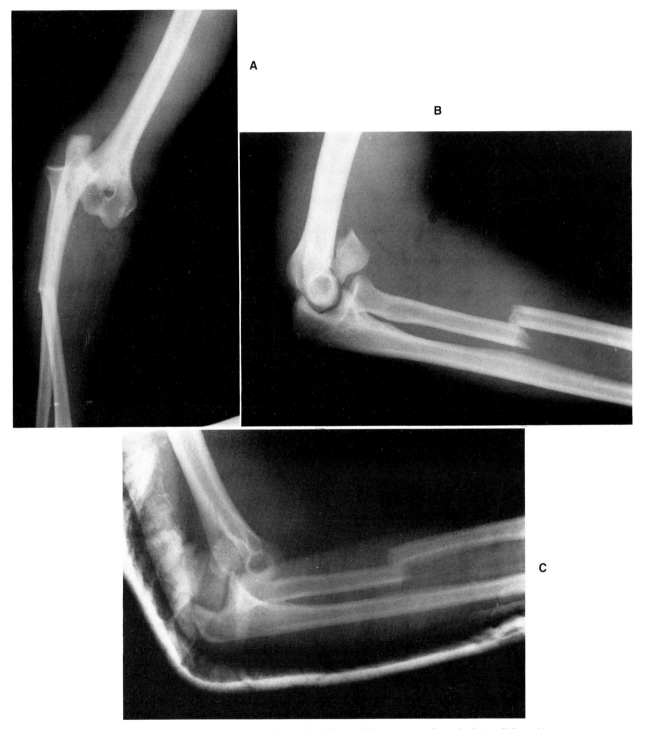

Fig. 9-8. A, Posterior dislocation elbow. **B,** Elbow dislocation reduced. **C,** Redislocation of elbow in cast.

ported series with a redislocation rate was that of Linscheid and Wheeler in 1965, with a 3% redislocation in plaster following reduction.[6] This is not true, however, when dislocations are associated with fractures, particularly fractures of the radial head. As can be seen in Table 9-2 the redislocation rate following a simple closed reduction in fracture dislocation is significant, varying from 10% to 14%. The highest redislocation rate is in those elbow dislocations associated with a radial head or radial neck fracture.[20]

Thus persistent instability following closed reduction of acute elbow dislocation does occur and can be a significant factor in acute fracture dislocations.[16]

MECHANISMS OF INSTABILITY

It is reasonable to question why some elbows are stable and others are not stable following a dislocation and simple reduction. The answer to that question may lie in the mechanism of dislocation itself. (Fig. 9-9)

Traumatic dislocation of the elbow is thought to be a hyperextension injury. As the elbow is extended and then hyperextended, the olecranon process impinges into the olecranon fossa and hinges open the anterior aspect of the joint, tearing the thin anterior capsule. As this occurs, the anterior oblique ligament must be either avulsed or torn. As the anterior oblique ligament fails, the trochlea rides superiorly over the top of the coronoid process and a dislocation occurs. Since the slope of the trochlea is lateral, the usual elbow dislocation is both posterior and lateral. In the process large translational forces are placed on the medial collateral ligament, causing its disruption or occasional avulsion of the medial epicondyle, particularly in younger patients.

Table 9-2. Redislocation rate (complex)

Conn and Wade (1961)	
Dislocation with fracture	9.0%
Dislocation with fracture of radial head	
and/or neck	14.0%
Roberts (1969)	
Dislocation with fracture	7.0%
Dislocation with radial head fracture	11.0%
Wheeler and Linscheid (1967)	13.0%

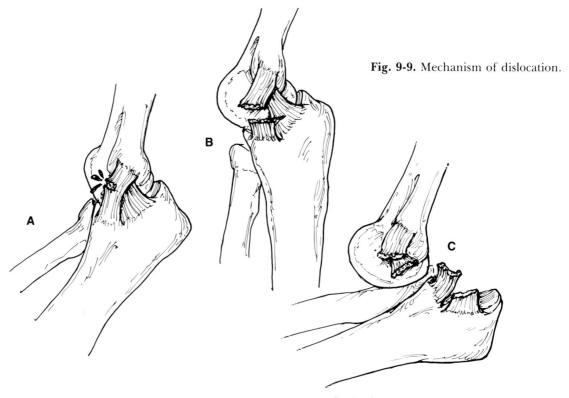

Fig. 9-9. Mechanism of dislocation.

Operative finding

If this hypothesis is true, than all simple elbow dislocations are associated with some degree of medial collateral ligament injury and related joint instability. To evaluate this theory, a surgical protocol for treatment of elbow dislocations within the Division of Orthopaedic Surgery at Baylor College of Medicine was developed.

This protocol consisted of the following: First, all elbow dislocations would be reduced with the patient under general anesthesia. Second, following reduction, valgus stress x-ray films and clinical examination for stability (Fig. 9-10a, 9-10b) would be obtained. Third, a surgical repair of the medial collateral ligament would be performed on all elbows that were clinically and radiographically unstable at the time of their stress x-ray examinations.

It was thought at the time at which this protocol was developed (based on prior clinical experience with elbow dislocations) that most relocated elbows would be stable to valgus stress and that there would be only a small percentage requiring surgical repair. However, this was not the case.

Postoperative care following medial collateral ligament repair included a posterior splint for 7 to 10 days followed by a cast brace for 8 to 12 weeks to allow flexion and extension but to prevent varus-valgus stress.

From 1980 to 1983, 37 elbow dislocations were seen by the Orthopaedic Trauma Service at Baylor College of Medicine. All were reduced with the patient under general anesthesia, and all underwent valgus stress x-ray studies. In 34 of the 37 dislocations, instability due to valgus stress was demonstrated by either the stress x-ray films, or clinical studies, or both. These findings are supported by the recent work of Josefsson and

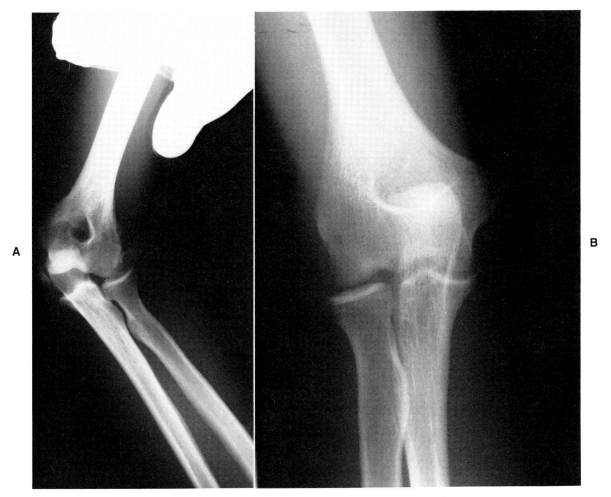

A

B

Fig. 9-10. A, AP reduced x-ray film of dislocation. **B,** X-ray: valgus stress test.

Table 9-3. Location of tear: anterior oblique ligament

16	Medial epicondyle
7	Proximal ulna
9	Mid substance

associates.[5] In 31 consecutive surgical explorations and operative repairs of simple elbow dislocations in adults, all had complete tears of the medial collateral ligament. Although similar tears also were seen in 18 of 31 cases explored laterally, only 8 of these lateral ligaments were associated with elbows that were clinically or radiographically unstable.

In our present series of 34 unstable dislocations, 16 had no associated fractures (simple dislocations). The remaining 18 were complex dislocations (elbow dislocations associated with one or more fractures).

All 34 unstable dislocations underwent surgical repair. In two instances an associated radial head fracture was present and was treated with a radial head spacer before exploration of the anterior oblique ligament. In these two instances the radial head spacer alone was sufficient to stabilize the elbow and no further surgery was performed. Thus 32 remaining patients underwent exploration of the anterior oblique ligament for proved radiographic and clinical evidence of anterior oblique disruption. The sites of the ligament tear are seen in Table 9-3.

Based on these observations the primary lesion in elbow dislocation is a tear of the anterior oblique ligament of the medial collateral ligament complex. Integrity of this ligament is necessary for stability. When the ligament is not intact, such as occurs in a spontaneous rupture during throwing[11] or with a traumatic dislocation, the elbow is unstable.

The role of the flexor forearm muscle mass

Instability of the elbow may be masked by spasm of the flexor forearm muscle mass. It is likely that the clinical stability manifested in the emergency room following reduction of an elbow dislocation is primarily dependent on the integrity of this muscle group. In Josefsson's experience (31 of 31) and our own (34 of 37), the act of dislocation ruptures the medial collateral ligament.

In contrast, of 31 dislocated elbows explored by Josefsson, only 19 had significant injury to the flexor forearm mass. However, all grossly unstable elbows had extensive damage to these muscles.

Therefore the medial collateral ligament is the dominant stabilizer to valgus stress, particularly the anterior oblique component. This is clear when muscle function and spasm are neutralized by general anesthesia. When the patient is awake, however, instability may be masked by spasm from an intact or a minimally damaged flexor forearm muscle group (Fig. 9-11, *A*). If the forearm muscle flexors are damaged extensively or ruptured, then there is no stability and this elbow is grossly unstable (Fig. 9-11, *B*).

The role of the lateral compartment

Although the medial side of the elbow may contain the primary stabilizer of the elbow joint (the medial collateral ligament and the flexor forearm mass), it is not the only area involved in joint stability. Under certain circumstances the lateral radio-capitellar joint can play a secondary role in joint stability, particularly in resisting valgus stress.[1,8]

When the anterior oblique ligament or the medial structures either are disrupted or attenuated, valgus stress can be transmitted across the joint from medial to lateral and produce compressive forces between the capitellum and the radial head (Fig. 9-12). These compressive forces can cause loose body formation as seen in professional athletes (Fig. 9-13).

More recently, the effects of the radial capitellar joint and radial head fractures on joint function and stability have been analyzed.[10] The use of a radial head spacer in dislocations of the elbow associated with radial head fractures has gained increasing popularity.[17,9] It was initially believed by us and others that the use of a radial head spacer would restore the secondary valgus support mechanism and thus provide sufficient stability so that the repair of the medial collateral ligament would not be necessary (Fig. 9-14). This, however, has not been our recent experience. Of nine fracture dislocations of the elbow associated with comminuted radial head fractures, only two have been stabilized successfully using a radial head spacer alone. In four, even after the use of a radial head spacer, the elbow continued to be unstable and repair of the anterior oblique ligament was necessary. In contrast, in three of the nine, repair of the anterior oblique ligament

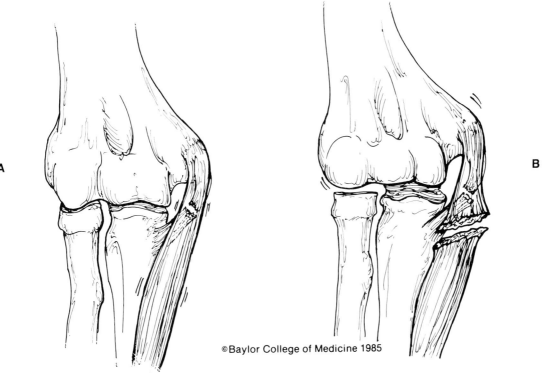

©Baylor College of Medicine 1985

Fig. 9-11. A, Elbow dislocation: Medial collateral ligament torn. Flexor muscle group intact and in spasm: stable. **B,** Elbow dislocation: Medial collateral ligament torn. Flexor muscle group ruptured: unstable.

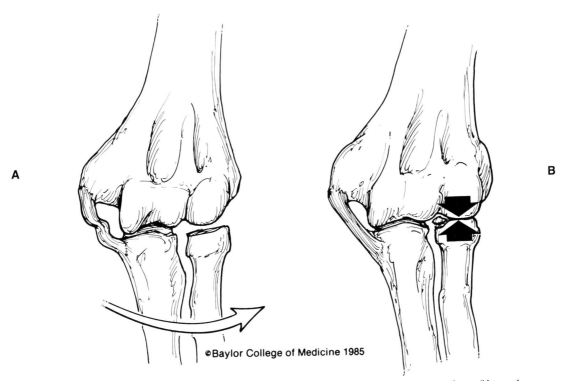

©Baylor College of Medicine 1985

Fig. 9-12. A, Attenuated medial collateral ligament, valgus stress, compression of lateral radiocapitellar joint. **B,** Loose body from capitellum.

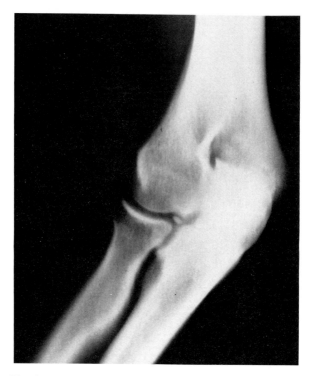

Fig. 9-13. X-ray film: Lateral radiocapitellar loose body.

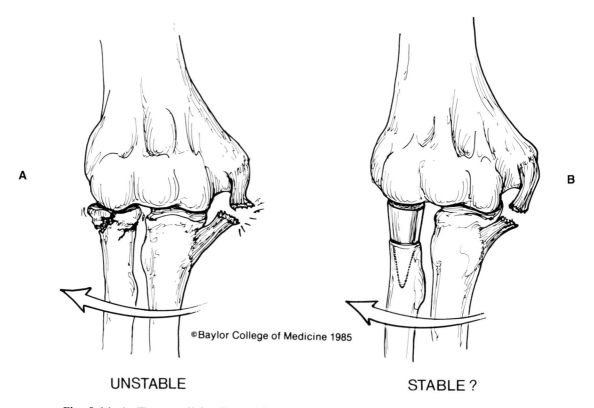

UNSTABLE

STABLE ?

©Baylor College of Medicine 1985

Fig. 9-14. A, Torn medial collateral ligament. Fracture radial head, unstable, valgus stress. **B,** Torn medial collateral ligament, radial head excision. Radial head spacer in place.

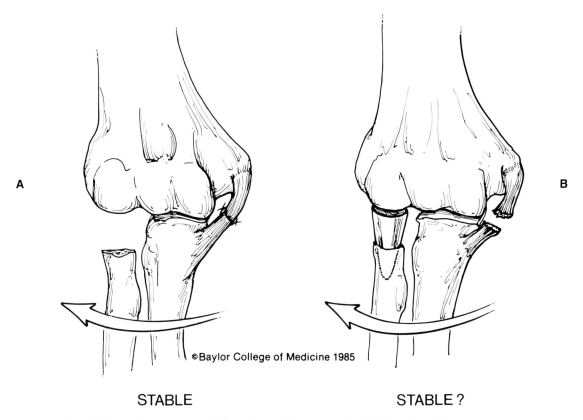

©Baylor College of Medicine 1985

STABLE   STABLE ?

Fig. 9-15. A, Repaired medial collateral ligament. Radial head excision, no spacer, stable to valgus stress. **B,** Medial collateral ligament torn. Radial head spacer, valgus stress.

alone was sufficient to stabilize the elbow even when a radial head spacer was not used.

Although these numbers are small, they suggest that the anterior oblique ligament is the primary stabilizer and that the lateral radiocapitellar joint is a secondary stabilizer. They also suggest that if instability is the primary concern, repair of the anterior oblique ligament alone is more likely to produce stability than the use of a radial head spacer alone (Fig. 9-15).

MEDIAL COLLATERAL LIGAMENT REPAIR: RESULTS OF ACUTE TREATMENT

Of the 32 elbow dislocations that underwent a medial collateral ligament repair 21 were available for follow-up of a year or longer.

The results of surgical repair can be compared to the more conventional closed treatment methods by using the grading system of Linscheid and Wheeler (Table 9-4). In cases of simple dislocation it is apparent that 80% of the patients in both the series of Linscheid-Wheeler and Roberts have experienced good or excellent results (Table 9-5).

Essentially the same statistics apply to the Baylor College of Medicine series, suggesting that open treatment results are equal to closed treatment. However, the series are not entirely comparable. Both the series of Linscheid-Wheeler and Roberts report a significant number of children with elbow dislocations. Since these children almost universally do well following a dislocation, their inclusion may slant the results of closed methods. If children are removed so that the series are comparable and adult elbow dislocations compared to adult elbow dislocations, the results of open repair may be more favorable. While these data are suggestive, they are not conclusive at this time.

However, when complex dislocations are reviewed, a different picture emerges. In the series by Linscheid-Wheeler, as well as by Roberts, good

Table 9-4. Grading system from Linscheid and Wheeler

	Composite loss of flexion and extension	Composite loss of pronation and supination	Complaints
Excellent	≤10°	≤10°	0
Good	≤30°	≤30°	0
Fair	≤60°	≤60°	Slight to mild discomfort or residual instability
Poor	>60°	>60°	Moderate pain

Table 9-5. Comparative results: simple dislocations

	Excellent (%)	Good (%)	Fair (%)	Poor (%)
Wheeler/Linscheid (1965) (Total = 62)	52	31	11	6
Roberts (1969) (Total = 37)	35	32	19	14
Baylor College of Medicine (Total = 6)	50	33	17	0

Table 9-6. Comparative results: complex dislocations

	Excellent (%)	Good (%)	Fair (%)	Poor (%)
Wheeler and Linscheid (1967) (Total = 32)	19	28	47	6
With radial head fracture (14)	21	21	43	15
With olecranon fracture (18)	17	33	50	0
Roberts (1969) (Total = 15)	13	13	27	47
Baylor College of Medicine (Total) (15)	80	13	0	7
With radial head fracture (7)	71	29	0	0
With olecranon fracture (3)	67	0	0	33

and excellent results are present only in some 30% to 40% of the cases. In our series with open repair of the medial collateral ligament, results are equal to those of the simple dislocations; that is, approximately 80% to 90% good and excellent results occurred (Table 9-6).[16]

COMPLICATIONS

Complications secondary to open repair of the medial collateral ligament have been minimal. There has been only one surgical failure where the repair of the anterior oblique ligament failed in an individual who had a massive fracture dislocation of the elbow (Fig. 9-16).

The incidence of heterotrophic bone formation has been reported at 4% to 8% in previous series of elbow dislocations treated conservatively.[6,13,18]

Since in this series 6% of the patients treated by open exploration had heterotrophic bone formation, surgical intervention does not seem to increase this risk.

No ulnar nerve injury or deficit that was not present preoperatively in the dislocated elbow occurred after open procedures.

SUMMARY

From these data it appears reasonable to advocate open repair of fracture dislocations of the elbow joint, particularly those associated with radial head fractures. In these instances improved functional results can be anticipated. In simple elbow dislocations in adults, it is possible that open repair of the medial collateral ligament will produce improved functional results. How-

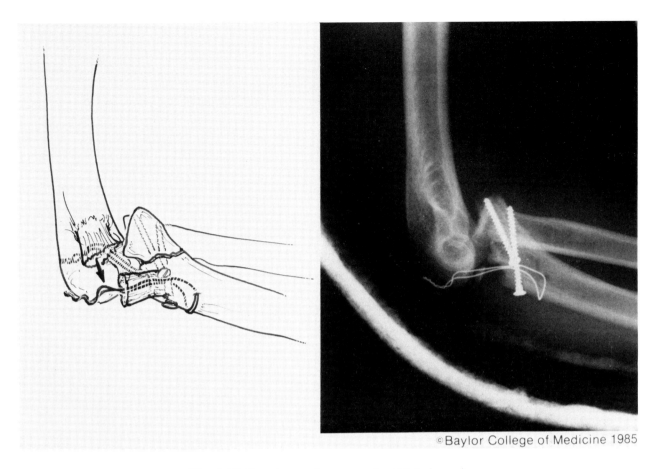

©Baylor College of Medicine 1985

Fig. 9-16. Drawing and x-ray study of failed repair.

ever, the data, although suggestive, are not conclusive at this time.

It is our belief that the indications for surgery in elbow dislocations can be summarized as follows.

1. Surgical intervention is indicated if spontaneous redislocation occurs, unless the arm is flexed above 90 degrees.

2. Surgery is indicated if a spontaneous redislocation of the elbow dislocation occurs with the arm in plaster.

3. Surgical repair of the medial collateral ligament is indicated in all instances of fracture dislocations of the elbow, particularly those associated with radial head fractures.

4. In adult simple elbow dislocations surgical repair of the anterior oblique ligament certainly does not impair elbow function at follow-up and indeed may lead to better results.

REFERENCES

1. An, K.N., and Morrey, B.F.: Biomechanics of the elbow. In Morrey, B.F., editor: The elbow and its disorders, Philadelphia, 1985, W.B. Saunders Co.
2. Bennett, J.B., and Tullos, H.S.: Ligamentous and articular injuries in the athlete. In Morrey, B.F., editor: The elbow and its disorders, Philadelphia, 1985, W.B. Saunders Co.
3. Eppright, R.H., and Wilkins, K.E.: Fracture dislocation of the elbow. In Rockwood, C.A., and Green, D.P., editors: Fractures, vol.1, Philadelphia, 1975, J.B. Lippincott Co.
4. Harrington, I.J., and Tountas, A.A.: Replacement of the radial head and the treatment of unstable elbow fractures, Injury **12:**405, 1981.
5. Josefsson, et al.: Ligamentous injuries and dislocations of the elbow joint, Clin. Orthop., 1985. (Submitted for publication.)
6. Linscheid, R.L., and Wheeler, D.K.: Elbow dislocations, **194:**1171, 1965.
7. Morrey, B.F.: Anatomy of the elbow joint. In Morrey, B.F., editor: The elbow and its disorders, Philadelphia, 1985, W.B. Saunders Co.

8. Morrey, B.F., and An, K.N.: Articulous and Ligamentous contributions to the stability of the elbow joint, Am. J. Sports Med. **11:**315, 1983.

9. Morrey, B.F., Askew, L.J., An, K.N., and Chao, E.Y.: A biomechanical study of normal functional elbow motion, J. Bone Joint Surg. **63A:**872, 1981.

10. Morrey, B.F., and Chao, E.Y.: Biomechanics study of the elbow following excision of the radial head, J. Bone Joint Surg. **61A:**63, 1979.

11. Norwood, L.A., Shook, J.A., and Andrews, J.R.: Acute medial elbow ruptures, Am. J. Sports Med. **9:**16-19, 1981.

12. Osborne, G., and Cotterill, P.: Recurrent dislocation of the elbow, J. Bone Joint Surg. **48B:**340, 1966.

13. Roberts, P.H.: Dislocation of the elbow, Br. J. Surg. **56:** 806-815, 1969.

14. Schwab, G.H., Bennett, J.B., Woods, G.W., and Tullos, H.S.: Biomechanics of elbow instability: The role of medial collateral ligament, Clin. Orthop. **146:**42-52, 1980.

15. Shepard, D.M., Bennett, J.B., and Tullos, H.S.: Acute elbow instability in the adult patient: Diagnosis and management, Orthop. Trans. **9**(1):45, 1985.

16. Shepard, D.M., Tullos, H.S., Bennett, J.B., Crouch, C.C., and Gartsman, G.M.: Dislocation of the elbow with radial head fractures: An unstable joint, Presented at the annual meeting of the American Academy of Orthopaedic Surgeons, Las Vegas, 1985.

17. Swanson, A.B., Jaeger, S.H., and LaRochelle, D.: Comminuted fracture of the radial head: The role of the silicone-implant replacement arthroplasty, J. Bone Joint Surg. **63A:**1039, 1981.

18. Thompson, H.C., III, and Garcia, A.: Myositis ossificans (aftermath of elbow injury), Clin. Orthop. **50:**129-134, 1967.

19. Tullos, H.S., Schwab, G., Bennett, J.B., and Woods, G.W.: Fractures of joints and elbow instability, Instructional course lectures: The American Academy of Orthopaedic Surgeons, vol. 30, St. Louis, 1981, The C.V. Mosby Co.

20. Wheeler, D.K., and Linscheid, R.L.: Fracture dislocation of the elbow, Clin. Orthop. 50-95, 1967.

Chapter 10

Physeal fractures of the distal humerus: avoiding the pitfalls

KAYE E. WILKINS

Because of the multiple ossification centers, evaluation of fractures involving the distal humeral physes can be difficult. The orthopaedist must have an accurate knowledge of when the various ossification centers appear and fuse. The anatomic structure of these secondary centers often determines the fracture patterns that occur. This monograph attempts to summarize these anatomic considerations and emphasize some of the common pitfalls that can occur in the treatment of these injuries.

ANATOMIC CONSIDERATIONS
Ossification process

The radiographic appearance of the ossification centers develops in a consistent manner (Fig. 10-1). The first center to develop is the center of the lateral condyle. It must be remembered that this ossification center extends into the lateral crista of the trochlea. This has an important significance regarding the types of fracture patterns involving the lateral condyle. The second ossification center to form is that of the medial epicondyle. Before the development of the ossification centers, a single physeal line forms in the distal humerus. This early common preosseous epiphysis includes the medial epicondyle. Around the age of 5 the medial epicondyle separates from this common epiphysis to become a separate apophysis.

The medial epicondyle is an extraarticular structure. Instead of being straight medial, the medial epicondyle lies somewhat posterior on the medial surface. Thus on a true lateral view of the distal humerus it may be visualized along the posterior surface. This apophysis is the last to fuse to the distal humerus, which accounts for the occurrence of separations of the medial epicondyle in the adolescent age-group.

The ossification center of the trochlea actually involves only the medial crista of the trochlea. Because of its unique blood supply, this center develops in a fragmented manner. These multiple ossification centers can simulate the appearance of a fracture (Fig. 10-2). The lateral epicondyle ossification center is actually a part of the lateral condyle. Its transient separate ossification center is the last to appear and may be confused with a small chip fracture. It is extremely rare for this ossification center to be involved as a separate fracture.

Blood supply

Because most of the distal humerus is articular cartilage, there are very few locations that permit the extraarticular entrance of vessels to supply nourishment to the secondary ossification center. The lateral condylar ossification center receives all of its blood supply through a very small area on the posterolateral aspect of the condyle (Fig. 10-3). In the surgical reduction of fractures involving this condyle, care must be taken to avoid this area to prevent the development of avascular necrosis of the lateral condyle.

The medial crista of the trochlea is supplied by two small separate vessels (Fig. 10-4). The one that supplies the lateral half of the crista actually must traverse the physis to enter its ossification center. This vessel can be injured in fractures that involve the entire distal humeral physis or in very

83

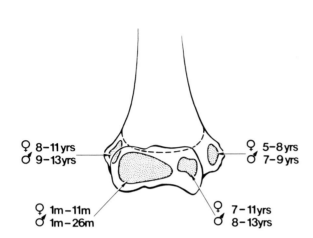

♀ 8–11yrs
♂ 9–13yrs

♀ 5–8yrs
♂ 7–9yrs

♀ 1m–11m
♂ 1m–26m

♀ 7–11yrs
♂ 8–13yrs

Fig. 10-1. The appearance of the ossification centers of the distal humerus. (From Rockwood, C.A., Wilkins, K.E., and King, R.E., editors: Fractures in children, Philadelphia, 1984, J.B. Lippincott Co.)

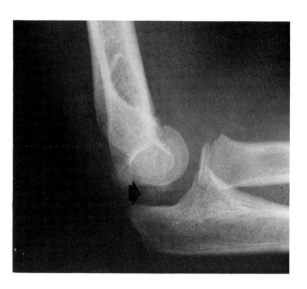

Fig. 10-2. The multiple ossification centers of the trochlea *(arrow)* may be mistaken for intraarticular fracture fragments. (From Rockwood, C.A., Wilkins, K.E., and King, R.E., editors: Fractures in children, Philadelphia, 1984, J.B. Lippincott Co.)

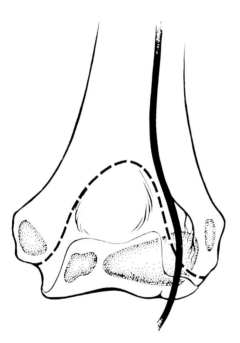

Fig. 10-3. The sole blood supply to the ossification center of the trochlea enters through the small posterolateral nonarticular area. (Redrawn from Haraldsson, S.: Acta Orthop. Scand. (Suppl.):38, 1959.)

Fig. 10-4. The ossification centers of the medial crista of the trochlea are supplied by a lateral transphyseal vessel and a medial extraarticular vessel. (Redrawn from Haraldsson, S.: Acta Orthop. Scand. (Suppl.):38, 1959.)

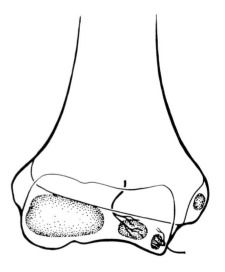

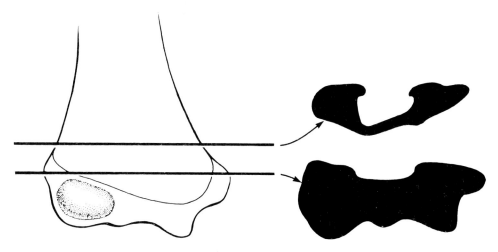

Fig. 10-5. The cross-sectional surface of the supracondylar area is much thinner than the cross-sectional area through the distal physis. (From Rockwood, C.A., Wilkins, K.E., and King, R.E., editors: Fractures in children, Philadelphia, 1984, J.B. Lippincott Co.)

distal supracondylar fractures. A second vessel enters through the extraarticular medial surface of the trochlea to supply a separate medial ossification center.

FRACTURES INVOLVING THE ENTIRE DISTAL HUMERAL PHYSIS

In infants there is a single transverse physeal line across the distal humerus. This forms the so-called common epiphysis, which includes the lateral and medial condyles and both epicondyles. In early infancy this common physeal line is more proximal and is actually at the proximal tip of the olecranon. Thus it is prone to separation with hyperextension injuries in this age-group.

As the individual grows, the common physeal line migrates distally. Around the age of 4 or 5, metaphyseal bone separates it from the extraarticular medial epicondylar apophysis. Later the medial and lateral condylar ossification centers become separated by a common central vertical physis that extends down to the center of the trochlear notch. In the older child, because of the more distal displacement of the physeal line, the surface area of these fracture fragments is larger than in the more narrow proximal supracondylar area (Fig. 10-5). This longer surface area is believed to help prevent the development of tilting of the distal fragment. Thus cubitus varus deformities occur much less commonly in fractures involving the common distal humeral physis than in those involving the more proximal supracondylar area.

Because of the lack of an ossification center, these fractures are often unrecognized when they occur in the very small infant. Although this fracture pattern was thought to be rare, I see about two to three cases per year in my practice.

There are some key clues to the recognition of this injury. First, the displacement of the distal fragment almost always is posterior and medial in relation to the distal humeral metaphysis.[1,2,3] A comparison film with the opposite elbow (Fig. 10-6) or an arthrogram may be helpful in establishing the diagnosis. Second, in the older child the shaft of the radius continues to maintain its relationship with the ossification center of the lateral condyle, even though the entire distal humeral physis is displaced posteriorly and medially (Fig. 10-7).

A very high incidence of this injury is related to child abuse in infants.[1] Consequently, the parents often delay seeking treatment. Many times the fragments may show early new periosteal bone formation around the distal metaphysis. In these cases no attempt should be made to change the position of the fragments.

In many cases there is a residual posterior and medial displacement of the distal fragment. The medial displacement will remodel rapidly with no residual deformity or loss of function. A residual varus or valgus tilt of the distal fragment will not remodel.

Treatment consists of performing a manipulative closed reduction in the fresh fractures. The distal fragment is more stable with the elbow

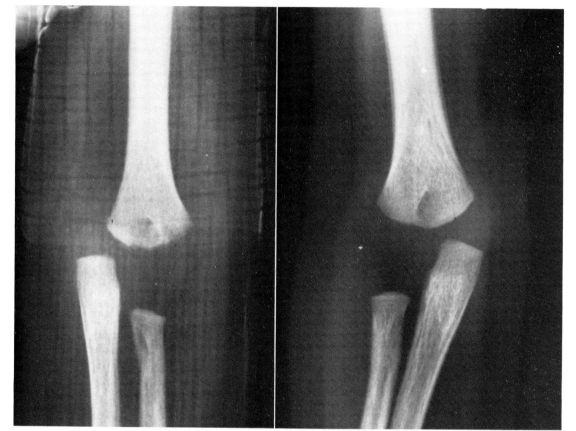

Fig. 10-6. A, In this young infant the posterior medial displacement of the left distal humeral physis along with the proximal radius and ulna **(A)** can be appreciated only when it is compared to the normal right elbow **(B).** (From Rockwood, C.A., Wilkins, K.E., and King, R.E., editors: Fractures in children, Philadelphia, 1984, J.B. Lippincott Co.)

hyperflexed and the forearm pronated. In cases where there is considerable swelling, or in older children, stability may be enhanced by percutaneous pins, a technique similar to that used for supracondylar fractures. Fractures that are seen late are treated best with simple external immobilization. Residual varus deformity can be treated later with a supracondylar osteotomy if necessary.

FRACTURES INVOLVING THE LATERAL CONDYLAR PHYSIS

After supracondylar fractures, fractures involving the lateral condylar physis are the most common elbow fractures in children.[5] Fractures of the lateral condyle rarely occur before the ossification center appears radiographically. Milch[8] has defined two separate fracture patterns involving the lateral condylar physis (Fig. 10-8).

Type I, the less common of the two, is a true Salter-Harris, Type IV, physeal fracture pattern. The distal fracture line emerges through the radiocapitellar groove. Because the lateral crista of the trochlea is intact, the elbow tends to remain stable. In this type of fracture an osseous bridge conceivably could develop between the epiphysis of the condyle and the metaphysis of the distal humerus with a resultant growth arrest. However, this rarely occurs. The Milch Type II is actually a Salter-Harris Type II fracture pattern in which a lateral metaphyseal fragment is situated posteriorly. The fracture line then courses along the physeal plate of the lateral condyle to emerge through the common physis with the medial condyle at the trochlear notch. Because the lateral crista is included with the fracture fragment, the elbow becomes unstable, with the proximal ulna translocating laterally.

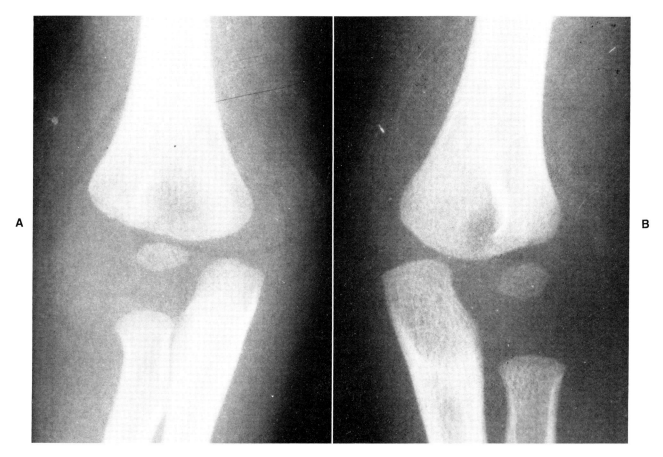

Fig. 10-7. When ossification of the lateral condyle is present, the posterior displacement of the right distal humeral physis **(A)** is easily seen when compared to the uninvolved left elbow **(B).** The relationship between the proximal radius and lateral condylar epiphysis remains intact. (From Rockwood, C.A., Wilkins, K.E., and King, R.E., editors: Fractures in children, Philadelphia, 1984, J.B. Lippincott Co.)

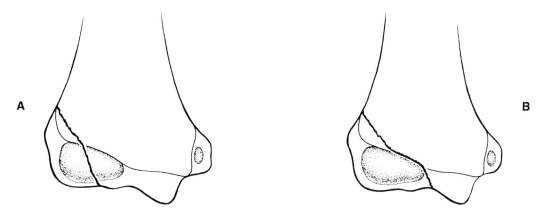

Fig. 10-8. Types of lateral condylar fractures. **A,** Milch Type I fracture pattern (Salter-Harris Type IV). (From Rockwood, C.A., Wilkins, K.E., and King, R.E., editors: Fractures in children, Philadelphia, 1984, J.B. Lippincott Co.) **B,** Milch Type II fracture pattern (Salter-Harris Type II). (Redrawn from Milch: J. Trauma **4:**592, © by Williams & Wilkins, 1964.)

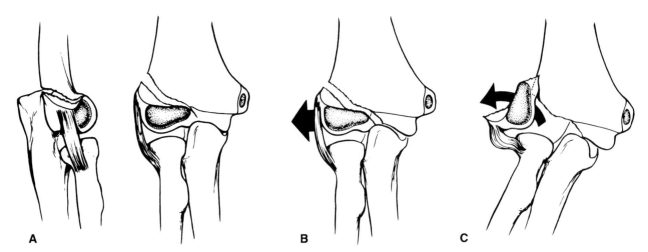

Fig. 10-9. Stages of lateral condylar displacement. **A,** Stage I, **B,** Stage II; **C,** Stage III. (Redrawn from Jakob, R.P., et al.: J. Bone Joint Surg. **57B:**430, 1975.)

Wadsworth and Jacob have described three stages of displacement for these fractures.[6,9] An understanding of these displacement patterns is essential for determining the appropriate treatment (Fig. 10-9). In stage I there is minimal displacement or rotation of the fracture fragment, and the articular surface remains intact. These fractures can be simply immobilized in a removable posterior splint. The triceps aponeurosis can be used to prevent further displacement. By hyperflexing the elbow and placing the forearm in full pronation, the triceps locks the distal fragment against the distal humeral metaphysis. The position of the fragment needs to be checked frequently with serial radiographs during the first 2 weeks of treatment to be sure that there is no further displacement.

In stage II, displacement of the articular surface is disrupted, and there is moderate displacement with some rotation of the distal fragment. If the fracture is fresh and the clot has not significantly organized, this fracture may be remanipulated into position by again hyperflexing the elbow and hyperpronating the forearm. Local digital pressure over the lateral condylar fragment may be necessary to effect the final reduction (Fig. 10-10). The lateral condyle fragment then is stabilized by two percutaneous pins. This manipulation requires a general anesthetic. An image intensifier greatly facilitates placing the pins across the fracture line.

In stage III of displacement the condylar fragment is rotated at least 90 degrees so that its articular surface is facing the raw metaphyseal bone. Because these fracture fragments are very difficult to reduce adequately closed, they require an open reduction with pin fixation. When performing the open reduction, it must be remembered that the dissection must be anterior, not posterior, to prevent injury to the blood supply to the ossification center.

Some specific problems involving fractures of the lateral condylar physis need to be addressed separately. In some cases there may be a delay in the union of the fragment with the distal humeral metaphysis (Fig. 10-11). This is actually a fibrous union that is not mobile and is often asymptomatic.[4] As long as it is not symptomatic, this delayed union is best left alone. With time, it ultimately will heal.[7]

In some cases there may be a delayed recognition of the fracture with a loose symptomatic lateral condylar fragment (Fig. 10-12). These fractures often have a considerable amount of callus or scar formation. Jacob and coworkers found that, in their cases that were treated longer than 3 weeks after fracture, there was such a high incidence of avascular necrosis, physeal arrest, and loss of elbow motion that they recommended leaving the fracture alone.[6] It has been my experience that if the dissection is meticulous and the posterior aspect of the condyle is avoided these complications can be prevented. Some reductions have been performed as late as 1 year after injury.

In an established nonunion with a cubitus

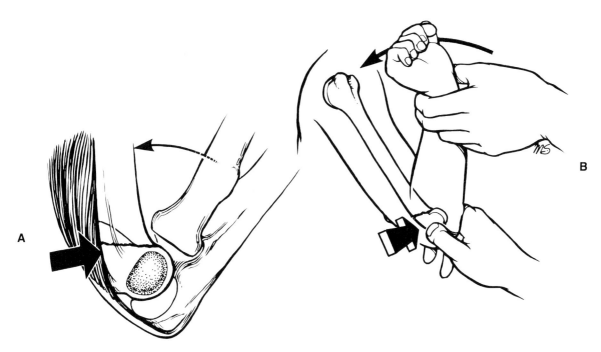

Fig. 10-10. Closed reduction of the lateral condylar fragment can be accomplished by hyperflexing the elbow with the forearm pronated, **(A)** and direct digital pressure over the fragment to complete the reduction **(B).** (From Rockwood, C.A., Wilkins, K.E., and King, R.E., editors: Fractures in children, Philadelphia, 1984, J.B. Lippincott Co.)

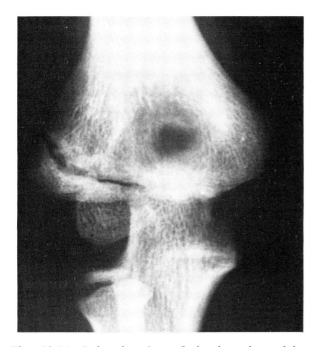

Fig. 10-11. Delayed union of the lateral condylar fragment. The fragment was immobile and the patient was asymptomatic. (From Rockwood, C.A., Wilkins, K.E., and King, R.E., editors: Fractures in children, Philadelphia, 1984, J.B. Lippincott Co.)

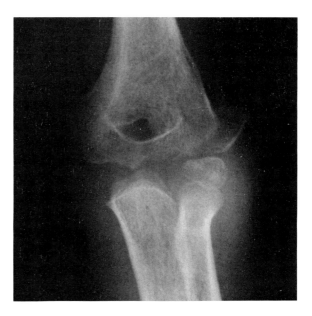

Fig. 10-12. A significantly displaced fracture of the lateral condyle that initially was seen 4 weeks after injury. The condylar fragment was still mobile and tender. This fracture was treated by delayed open reduction and internal fixation. (From Rockwood, C.A., Wilkins, K.E., and King, R.E., editors: Fractures in children, Philadelphia, 1984, J.B. Lippincott Co.)

valgus deformity, treatment requires a complex translocating osteotomy as described by Milch.[8] After this osteotomy there is often some resultant loss of elbow extension and flexion. Union of the condylar fragment is many times difficult to achieve. Whether this complex osteotomy prevents the development of tardy ulnar nerve palsy has not been well defined.

A mild cubitus varus deformity can occur after a lateral condylar fracture. Individuals who have no carrying angle are more prone to the development of some varus. This occurs in those fractures with a stage I of displacement (Fig. 10-13). The displaced metaphyseal fragment often may stimulate the formation of a lateral spur, which produces a lateral prominence of the distal humerus. This lateral prominence, in an individual with no carrying angle, may produce a "pseudovarus" appearance of the elbow. Even in those

fractures that are anatomically reduced, this pseudovarus may still occur. In some minimally displaced fractures there may be lateral overgrowth that may produce a true varus. Thus, in children who have no clinical carrying angle on the uninvolved extremity, the parents need to be warned beforehand that some true or pseudovarus may develop.

Finally, in the very young infant there may be some difficulty in differentiating a fracture of the lateral condylar physis from that involving the entire distal humeral physis. In these cases an arthrogram may help. In fractures involving the lateral condyle only, there is loss of the relationship of the proximal radius to the lateral condylar ossification center. The proximal ulna and radius are more likely to be displaced posteriorly and laterally rather than posteriorly and medially as with fractures of the entire distal humeral physis.

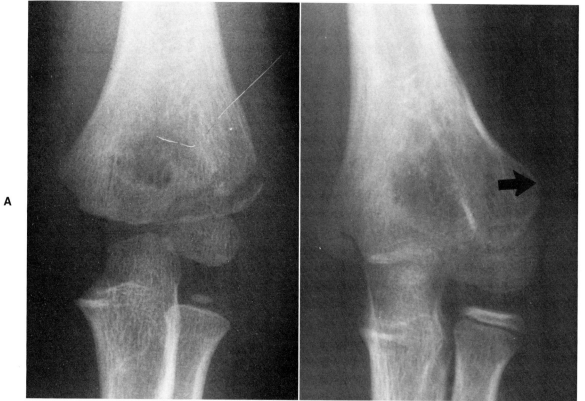

Fig. 10-13. A, The initial radiograph of a minimally displaced lateral condyle that was treated by simple immobilization. **B,** 3 years later there was residual cubitus varus deformity. The varus deformity was accentuated by the lateral spur formation *(arrow).* (From Rockwood, C.A., Wilkins, K.E., and King, R.E., editors: Fractures in children, Philadelphia, 1984, J.B. Lippincott Co.)

In this latter fracture the relationship between the proximal radius and lateral condylar ossification center is maintained.

FRACTURES INVOLVING THE MEDIAL CONDYLAR PHYSIS

Next to the extremely rare fractures of the lateral epicondyle, fractures involving the medial condyle are the most rare. They are commonly unappreciated because the medial crista of the trochlea does not ossify until late. Because they often are missed and because the fracture line exits through the trochlear notch, these fractures can produce significant elbow disability.[13,14] The deformity is accentuated because the forearm flexor muscles pull the loose fragment anteriorly and medially (Fig. 10-14).

The major pitfall with this fracture is the failure to make the correct diagnosis. In younger individuals, where the medial epicondyle is ossified but the medial trochlear crista is not yet ossified, it is difficult to appreciate the true course

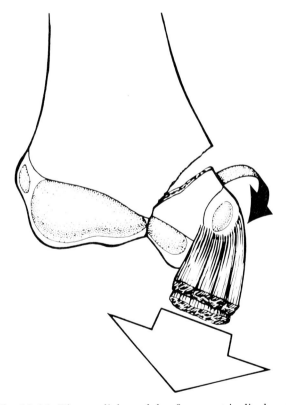

Fig. 10-14. The medial condylar fragment is displaced anteriorly and medially by the origin of the forearm flexor muscles. (From Rockwood, C.A., Wilkins, K.E., and King, R.E., editors: Fractures in children, Philadelphia, 1984, J.B. Lippincott Co.)

of the fracture line. In fact, this injury may be mistaken for a simple fracture involving only the medial epicondyle.[10,12] If there is any metaphyseal bone seen accompanying the displaced medial epicondyle, it is up to the treating physician to prove that this does not involve the media crista of the trochlea. Again, an arthrogram may be helpful in making that differentiation.

Failure to recognize this injury can result in the development of an unstable elbow with progressive cubitus varus from either nonunion or avascular necrosis of the trochlea. Prompt recognition with appropriate open reduction and internal fixation can produce a good cosmetic and functional result.

AVASCULAR NECROSIS OF THE TROCHLEA

Avascular necrosis of the trochlea has been recognized only recently as a sequela of elbow injuries in children.[15] It occurs when there is disruption of the blood supply to the medial crista of the trochlea. Two distinct patterns of necrosis can occur. The first occurs when there is disruption of the transphyseal vessels that supply the lateral ossification center of the lateral crista (Fig. 10-15, *A*). This results in a central defect that accentuates the depth of the trochlear notch to produce the "fish mouth" deformity (Fig. 10-15, *B*).

Such a deformity can occur after a simple undisplaced but very distal supracondylar fracture that disrupts these critical transphyseal vessels. No angular deformity is associated with this defect. The result is simple early degenerative joint disease with subsequent loss of elbow motion. There is no specific treatment for this pattern of avascular necrosis.

In the second form both arteries are disrupted with total loss of blood supply to the medial crista and to some of the metaphysis as well (Fig. 10-16, *A*). This results in a progressive varus deformity with considerable loss of elbow motion (Fig. 10-16, *B*). A valgus osteotomy can improve the angular deformity. However, the stiffness may remain because of the disruption of the articular surface.

Because the damage to these critical vessels occurs at the time of injury, there is no adequate method of prevention of the avascular necrosis. It is wise, however, to warn of its possible occurrence in the very distal fractures that can affect the blood supply to these areas.

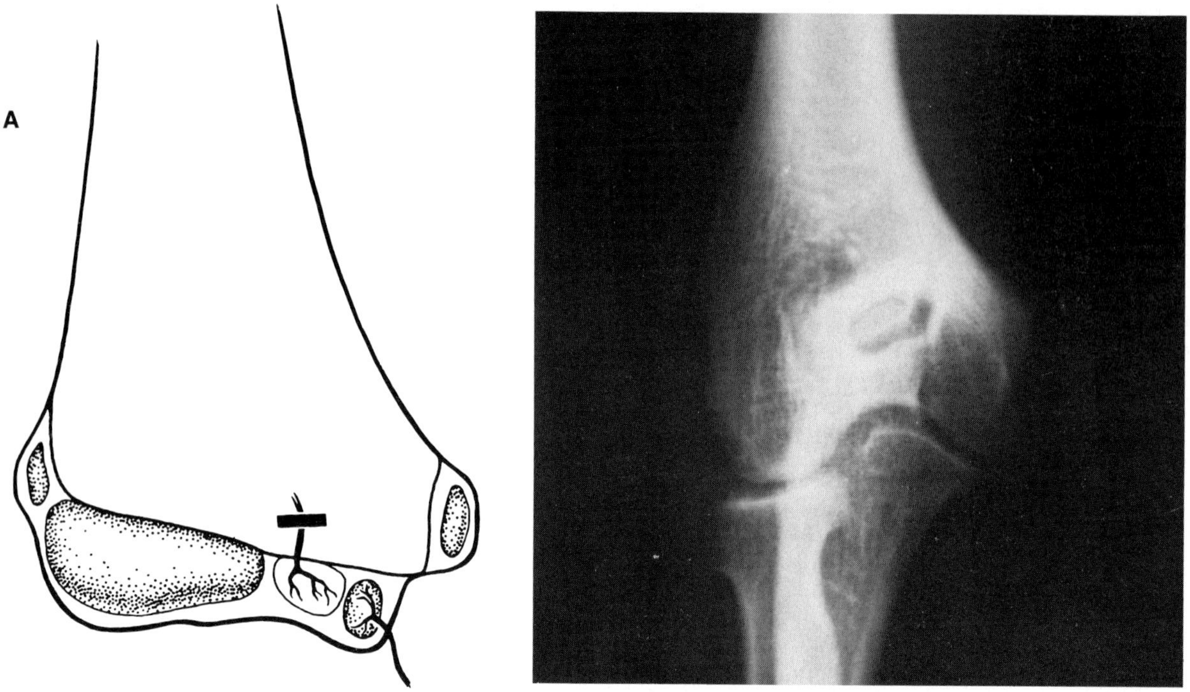

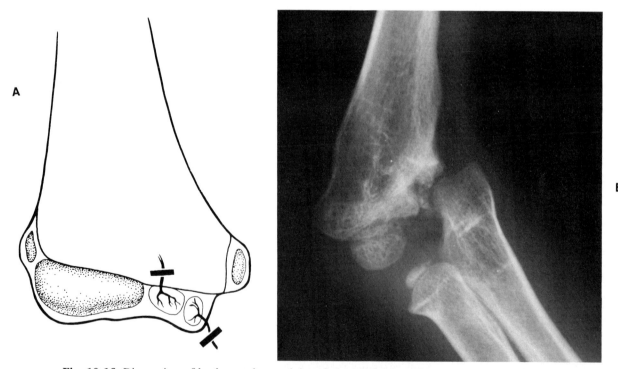

Fig. 10-15. Disruption of the lateral transphyseal vessel to the medial crista **(A)** can result in a central defect producing a "fish mouth" deformity of the distal humeral articular surface **(B)**. (From Rockwood, C.A., Wilkins, K.E., and King, R.E., editors: Fractures in children, Philadelphia, 1984, J.B. Lippincott Co.)

Fig. 10-16. Disruption of both vessels supplying the medial crista **(A)** can result in total destruction of the medial side of the distal humerus, producing a severely disabling cubitus varus deformity **(B)**. (From Rockwood, C.A., Wilkins, K.E., and King, R.E., editors: Fractures in children, Philadelphia, 1984, J.B. Lippincott Co.)

REFERENCES

Distal humeral physis

1. De Lee, J.C., Wilkins, K.E., Rogers, L.F., and Rockwood, C.A.: Fracture separation of the distal humerus epiphysis, J. Bone Joint Surg. **62A:**46-51, 1980.
2. Holda, M.E., Monole, A., and LaMont, R.L.: Epiphyseal separations of the distal end of the humerus with medial displacement, J. Bone Joint Surg. **52A:**52-57, 1980.
3. Mizuno, K., Hirakata, K., and Kashiwogi, D.: Fracture separation of the distal humeral epiphysis in young children, J. Bone Joint Surg. **61A:**570-573, 1979.

Lateral condylar physis

4. Flynn, J.D., and Richards, J.F.: Non union of minimally displaced fractures of the lateral condyle of the humerus in children, J. Bone Joint Surg. **53:**1096-1101, 1971.
5. Hardacre, J.A., et al.: Fracture of the lateral condyle of the humerus in children, J. Bone Joint Surg. **53:**1983-2095, 1971.
6. Jacob, R., et al.: Observations concerning fractures of the lateral humeral condyle in children, J. Bone Joint Surg. **57B:**430-436, 1975.
7. Jeffrey, C.C.: Non union of epiphysis of the lateral condyle of the humerus, J. Bone Joint Surg. **40:**396-405, 1958.
8. Milch, H.E.: Fracture and fracture dislocations of the humeral condyles, J. Trauma **4:**592-607, 1964.
9. Wadsworth, T.B.: Injuries of the capitular epiphysis, Clin. Orthop. **85:**127-142, 1972.

Medial condylar physis

10. Cathay, P.M.: Injury to the lower medial epiphysis of the humerus before development of the ossific center, J. Bone Joint Surg. **49:**766-767, 1967.
11. Chacha, P.B.: Fractures of the medial condyle of the humerus with rotational displacement, J. Bone Joint Surg. **52A:**1453-1458, 1970.
12. Fahey, J.J., and O'Brien, E.T.: Fracture separation of the medial humeral condyle in a child confused with fracture of the medial epicondyle, J. Bone Joint Surg. **53A:**1102-1104, 1971.
13. Fowles, J.V., and Kassab, M.T.: Displaced fractures in the medial humeral condyle in children, J. Bone Joint Surg. **62A:**1159-1163, 1980.
14. Kifoyle, R.M.: Fractures of the medial condyle and epicondyle of the elbow in children, Clin. Orthop. **41:**54-50, 1965.

Avascular necrosis trochlea

15. Morrissy, R.T., and Wilkins, K.E.: Deformity following distal humeral fracture in childhood, J. Bone Joint Surg. **66A:**557-562, 1984.

Chapter 11

Tennis elbow

RALPH W. COONRAD

The symptoms of tennis elbow were originally described in a discussion of lawn tennis by Major in 1883.[12] Subsequently the term *tennis elbow* has become accepted as a descriptive, diagnostic term for a syndrome of pain and point tenderness localized to either the extensor or flexor epicondylar origin at the elbow. Although 95% of the reported cases occur in other than tennis players,[4] it is estimated that from 10% to 50% of people who regularly play tennis experience the symptoms of tennis elbow in varying degree sometime during their tennis lives.[14]

OCCURRENCE

The occurrence of tennis elbow is about equal in men and women, but among regular tennis players it is more common in the male. It is rare in black persons; in fact, in one series of 1000 patients in the South, in an area of equal racial distribution, occurrence was limited to Caucasians.[4] It is a common office problem in orthopaedics and, although more frequently seen in the age-group of 30 to 50, occurs four times more commonly in the fourth decade. There is a peak incidence at the age of 42 in my experience, and it involves the lateral epicondylar origin seven to ten times more frequently than the medial.

ETIOLOGY

The etiology of tennis elbow is actually unknown, but it appears to be multifactorial in origin. Although often termed *epicondylitis*,[10] *tendonitis*, or *bursitis*, no pathologic studies at the time of early symptoms have been reported.

In 1936 Cyriax[5] and, later, others theorized without pathologic or surgical documentation that microscopic or macroscopic tears of the common extensor origin were the likely cause of symptoms. In an extensive monograph on the subject in 1964, Goldie[9] reported the first pathologic studies associated with the syndrome with a description of granulation tissue in the subtendinous space, but he described no actual tendinous tears. Macroscopic tendon tears of extensor origin and associated pathologic changes first were reported in 1973[4] and later confirmed by Nirschl and Pettrone[16] and others with similar findings and microscopic descriptions of the pathology.

Although it would appear the initial inciting factor is actually a microscopic or macroscopic tear, it has been suggested by Nirschl[15] that findings concerning tennis elbow are comparable to McNab's theory relating to the origin of shoulder rotator cuff tears. The likely sequence of events is: "Avascular compromise, an altered nutritional state, and force overload cause angiofibroblastic changes and then ultimate rupture of these vulnerable tissues." Pathologic changes in the conjoined tendon and peritendinous area at the time of surgery often show evidence of granulation and scar tissue attempts at healing degenerative or already scarred tendon from prior insult.[15] It is my opinion that the synovitis and effusion often associated with long-standing symptoms from tennis elbow result from ligamentous stress associated with poor muscle control. Macroscopically, tears of either the flexor or extensor tendinous origin can be superficial or deep. When deep, the superficial tendon attachment to bone may be undisturbed, totally hiding the pathology beneath it (Fig. 11-1).

The onset of symptoms can be sudden or gradual. Although a history of repetitive activity,

94

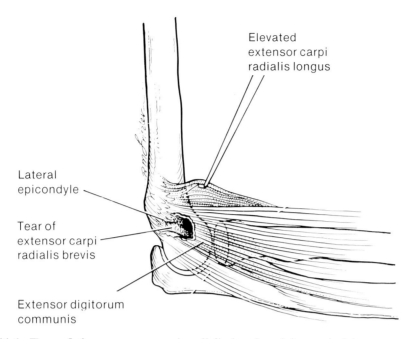

Elevated
extensor carpi
radialis longus

Lateral
epicondyle

Tear of
extensor carpi
radialis brevis

Extensor digitorum
communis

Fig. 11-1. Tear of the extensor carpi radialis brevis origin, underlying a marginal portion of the extensor carpi radialis longus origin.

overuse, or sudden overt force often can be obtained, in many instances no predisposing activity can be determined. Pain and a feeling of subjective weakness of the wrist and digital extensors are present with lateral symptomatology, and, by examination, there is point tenderness characteristically over the extensor carpi radialis brevis origin at the mid-lateral epicondyle. Less commonly, tenderness may be present over the origin of the extensor longus or common digital extensors. The "coffee cup test," that is, picking up a full cup of coffee with associated localized pain at the lateral epicondylar origin, is almost pathognomonic. Similarly, testing wrist extension with resistance when the forearm is in pronation also reproduces pain at the same location. Conversely, medial epicondylar symptoms when flexing the wrist against resistance in forced or full supination usually will reproduce localized pain at the medial epicondylar flexor origin. If tenderness is localized more distal than one to two cm from the medial epicondyle with flexor symptoms, or more distal than the radial head, or in the extensor muscle mass laterally with extensor symptoms, other causes should be evaluated as a basis for the syndrome.

DIFFERENTIAL DIAGNOSIS

Associated or separate problems that need to be considered in a differential diagnosis include radial or median nerve entrapment, localized pathology within the elbow joint, or referred pain from cervical root irritation.

The radial nerve and posterior interosseous or superficial radial nerve branches are vulnerable to compression from distal to the level of the lateral head of the triceps through the arcade of Frohse. Pain at this level of the elbow may be difficult to differentiate from lateral epicondylar origin pain. Because point tenderness with nerve entrapment is usually localized directly over the area of nerve entrapment, EMG and nerve conduction studies may be helpful in differentiation if a motor segment is involved. Conduction delays and fibrillation potentials are not seen with tennis elbow. It must be remembered that electrodiagnostic testing of the supinator muscle can be normal when posterior interosseous nerve branch compression is beyond the arcade of Frohse. Adhesions of the anterior aspect of the distal humerus, muscular or vascular anomalies, fibrous bands, tumors, and many other causes of compression have been reported in the region of the supinator and proximal extensor muscles. Compression of the posterior interosseous nerve as it passes through the arcade of Frohse, however, is the most common site of entrapment,[18] and an illustration of the proximity to the lateral epicondyle and brevis origin is shown in Fig. 11-2. Pain on resistive extension testing of the long finger often is an associated characteristic finding of posterior interosseous nerve compression.[19]

The median nerve is vulnerable to entrapment and compression between the ligament of Struthers and the superficialis muscle arcade in the proximal forearm.[18] Pain in this area can be confused with medial epicondylar flexor origin symptoms. Point tenderness usually is present over the site of nerve entrapment rather than over the pronator or flexor origin at the epicondyle. Peripheral neurologic findings, positive EMG and nerve conduction studies, and sometimes resistance to long finger flexion testing, usually will localize pain at the superficialis arch.

Nirschl has reported 60% associated ulnar nerve findings of neuropraxia with medial epicondylar flexor origin symptoms, and 15% in those with combined medial and lateral epicondylar involvement.[15] In a follow-up of 339 of 1000 patients with tennis elbow, I have not found this clinical association. However, the physician should be aware of ulnar nerve damage when findings and symptoms on the medial side are adjacent to the ulnar groove, particularly when medial collateral ligament instability is present.

A neural lesion at the cervical foraminal level may occur with either medial or lateral elbow pain. The lesion usually is associated with painful restriction of movement in the neck, positive foraminal compression testing, and absence of point tenderness about the elbow. Electromyographic and nerve conduction studies usually are positive, in addition to peripheral neurologic changes. Nirschl reported normal electromyographic findings in 20 unselected patients with classic tennis elbow findings.[15]

X-RAY STUDIES

Routine AP and lateral x-ray studies are usually of little help in the diagnosis of tennis elbow. However, a "gunsight" oblique view of the medial or lateral epicondyle often will show irregularity

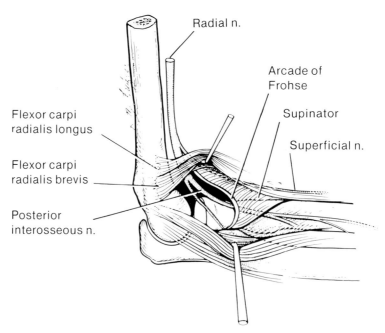

Fig. 11-2. Illustration of the proximity of the origin of the extensor carpi radialis brevis and the arcade of Frohse on the lateral aspect of the elbow.

or punctate calcification. Calcification of some degree has been reported in 22% of one series of cases.[15] Gross calcification or avulsion-type ossification can sometimes be seen over the epicondylar region on routine x-ray films.

ANATOMY

A knowledge of medial and lateral epicondylar anatomy and the location and functional importance of the medial and lateral collateral ligaments is important in understanding the pathology and stress features associated with the symptoms of tennis elbow.

The extensors of the wrist and fingers arise from a common tendinous origin at the lateral epicondyle. In reporting macroscopic tears of the lateral conjoined tendon, superficial or deep pathologic changes most frequently are noted at the origin of the extensor carpi radialis brevis. The tear is not always isolated to the brevis origin but also may involve the adjacent extensor digitorium communis or extensor carpi radialis longus as well. (Figs. 11-3 and 11-4). The extensor carpi radialis longus arises from the lower supracondylar ridge of the humerus and seldom shows isolated involvement. The extensor brevis arises from the central and proximal portion of the lateral epicondyle and from the radial collateral ligament that attaches to the orbicular ligament. No definite pathology of either of these latter two structures has been reported; therefore there is no rationale for surgically disturbing

them. The extensor digitorium communis sometimes shares involvement as it originates distal to and sometimes overlies a portion of the brevis origin on the epicondylar ridge. In instances where pathology at the tendon origin is found, exploration of the elbow joint has been unnecessary and unrewarding.

On the medial aspect of the elbow, the pronator, flexor carpi radialis, flexor digitorium communis, palmaris, and a portion of the sublimis originate with a common tendon of origin, and pathology is usually demonstrated either deep or superficially and involves the pronator teres or flexor carpi radialis. In my experience, the sublimis, palmaris, and flexor carpi ulnaris origin are less commonly involved.

CONSERVATIVE TREATMENT

The patient with a tennis elbow usually has a history of several weeks or months of pain and associated functional disability, involving either the extensor or flexor origin at the elbow. In the nonathlete and non–tennis player, elimination of activities that are painful is of utmost importance. For extensor symptoms, avoidance of grasping in pronation and substituting supination lifting instead immediately relieves much of the symptomatology. Rest and use of aspirin or other antiinflammatory medications may be helpful.

Once rest and avoidance of chronic abuse or overuse have been instituted, a graduated program of strengthening exercise is effective in a

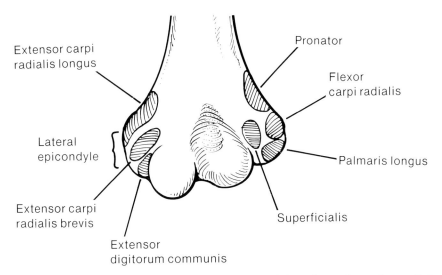

Fig. 11-3. Relative representation of the tendinous origins of muscles at the medial and lateral epicondyles of the elbow.

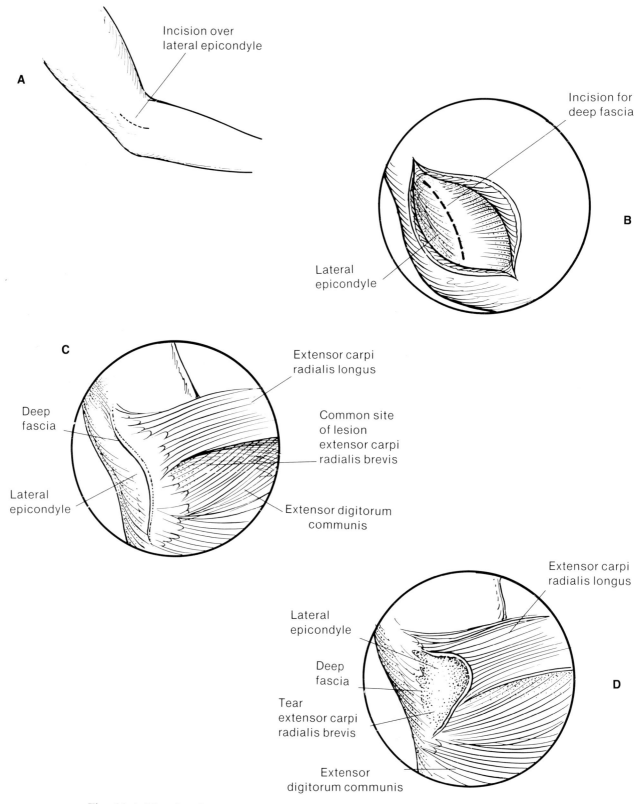

Fig. 11-4. The drawings **A** through **D,** The anatomy and exposure of the conjoined tendon, lying beneath the superficial fascia at the lateral epicondyle of the elbow.

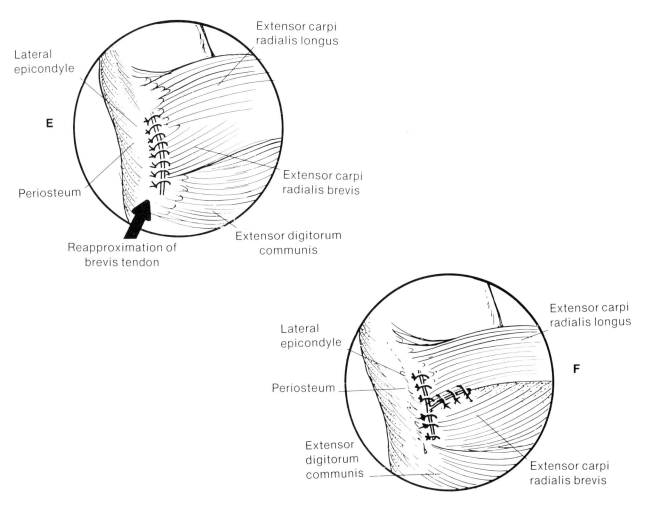

Fig. 11-4, cont'd. E and **F,** The type of alternative reapproximation of the extensor brevis tendon after excising torn or scarred portions of tendon.

large number of patients. Grip strength can be monitored at a less than painful level, and resistive strength and endurance exercises may be initiated and monitored through a full rehabilitation program. Isotonic exercises, using graduated weights in the hand and through the arc of wrist motion, and isometric exercises without any arc of motion are best. Progressive repetitions on a daily basis should be increased gradually as long as the program is kept below a painful level. It should be stressed that the program should include strengthening exercises for the *entire* involved upper extremity, including the shoulder, elbow, wrist, and hand. If pain recurs during such an exercise program, a return to either a lower level of exercise, use of an antiinflammatory agent, or a rest regime will be mandatory. Athletes or tennis players may need to modify their

techniques. The manner of using the flexed or extended wrist may need to be varied in positions of pronation or supination that are painless. This is particularly important in patients with occupational activities that require overuse, such as gasoline station attendants, assembly line workers, typists, and hand-shaking politicians or morticians. The tennis player should consider reducing racket string tension, enlarging the grip, avoiding heavy tennis balls, and using a wide, nonelastic band or strap[6] designed to fit the conical forearm, as described by Froimson and Nirschl.[15,7] The band tends to produce a counterforce in concept, which limits full muscular expansion. A detailed rehabilitation program for the tennis player and athlete has been described by Nirschl.[15]

The use of injectable steroids should be deferred *as long as possible* and employed only for resistant cases of tennis elbow that have not responded to more conservative measures. A good rule of thumb is to avoid steroid injections until the level of incapacitation warrants consideration of surgery. In this case up to three injections of steroid over a period of a year should not produce enough tendon atrophy to further contribute to microscopic or macroscopic rupture. If an injection of steroid is to be used at the elbow, only a small amount should be used (probably not more than 10 mg of triamcinolone mixed with 0.5 ml of lidocaine) and injected below the extensor brevis, directly over the point of maximum tenderness, preferably not into the tendon substance itself.

Historically, in my experience the use of ultrasound, periods of immobilization, bracing and other modalities have not been successful.

SURGICAL TREATMENT

Surgical treatment rarely is indicated with less than a year of symptomatology. Many types of surgical procedures described for the relief of tennis elbow have not been directed at the pathologic anatomy more recently described with this syndrome. Since only extraarticular pathology has been demonstrated in tennis elbow, procedures involving intraarticular structures would appear to have no basis. Synovitis and effusion are usually stress induced and commonly associated with chronic and long-standing tennis elbow, and they will resolve after extensor origin repair. Earlier intraarticular operations such as described by Bosworth[1,2] usually were associated with elevation of the extensor origin in the surgical approach, explaining the reason for some of the successes attributed to those procedures. Neurectomy of the sensory branch to the lateral aspect of the elbow, which has been reported in only three cases,[11] and decompression of an associated posterior interosseous nerve entrapment are not directly related to the pathology of tennis elbow and will not be discussed here.

The primary extraarticular procedures described for relieving tennis elbow are of two types: (1) those that reduce tension at the origin by proximal fasciotomy,[13,17] or distally by lengthening the tendon of the extensor carpi radialis brevis[8] and (2) those that excise the torn portion of the tendon origin proximally and repair or reattach the origin to the epicondyle.[4,7] Distal lengthening of the extensor carpi radialis brevis tendon was unsuccessful in 50% of the cases reported by Carroll[3] and in others I have observed. Fasciotomy by either open or closed methods and complete extensor origin release without repair have been reported to produce loss of strength in some patients and may be disabling in athletes.[15] It is also difficult to rationalize an unrestricted fasciotomy or extensor origin release when the pathology is confined to a much smaller area of the tendon origin or when treatment directed at the localized area of involvement has been successful in a high percentage of cases reported by many authors.

The operative approach that I have found reliable in over 125 cases followed up during the past 25 years includes elevation of only that portion of the conjoined tendon contributed by the extensor brevis and overlying extensor longus tendon; the excision of avulsed and fimbriated tendon margins, scar tissue, and any calcification present; freshening the epicondyle or even lightly excising a small portion of it with reattachment of freshened tendon over exposed bone adjacent to the periosteum and soft tissue. Exposure during elevation of the tendon origin usually extends to the underlying synovium and may include opening of the joint when no implicating pathology is found.

OPERATIVE TECHNIQUE

Using a tourniquet for a bloodless field and with the patient supine and arm across the chest, a 2 to 3 cm incision is made in a curvilinear fashion over the lateral epicondyle, exposing the common extensor origin (Fig. 4). The tendon lesion is found best by carefully identifying the precise point of tenderness preoperatively with a skin mark, and, with the patient under local or regional anesthesia, inserting a long, 25-gauge needle at that point and following it during the exposure. The deep, antibrachial fascia is incised directly over the epicondyle, exposing the fibers of the common tendon origin beneath it and identifying both the superior and inferior margins of the epicondyle. If a tear or scar tissue replacement is not identified in the superficial fibers of the extensor brevis, which usually lie partially covered by the fibers of the extensor longus, the common extensor origin should be elevated more deeply, but *only* in the small area directed toward the synovium and in the direction of the point of maximum tenderness identified preoperatively. I have found scar tissue replacement or fimbriated ends of torn tendon in more than 50% of the cases, and Nirschl[15] has reported a 35% incidence.

In those cases where actual tearing or scar tissue replacement is not identified, calcification should be looked for adjacent to the osseous attachment and a little larger area of extensor origin elevated from the epicondyle. It is not necessary to elevate the entire extensor origin; however, if this is carried out, careful reattachment must be achieved and a longer period of immobilization anticipated. A degenerative portion of tendon, scarred tendon replacement, or fimbriated torn ends of tendon may be excised either in a V-shaped fashion if it is small or excised in a scalloped fashion if it is larger. The adjacent tendon then is pulled together longitudinally. The use of magnifying loops or glasses is helpful in identifying tendon changes and differentiating scar and granulation tissue. A small osteotome may be used to denude lightly the bone surface of the epicondyle, producing raw, cancellous surface over which the tendon can be reattached firmly to adjacent periosteum and soft tissue. Damage to the radial collateral ligament should be avoided and the ligament protected during the exposure.

Exposure of the medial epicondyle for a flexor origin tennis elbow also requires localization of the point of tenderness with a skin marker and optional insertion of a needle as an exposure guide. The tendon origin of the pronator or a portion of the flexor carpi radialis is elevated similarly with the exposure directed toward the synovium of the elbow joint. Excision of torn or scarred tissue and repair are similar to that described for the lateral epicondyle. Identification of the ulnar nerve is mandatory, although transposition of the ular nerve or neurolysis is not necessary ordinarily unless associated with evidence of neuropathy.

Postoperative immobilization is carried out with six layers of sheet cotton and a light circumferential long arm cast with the elbow at ninety degrees and the wrist in functional position. Total elevation of the extremity above shoulder level for 3 days after the operation will offer significant relief of pain. Mobilization is initiated at 5 days out of the cast with a light dressing, and a graduated exercise program of activity is initiated at 4 weeks. Restrictive exercises with dumbbell weights or isotonic exercise might be initiated with the younger patient at 6 to 12 weeks on a very graduated basis. Resumption of tennis and other sports may be initiated selectively in 3 to 6 months along with other graduated activity.

REFERENCES

1. Bosworth, D.M.: The role of the orbicular ligament in tennis elbow, J. Bone Joint Surg. **37A:**527-533, 1955.
2. Bosworth, D.M.: Surgical treatment of tennis elbow: A follow-up study, J. Bone Joint Surg. **47A:**1533-1536, 1965.
3. Carroll, R.E., and Jorgensen, E.C.: Evaluation of the Garden procedure for lateral epicondylitis, Clin. Orthop. **60:**201-204, 1968.
4. Coonrad, R.W., and Hooper, W.R.: Tennis elbow: Its courses, natural history, conservative and surgical management, J. Bone Joint Surg. **53A:**1177-1182, 1973.
5. Cyriax, J.H.: The pathology and treatment of tennis elbow, J. Bone Joint Surg. **18:**921-940, 1936.
6. Froimson, A.I.: Treatment of tennis elbow with forearm support band, J. Bone Joint Surg. **53A:**183-184, 1971.
7. Froimson, A.I.: Tenosynovitis and tennis elbow. In Green, D.P.: Operative hand surgery, New York, 1982, Churchill Livingstone, Inc.
8. Garden, R.S.: Tennis elbow, J. Bone Joint Surg. **43B:**100-106, 1961.
9. Goldie, I.: Epicondylitis lateralis humeri (epicondylalgia or tennis elbow), Acta Chir. Scand. Suppl. **339:**1-119, 1964.
10. Hohl, M.: Epicondylitis—tennis elbow, Clin. Orthop. **19:**232-238, 1961.
11. Kaplan, E.B.: Treatment of tennis elbow (epicondylitis) by denervation, J. Bone Joint Surg. **41A:**147-151, 1959.
12. Major, H.P.: Lawn-tennis elbow, Br. Med. J. **2:**557, 1883.
13. Michele, A.A., and Krueger, F.J.: Lateral epicondylitis of the elbow treated by fasciotomy, Surgery **39:**277-284, 1956.
14. Nirschl, R.P.: Tennis elbow, Orthop. Clin. North Am. **4**(3):787, 1973.
15. Nirschl, R.P.: Muscle and tendon trauma: tennis elbow. In Morrey, B.F., editor: The elbow and its disorders, Philadelphia, 1985, W.B. Saunders Co.
16. Nirschl, R.P., and Pettrone, F.: Tennis elbow: The surgical treatment of lateral epicondylitis, J. Bone Joint Surg. **61A:**832, 1979.
17. Spencer, G.E., and Herndon, C.H.: Surgical treatment of epicondylitis, J. Bone Joint Surgery, **35A:**421-424, 1953.
18. Spinner, M., and Linscheid, R.L.: Nerve entrapment syndromes. In Morrey, B.F., editor: The elbow and its disorders, Philadelphia, 1985, W.B. Saunders Co.
19. Werner, C.O.: Lateral elbow pain and posterior interosseous nerve entrapment, Acta Orthop. Scan. Suppl. **174:**1-62, 1979.

Chapter 12

Arthroscopy of the elbow

B.F. MORREY

The technical ability to perform arthroscopy has expanded to joints other than the knee for quite some time, but the application of this technique to disorders of the elbow has been limited. This might be explained by the unique anatomy of this joint, which results in such a high degree of congruency that attaining the technical ability to perform elbow arthroscopy is somewhat difficult. A second explanation is the fact that specific disorders associated with this joint usually may be diagnosed by routine clinical assessment and radiographs. It is therefore important to understand that a detailed knowledge of the anatomy and pathology of the elbow joint and a general technical proficiency in arthroscopy are crucial to successfully perform arthroscopy of the elbow joint.

TECHNIQUE

The technique of elbow arthroscopy should not be discussed without a review of the relevant anatomy. The tightly constrained joint precludes marked distension, and in most instances manipulation of the joint does not allow a significant improvement in visualization. Furthermore, the proximity of the neurovascular bundle causes major problems with respect to the use of multiple portals of entry. The ulnar nerve limits the use of posterior medial insertion sites, and the median nerve similarly limits the use of anterior medial insertion sites. In addition, the radial nerve is in jeopardy with anterior lateral puncture sites.

Finally, an understanding of the appearance of the pathologic processes gained from experience at arthrotomy is helpful to interpret arthroscopic observations adequately.

Although several arthroscopic techniques may be used with the elbow,[1-7] I prefer to have the patient lying supine on the table with a sandbag under the shoulder. The arm is prepared as for any open procedure and draped so that the extremity may be manipulated at the time of surgery.

Portals. Several portals have been described, but in my estimation the most useful is the midlateral portal, which is in the middle of the triangle formed by the lateral epicondyle, radial head, and tip of the olecranon (Fig. 12-1). This insertion site allows visualization of the ulnohumeral joint, anteriorly (Fig. 12-2) and posteriorly (Fig. 12-3) and the radial humeral joint (Fig. 12-4). Supplemental insertions may be made anterior to the radial humeral joint that allow visualization of the coronoid, this is an excellent approach for anterior loose bodies. Olecranon fossa approaches are helpful for isolation and removal of loose bodies that often lodge in the fossa.

I do not maintain overhead suspension of the arm during the procedure but do position the elbow according to the dictates of the procedure. The use of a camera and monitor is routine (Fig. 12-5). Since the small confines of the joint do not allow a great number of instruments in the joint at any one time, I do not use continuous irrigation routinely. Instead, I use intermittent distension with ingress through the arthroscope. Intermittent engress through the arthroscope is routine.

Operative insertion portals are most frequently in the midlateral area just adjacent to the arthroscope. The posterior olecranon fossa insertion may be used for ingress or for surgical instru-

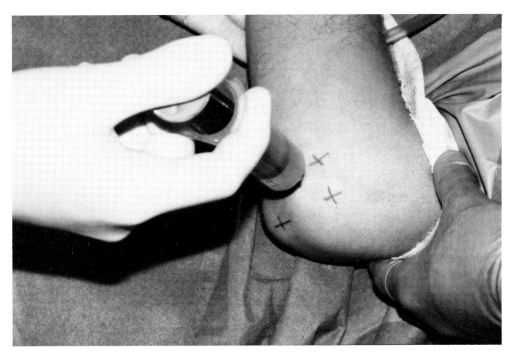

Fig. 12-1. The most commonly performed insertion for elbow arthroscopy is in the center of the triangle formed by the lateral epicondyle, olecranon, and radial head.

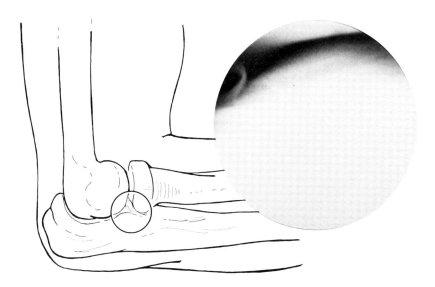

Fig. 12-2. With the demonstrated midlateral insertion site, the anterior ulnohumeral joint is readily visualized.

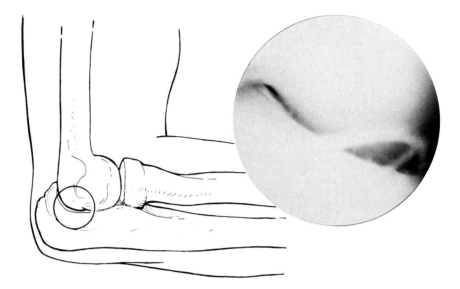

Fig. 12-3. The midlateral insertion also provides visualization of the posterior ulnohumeral joint.

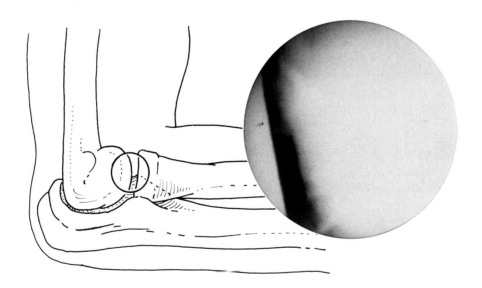

Fig. 12-4. The radial head articulation with the capitellum as visualized through the midlateral portal.

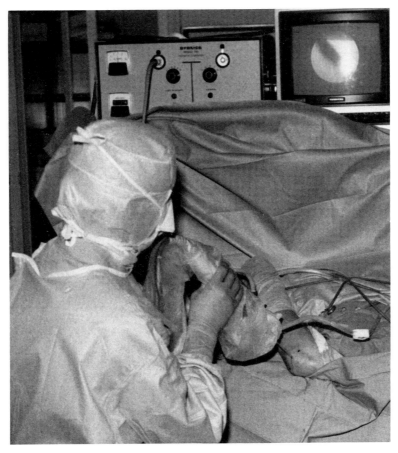

Fig. 12-5. The elbow joint is not amenable to manipulation as readily as the knee and shoulder with the exception of the radiocapitellar articulation, which is aided by pronation and supination of the forearm.

ments. I rarely have used any of the medial approaches, because I believe that the risk of complication exceeds the potential benefits in most instances.

INDICATIONS

The indications for arthroscopy of the elbow may be separated broadly into diagnostic and operative.

Diagnostic indications. The indications to perform a diagnostic arthroscopy are often found in that clinical setting in which the symptoms exceed the clinical findings. This is seen in instances of:
1. Nontraumatic dysfunction that results in pain of uncertain etiology
2. A loss of elbow motion, usually a lack of extension, that cannot be explained by a pathologic event or process
3. When the cause of the symptoms is known but the pain and dysfunction exceeds that anticipated from the clinical findings

Operative indications. The best established indication for operative arthroscopy is the identification and removal of a symptomatic loose body of the joint. This may be a relatively easy procedure if a loose body resides in the olecranon fossa, which is the typical case. However, in those instances when the loose body is in the anterior or medial aspect of the joint, the identification and retrieval can be more difficult (Fig. 12-6).

A second indication for operative arthroscopy is the debridement of cartilage defects, which in my experience is usually associated with a radial head fracture that does not justify radial head excision but that is significantly symptomatic. Osteochondritis dissecans also is amenable in some instances to debridement through the arthroscope.

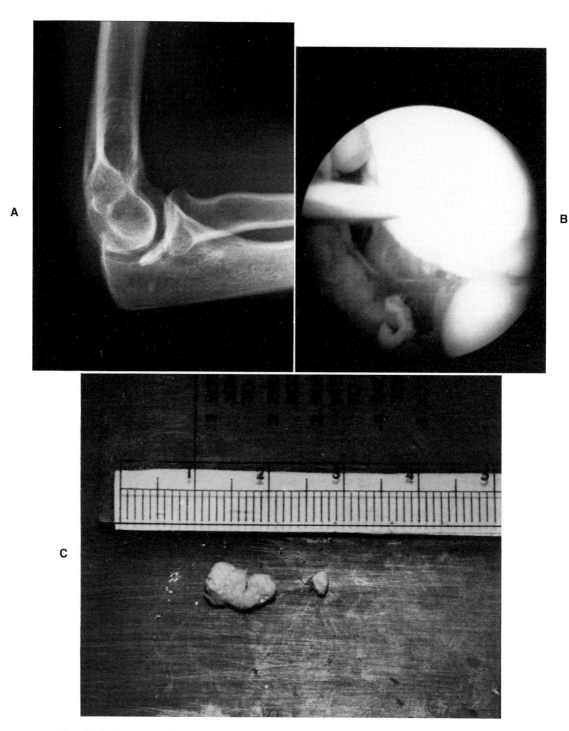

Fig. 12-6. Symptomatic loose bodies visualized on the lateral radiograph of the elbow **(A).** Identification of loose bodies through the arthroscope and localization with spinal needle **(B).** Removal of large and small loose bodies with limited incision under arthroscopic control **(C).** The removal of loose bodies constitutes the best operative indication for elbow arthroscopy.

A third indication is the limited soft tissue debridement, for example, partial synovectomy for rheumatoid arthritis or in posttraumatic synovitis.

The use of arthroscopy to relieve a soft tissue contracture is not a reliable procedure. Elbow contractures are a complex process involving intrinsic and extrinsic mechanisms, and arthroscopy does not begin to address the pathology in any adequate manner. Thus this procedure is primarily of diagnostic value.

RESULTS

The following is an assessment of experience with 30 elbow arthroscopies over the last 4 years. The procedure constitutes about 10% of this elbow surgical practice.

Diagnostic accuracy. During this time, the diagnostic accuracy accomplished the following:

1. Confirmed clinical presentation in 31%
2. Expanded a clinical diagnosis in 38%
3. Provided the initial diagnosis in 10% of these cases

Thus the procedure was believed to have been helpful with 79% of the patients in this group.

The examination was of no benefit in three groups of patients:

1. Indeterminate examination in 14%
2. In one patient (3%), 24 hours after radial head fracture, an adequate assessment could not be obtained because of hemarthrosis
3. In one patient (3%) this was the third procedure performed, and an incorrect impression was obtained from the arthroscopy when arthrotomy revealed a chondral lesion of the medial capitellum

In summary the properly selected patient arthroscopy will be of some diagnostic value in about 80% of cases. Based on these data, the major diagnostic value is to expand a diagnosis that is suggested by the clinical assessment.

TREATMENT

Treatment was influenced by arthroscopy in 19 patients (62%). Tentative plans for arthrotomy were changed in 5 (17%) as a result of arthroscopic data. Arthrotomy was performed in 6 patients, (20%) specifically because of information obtained at arthroscopy. Nonoperative treatment was rendered with 2 patients, and operative arthroscopy was performed with the remaining 6 patients.

Operative arthroscopy. Treatment by arthroscopy was rendered in 6 patients (20%). Localization and removal of a loose body (with 3 patients or 10%) was the most frequently performed arthroscopic procedure. Cartilage debridement after a Mason I radial head fracture was accomplished in 2 patients with satisfactory results. A limited debridement has been done in 2 additional patients with gratifying success in one and no benefit in the second.

COMPLICATIONS

If lateral portals are used, complications are relatively rare. I have observed one incidence of a temporary radial nerve palsy affecting motor, but not sensory, function following an anterior lateral insertion of the arthroscope. This probably relates to the extravasation of the local anesthetic injected in the joint after the procedure. The complication completely and spontaneously resolved in 12 hours. There have been no other complications in this experience. A similar complication has been observed by Andrews and Carson,[1] and none have been reported in the literature.

SUMMARY

Elbow arthroscopy is a valuable adjunctive means to diagnose difficult elbow problems and is a relatively atraumatic means to remove loose bodies. It is also helpful with the patient in whom the objective findings do not coincide with persistent and significant subjective complaints. However, the use of elbow arthroscopy in a routine fashion is to be avoided, and the procedure should have limited indications at this time. Ideally it should be done primarily only by those experienced in the technique of arthroscopy who possess a significant knowledge of elbow anatomy and pathology.

REFERENCES

1. Andrews, J.B., and Carson, W.G.: Arthroscopy of the elbow, Arthroscopy **1**:97, 1985.
2. Cofield, R.H.: Arthroscopy of the shoulder, Mayo Clin. Proc. **58**:501, 1983.
3. Johnson, L.L.: Diagnostic and surgical arthroscopy: The knee and other joints ed. 2, St. Louis, 1981, C.V. Mosby Co.
4. McGinty, J.B.: Arthroscopic removal of loose bodies, Orthop. Clin. North Am. **13**:313, 1982.
5. Morrey, B.F.: Arthroscopy of the elbow. In Morrey, B.F., editor: The elbow and its disorders, Philadelphia, 1985, W.B. Saunders Co.
6. Watanabe, N., Takeda, S., and Ikeuchi, H.: Atlas of arthroscopy, ed. 3, Tokyo, 1979, Igaku-Shoin, Ltd.
7. Zarins, B.: Arthroscopic surgery in a sports medicine practice, Orthop. Clin. North Am., **13**:415, 1982.

Chapter 13

Reconstruction of complex elbow problems

FREDERICK C. EWALD

Almost all of the difficult reconstructive problems in the elbow arise from failed posttraumatic osteoarthritis and rheumatoid arthritis. Primary osteoarthritis in the elbow is as rare as it is in the ankle joint. The elbow joint and ankle joint share a common anatomic feature that enables them to distribute and handle forces in a very efficient manner. Both of these joints have an interosseous membrane that acts as a shock absorber to dissipate joint reactive forces.

FAILED POSTTRAUMATIC OSTEOARTHRITIS
Distraction-resection arthroplasty

In 1975 Volkov and Organesian[6] published a novel way of restoring function in both knees and elbows with a hinge-distractor apparatus. This device was used for failed treatment of posttraumatic elbows, old sepsis, and old dislocations. Walker[1] designed a lighter, more compact and efficient distractor, which has been used at our institution to salvage these difficult problems, particularly in the young, active patient (Fig. 13-1). For example, a young male in his twenties with a severe comminuted fracture of the elbow joint may develop a stiff, painful joint with exuberant new bone formation after treatment. In these patients, particularly those with limited motion, a partial resection arthroplasty can be performed, the distraction apparatus applied, the joint surfaces held in constant distraction, and motion achieved through physiotherapy at the same time (Figs. 13-2 and 13-3). It is a way of performing an interpositional membrane arthroplasty using the patient's own fibrous tissue that is mobilized to provide functional motion. Since no prosthetic devices are used and no bone cement is used, the operation is particularly helpful with young patients. In addition, stability, which is a reported problem with the older interpositional membrane arthroplasties such as a fascial arthroplasty, can be maintained.

The distraction resection arthroplasty is also useful to salvage a failed total elbow replacement, particularly of the nonconstrained resurfacing type where the olecranon is intact. With an intact olecranon the patient has a fulcrum to flex against, and the elbow remains stable during flexion. This concept also can be used to salvage septic elbows, particularly those that end with limited motion.

The only other option for this group of young patients with failed posttraumatic elbows is an elbow fusion. However, an elbow fusion will result in unsatisfactory function, particularly in a dominant extremity, because there is no satisfactory fusion position for good elbow function. An elbow fusion at 90 degrees may be the most satisfactory from a cosmetic standpoint, but very few activities of daily living are performed with the elbow at exactly 90 degrees. Most hand functions are performed with the elbow at approximately 30 to 45 degrees of elbow flexion or with the elbow flexed 110 to 125 degrees. The elbow only passes through 90 degrees of flexion to move from the extended functional position to the flexed functional position. Elbow fusion generally is not recommended as a primary salvage procedure unless the patient has had a functional elbow fusion of a nondominant extremity for many years and has accepted the limitation of motion. The inability to place one's hand in space after an elbow fusion often is extremely frustrating to the patient, and, despite the absence of

108

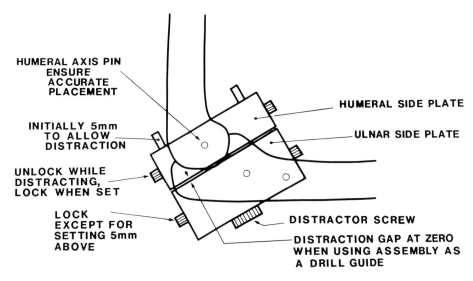

Fig. 13-1. Schematic diagram of hinge-distractor illustrating principles of fixation with transverse wire through center of rotation of trochlear and capitellum.

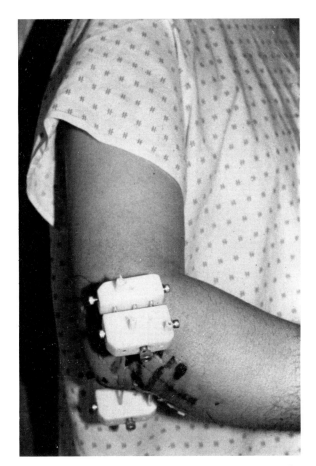

Fig. 13-2. Hinge-distractor in place on patient undergoing active physical therapy during the 6-week postoperative period of use.

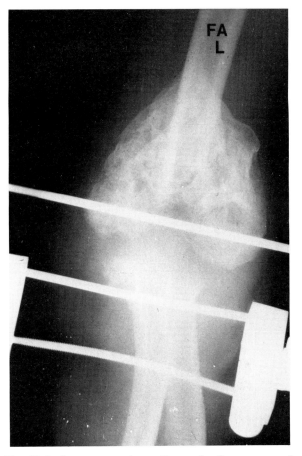

Fig. 13-3. Anteroposterior radiograph of posttraumatic elbow showing distraction of joint surfaces.

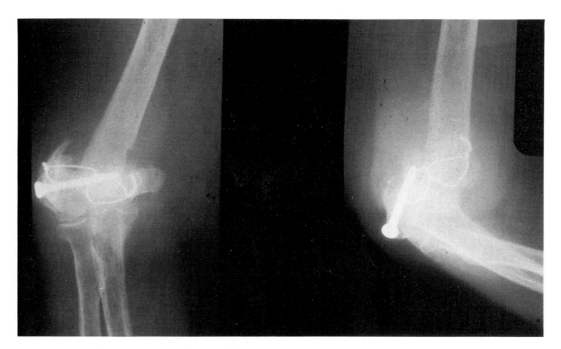

Fig. 13-4. Failed comminuted supracondylar T fracture with nonunion, pain, and limited motion in the dominant arm of an elderly patient.

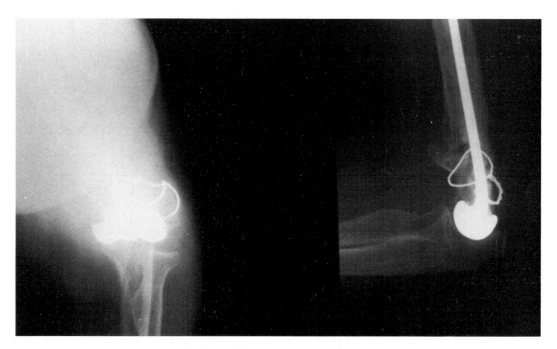

Fig. 13-5. Long-stem resurfacing humeral component inserted with circlage wire to reduce separated epicondyles and bone graft added to give a satisfactory clinical result.

pain combined with good stability, many patients desire to have the fusion taken down to restore motion.

Total elbow resurfacing arthroplasty

If the failed posttraumatic elbow is in an older, low-demand patient, if the olecranon bone stock is relatively intact, and if there is remaining trochlear and capitellum, then the elbow joint can be resurfaced with a nonconstrained prosthesis such as the capitellocondylar.[2,3] This alternative should be avoided with young patients, because their high demands may lead to early failure seen with the constrained hinged-type total elbow replacements. An example of a low-demand patient would be a retired individual who does not do any heavy labor and who would not lift anything heavier than 25 pounds. If the bone stock is deficient or there is not enough bony tissue to get effective three-point fixation of the resurfacing device, then one of the loose or sloppy hinged-type devices may be useful. Two of the best examples are the triaxial[4] loose hinge or the Mayo modification of the loose Coonrad[5] hinge joint. Both of these devices can be used with deficient bone stock, but I still would recommend and limit their use to the older, low-demand patient. A history of sepsis is an absolute contraindication unless the infection has been cleared completely by a course of antibiotics after joint debridement. In these cases a distraction resection arthroplasty may be a better choice.

Hemiarthroplasty

Occasionally the failed posttraumatic osteoarthritic elbow may involve only the humeral portion of the elbow joint. This is seen in the comminuted T fractures without olecranon involvement and without elbow dislocation or radial head fracture (Fig. 13-4). In these cases a nonconstrained resurfacing type of stemmed arthroplasty should be considered. This type of treatment is similar to a bipolar hemiarthroplasty for a fractured femoral neck or a Neer-type prosthesis for a four-part humeral head fracture. A custom long-stem can be used for fixation with or without cement, depending on the age of the patient, and the distal humerus can be internally fixed and bone grafted if a nonunion exists (Fig. 13-5). In all of these cases the olecranon must be intact, and there must be salvageable remaining articular cartilage on the trochlear notch of the olecranon.

FAILED POSTTRAUMATIC RHEUMATOID ARTHRITIS
Distraction-resection arthroplasty

In rheumatoid arthritis as in posttraumatic osteoarthritis, the distraction-resection arthroplasty designed by Walker can be used to salvage a failed total elbow replacement for sepsis, loosening, or recurrent dislocations. The distraction resection arthroplasty works best if the olecranon fossa is intact to provide a fulcrum for flexion.

Total elbow replacement

Patients with rheumatoid arthritis who have elbow fractures should be treated initially as one would treat a patient with an otherwise normal traumatic elbow (Fig. 13-6). However, if the treatment fails and the elbow undergoes degeneration either secondary to the injury or because of progression of the rheumatoid arthritis (Fig. 13-7), then a total elbow resurfacing arthroplasty is recommended at any age, provided the bone stock is sufficient to allow resurfacing (Fig. 13-8). If the bone stock is deficient, then a flexible hinge-type prosthesis should be selected. A hemiarthroplasty for rheumatoid arthritis is not recommended.

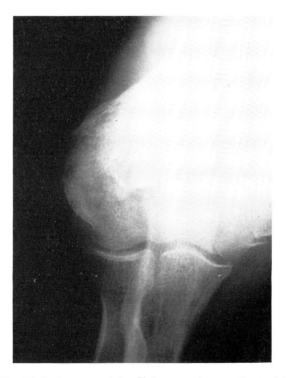

Fig. 13-6. Supracondylar T fracture in a patient with rheumatoid arthritis.

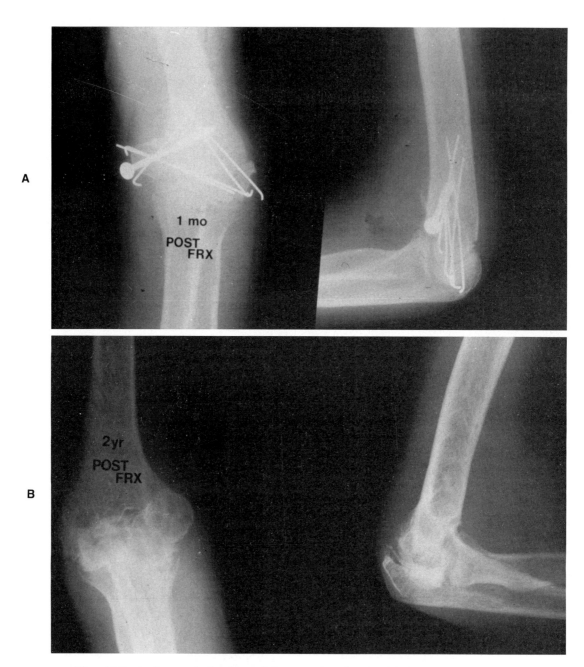

Fig. 13-7. A, Internal fixation of fracture in Fig. 6 with loss of initial anatomic reduction. **B,** Internal fixation removed and joint completely destroyed 2 years after injury with intractable pain and limited motion.

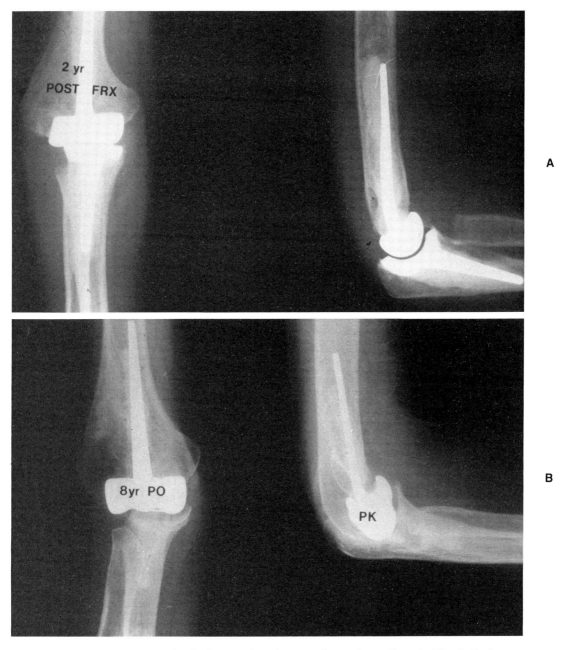

Fig. 13-8. A, Nonconstrained elbow arthroplasty performed on elbow in Fig. 6. **B,** 8-year follow-up of total elbow arthroplasty on opposite elbow of patient in Fig. 6 with a pristine bone-cement interface.

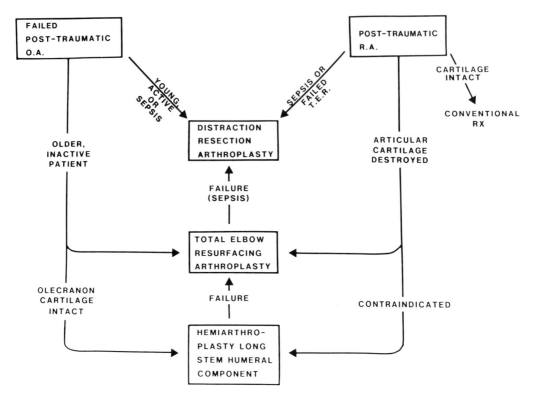

Fig. 13-9. Treatment flow sheet for failed posttraumatic osteoarthritis and rheumatoid arthritis.

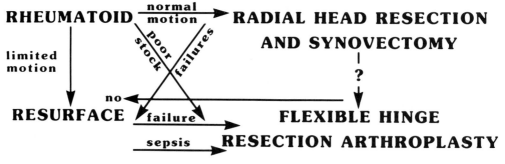

Fig. 13-10. Treatment flow sheet for primary rheumatoid arthritis and failed rheumatoid arthritis.

A summary of these treatment options is seen in Fig. 13-9 for both the posttraumatic failed osteoarthritic elbow and the posttraumatic elbow with rheumatoid arthritis. Fig. 13-10 is a flow sheet of treatment for the rheumatoid elbow with complete radiographic destruction and intractible pain. In general if the rheumatoid elbow has normal motion and relatively intact subchondral bone with cartilage loss then a radial head resection with synovectomy is indicated. If this fails, a flexible hinge or a resurfacing type of arthroplasty can be performed easily. If the initial rheumatoid elbow joint has limited motion, a radial head resection and synovectomy is not indicated, and resurfacing with a nonconstrained prosthesis is recommended. If the resurfacing arthroplasty fails, then a distraction-resection arthroplasty can be performed—especially in the case of sepsis—or a flexible hinge can be performed.

These are extremely difficult problems to salvage. The preceding recommendations are designed to be as conservative as possible, avoiding the problems of the past and attempting to preserve—at all costs—bone stock.

REFERENCES

1. Deland, J.T., Walker, P.S., Sledge, C.B., and Faberov, A.: Treatment of post-traumatic elbows with a new hinge-distractor, Orthopaedics 1983.
2. Ewald, F.C., and Jacobs, M.A.: Total elbow replacement, Clin. Orthop. **182:**137-142, 1984.
3. Ewald, F.C., and Scheinberg, R.D., Poss, R., Thomas, W.H., Scott, R.D., and Sledge, C.B.: Capitello-condylar total elbow arthroplasty, J. Bone Joint Surg. **62A:**1259-1263, 1980.
4. Inglis, A.E., and Pellicci, P.M.: Total elbow replacement, J. Bone Joint Surg. **62A:**1252-1258, 1980.
5. Morrey, B.F., Bryan, R.S., Dobyns, J.H., and Linscheid, R.L.: Total elbow arthroplasty: A five-year experience at the Mayo Clinic, J. Bone Joint Surg. **63A:**1050-1063, 1981.
6. Volkov, M.D., and Organesian, O.V.: Restoration of function in the knee and elbow with a hinge-distractor apparatus, J. Bone Joint Surg. **57A:**591-600, 1975.

TOTAL HIP ARTHROPLASTY

Chapter 14

Osteoarthritis of the young adult hip: etiology and treatment

JAMES ARONSON

Contrary to popular belief, a significant number of young adults suffer from the insidious yet progressive disability caused by osteoarthritis of the hip.* *Young adults* can be defined as those patients too old for the pediatric orthopaedist and too young for the prosthetic hip specialist. Since skeletal maturation varies with the individual and some pediatric orthopaedists follow their patients beyond adolescence, the lower age limit of the young adult averages 20 years. When the best reported longevity of current prosthetic hip replacement (25 years)[38] is subtracted from the current life expectancy (75 years),[57] the upper age limit averages 50 years. A growing concern that prosthetic hip replacement fails more frequently in the young adult[10,18] leaves these patients with no choice but to palliate pain and compromise their activities until their remaining life expectancy equals the expected longevity of current prosthetic hip technology.

Three myths have induced complacency among orthopaedists toward taking this problem more seriously. The first myth, perpetuated over the last two decades, indicates that treatment of childhood hip disorders usually results in normal hips.[19,21,44] The second myth promotes total hip replacement as the panacea for adult hip disease,[43,51] especially with regard to the third myth that relegates osteotomy to rare, specific indications because of unpredictability.[22,34,35,45,48] In reality these myths are not so bluntly stated in the literature, but in effect they are transmitted to the public.

The facts no longer support these myths. Several recent studies provide information on the prognosis of childhood hip deformities through the sixth decade.[13,30,53] By combining these data with etiologic and epidemiologic studies, it is possible to accurately project the magnitude of resultant hip disability in our society.

Likewise, 10-year follow-ups on major treatment options (osteotomies[20,34,45,47,48] and prosthetic hip replacement[31,50,55]) for osteoarthritic hips now provide the essential facts to compare long-term results. By using common denominators of success and failure, we can define reliably the indications for current reconstructive procedures.

ETIOLOGY

Osteoarthritis is a term occasionally used to include any joint affliction that leads to destruction of hyaline cartilage by local or systemic disease.[42] This broad definition does not take into account the host response that is integral to the process of osteoarthritis, that is, bony sclerosis and fibrocartilaginous osteophyte formation. It is important to realize that osteoarthritis is a process of degeneration and repair, thereby differentiating it from osteoporosis and rheumatoid arthritis; the latter rarely mount a reparative response.[32] Osteoarthritis results from mechanical disequilibrium between articular force transmission (pressure) and host tissue resistance.[40] Within a joint, pressure can easily reach pathologic magnitude if maldistributed (for example, incongruity);[52] similarly, an entire joint can be overstressed to pathologic magnitude by external forces.[5,40]

---

*References 10-15, 19, 21, 29, 30, 39, 44, 48, 49, 51, 53, 60.

119

Table 14-1. Etiology of endstage osteoarthritis*

Author (year)	CDH	SCFE	LCP	Idiopathic
Wiberg[60] (1939)	26%	6%	5%	
Lloyd-Roberts[27] (1955)	21%	6%	2%	59%
Adam[1] (1958)	21%	5%	5%	66%
Gudmundsson[22] (1970)	12%	6%	6%	55%
Ranawat[43] (1984)	19%	4%		57%
Averages	20%	5.4%	4.5%	59%
Modified†	43%	11%	22%	12%

CDH, congenital dysplasia of the hip; SCFE, slipped capital femoral epiphysis; LCP, Legg-Calvé-Perthes.
*Endstage osteoarthritis in all of these series is equated with pain requiring prosthetic hip replacement.
†To match incidence and prognosis figures (see text).

Table 14-2. Congenital hip dysplasia results by age fifty*

Author (year)	Number of hips at follow-up	Painful osteoarthritis
Mardem-Bey[29] (1982)	134	11% second decade
Wiberg[60] (1939)	38	37% third decade 50% fifth decade*
Cooperman[13] (1983)	32 (mild dysplasia)	12% fifth decade* 38% sixth decade 66% seventh decade
Cooperman[12] (1980)	30 (aseptic necrosis)	80% fourth decade

*Wiberg's patients had severe CDH, whereas Cooperman's patients (1983) had only mild acetabular dysplasia. Note that the overall incidence increases with age. Iatrogenic aseptic necrosis in CDH carries a significant risk for painful osteoarthritis.

Childhood diseases such as congenital dislocated hip and Legg-Calvé-Perthes disease (LCP) often leave the joint surface deformed at skeletal maturity; slipped capital epiphysis can lead to either cartilage destruction (chondrolysis), joint incongruity (aseptic necrosis), or simply joint malorientation (slip itself). One would expect patients with these conditions to develop osteoarthritis over time.

Congenital dysplasia of the hip. Congenital hip dysplasia (CDH) in the form of subluxable, dislocatable, or dislocated neonatal hips is one of the five most common multifactorial inherited diseases at birth. Recent large-scale screening projects totaling almost 50,000 newborns support the traditionally quoted incidence of 1% of all live births.[33,56] It is no wonder that this diagnosis results in endstage osteoarthritis more frequently than the other childhood diseases (Table 14-1). After CDH treatment some residual deformity often persists into adult life.[5,60] The mechanical imbalance created by a narrow, tilted acetabular roof leads to predictable osteoarthritis that is proportional to time[5,13,60] (Table 14-2). A significant number of these hips causes painful disability by age 50, from 12% to 80% depending upon complications of treatment and severity of the dysplasia. It is safe to say that 25% to 50% of these patients will suffer by the end of the fifth decade despite current treatment techniques.

Legg-Calvé-Perthes disease. Perthes (LCP, coxa plana) is really a transient dysplasia of the growing femoral head and neck induced by ischemic episodes. The ultimate deformity correlates most closely with age of onset[30,44,53]; older children seem to have less potential for remodeling the deformity. In an elegant epidemiologic study, Molloy and MacMahon[35] identified the annual incidence of LCP in Massachusetts. The cumulative incidence or attack rate then was calculated to be only 0.08% or 1 in 1200 live births. CDH is 12 times more common. Yet, at endstage osteoarthritis CDH is represented only four to five times more frequently than LCP (see Table 14-1). The

Table 14-3. Legg-Calvé-Perthes results by age 50*

Author (year)	Number of hips at follow-up	Painful osteoarthritis
Danielsson[15] (1965)	35	20% fourth decade
Ratliff[44] (1967)	34	25% fourth decade
Gower[21] (1971)	36	50% fifth decade
Stulberg[53] (1981)	99	50% sixth decade
McAndrew[30] (1984)	37	60% sixth decade

*McAndrew reexamined several of Gower's patients over 10 years later, finding further deterioration. Ratliff emphasizes the positive results in his article.

prognosis for treated LCP is somewhat worse than CDH as seen in Table 14-3. Clearly 50% of these patients will demonstrate painful osteoarthritis in the sixth decade; many cases are being diagnosed earlier.[11] The osteoarthritis process is clearly time-related (Table 14-3).

Slipped capital femoral epiphysis. Slipped capital femoral epiphysis (that is, SCFE, epiphyseolysis) results in simple limitation of joint mobility as a result of articular maldirection of varying severity. The actual joint surfaces remain undisturbed unless complicated by chondrolysis or aseptic necrosis. The cumulative incidence, which is reported between 0.05% and 0.07%,[23,25] or 1:1500 live births, is similar to that of LCP. However, long-term studies of SCFE reveal that only 15% to 20% of these patients have painful osteoarthritis by age 50. There is a direct relationship between severity of slip and onset of osteoarthritis,[8,39,61] but not enough to account for equal representation with LCP at endstage hip review (see Table 14-1).

Idiopathic osteoarthritis. Primary or idiopathic osteoarthritis (OA) is a diagnosis of exclusion, since no known cause has been identified. Given the limitations of retrospective studies, it is understandable that OA is by far the most common etiology reported for endstage osteoarthritis (see Table 14-1). A critical investigation was undertaken by Stulberg and associates in 1975[54] to clarify the etiology of OA. The majority of cases originally called idiopathic could be reclassified by using strict criteria and reproducible measurements as either mild acetabular dysplasis (39%) or pistol grip deformity (40%). The latter term refers to a common pathway of degeneration found in both LCP and SCFE. If these estimates are correct, then Table 14-1 could be modified to account for less idiopathic (12%) and more CDH (43%). The additional cases of pistol grip defor-

Table 14-4. Slipped capital femoral epiphysis results by age 50

Author (year)	Grade of slip	Painful osteoarthritis*		
Boyer[8] (1981)	I	0%		
(149 hips)	II		15%	
	III			30%
Ordeberg[39]				
(1984)	I	5%		
(77 hips)	II		8%	
	III			17%

*Painful osteoarthritis is proportional to the degree of slip in both series.

mity could account for any discrepancy between the etiologic projections and the reported incidence-prognosis figures for LCP and SCFE (see Table 14-1).

Primary OA may, in fact, be a biologic disease without apparent mechanical deformity, since joint degeneration and reparative processes typical of osteoarthritis and secondary to CDH, SCFE, and LCP can occur in previously normal hips. In 234 such cases that were identified from a larger series of endstage hips,[28] no local or systemic disease could be identified. The onset of bilateral hip pain with flexion contracture peaked in the sixth decade for males and in the seventh decade for females. Radiographic degeneration followed the usual pattern of lost joint space and cysts, followed by reactive sclerosis and osteophytes. On the average, progression was rapid over 5 years and lead to debilitating pain. At prosthetic hip replacement the superolateral quadrant of the femoral head was commonly eburnated. In a small percentage the pain spontaneously abated with osteophytes and reappearance of a joint space. Primary or idiopathic OA rarely is seen in the young adult.

Table 14-5. Etiology of endstage coxarthrosis*

Author (year)	Number of hips for THR	OA	RA	ASN	Failed prosthesis	Other
Lloyd-Roberts[27] (1955)	124	88%				12%
Amstutz[2] (1982)	860	44%	13%	13%		30%
Stauffer[50] (1982)	231	61%	7%	4%	26%	2%
Ranawat[43] (1984)	103	80%		11%		9%
Aronson[3] (1985)	100	43%	19%	23%	12%	3%

THR, total hip replacement; OA, Osteoarthritis; RA, rheumatoid arthritis; ASN, aseptic necrosis.
*Coxarthrosis implies all etiologies for the endstage hip. Osteoarthritis is still the most common etiology over the last three decades.

Childhood hip disease. Since the three most common diseases of the child's hip (CDH, LCP, and SCFE) occur in 1.1% of the young adult population, approximately 1 million of the 97 million young adults (20 to 50 years old)[57] are at risk. As each generation reaches age 50, at least 25% (8000 per year) will be disabled by painful osteoarthritis (Tables 14-2, 14-3, 14-4). In 1980 3.6 million live births were reported[57]; therefore 36,000 new cases of CDH, LCP, and SCFE could occur each year. Unless treatment techniques for these childhood diseases improve significantly, 9000 new cases of osteoarthritis by age 50 could continue each year.

The number of patients with endstage coxarthrosis who require prosthetic hip replacement is astounding. Osteoarthritis has continued to be the most common etiology for all coxarthrosis over the last three decades (Table 14-5). Since two thirds of all osteoarthritis is estimated to originate from childhood hip disorders (Table 14-1), the magnitude of this problem in young adults cannot be overlooked.

TREATMENT

Natural history. Ironically, the belief that treatment of childhood hip disorders usually results in normal hips has provided good impetus to observe the natural history of many patients with secondary osteoarthritis of the hip. Most patients who are fortunate enough to continue their care at the same institution for 40 to 50 years[8,15,21,44] develop loyalties that naturally bias toward success of early treatment. The tremendous investment of time and energy by the treating physician also biases toward optimism. This arrangement is advantageous for learning the natural history of a disease process, since only the most severe problems merit surgical intervention.

Periodic prospective follow-up studies routinely lose track of many patients, however, they are valuable for the few individuals who can help reconstruct their own symptoms and activities over several decades. As independent examiners take over these study groups, the patients tend to admit more severe symptoms. [11-13,30,53]

The natural history of osteoarthritis is the basic standard to which all methods of treatment must compare. Few patients improve spontaneously. Schneider[48] observed 100 patients over an average of 1½ years; all 100 noted worsening pain despite limiting activities and an average 23-degree loss in total motion. Macys[28] reviewed the clinical and radiographic course of 234 patients for an average of 5 years. All of these patients underwent steady deterioration. In a small group 10% actually experienced spontaneous pain relief 7 to 10 years later with the development of osteophytes. Activity levels and mobility of the hips remained severely impaired. Cooperman and associates[13] followed patients with mildly dysplastic hips for 20 years only to find that greater than 90% developed moderate to severe osteoarthritis, thus confirming Wiberg's[60] earlier observations. Danielsson[14] followed 140 patients for an average of 10 years. Half had severely limited their activities, but 35% were pain free at an average age of 69 years. Bombelli[5] made the same observation that a few patients with osteoarthritis experienced spontaneous resolution of pain. His ingenious realization that certain osteophyte patterns were associated with pain relief and joint space reappearance led him to exploit osteophytes for actual treatment.

Osteophytes generally do not appear before age 40,[5,44,53] and painful osteoarthritis also is much less common before then (see Tables 14-2 and 14-3), although some cases have been reported.[11] Radiographic abnormality often precedes symptoms.[8,13,15,61] Severe joint incongruity often goes unnoticed by patients under thirty. The primary symptom, pain, responds initially to limitation of activity and nonsteroidal antiinflammatory agents.[49] In the younger adult a subtle limp goes unnoticed, an ache is attributed to muscle strain, and the childhood hip disease is often forgotten, "cured" like an earache. The young adult is career- and family-oriented with little time or money to consider medical attention. Initially the disability can be hidden, but before age 50 it becomes painfully apparent, possibly forcing vocational change or even retirement when life-style demands may be greatest.

Unfortunately, patients rarely seek medical attention to prevent this catastrophe. Pain that is refractory to rest or medication is the usual motivator. Limited function is the next most common complaint. When these young adults request treatment, tremendous demands are placed on the orthopaedist to relieve pain, restore normal function, and ensure longevity.

Surgical management. It is not my purpose to review the historical evolution of treatment (for example, Voss, Girdlestone, Colonna) that is fully discussed by others.[4,5,42] There are basically three treatment options currently considered viable: arthrodesis, osteotomy, and prosthetic hip replacement. The indications for hip arthrodesis are specific and limited to a small minority of patients. Based on a review of 525 hip arthrodeses, Leichti[26] found the best results in patients employed at heavy labor with a unilateral painful, stiff hip and normal lumbar spine, ipsilateral knee, and contralateral hip. Contraindications include sedentary work, mild to moderate osteoarthritis, females desiring natural childbirth, and ipsilateral knee valgus or varus. Of all adult hip operations in St. Gall, Switzerland, between 1961 and 1971 these 525 arthrodeses represented 10%. During this 10-year period the 10% figure remained relatively constant. During the same period the percentage of intertrochanteric osteotomies peaked in 1966, although prosthetic hip replacements peaked in 1972. When osteoarthritis of the hip was studied in all of Switzerland (1955 to 1976), similar proportions were found.[36] In fact, as prosthetic hip replacements peaked, the osteotomies fell to a proportionate nadir. By 1976 the Swiss group[36] began to approach a steady state of four prosthetic hips for every

Table 14-6. 10-year results of prosthetic hip replacement

Author (year)	Number of hips at follow-up	Failure*	Impending failure
Sutherland[55] (1982)	100	32.0%	40%
Stauffer[50] (1982)	231	7.4%	30%
McBroom[31] (1984)	1030	14.0%	

*Failure means painful mechanical loosening requiring reoperation. Impending failure means progressive radiolucency around either or both components but not yet revised.

osteotomy performed. Specific indications have been elaborated.

In the United States patient demands for a panacea were met as prosthetic hip replacement has all but supplanted osteotomy in these patients. As a consequence, several centers now are reporting results of prosthetic hip replacement in young adults.[10,18,43]

The controversy stemming from the second and third myths has been sparked by recent reports of high failure rates for prosthetic hip replacements in young adults.[10,18] Let us judge the facts.

Prosthetic hip replacement. Initial response to the prosthetic hip replacement was encouraging, since a painless mobile hip resulted with a minimum period of rehabilitation. This technological triumph, of course, pleased the American public. Even at 7-year follow-up some highly skilled surgeons have reported a relatively low failure rate, 10%, mostly attributed to technical problems that have since been solved.[43] The nagging problem that remained was a 30% incidence of radiographic loosening. Would these hips soon be failures?

At 10-year follow-up the average failure rate approximates 15% with a range from 7% to 32% (Table 14-6). Failure means painful loosening and does not include infection that requires reoperation. Impending failures imply progressive radiographic lucency around the prostheses with minimal pain. The reported incidence, 30% to 40% of impending failure, is frighteningly high at 7- to 10-year follow-ups, not even close to the 25-year mark.

The solution might have been to revise the prosthesis at a second operation, but these attempts are meeting early disaster. The revision

Table 14-7. Early results of revision prosthetic hip replacement

Author (year)	Number of hips at follow-up	Average follow-up	Failure*	Impending failure
Amstutz[2] (1982)	67	2 years	9%	20%
Pellicci[41] (1984)	139	3½ years	33%	12%

*Failure and impending failure are defined as in Table 14-6.

Table 14-8. 5-year results of prosthetic hip replacement in young adults

Author (year)	Number of hips at follow-up	Average age at operation	Failure*	Impending failure
Chandler[10] (1981)	33	23 years	21%	57%
Dorr[18] (1983)	108	30 years	19%	28%

*Failure and impending failure are defined as in Table 14-6. See a recent article by Perrin, Dorr, Perry, and Gronley in Clin. Orthop. **195:**252, 1985 for further complimentary data on the high failure rate of prosthetic hip replacement in young adults.

operations are demanding technically and often fraught with problems of severe bone loss. Custom-made prostheses and allograft bone replacements frequently must be used. Early reports of revision prosthetic hip replacement cite alarmingly high failure rates at less than 5-year follow-up (Table 14-7). Again, impending failure rates are significant.

An explanation for these failures might revert to the original admonitions of Charnley that overuse or high-level activity by these patients might result in mechanical loosening.[43] Better results could be expected in more elderly, sedentary individuals. When the results are reviewed in young, active adults this explanation seems quite plausible. For example, 5-year follow-ups list 20% failure rates with 30% to 60% impending (Table 14-8).

Prosthetic hip replacement succeeds with great reliability in restoring a painless mobile hip in a very high percentage of patients. However, if this result is to last, activities must be severely curtailed. Herein lies the problem facing the young adult with osteoarthritis. The problem is further complicated by as yet unsolved complications of bone loss during revision surgery. With many patients facing this potential crisis, many orthopaedists are reexamining the role of a biologic alternative, the osteotomy.

Intertrochanteric osteotomy. The reputation of unpredictability bestowed on treatment by osteotomy derives from fact. Recently, failure rates are reported between 40% to 50%.[34,45] Fortunately these results reflect primarily the early technique

as described by McMurray.* The majority of these operations attempted to displace medially the distal fragment under the acetabulum to unload the hip. Spica casting was common and valgus or varus angulation occurred only by accident. It is incredible that this operation even improved the prognosis of the natural history. At 5-year follow-ups, the McMurray osteotomy generally succeeded in significant pain relief (80%) with acceptable failure rates (Table 14-9). The shortcoming was relatively immobile hips that limited activity levels. The trend worsened in time so that 10-year results had deteriorated (Table 14-10). These facts clearly led to the third myth. It is understandable that prosthetic hip replacements became a panacea for surgeons frustrated by the results of the McMurray osteotomy.

A few surgeons in Europe continued to explore the potential of a biologic solution. The monumental works of Wolff, Braune, and Fischer before the turn of the century and Fick shortly thereafter lay dormant nearly 50 years until Pauwels synthesized a theory of hip biomechanic.[5,40] Wolff originally inferred the role of physical stress in stimulating and maintaining bone structure. Braune and Fischer (1889 to 1899) laboriously calculated the center of gravity in the human body by examining soldiers and cadavers.[5,9] They went on to plot the center of gravity through 31 phases of gait. Fick (1910) estimated a common vector for hip abductors[5]

---

*References 20, 22, 24, 34, 45, 46.

Table 14-9. 5-year follow-up of McMurray osteotomy

Author (year)	Number of hips at follow-up	Average follow-up	Average age at operation	Failure*	Functional pain relief†	Unlimited activity‡
Gudmundsson[22] (1970)	107	5 years	59 years	28%	80%	61%
Salenius[46] (1971)	209	5½ years	52 years	18%	82%	56%
Reigstad[45] (1984)	98	5 years	58 years	25%	50%	50%
Harris[24] (1964)	71	4 years	61 years	22%	92%	

*Osteotomy required reoperation usually for pain and occasionally for stiffness or malposition of the leg. Nonunion was more frequent in these patients treated in spica cast without internal fixation.
†Pain completely resolved or only a minor ache occurred that in no way limited activities.
‡Patient participated in all desired activities without needing a cane or other aid.

Table 14-10. 10-year results of McMurray osteotomy

Author (year)	Number of hips at follow-up	Failure	Functional pain relief	Unlimited activity
Goldie[20] (1973)	81	23%	67%	53%
Reigstad[45] (1984)	78	40%		
Meigel[34] (1984)	67	51%	25%	9%

Failure, functional pain relief, and unlimited activity are defined as in Table 14-9.

Table 14-11. 5-year follow-up of Pauwels osteotomy

Author (year)	Number of hips at follow-up	Average follow-up	Average age at operation	Failure	Functional pain relief	Unlimited activity
DePalma[16] (1970)	29	4 years	57 years	16%	87%	31%
Detenbeck[17] (1972)	59	2½ years	57 years	20%	93%	80%
Swiss Group[36] (1970)	2251	4 years	54 years	18%	84%	61%
Bombelli[6] (1984)	816	5½ years	42 years	8%	92%	78%

Categories defined as in Table 14-9.

through anatomic dissections. Pauwels then integrated these works to explain osteoarthritic patterns of sclerosis on the basis of coronal plane biomechanical vectors.[5,40] His treatment, in the form of valgus or varus osteotomy based on these theories, is well-documented,[40] but it could not be reproduced universally.

Two further developments were essential in the evolution of the modern osteotomy: stable internal fixation and an understanding of osteophytes. Although Blount (1945)[4] is credited with the first reliable fixation plate, the art of rigid internal fixation for osteotomy was not perfected until Müller[37] and the Swiss group popularized their technique and instrumentation.

As alluded to earlier, Bombelli[5] realized the natural role of the osteophyte as an insensate host reparative mechanism. His osteotomies exploit osteophytes for pain relief (load-bearing surface) and improved biomechanics.[5,6,7] Bombelli expanded Pauwels' theory to include a three-dimensional analysis of gait, thereby realizing the additional importance of adding flexion or extension (sagittal plane) to the coronal plane osteotomies. Let us examine the results of the modern osteotomy.

At 5-year follow-up of Pauwels' technique, the failure rate of 20% is lower than the McMurray failure rate and reliable pain relief is greater (Table 14-11). Bombelli's own results are better yet with only 8% failure rate and 92% functional pain relief in over 800 patients. In three of these

Table 14-12. 10-year results of Pauwels osteotomy

Author (year)	Number of hips at follow-up	Failure	Functional pain relief	Unlimited activity
Santore[47] (1983)	45	8%	82%	40%
Schneider[48] (1984)	35	6%	94%	

Categories defined as in Table 14-9.

Table 14-13. Bombelli experience in patients under 40[7]

Osteotomy	Number of hips at follow-up	Average follow-up	Average age at operation	Failure	Functional pain relief	Unlimited activity
Varus	59	7 years	31 years	3%	97%	92%
Valgus	139	7 years	34 years	14%	95%	91%

Categories defined as in Table 14-9. Varus and valgus osteotomies were often supplemented by flexion or extension along with appropriate medial or lateral displacement.

series more than half of the patients were able to engage in full, unlimited activity (See Table 14-11). At 10 years the results did not deteriorate, except in the category of unlimited activity (Table 14-12). Bombelli's patients are among a consecutive series reviewed by an independent observer.[47] The best overall results are reported by Bombelli in young adults (Table 14-13). The modern osteotomy is not a panacea; improved hip motion is not the rule even though pain relief and full activity are reliable results. Careful planning and mature physician-patient rapport are critical.

Planning an osteotomy for osteoarthritis. Certain technical features are common to all successful osteotomies. I have attempted to unify the basic concepts into five major areas: joint surfaces, overall hip joint force, mechanical axis of the limb, leg length discrepancy, and capsulotomy. For a more detailed discussion of these techniques as well as the methods of internal fixation, see the original texts.*

Available *joint surfaces* must be studied for congruency (arthrograms under fluoroscopy are helpful). Improved congruency decreases stress per unit area.[40] Mobility must be assessed to ensure that appropriate weight-bearing position is attainable after osteotomy[4,37] (examination under anesthesia occasionally is necessary). Hyaline surfaces are preferred to secondary fibrocartilage when available, usually in patients under 40. When present, fibrocartilaginous osteophytes

serve as insensate force-bearing structures that decompress painful incongruencies, increase contact area, and medialize the center of rotation.[5]

Overall hip joint force is a function of the patient's weight and activity level.[5] Osteotomy can modify this internally by two separate options. First, the center of rotation can be medialized either within the joint (for example, valgus osteotomy creating contact between the capital drop osteophyte and curtain osteophyte)[5,6,7] or by medializing the entire joint (Chiari osteotomy).[58] Either maneuver decreases the load arm.[59] Second, the effort arm[59] can be lengthened by lateralizing the greater trochanter.[59] A valgus osteotomy can be combined with a greater trochanteric osteotomy to achieve both.[5,6,7] Wagner[58,59] sometimes combines these with a Chiari osteotomy to maximize this effect.

The normal *mechanical axis of the limb* must be maintained or corrected if it is abnormal.[37] To avoid abnormality the distal fragment is lateralized with a valgus osteotomy and medialized with a varus osteotomy.[5,37] If concomitant gonarthrosis exists, the knee can be unloaded with the appropriate intertrochanteric osteotomy.[37] Full-length standing radiographs assist proper planning of limb axis.

Leg length discrepancy can be normalized either by opening or closing wedge osteotomies. Bombelli[5] and Wagner[58] commonly use opening wedge rather than the classical closing wedge[37] to improve leg-length discrepancies.

Capsulotomy is important for three reasons. First, it facilitates visualization for proper joint

---

*References 5-7, 36, 37, 40, 42, 47, 48, 58, 59.

realignment and internal fixation placement.[6] Second, it releases frequent flexion contracture.[5] Third, it hypothetically decompresses intracapsular hypertension seen in active synovitis in some patients.[36,42]

SUMMARY

1. Childhood hip disorders contribute to a significant proportion of young adults with painful osteoarthritis of the hip.

2. Prosthetic hip replacement rarely is indicated for active young adults with osteoarthritis of the hip because of high failure rates without subsequent solutions.

3. Modern osteotomies provide a viable alternative for these individuals. Recently published data indicate that the osteotomy can have reliable results with more modest expectations.* Four requirements must be met. (1) The orthopaedist should grasp the modern principles of osteotomy and be willing to carry out more involved operative planning. (2) The patient should exhibit a mature understanding of alternatives and long-range goals of treatment. (3) Both orthopaedist and patient should commit themselves to a long-term relationship, beyond the 6-month rehabilitation period. (4) The patient should be willing to compromise some motion (hip mobility) for pain relief and increased function.

REFERENCES

1. Adam, A., and Spence, A.J.: Intertrochanteric osteotomy for osteoarthritis of the hip, J. Bone Joint Surg. **40B:**219, 1958.
2. Amstutz, H.C., Steven, M., Jinnok, R.H., and Mai, L.: Revision of aseptic loose total hip orthroplasties, Clin. Orthop. **170:**21, 1982.
3. Aronson, J., Lytle, J., and Nelson, C.: Etiology of coxarthrosis in 100 consecutive prosthetic hip replacements, Unpublished data, 1985.
4. Blount, W.P.: Osteotomy in the treatment of osteoarthritis of the hip, J. Bone Joint Surg. **46A:**1297, 1964.
5. Bombelli, R.: Osteoarthritis of the hip, New York, 1983, Springer-Verlag.
6. Bombelli, R., and Aronson, J.: Biomechanical classification of osteoarthritis of the hip with special reference to treatment technique and results. In Schatzker, J., editor: The intertrochanteric osteotomy, New York, 1984, Springer-Verlag.
7. Bombelli, R., Gerundini, M., and Aronson, J.: The biomechanical basis for osteotomy in the treatment of osteoarthritis of the hip: Results in younger patients. In Welch, Richard B., editor: The hip, proceedings of the

twelfth open scientific meeting of The Hip Society, Vol. 12, St. Louis, 1984, The C.V. Mosby Co.
8. Boyer, D., Michelsson, M., and Ponseti, I.: Slipped capital femoral epiphysis, J. Bone Joint Surg. **63A:**85, 1981.
9. Braune, W., and Fischer, O.: On the centre of gravity of the human body, New York, 1985, Springer-Verlag.
10. Chandler, H., Reineck, T., Wixson, M., and McCarthy, J.: Total hip replacement in patients younger than thirty years old, J. Bone Joint Surg. **63A:**1426, 1981.
11. Clarke, N., and Harrison, M.: Painful sequelae of coxa plana, J. Bone Joint Surg. **65A:**13, 1983.
12. Cooperman, D., Wallensten, R., and Stulberg, S.: Post-reduction avascular necrosis in congenital dislocation of the hip, J. Bone Joint Surg. **62A:**247, 1980.
13. Cooperman, D., Wallensten, R., and Stulberg, S.: Acetabular dysplasia in the adult, Clin. Orthop. **175:**79, 1983.
14. Danielsson, L.: Incidence and prognosis of coxarthrosis, Acta Orthop. Scand. Suppl. **66:**9, 1964.
15. Danielsson, L., and Hernborg, J.: Late results of Perthes' disease, Acta Orthop. Scand. **36:**70, 1965.
16. DePalma, A., Rothman, R., and Klemek, J.: Osteotomy of the proximal femur in degenerative arthritis, Clin. Orthop. **73:**109, 1970.
17. Detenbeck, L., Coventry, M., and Kelly, P.: Intertrochanteric osteotomy for degenerative arthritis of the hip, Clin. Orthop. **86:**73, 1972.
18. Dorr, L., Takei, G., and Conaty, T.: Total hip arthroplasties in patients less than forty-five years old, J. Bone Joint Surg. **65A:**474, 1983.
19. Eaton, G.: Long-term results of treatment in coxa plana, J. Bone Joint Surg. **48A:**1031, 1967.
20. Goldie, I., Andersson, G., and Olsson, S.: Long-term follow-up of intertrochanteric osteotomy in osteoarthritis in the hip joint, Clin. Orthop. **93:**265, 1973.
21. Gower, W., and Johnston, R.: Legg-Perthes disease, J. Bone Joint Surg. **53A:**759, 1971.
22. Gudmundsson, G.: Intertrochanteric displacement osteotomy for painful osteoarthritis of the hip, Acta Orthop. Scand. **41:**91, 1970.
23. Hagglund, G., Hansson, L., and Ordeberg, G.: Epidemiology of slipped capital femoral epiphysis in southern Sweden, Clin. Orthop. **191:**82, 1984.
24. Harris, N., and Kirwan, E.: The results of osteotomy for early primary osteoarthritis of the hip, J. Bone Joint Surg. **46B:**477, 1964.
25. Kelsey, J., Keggi, K., and Southwick, W.: The incidence and distribution of slipped capital femoral epiphysis in Connecticut and southwestern United States, J. Bone Joint Surg. **52A:**1203, 1970.
26. Liechti, R.: Hip arthrodesis and associated problems, New York, 1978, Springer-Verlag.
27. Lloyd-Roberts, G.: Osteoarthritis of the hip, J. Bone Joint Surg. **37B:**8, 1955.
28. Macys, J.R., Bullough, P.G., and Wilson, P.D.: Coxarthrosis: A study of the natural history based on a correlation of clinical, radiographic and pathological findings, Semin. Arthritis Rheum. **10:**66, 1980.
29. Mardem-Bey, T., and MacEwen, G.D.: Congenital hip dislocation after walking age, J. Pediatr. Orthop. **2:**478, 1982.
30. McAndrew, M., and Weinstein, S.: A longterm follow up of Legg-Calvé-Perthes disease, J. Bone Joint Surg. **66A:**860, 1984.

---

*References 5-7, 36, 42, 47, 48.

31. McBroom, R., and Muller, M.: Aseptic loosening in 1,030 consecutive total hip replacements at 10-15 years follow-up, J. Bone Joint Surg. **66B:**300, 1984.

32. McEwen, C.: A logical approach to the differential diagnosis of arthritis. In Hollander, J.L., editor: The arthritis handbook, West Point, Pa., 1974, Merck, Sharp & Dohme.

33. McKinnon, B., Bosse, M., and Browning, W.: Congenital dysplasia of the hip: The lax (subluxable) newborn hip, J. Pediatr. Orthop. **4:**422, 1984.

34. Meigel, R., and Harris, W.: Medial displacement intertrochanteric osteotomy in treatment of osteoarthritis of the hip, J. Bone Joint Surg. **66A:**878, 1984.

35. Molloy, M., and MacMahan, B.: Incidence of Legg-Perthes disease (osteochondritis deformans), N. Engl. J. Med. **275:**988, 1966.

36. Morscher, E., and Feinstein, R.: Results of intertrochanteric osteotomy in the treatment of osteoarthritis of the hip. In Schatzker, J., editor: The intertrochanteric osteotomy, New York, 1984, Springer-Verlag.

37. Müller, M.E.: Intertrochanteric osteotomy: Indication, preoperative planning, technique. In Schatzker, J., editor: The intertrochanteric osteotomy, New York, 1984, Springer-Verlag.

38. Müller, M.: ASIF/AO basic course on total hip replacement, sponsored by University of South Florida Division of Orthopedic Surgery and AO International, San Diego, April 1980.

39. Ordeberg, G., Hansson, L., and Sandstrom, S.: Slipped capital femoral epiphysis in southern Sweden, Clin. Orthop. **191:**95, 1984.

40. Pauwels, F.: Biomechanical principles of varus/valgus intertrochanteric osteotomy in the treatment of osteoarthritis of the hip. In Schatzker, J., editor: The intertrochanteric osteotomy, New York, 1984, Springer-Verlag.

41. Pellicci, P., Callaghan, J., Wilson, P.D., Sledge, C., Salvati, E., Ranawat, C., and Poss, R.: Results of revision total hip replacement. In Welch, Richard B., editor: The hip, proceedings of the twelfth open scientific meeting of The Hip Society, vol. 12, St. Louis, 1984, The C.V. Mosby Co.

42. Poss, R.: The role of osteotomy in the treatment of osteoarthritis of the hip, J. Bone Joint Surg. **66A:**144, 1984.

43. Ranawat, C., Atkinson, R., Salvati, E., and Wilson, P.: Conventional total hip arthroplasty for degenerative joint disease in patients between the ages of forty and sixty years, J. Bone Joint Surg. **66A:**745, 1984.

44. Ratliff, A.: Perthes disease, J. Bone Joint Surg. **49B:**102, 1967.

45. Reigstad, A., and Gronmark, T.: Osteoarthritis of the hip treated by intertrochanteric osteotomy, J. Bone Joint Surg. **66A:**1, 1984.

46. Salenius, P., Langenskiold, A., and Osterman, K.: Intertrochanteric displacement osteotomy in the treatment of osteoarthritis of the hip, Acta Orthop. Scand. **42:**63, 1971.

47. Santore, R., and Bombelli, R.: Long term follow-up of the Bombelli experience with osteotomy for osteoarthritis: Results at 11 years. In Hungerford, David S., editor: The hip, proceedings of the eleventh open scientific meeting of The Hip Society, vol. 11, St. Louis, 1983, The C.V. Mosby Co.

48. Schneider, R.: Intertrochanteric osteotomy in osteoarthritis of the hip joint. In Schatzker, J., editor: The intertrochanteric osteotomy, New York, 1984, Springer-Verlag.

49. Shulman, L.: Degenerative joint disease. In Wintrobe, Thorn, Adams, Bennett, Braunwald, Isselbacher, and Petersdorf, editors: Harrison's principles of internal medicine, ed. 6, New York, 1970, McGraw-Hill Book Co.

50. Stauffer, R.: Ten-year follow-up study of total hip replacement, J. Bone Joint Surg. **64A:**983, 1982.

51. Stevens, M., and Townes, A.: Degenerative joint disease. In Harvey, Johns, Owens, and Ross, editors: The principles and practice of medicine, ed. 18, New York, 1972, Prentice-Hall Inc.

52. Straub, L.: An overview of surgical procedures in arthritis. In Hollander, J.L., editor: The arthritis handbook, West Point, Pa., 1974, Merck, Sharp, & Dohme.

53. Stulberg, S., Cooperman, D., and Wallensten, R.: The natural history of Legg-Calvé-Perthes disease, J. Bone Joint Surg. **63A,**1095, 1981.

54. Stulberg, S., Harris, W., and MacEwen, G.D.: Unrecognized childhood hip disease: A major cause of idiopathic osteoarthritis of the hip, The hip, proceedings of the third open scientific meeting of The Hip Society, vol. 3, 1975, St. Louis, The C.V. Mosby Co.

55. Sutherland, C., Wilde, A., Borden, L., and Marks, K.: A ten-year follow-up of one hundred consecutive Muller curved-stem total hip replacement arthroplasties, J. Bone Joint Surg. **64A:**970, 1982.

56. Tredwell, S., and Bell, H.: Efficacy of neonatal hip examination, J. Pediatr. Orthop. **1:**61, 1981.

57. U.S. Bureau of the Census: Statistical abstract of the United States, 1985, ed. 105, Washington, D.C., 1984.

58. Wagner, H.: Experiences with spherical acetabular osteotomy for correction of the dysplastic acetabulum, Progress in Orthopaedic Surgery, vol. 2, New York, 1978, Springer-Verlag.

59. Wagner, H., and Holder, J.: Treatment of osteoarthritis of the hip by corrective osteotomy of the greater trochanter. In Schatzker, J., editor: The intertrochanteric osteotomy, New York, 1984, Springer-Verlag.

60. Wiberg, G.: Acetabular dysplasia and osteoarthritis, Acta Chir. Scand. **83:**(Suppl. 58):5, 1939.

61. Wilson, P., Jacobs, B., and Schecter, L.: Slipped capital femoral epiphysis, J. Bone Joint Surg. **47A:**1128, 1965.

Chapter 15

Intertrochanteric osteotomy in osteoarthritis of the hip

ROBERT POSS

There are three major goals of reconstruction surgery: first, to relieve pain and improve function; second, to preserve bone stock; and third, to address the question of how many operations will be required per lifetime to satisfy the patient's *immediate and future* needs. The results of total hip arthroplasty are the benchmark with which any alternative procedure must be compared. For patients older than 70 the likelihood of a definitive result from conventional total hip arthroplasty (THA) is so great that alternative procedures must be considered with great caution. Conversely, the results of conventional THA in patients younger than 50 have not proved to be long lasting, therefore a biologic alternative such as osteotomy is attractive. For patients between the ages of 50 and 70 the choice of the most appropriate operation becomes more difficult. One must weigh the patient's physiologic age and activity requirements against the short-term and long-term prognosis of the proposed surgical procedure.

Osteotomy offers the following advantages: preservation of bone stock; dramatic pain relief; potential healing of overloaded cartilage and bone; and if initially successful, the likelihood of a good result for 10 to 20 years. Its disadvantages in comparison to total hip arthroplasty are that proper patient selection is more difficult, thereby rendering the results to be less predictable; the convalescence and rehabilitation period is long,

and eventual revision to THA may be difficult if the proximal femur has been altered radically. The rationale for choosing a biologic alternative such as osteotomy is that in the proper patient the restorative potential of bone and cartilage can be realized.

Bone and cartilage function within a biologic range of mechanical load. Pauwels calculated that in the hip the unit load is 23 kg/cm^2.[7] Calculations for other human joints have shown this to be a remarkably constant unit load.[2] Although we cannot presently quantify the lower or upper limits of this physiologic stress window for chondrocyte and osteocyte function, the consequences of underloading or overloading a joint can be observed radiographically.

When bone is underloaded (understressed or understrained), resorption occurs. When the upper limits of the window are exceeded, adaptive bone deposition in the areas transmitting increased load and localized cartilage space narrowing result. As the adaptive response is overwhelmed, cyst formation and bony collapse follow (Fig. 15-1). Thus mechanical failure occurs in a joint when the unit load (kg/cm^2) exceeds the adaptive capacity of cartilage and bone.

Cartilage degeneration can be arrested and perhaps reversed by decreasing the unit load, altering the load transmission pattern, and restoring a functional arc of motion. These then are the goals of modern approaches to osteotomy. In this paper I seek to define those patients who are candidates for osteotomy and then to describe the critically important technical aspects of this procedure. Before so doing, it is useful to address

Supported in part by NIH Fogerty Senior International Fellowship, #F06TW00709-01.

129

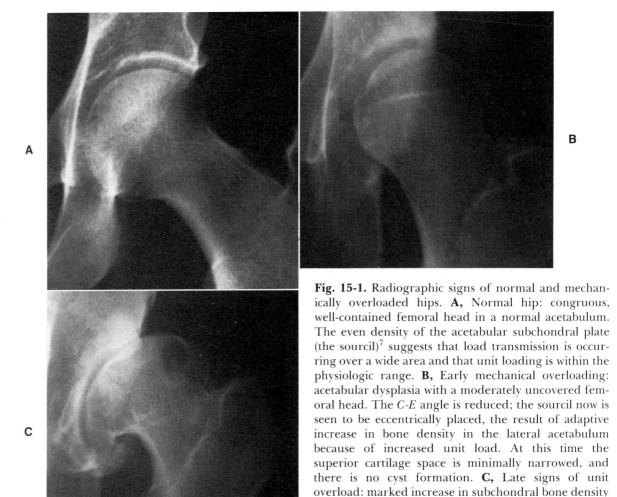

Fig. 15-1. Radiographic signs of normal and mechanically overloaded hips. **A,** Normal hip: congruous, well-contained femoral head in a normal acetabulum. The even density of the acetabular subchondral plate (the sourcil)[7] suggests that load transmission is occurring over a wide area and that unit loading is within the physiologic range. **B,** Early mechanical overloading: acetabular dysplasia with a moderately uncovered femoral head. The *C-E* angle is reduced; the sourcil now is seen to be eccentrically placed, the result of adaptive increase in bone density in the lateral acetabulum because of increased unit load. At this time the superior cartilage space is minimally narrowed, and there is no cyst formation. **C,** Late signs of unit overload: marked increase in subchondral bone density that is localized superolaterally. There is marked narrowing of the cartilage space and prominent cyst formation in the femoral head. Adaptive osteophytes in both the acetabulum and femoral head have rendered the joint incongruous.

some pertinent aspects regarding the evolution of osteotomy.

TYPES OF OSTEOTOMY

Historically, osteotomies have been divided into two types: displacement and angulation. These distinctions are now somewhat artificial because modern osteotomy usually combines angulation in one or two planes with displacement.

Displacement. In 1935 McMurray presented his results of medial displacement osteotomy.[8] Subsequent series reported by MacFarland,[8] Nigel Harris and Kirwan,[3] and Miegel and William Harris[4] report that long-term pain relief and

improved function are achieved with approximately 80% of patients. Nigel Harris and Kirwan found that the best clinical results occurred in patients with the least preoperative derangement in radiographic anatomy. Thus the presence of a spherical head, intact Shenton's line, and a 90-degree flexion arc constituted the best prognostic group. In William Harris's series, the mean interval between osteotomy revision and total hip replacement was 8½ years. Some patients had good results with osteotomy for at least 15 years postoperatively. The mechanism of improvement following displacement osteotomy is unknown, but most would agree that the immediate symptomatic improvement is related in some way to altering the hemodynamics of the proximal femur and/or changing the orientation of trabecular support, thus inducing bone remodeling.[8] It is of interest that Harris and Kirwan suggested that their best results were obtained in those patients who had inadvertent varus angulation. The theoretic advantages of angulation osteotomy (maximizing surface contact areas while unloading the hip) suggest that its choice is preferable to that of pure displacement in the majority of patients.

Angulation osteotomy. The father of the modern angulation osteotomy is Pauwels,[7] whose view of the pathogenesis of osteoarthritis led to his formulation of a surgical rationale aimed at reversing the progression of disease. The pathogenesis of osteoarthritis can be viewed as the inability of competent chondrocytes and osteocytes to function under increasing mechanical loads. If, as in acetabular dysplasia, the unit load is increased, bone and cartilage can respond and continue to function up to a point. When the unit load exceeds the adaptive capacity of these tissues, then cartilage failure and bony changes, including collapse, and cyst formation occur. Pauwels stated that a disease, the pathogenesis of which could be explained on a mechanical basis, should be reversible if the mechanical derangement were reversed, that is, if the unit load were decreased. Thus deterioration of an overloaded hip could be reversed by decreasing the load or increasing the weight-bearing surface.

One should be able to identify candidates for osteotomy by their radiographic anatomy. Radiographic signs of mechanical overload include a localized decrease in cartilage space, increased subchondral density, particularly laterally in the acetabulum, and the appearance of cysts (see Fig. 15-1). Many authors have stated that clinical improvement parallels improvement in the radiographic appearance.[8] It follows that patients who do not have signs of mechanical overload, as, for example, in inflammatory or metabolic bone diseases, or patients whose bone cannot mount an adaptive response, that is, atrophic bone,[1] will not benefit from osteotomy.

Varus osteotomy

The classic radiographic candidate for varus osteotomy is a patient whose hip has a spherical femoral head, moderate or absent acetabular dysplasia (a center-edge angle of 15 to 20 degrees), signs of lateral overloading of the sourcil (the acetabular subchondral plate), and a valgus neck-shaft angle of more than 135 degrees. (see Fig. 15-1, *B*) If radiographs in hip abduction demonstrate improved congruity of the hip, then varus osteotomy is indicated. By performing varus osteotomy with iliopsoas release and medial shaft displacement, the abductors, psoas, and adductors are relatively relaxed, thus "unloading" the hip joint, and the weight bearing surface is increased. Medial shaft displacement of 10 to 15 mm is desirable not only to decrease the force of the adductors but also to keep the ipsilateral knee centered under the femoral head.

In various series well-selected candidates achieved long-term, good to excellent results in more than 90% of cases.[8] Varus osteotomy carries with it, however, the certainty of approximately 1.5 cm of shortening, the presence of a Trendelenburg gait for approximately 1 year, and a prominent greater trochanter. Patients must be aware of the longer convalescent period intrinsic with this operation.

Valgus osteotomy

When the femoral head is no longer spherical, the goals of decreasing the unit load and improving congruence can be achieved by a valgus osteotomy. Osteophytes that form in predictable locations on the femoral head and acetabulum[1] are exploited to achieve the desired result (Fig. 15-2). The capital drop and inferior cervical osteophytes of the femoral head are brought into contact with the floor osteophytes of the acetabulum by adduction of the hip. With these osteophytes now serving as a fulcrum, the superior and lateral joint space is widened. An assessment of the magnitude of correction required can be obtained by examination under fluoroscopy, tracings, or radiographs obtained in various degrees of hip adduction. Sufficient valgus correction should be done so that lateral traction on the superior capsule results in the stimulation of formation of the roof osteophyte.[1] Pain relief is achieved by: (1) unloading the hip joint (abductor and psoas relaxation), (2) changing the bone on bone contact from the painful innervated superior femoral head and acetabulum to noninnervated medial osteophytes, (3) decreasing the lever arm of body weight by shifting it medially to the new center of rotation of the femoral head, the osteophytes, and (4) improving the congruity of the joint and thus increasing the weight-bearing

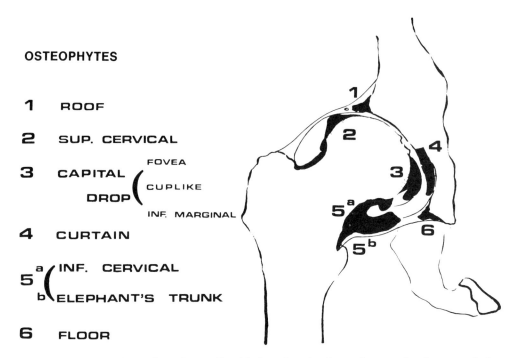

OSTEOPHYTES

1 ROOF

2 SUP. CERVICAL

3 CAPITAL $\Big($ FOVEA
CUPLIKE
DROP $\Big($ INF. MARGINAL

4 CURTAIN

5 $\begin{cases} a & \text{INF. CERVICAL} \\ b & \text{ELEPHANT'S TRUNK} \end{cases}$

6 FLOOR

Fig. 15-2. Osteophytes form in predictable locations in the pathogenesis of osteoarthritis. The capital drop and curtain osteophytes are exploited in valgus osteotomy to form the furcrum (new contact area). The roof osteophyte seen after valgus osteotomy increases the surface area of the acetabulum (see text). (From Bombelli, R.: Osteoarthritis of the hip, ed. 2, New York, 1983, Springer-Verlag.)

surface. Further long-term improvement may come with formation of the roof osteophyte, which further increases the weight-bearing surface, and cartilage healing.[1]

RESULTS OF OSTEOTOMY

The long-term results from different European centers suggest good to excellent results in approximately 70% of patients.[8,9] It must be remembered that these long-term results represent an era when patient selection was not as stringent as is possible today with arthroplasty as a viable alternative. It is important to note that good early results do not seem to deteriorate with time. Clinical improvement is seen to correlate with radiographic improvement.[5,8,9]

SURGICAL PLANNING

In the surgical planning of an osteotomy, the most important task is to determine whether the patient is an appropriate candidate. Determining factors are the patient's age, activities, goals, radiologic assessment, range of motion, leg lengths, and status of the ipsilateral knee. Techni-

cal preparation includes examination under fluoroscopy, tracings, and choice of instrumentation and fixation devices.

PATIENT SELECTION

The ideal candidate for intertrochanteric osteotomy is generally younger than 50 but can be somewhat older if all other criteria are met. Ideally, the patient should not be obese and preferably is a sedentary worker rather than one who engages in heavy physical labor.[5] It is essential that a mechanical pathogenesis be demonstrated on radiographs. If cartilage and bone demonstrate radiographically a capacity to respond to mechanical overload, then by inference these tissues are capable of a healing process once a proper mechanical environment has been restored. The radiologic criteria demonstrated by an ideal candidate are those of excessive unit load, a localized increase in radio density, localized joint narrowing, and cyst formation. If there is incongruity, then improved congruency must be demonstrated on examination under fluoroscopy.

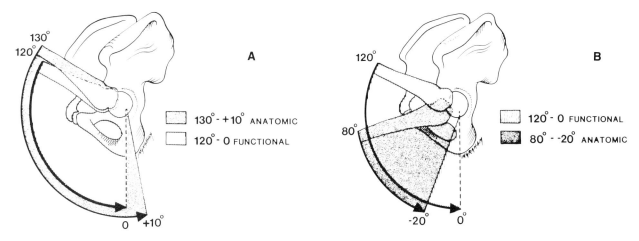

Fig. 15-3. Anatomic and functional arcs of hip motion in the sagittal plane. **A,** In the normal hip the functional arc of motion is well within the anatomic arc, but in osteoarthritis **B** the restricted anatomic arc is less than that required for normal hip function. An important source of pain in osteoarthritis is the impingement produced by this restricted motion.[10] An extension osteotomy can eliminate a fixed flexion contracture and thus remove a source of impingement and pain (see text).

Patients who undergo osteotomy usually neither gain nor lose overall hip motion. A minimum of 80 degrees of flexion arc is preferred.[5,6] The magnitude of angular correction in the coronal plane should not significantly exceed the patient's abduction to adduction arc. For example, if a 30-degree valgus osteotomy is performed in a patient who can only adduct 10 degrees, the patient may walk in abduction and experience severe valgus strain in the knee.

EXTENSION

In addition to angular correction in the coronal plane, correction in the sagittal plane can increase the effectiveness of osteotomy. Biplane correction is desirable for two reasons: (1) In acetabular dysplasia, the femoral head is uncovered not only laterally (the frontal plane) but anteriorly (the sagittal plane). Better coverage is achieved by correction in both planes.[1] (2) Fixed flexion contractures can be eliminated by extension correction to a degree at least equal to the magnitude of the flexion contracture. By so doing, the functional arc of motion is returned to within the anatomic arc, and an important source of pain and impingement is removed (Fig. 15-3).[10]

The use of the term *extension* is often confusing. Extension refers to the angular correction of the femur in the sagittal plane after osteotomy. Thus, with extension, the apex of the angle is directed anteriorly. To achieve this correction, the femur is flexed to the desired degree, the osteotomy performed, and the distal femoral fragment brought parallel to the floor. Thus the proximal fragment is flexed, but the final angular correction of the femur is said to be extended (see Fig. 15-9).

ROTATION

Patients with dysplastic hips usually have a constellation of anatomic variations in the pelvic and femoral sides of the hip joint. The acetabulum is deficient both laterally and anteriorly, the femoral neck is in excess valgus (greater than 135 degrees), and anteversion is increased. The true degree of femoral anteversion (and hence the true neck shaft valgus) and be determined by fluoroscopic or other methods. It is likely that a neck shaft angle of 150 degrees seen on AP radiograph is in reality a combination of 140- to 145-degree neck shaft angle, and 25-degree femoral anteversion. Preoperative planning for a varus-extension osteotomy should allow for 10 to 15 degrees of derotation (leave 115 degrees of residual internal rotation to allow for a normal gait) and varus correction of 10 to 15 degrees.

LIMB ALIGNMENT AND LIMB LENGTH

The planning of the intertrochanteric osteotomy must include an assessment of leg lengths and the effect os osteotomy on the mechanical

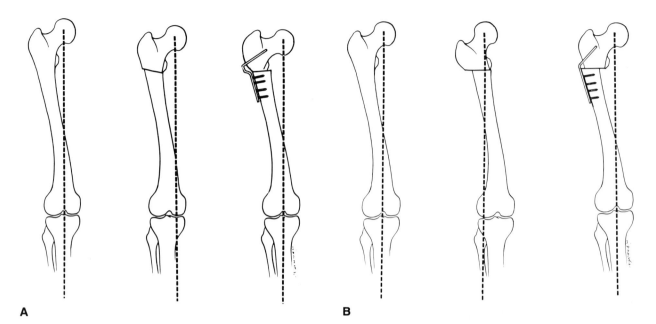

A   **B**

Fig. 15-4. Angulation osteotomy of the proximal femur changes the mechanical axis of the lower extremity. Shaft displacement is required so that the mechanical axis does not pass eccentrically through the knee and ankle. **A,** Varus osteotomy must be accompanied by medial shaft displacement. **B,** Valgus osteotomy must be accompanied by lateral shaft displacement.

axis of the limb. Of particular importance is the effect of hip realignment on the ipsilateral knee. When varus osteotomy is performed, medial shaft displacement is required so that the mechanical axis of the extremity remains through the center of the knee. Similarly, in valgus osteotomy lateral shaft displacement is required (Fig. 15-4). With varus osteotomy shortening of the limb by approximately 0.5 to 1.5 cm is inevitable. With valgus osteotomy up to 2.0 cm of length can be gained if necessary, or the limb can be shortened by appropriate wedge resection.

TECHNICAL PLANNING

In planning the direction and magnitude of angular correction, fluoroscopy is invaluable. Under fluoroscopic examination the exact degree of desired adduction (or abduction), rotation, and extension correction can be determined. Appropriate spot films document the corrections obtained in various ranges of motion (Fig. 15-5). Once the degree of angular correction in the coronal plane has been determined, tracings are very helpful in planning the site of osteotomy, the

site of chisel and blade insertion, and the amount of wedge resection and shaft displacement. Tracings also help the surgeon anticipate the configuration of the femur during and after surgery (Fig. 15-6).

THE OPERATION

The extent to which the procedure is done preoperatively greatly facilitates the technical procedure that is performed in the operating room. It is critical that the osteotomy be performed just at the proximal border of the lesser trochanter. The second critical point is that a cortical bridge of 1.5 to 2.0 cm be preserved between the site of blade insertion and the osteotomy site. The angle at which the chisel is introduced and the site of insertion can be accurately planned on the preoperative radiograph (Fig. 15-7). The plan is accurately effected at the time of surgery by use of A0 fixed-angled blade plates and A0 measuring triangles.[6] For valgus osteotomy a 130-degree A0 blade plate is used.[1] For varus osteotomy, a 90-degree A0 blade plate is used.[6] By using 60- through 90-degree triangles

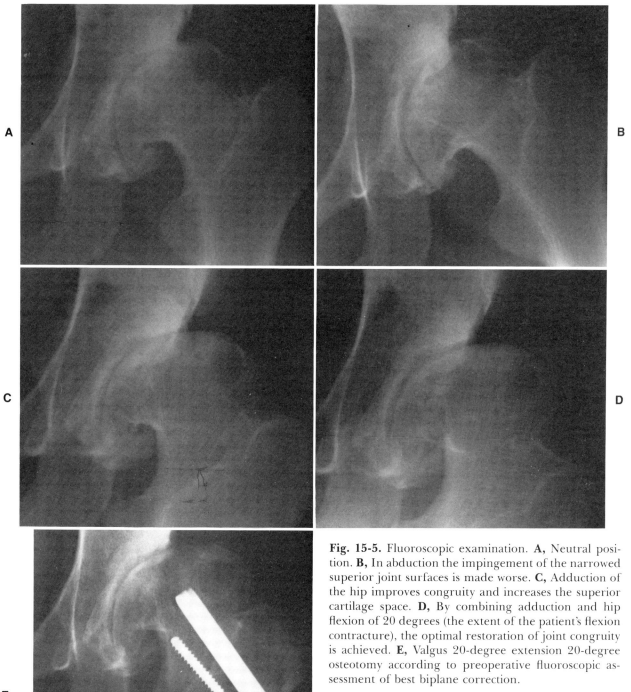

Fig. 15-5. Fluoroscopic examination. **A,** Neutral position. **B,** In abduction the impingement of the narrowed superior joint surfaces is made worse. **C,** Adduction of the hip improves congruity and increases the superior cartilage space. **D,** By combining adduction and hip flexion of 20 degrees (the extent of the patient's flexion contracture), the optimal restoration of joint congruity is achieved. **E,** Valgus 20-degree extension 20-degree osteotomy according to preoperative fluoroscopic assessment of best biplane correction.

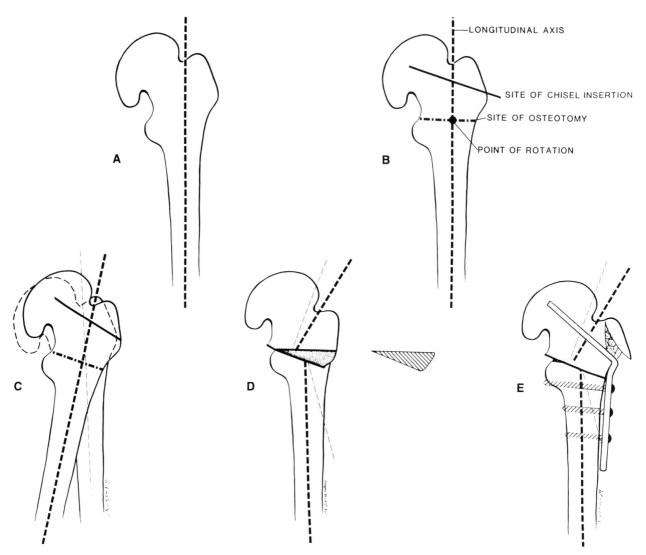

Fig. 15-6. Tracings as an aid to planning osteotomy. The magnitude of biplane correction has been determined by fluoroscopic examination. In this example we will plan for valgus extension osteotomy of 25-degree valgus, 20-degree extension. **A,** Make a tracing of the AP radiograph, and draw the longitudinal axis of the femur. **B,** Make a second tracing of the AP radiograph, and include the longitudinal axis of the femur, the site of osteotomy (perpendicular to the axis at the proximal border of the lesser trochanter), and the track of the chisel insertion. The distance between the osteotomy and site of chisel insertion must be at least 1.5 to 2.5 cm to ensure a sufficient cortical bridge for stability of fixation. Superimpose the two tracings. **C,** At the intersection of the osteotomy and longitudinal axis (point of rotation) rotate the second tracing to achieve 25 degrees of valgus. Tape the proximal femur in the corrected position, and cut along the osteotomy line with scissors. **D,** Bring the distal fragment parallel to the original longitudinal axis, and displace it laterally 1 cm. Where the two fragments overlap denotes the size of the wedge that will be resected at surgery. Note that with this degree of valgus correction, the greater trochanter is not sufficiently lateral to the femoral head to restore effective abductor power. Also note the importance of retaining the lesser trochanter and the medial cortex as a medial buttress. This is achieved by taking less than a full wedge from the distal fragment. **E,** Final preoperative plan for osteotomy: excellent medial buttress; lateral displacement of shaft; sufficient cortical bridge between the osteotomy site and site of chisel insertion; greater trochanteric osteotomy to restore a more normal proximal femoral anatomy. The resected wedge is used as a graft for the trochanteric bed.

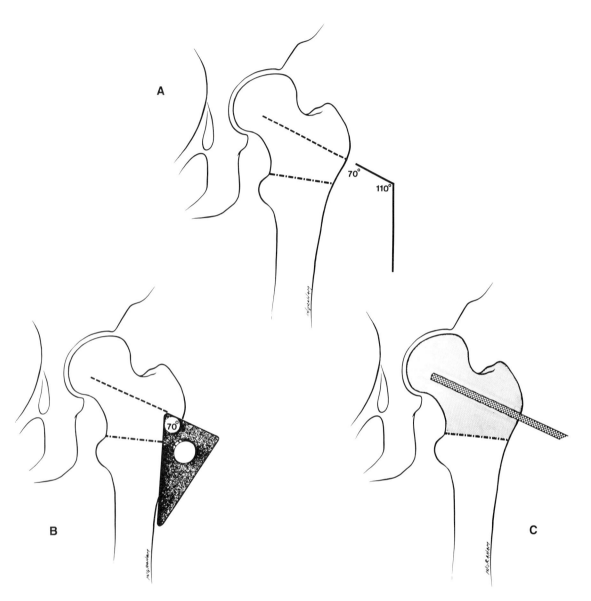

Fig. 15-7. Planning the osteotomy from the preoperative AP radiograph. Using the AP radiograph and a goniometer, the critical sites for osteotomy can be determined. In this example we can plan for either 20-degree valgus or 20-degree varus correction using the same measurements (see Table 15-1). **A,** Draw the site of osteotomy on the radiograph. For 20-degree correction draw a line 70 degrees to the longitudinal axis of the femur so that it is at least 1.5 to 2.5 cm proximal to the osteotomy site, and engages the head, optimally in the inferior and posterior quadrants. This is the site of chisel insertion. An estimate of the length of blade to be used can be made by measuring the depth of chisel insertion. **B** and **C,** At surgery this point of entrance can be found (usually just proximal to the vastus tubercle) and confirmed by fluoroscopy. The chisel is directed into the neck parallel to an A0 70-degree triangle.

Continued.

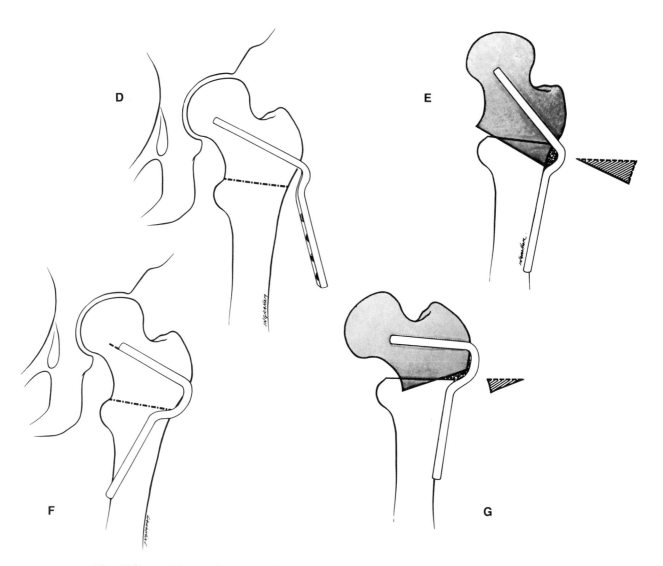

Fig. 15-7, cont'd. D and **E,** For valgus osteotomy of 20 degrees a 130-degree blade plate is inserted into the chisel track (see Table 15-1). **F** and **G,** For varus osteotomy of 20 degrees, a 90-degree blade plate is inserted into the chisel track (see Table 15-1).

Table 15-1. Determining angular corrections achieved with AO triangles

	Triangle (degrees)	Valgus correction (degrees)	Varus correction (degrees)
For 130-degree blade plate (Valgus osteotomy)	50*	0	
	60	10	
	70	20	
	80	30	
	90	40	
For 90-degree blade plate (Varus osteotomy)	60		30
	70		20
	80		10
	90		0

*See Fig. 15-8.

and the appropriate fixed angled blade plate, the corrections in either valgus or varus can be determined accurately (Table I and Fig. 15-8).

TECHNIQUE OF VALGUS EXTENSION OSTEOTOMY (AFTER BOMBELLI)
Position

The patient is supine with a small roll under the buttock; the extremity is draped free. A radiolucent operating room table extension is used to permit easier use of the C-ARM.

Approach

The approach is anterolateral. The incision is centered at the posterior proximal tip of the

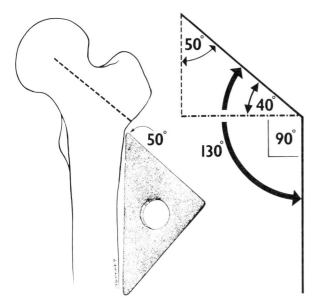

Fig. 15-8. Determining angular correction for a 130-degree blade plate. To insert a 130-degree blade plate and achieve *no* angular correction, the blade is inserted at an angle 50 degrees to the longitudinal axis of the femur. Therefore angular correction in valgus is achieved by inserting this fixed blade plate from 60 to 90 degrees to the femoral longitudinal axis (see Table 15-1).

greater trochanter with the leg in the neutral position. The proximal limb of the incision extends toward the anterosuperior iliac spine approximately 10 cm. The distal limb extends from the greater trochanter approximately 15 cm along the posterior border of the femoral shaft. The subcutaneous tissue and iliotibial band are incised in the line of the incision. With upward retraction of the anterior iliotibial band flap, the anterior border of the gluteus medius is readily seen. The fat between the tensor and the gluteus medius is incised carefully, and branches of the lateral femoral circumflex artery are ligated. The hip capsule then is readily exposed, allowing direct visualization of the anterior neck of the femur. Arthrotomy can be performed easily.

Biplane osteotomy (Fig. 15-9)

Extension. The degree of ultimate extension correction (determined preoperatively) is achieved by flexing the extremity to the desired degree of hip flexion and maintaining that flexion with dry goods under the knee. The seating chisel is inserted perpendicular to the floor, thus secur-

ing the proximal femur in the desired degree of hip flexion. (The term extension refers to the final angulation of the femur. Thus, for 20 degrees of extension correction, the hip is flexed 20 degrees, the osteotomy performed, and the distal fragment then brought parallel to the ground.) Thus the proximal fragment has been flexed 20 degrees, delivering the anterior femoral head into the acetabulum, but overall correction of the femur is said to have been in extension.

Valgus. A 130-degree blade plate is used. Preoperative planning should establish the site of chisel insertion, the length of the blade required, and the angle at which the chisel will be inserted. The optimal site of chisel placement is in the inferior quadrant of the femoral head. The chisel placement site must allow at least 1.5 to 2.0 cm cortical bridge distally, so that the osteotomy can be performed at the proximal border of the lesser trochanter. In valgus osteotomy lateral shaft displacement is required, thus a blade approximately 1.0 cm longer than the desired depth of insertion should be chosen. By leaving the blade 1.0 cm, the distal shaft can be brought laterally to the plate, ensuring lateral shaft displacement.

The center of the femoral neck in the sagittal plane can be judged under direct vision because the anterior surface of the neck has been exposed. Placement of the chisel is anterior to the midtrochanteric line (the greater trochanter is a posterior structure, and if the chisel is inserted in the midtrochanteric line the blade will perforate the posterior femoral neck).[6] For varus osteotomy, chisel insertion is made easier by multiple drill holes in the cortex. In valgus osteotomy a thin trochanteric osteotomy usually is performed. This trochanteric osteotomy should hinge superiorly on the soft tissues and should not disrupt the capsule. In valgus osteotomy, trochanteric osteotomy allows relaxation of the abductors and establishes a more normal neck-shaft angle. The cancellous bed of the greater trochanter then is used as the site of entrance of the chisel. This entrance site can be confirmed by placing a Kirschner wire in the soft tissues at the estimated site and angle of correction and checking its position under fluoroscopy. With the extremity fixed in the desired degree of flexion, the chisel is introduced at the desired site and angle of correction in the coronal plane and advanced to the intended depth. Its path can be checked in two planes by abducting and externally rotating the extremity and obtaining a frog lateral in addition to an AP view.

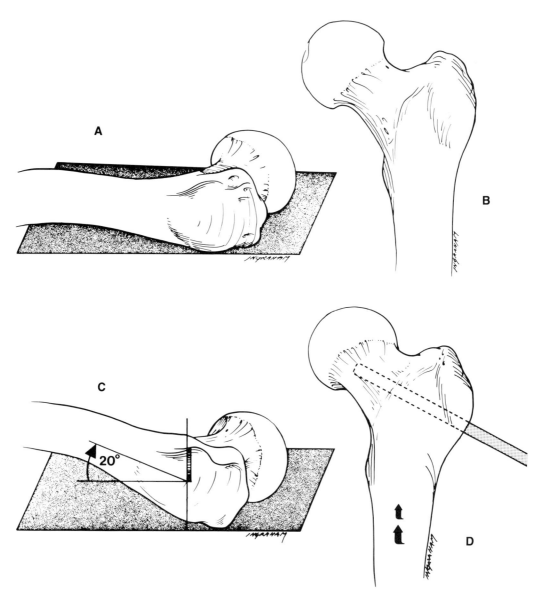

Fig. 15-9. Surgical technique of valgus 20 degrees—extension 20 degrees osteotomy (see text). **A** and **B,** The proximal femur viewed from the sagittal and the coronal planes. **C** and **D,** The femur is flexed 20 degrees and maintained in this position with dry goods under the knee. The chisel, however, is inserted perpendicular to the floor and just posterior to the anterior femoral neck. (The greater trochanter is a posterior structure. Perforation of the posterior femoral neck will occur if the chisel is inserted at the midtrochanteric level rather than just under the anterior femoral neck).[6] In the coronal plane the chisel is inserted 70 degrees to the longitudinal axis of the femur. **E** and **F,** The osteotomy is performed just proximal to the lesser trochanter and perpendicular to the femur in *both* planes. **G** and **H,** The distal fragment is delivered, the iliopsoas tendon released, and a biplane wedge of 20 degrees in each plane is resected. The lesser trochanter and medial cortex of the distal fragment should be retained to ensure a stable medial buttress. **I,** After the chisel is removed, a 130-degree blade plate is inserted into the chisel tract. Dry goods are removed from under the knee and the osteotomy site is reduced (*dotted line*) with the femur now extended and the patella in neutral rotation. A portion of the resected wedge is placed under the trochanteric osteotomy (*solid line*).

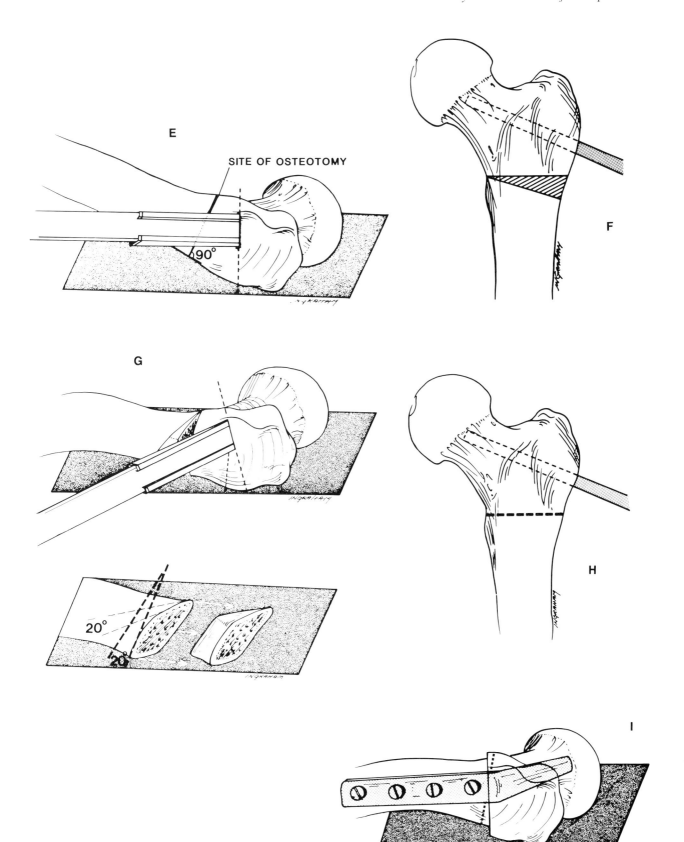

E

SITE OF OSTEOTOMY

90°

F

G

20°

20°

H

I

The osteotomy

The ideal site for osteotomy is at the proximal border of the lesser trochanter. After satisfactory positioning of the chisel, the femur is transected 1.5 to 2.0 cm distal to the site of the chisel insertion and perpendicular to the long axis of the femur in both planes. A biplane wedge then is removed from the distal fragment. For example, if one is performing a valgus extension osteotomy of 20 degrees in each plane, then a 20-degree wedge is fashioned in the anteroposterior plane; in addition, a posteriorly based wedge is fashioned from the lateral surface of the femur. The wedge is preserved and will be used later as a bone graft in the trochanteric bed. The distal osteotomy fragment is delivered into the wound, and the insertion of the iliopsoas tendon is resected. If lateral displacement is difficult, the pectineus insertion also can be released.

Reduction of the osteotomy

Immediately following chisel removal, the blade is inserted into the chisel tract by hand and advanced to its final depth by attachment of the blade plate holder and the use of a mallet. The osteotomy then is reduced by removing the dry goods under the knee and bringing the distal fragment in apposition to the proximal fragment so that the plate lies against the lateral surface of the femur. Lateral displacement should be achieved readily because of the lateral extension allowed by the additional 1.0 cm of blade length. The Homan retractor, elevating the distal fragment, is useful in holding position until the bone-holding clamp has secured the plate to the femur. The external compression device, with about 50% of the compression, is applied. At this point, it is useful to place a cortical screw into the proximal fragment to enhance blade fixation proximally. Following this, compression is completed and then four A0 cortical screws are inserted in the usual fashion. Excellent fixation and greater than 70% apposition of cancellous surfaces are usually achieved in this manner. If for reasons of leg length discrepancy no wedge has been taken, satisfactory stability can be achieved by interposing and impacting the osteotomy surfaces into each other. The wedge is inserted underneath the hinged greater trochanter fragment and secured by a careful suturing of the vastus lateralis origin to the greater trochanter. Final positioning and fixation are checked by fluoroscopy.

SURGICAL TECHNIQUE: VARUS EXTENSION OSTEOTOMY

The operative technique and preparation for varus extension osteotomy are similar to that for valgus osteotomy. The following differences are noted.

Varus osteotomy results in elevation of the greater trochanter. So that abductor mechanics are not excessively compromised, the tip of the greater trochanter should be no more proximal than the midpoint between the center of rotation of the femoral head and the subchondral bone plate after correction.[10] Most varus osteotomies accomplish the goal of improved congruence and satisfactory trochanter–center of rotation relationships with correction of no more than 15 to 20 degrees. Because extension increases the magnitude of varus correction, excessive varus correction may occur if the contribution of extension to varus is ignored.[1] In varus osteotomy approximately one-half shaft diameter medial displacement is desired; therefore a 90-degree osteotomy blade with either 10, 15, or 20 mm medial displacement can be chosen preoperatively.[6] The configuration of the 90-degree plate allows accurate displacement.

If the femoral neck is of sufficient length, I prefer to take the wedge from the proximal fragment.[6] A minimal wedge resection of the medial half of the proximal fragment is taken. Its direction is parallel to the chisel in both planes. This results in maximal surface contact with the final plane of osteotomy being transverse (that is, in compression rather than in shear). The wedge is used as bone graft inserted into the elbow of the plate. Rapid incorporation occurs. If derotation is desired, the order of steps is as follows:

1. Obtain extension as desired with dry goods under the knee.

2. Internally rotate the femur to correct excessive anteversion, but leave approximately 10 to 15 degrees of residual anteversion. This can be assessed accurately by direct inspection of the anterior surface of the femoral neck.

3. Introduce the chisel perpendicular to the floor, diverging 10 degrees posteriorly from the plane of the femoral neck. This must be done with extreme care because of the possibility of violating the posterior neck with the chisel. It must be remembered that the site of chisel insertion must be just under the

anterior cortex of the neck, rather than in the midtrochanteric line.

4. After the osteotomy, rotate the distal fragment to neutral (patella straight up), do appropriate wedge resection, and then fix the osteotomy.

EXPERIENCE WITH INTERTROCHANTERIC OSTEOTOMY AT BRIGHAM AND WOMEN'S HOSPITAL 1982-1984

Between 1982 and 1984, 37 osteotomies were performed at the Brigham and Women's Hospital: 26 were performed for a diagnosis of osteoarthritis, usually secondary to acetabular dysplasia; 5 were performed for osteonecrosis; and 6 other osteotomies were performed for a variety of reasons; for example, trochanteric advancement and revision of nonunion secondary to intertrochanteric fractures. The mean age of 26 patients undergoing osteotomy for osteoarthritis was 40 years old. There were 11 osteotomies in patients 21 to 30, 3 in patients 31 to 40, 7 in patients 41 to 50, and 5 in patients 51 to 57 years old.

During the same 3-year period, 1982 to 1984, 900 primary total hip arthroplasties were performed at BWH. Of these procedures, 518 were performed for a diagnosis of osteoarthritis. Only 36 hip arthroplasties were performed for osteoarthritic patients who were younger than 50 years of age.

These figures reflect the increasing recognition at our institution that younger patients with a diagnosis of osteoarthritis are often excellent candidates for osteotomy. It is also important to note that a somewhat larger number of patients in this age-group were believed *not* to be candidates for osteotomy, and so they were treated with arthroplasty. When one considers the major goals of reconstructive hip surgery stated earlier, there appear to be a significant number of younger osteoarthritic patients for whom osteotomy is the procedure of choice.

REFERENCES

1. Bombelli, R.: Osteoarthritis of the hip, ed. 2, Berlin, 1983, Springer-Verlag.
2. Ewald, F.C., Poss, R., Pugh, J., Schiller, A.L. and Sledge, C.B.: Hip cartilage supported by methacrylate in canine arthroplasty, Clin. Orthop. **171:**273, 1982.
3. Harris, N.H., and Kirwan, E.: The results of osteotomy for early primary osteoarthritis of the hip, J. Bone Surg. **46B:**477, 1964.
4. Miegel, R., and Harris, W.H.: Medial displacement intertrochanteric osteotomy in osteoarthritis of the hip, J. Bone Joint Surg. **66A:**878, 1984.
5. Morscher, E.W.: Intertrochanteric osteotomy in osteoarthritis of the hip. In: The hip, proceedings of the eighth open scientific meeting of The Hip Society, St. Louis, 1980, The C.V. Mosby Co.
6. Muller, M.E.: Intertrochanteric osteotomies in adults: Planning and operating technique. In Cruess, R., and Mitchell, N.: Surgical management of degenerative arthritis in the lower limb, Philadelphia, 1975, Lea & Febiger.
7. Pauwels, F.: Biomechanics of the normal and diseased hip, Berlin, 1976, Springer-Verlag.
8. Poss, R.: The role of osteotomy in the treatment of osteoarthritis of the hip (Current Concepts Review), J. Bone Joint Surg. **66A:** Jan. 1984.
9. Schatzker, J.: The intertrochanteric osteotomy, Berlin, 1984, Springer-Verlag.
10. Wagner, H.: Osteotomy of the hip and knee, Unpublished paper presented to Postgraduate Students, (Michael Millis and Robert Poss, Directors), Boston, May 1984, Harvard University School of Medicine.

Chapter 16

Mechanical properties of porous metal total hip prostheses

ROY D. CROWNINSHIELD

The fatigue strength of porous metal total hip prostheses is of increasing importance, since many of these prostheses are used in young and physically active patients. The processes used in implant fabrication can have a profound effect on the microstructure and mechanical properties of the implant material. This paper reports on the mechanical properties of the orthopaedic alloys used in porous total hip prostheses.

MANUFACTURING PROCESSES AND MATERIAL PROPERTIES

The microstructure and mechanical properties of devices made from cobalt-chromium-molydenum (Co-Cr-Mo) and titanium-aluminum-vanadium (Ti-6Al-4V) alloys in large part are determined by the processes used in their manufacture. The processes most widely used to produce orthopaedic implants are investment casting, forging, and machining.

Investment casting

All alloys used to produce implants are formed initially by melting and casting. As the molten metal cools below its melting point, solid grains begin to grow. These grains typically become quite large before the metal is totally solidified. Metal alloys also develop chemical segregation as a result of changes in composition as the metal solidifies. Metal bars used for machining or forging have the grain size refined by working large (for example, 18-inch diameter) cast ingots into suitably sized (for example, 2-inch diameter) bar stock. This working also reduces the extent of chemical inhomogeneity. These refinements are not present in investment cast prostheses.

Investment casting has been used widely to produce geometrically complex components. The large grains observed in cast Co-Cr-Mo are shown in Fig. 16-1. Castings also may include small amounts of porosity and small foreign particles (inclusions). These structural features lead to tensile and fatigue properties that are not as high as the properties of fine-grain materials produced by other techniques. Cast Co-Cr-Mo alloy with the microstructure shown in Fig. 16-1 was used commonly in total hip femoral components during much of the 1970s.

Forging

Forging is another conventional metal-forming technique. The forging process involves forming metal by mechanical force. Generally, this is done with the metal heated to a temperature at which it can be shaped more easily when hammered under force. This reduces the force needed to shape the material and increases the ability for the metal to deform into the desired shape. In forging an orthopaedic device such as hip stems, a series of shaped cavities (dies) is used which gradually forms the material to the desired shape. Proper control of metal temperature and die design produces fine-grained, high-strength material.

Fig. 16-2 shows the fine grain microstructure of forged Co-Cr-Mo alloy. The fatigue strength of this forged alloy is considerably higher than that of the cast alloy. By the late 1970s, forging became one of the preferred methods of manufacturing Co-Cr-Mo alloy total hip femoral components. These forged total hip femoral components are of considerably higher strength than

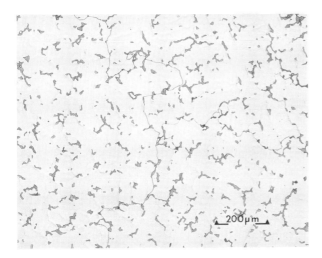

Fig. 16-1. The coarse grain structure of investment cast Co-Cr-Mo.

Fig. 16-2. Microstructure of forged low carbon Co-Cr-Mo. The forged material exhibits much finer grain size than the cast material shown in Fig. 16-1.

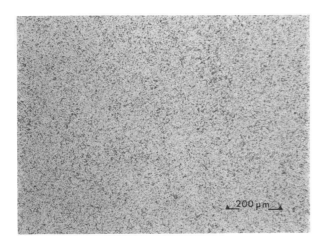

Fig. 16-3. Microstructure of wrought Ti-6A1-4V bar usable in machined total hip femoral components.

otherwise similar investment cast prostheses and have successfully served to substantially reduce the incidence of femoral component fracture.

Machined implants from wrought material

Machining implants from wrought, fine-grain bars of the desired material is another common manufacturing method. The machining stock bars are formed by forging techniques similar to those previously described. Modern machining techniques such as computer numerical control (CNC) and computer aided design/computer aided manufacturing (CAD/CAM) can rapidly produce parts directly from drawings, saving the time needed to produce forging dies or tools to make investment casting waxes.

There are essentially no metallurgic changes during conventional machining. Therefore the mechanical properties of machined parts are identical to the properties of the forged bar from which it was machined. Machining of titanium alloy is relatively easy; therefore machined Ti-6Al-4V alloy implants are fairly common. Because machining of Co-Cr-Mo is much more difficult, machined Co-Cr-Mo devices are uncommon. Fig. 16-3 demonstrates the microstructure of wrought Ti-6Al-4V. This material is a fine-grained material that can be used in high-strength implant production.

POROUS COATING APPLICATION TECHNIQUES

The techniques used to apply porous metal coatings to implants can have a dramatic influence on the material's microstructure and the implant's mechanical properties. Porous surfaces are not made as integral parts of porous implants; instead, the porous surface is preformed and later attached to the implant substrate. This porous surface attachment is accomplished by sintering. Sintering is a temperature-activated metallurgic bonding of the porous surface to the implant. Gravity sintering and diffusion bonding are two sintering methods commonly used in orthopaedic implant manufacture. These two methods of sintering have important differences.

Gravity sintering

Gravity sintering is carried out at temperatures quite close to the melting temperature of the implant. This process typically is used to attach spherical beads to Co-Cr-Mo alloy implants. Exposing fine-grain forged or wrought Co-Cr-Mo to temperatures near their melting points (as required in gravity sintering) results in grain growth and microstructural modifications. Since exposure to gravity-sintering conditions transforms fine-grain structures to the grain size of cast Co-Cr-Mo alloy material, forged implants generally are not used as substrates for porous coating. Most porous Co-Cr-Mo implants are investment cast devices.

The effect of the high sintering temperatures on cast Co-Cr-Mo is rather different. Cast Co-Cr-Mo already exhibits a coarse grain structure and contains carbide second phase particles that have a different composition from the bulk material. This chemical inhomogeneity is important in sintering, because local inhomogeneities exhibit lower melting points than the bulk material. Thus it is not unusual to observe melted areas in cast Co-Cr-Mo implants with sintered bead coatings. This effect, known as incipient melting, is shown in Fig. 16-4. The extent of incipient melting in such implants depends on variables such as casting quality and sintering temperature control. Incipient melted regions in an implant can occur anywhere.

The fatigue strength of Co-Cr-Mo alloy produced by different manufacturing methods is shown in Fig. 16-5. Investment cast Co-Cr-Mo alloy is less than one half the strength of forged alloy. The heat treatment required to gravity sinter beads onto the alloy further reduces its strength. The strength loss of sintered Co-Cr-Mo compared to forged Co-Cr-Mo is a generalized condition that occurs throughout the implant.

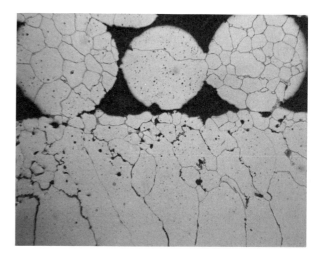

Fig. 16-4. Gravity sintered Co-Cr-Mo alloy. This coarse grain structure can have localized melting of chemically segregated regions.

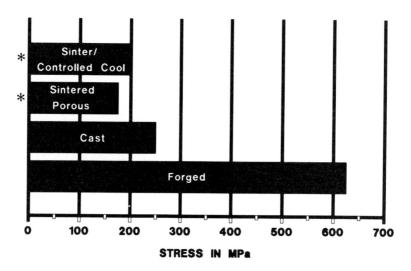

Fig. 16-5. The reverse bending fatigue strength of Co-Cr-Mo alloy produced by different manufacturing techniques.

Diffusion bonding

In the process of diffusion bonding, pressure and temperature are used to bond the porous coating. This combination enables the use of much lower temperatures. The temperatures required to diffusion bond commercially pure titanium fiber metal pads to Ti-6Al-4V cause only subtle changes in the fine-grain, high strength structure of wrought Ti-6Al-4V (Fig. 16-6). The

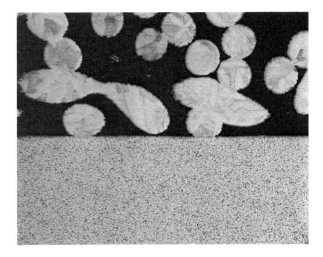

Fig. 16-6. A diffusion-bonded, commercially pure titanium porous surface on a wrought Ti-6Al-4V implant. The implant's microstructure is similar to wrought Ti-6Al-4V (Fig. 16-3).

fatigue limit of wrought/forged Ti-6Al-4V exposed to diffusion bonding conditions (Fig. 16-6) is typically about 5% to 10% less than wrought/forged material.

Notch effect

Porous coatings locally influence the properties of implants, because they alter the implant's surface geometry in the region of the porous coating. The bond sites between the coating and implant have irregular geometries that can act as stress concentrators. This is sometimes referred to as a notch effect. The fatigue strength of both Co-Cr-Mo and Ti-6Al-4V is reduced in the presence of the notches provided by porous metal coatings.

This notch effect is an important consideration in the design of titanium alloy implants. The strength of porous coated titanium alloy (Fig. 16-7) is *considerably* lower than that of the wrought/forged titanium alloy. This notch effect is a localized condition that affects implant strength in the region of the porous coating. Implant design must take this notch effect into account by placing the porous coating in low stress regions of the implant.

SUMMARY

The forged condition is the strongest form of the Co-Cr-Mo and Ti-6Al-4V alloys used in orthopaedics. Both the Co-Cr-Mo alloy and the

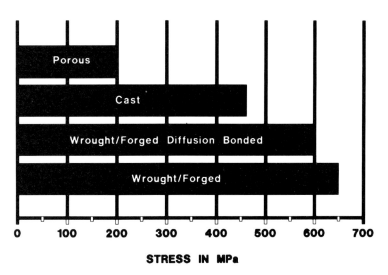

Fig. 16-7. The reverse bending fatigue strength of Ti-6Al-4V alloy produced by different manufacturing techniques.

Ti-6Al-4V alloy lose strength when incorporated into porous implants.

The strength loss in the Co-Cr-Mo alloy is a generalized condition and is largely a result of the microstructure of these cast and then gravity-sintered prostheses. The greatest fatigue strength achieved throughout these porous Co-Cr-Mo implants is that of the cast alloy. The strength loss in diffusion-bonded, porous titanium—alloyed implants is largely a result of notch sensitivity. This strength loss is not a generalized condition; it is localized on the implant to regions of porous coating attachment. In implant regions apart from the porous coatings, these titanium implants can have the strength of other wrought or forged titanium alloy implants.

To achieve a functionally strong implant, porous implant design needs to account for these losses in material strength. Implant strength should be verified experimentally and communicated to the orthopaedic surgeon for assessment of implant adequacy for a particular patient. Patient weight, activity, and life expectancy are important elements in judging the adequacy of an implant's strength.

REFERENCE

1. Pilliar, R.M.: Powder metal-made orthopaedic implants with porous surface for fixation by tissue ingrowth, Clin. Orthop. **176**:42-46, 1983.

Chapter 17

Revision total hip arthroplasty for aseptic component loosening, tilting, and/or migration

Part A

Introduction

P.D. WILSON, JR.

For the past 3 years this course has featured eight different authors speaking on various aspects of the problem of revision arthroplasty. Five of the presentations are here reproduced.

The first, by Pellicci, deals with comparative retrospective follow-up studies of revision total hip arthroplasties at two institutions. The second, by Collis, deals with conventional revision of the femoral side using cemented devices. The third, by Johnston, presents conventional recementing approaches to acetabular side revisions. The fourth, by Gustilo, presents a short term experience and follow-up study of femoral side revisions done with a customized "ingrowth" femoral component and autologous bone grafts. The last, by Murray, deals with unique "salvage" approaches for difficult problems that use various prosthetic devices such as spacers to avoid the extreme shortening and instability consequent to mere removal and debridement.

The most noticeable lack in these papers is that of a presentation on the current status of adjunctive bone grafting as a method of supplementing lost acetabular and pelvic wall bone stock when revising loosened migrated socket components. Although much remains to be learned about the longer term fate of autografts and particularly of allografts in such situations, a body of experience has accumulated that deserves recognition in a symposium of this kind. Techniques and principles governing their clinical indications and appli-

cations are widely accepted. For some insight into this aspect of total hip revision surgery refer to the following articles and abstracts.

Ganz, R.: Bone grafting: Revision arthroplasty, vol. 2, Proceedings of a symposium held in Harrogate, England, March 1983.

Harris, W., Allografting in total hip arthroplasty, Clin. Orthop. **162:**150-164, 1982.

Harris, W.: Autografting and allografting in aseptic failure of total hip replacement, In Welch, R.B., editor: The hip: Proceedings of the twelfth open scientific meeting of The Hip Society, St. Louis, 1984, The C.V. Mosby Co.

Marti, R.K., and Besselaar, P.P.: Reconstruction of the acetabular roof and other bone grafts in total hip replacement and total hip revision, J. Bone and Joint Surg. **63B:**283, 1981.

This introduction would not be complete without emphasizing the extreme difficulty of this type of orthopaedic surgery. I know of no other type of orthopaedic surgery where careful preoperative workup and planning are as essential. But even then there is a need for optimal facilities in which to carry out such surgery. The facilities must include the availability of a well-trained team of assistants for difficult preoperative and postoperative care regimens, as well as for intraoperative assistance; extensive backup of devices, banked bone, special orthoses, and the like; ready access to customizing facilities

149

for special prostheses and equipment, including adequate radiologic workup capabilities from which to plan them; and excellent bacteriologic, blood replacement-banking, and anesthesiologic backup.

At least one other point deserves emphasis before proceeding with the papers. Orthopaedic surgeons very rightly tend to advise surgery only when symptoms and impairment are disabling enough to counterbalance the inherent risks involved. However, an exception to this rule is justified when radiologic studies show important bone stock absorption despite the absence of distressing pain or disabling impairment. Although this occurs infrequently, it should be looked for, and all patients with endoprostheses, whether cemented or not, should be subjected to periodic standardized evaluations, since there is no better way to recognize impending serious bone stock loss than by the comparison of serial x-ray films over time. Serious bone stock loss is certainly as important an indication for reoperation as is pain or impairment.

I will close this introduction by stating that the faculty of this course has unanimously endorsed the need for a wide exposure and for a thorough debridement of scar and reactive tissue as primary steps in their surgical revision techniques.

Part B

Results of revision total hip replacement

PAUL M. PELLICCI

Revision total hip replacement has assumed increasing importance over the past decade as the number of patients with failed hip replacement has grown. At The Hospital for Special Surgery the number of revision total hip replacements performed in 1984 increased 22-fold over the number performed in 1972 (Fig. 17-1).[1]

In 1980 we reviewed those patients who had undergone revision total hip replacements at The Hospital for Special Surgery and the Robert B. Brigham Hospital. The results were reported to The Hip Society in Las Vegas in 1981.[2] Briefly summarizing that study, 110 hips were followed for an average of 3.4 years. Time to failure averaged 3.5 years. The infection rate was 3.6%,

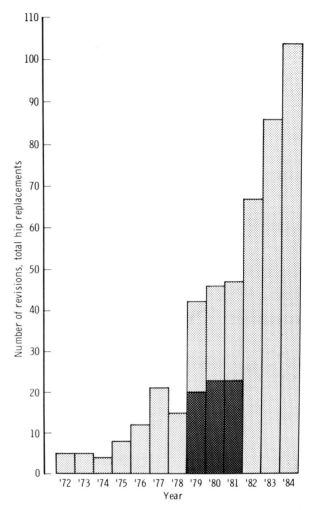

Fig. 17-1. Number of revision total hip replacements performed at The Hospital for Special Surgery on a yearly basis. Shaded areas represent patients in whom the index of total hip replacement was also performed at The Hospital for Special Surgery. As a percentage of all total hip replacements performed at The Hospital for Special Surgery, there was a tenfold increase over the years noted, from just over 1% in 1972 to just over 12% in 1984.

over twice that reported in the literature for primary total hip replacement. Trochanteric problems occurred in 13% of hips, nearly three times that published for primary replacement. There was also a higher incidence of mechanical failure at 14%. A second revision for loosening was performed in 5.8% of cases, again between two and three times that reported for primary replacement. Furthermore, an additional 8.2% of the revision arthroplasties were loose both clinically and radiographically. Of further concern was the finding that of those hips causing no symptoms, 26% had progressive radiolucent zones between cement and bone on serial radiographs.

A second group of patients whose revisions were performed at The Hospital for Special Surgery between 1979 and 1981 has recently been reviewed.[1] Follow-up, which averaged 3.6 years, was obtained in 139 hips in 136 patients. The minimum follow-up was 2 years. The patients' average age was 65.7 years. Females slightly outnumbered males. Time to failure averaged 5.8 years. Infections occurred in 5.5% of hips. Trochanteric complications occurred in 6.2% of hips. The dislocation rate was 8%, and the incidence of mechanical failure was 15.1%. Only one third of the failures have been revised. Initial x-ray studies taken in the recovery room or during the first postoperative week revealed acetabular or femoral radiolucencies of 1 mm or less in 70% of cases. In summary, only 56% of patients had what would be considered to be an excellent result, that is, the complete absence of symptoms and nonprogressive radiolucencies on serial radiographs.

Results were classified as good if the hip was causing only mild symptoms, if it was not significantly decreasing activity level, and if there were no progressive radiolucencies on serial radiographs. Of the patients reviewed, 7.6% had good results and 17% had fair results; that is, they were asymptomatic, but there were progressive radiolucencies on serial radiographs. The results of the two studies were therefore quite similar. However, we wished to obtain a longer term follow-up to determine the durability of these results. We went back to examine the original group of patients first reported in 1981.

Information was obtained on 99 hips in 97 patients, a 91% retrieval rate. There were 40 men and 57 women whose average age was 60 years. The average length of follow-up was 8.1 years with a range of 5 to 12.5 years.

There were 58 hips at the time of follow-up in 1980 that were producing no symptoms and were stable on serial radiographs. At long-term follow-up recently, 74% were still asymptomatic with stable interfaces, and 16% were still asymptomatic but had developed progressive radiolucencies on one or both sides of the arthroplasty. In addition, 5% had become clinically and radiographically loose but had yet to be revised. All were femoral loosenings. Two hips, or 3%, had come to revision, a loosened femoral component and a frac-

tured femoral shaft. One patient developed what was believed to be a delayed primary infection with *Staphylococcus epidermidis*. The hip was not revised. Treatment consisted of suppression with antibiotics.

At the time of the study in 1980 there were 24 hips that were producing no symptoms. Although they had demonstrated progressive radiolucencies on serial radiographs at one or both interfaces, 50% of these remained asymptomatic with interfaces that seemed to have stabilized. An additional 8% remained asymptomatic, although the radiolucencies continued to progress. Finally, 42% became loose clinically and radiographically. Half of them had been revised at the time of final follow-up. Time to failure averaged 6.2 years. There were five femoral, three acetabular, and two combined loosenings.

Fifteen hips were classified as mechanical failures at follow-up in 1980 (six had already come to revision at that time). Six more have been revised since; all were femoral component loosenings. Two hips remain unchanged and have not been revised. One hip has improved in that it has become much less symptomatic.

Six hips had been revised a second time by the time of the 1980 study. Two are asymptomatic without progressive radiolucencies. Two have "tolerable" symptoms with stable interfaces. Two are loose and painful, but neither has been revised a third time.

REFERENCES

1. Callaghan, J.J., Salvati, E.A., Pellicci, P.M., Wilson, P.D., Jr., and Ranawat, C.S.: Two to five year results of revision total hip replacement: Have we improved, J. Bone Joint Surg. (In press.)
2. Pellicci, P.M., Wilson, P.D., Jr., Sledge, C.B., Salvati, E.A., Ranawat, C.S., and Poss, R.: Revision total hip arthroplasty, Clin. Orthop. **170:**34, 1982.

Part C

Revision of aseptic, loose, broken femoral components

DENNIS K. COLLIS

This portion of the instructional course will cover revision of the aseptic, loose or broken, cemented femoral hip component. The section will be divided into five areas: indications, preoperative planning, cement and prosthesis removal, reinsertion of new components, and postoperative care.

Indications. The two basic indications for revision of the femoral component are disabling pain and progressive bone loss. (Infrequent other indications include prosthesis malposition resulting in incapacitating instability of the hip and a rare femoral fracture that can be stabilized best by a new prosthesis.) Assessment of the patient's pain must be accomplished by a careful history and physical examination. Roentgenographic findings of lucency are not diagnostic of loosening, and they alone do not constitute an indication for surgery unless there is also progressive bone loss. Simultaneous study of serial hip x-ray examinations taken over several years' time permits measurement of the amount of bone loss. Many hips will show an initial, progressive loss of bone proximal to the lesser trochanter. This process often stops and does not indicate loosening of the prosthesis. If bone resorption progresses into the lesser trochanter, major femoral cortical thinning is noted, or distal prosthetic component migration within the femoral shaft occurs, consideration of revision surgery is appropriate.

Blood studies and cultures of a hip aspiration are helpful measures to rule out infection. Differential bone scanning can be useful. In loosening, the technetium scan characteristically shows increased activity, although the gallium scan usually is inactive. Arthrograms, fluoroscopy, and push-pull roentgenograms also are occasionally helpful.

Preoperative planning. Revision cases require more planning than primary total hip replacement and involve assembling an appropriately skilled surgical team, special instruments for prosthetic and cement removal, and a variety of prostheses for reinsertion. Careful study of the previous operative report can often give the surgeon specific information that will be helpful during the revision surgery. Preoperative assessment of the acetabular component should be made, since, if the cup is of appropriate design and not loosened, worn, or malpositioned, it should not be removed. An appropriate matching femoral component should be available for insertion. Custom prostheses that are computer designed and computer manufactured are available from several sources but are rarely necessary. They often require several week's preparation

time and cost considerably more than standard prostheses. Despite their careful design and manufacture, they still may not fit exactly, necessitating "force fitting" because this special prosthesis may not fit the femur of any other patient. It is imperative to have extra-long neck prostheses available at the time of surgery, since bone of the proximal aspect of the femur usually is absent or of poor quality. Noncustom calcar replacement-type prostheses may even be needed.

Some planning with the anesthesiologist is useful. Hypotensive general anesthesia can significantly lower the blood loss in these lengthy operations and also improve the surgeon's visualization of the internal aspect of the femoral canal.

In my opinion a carefully planned trochanteric osteotomy is essential for these taxing operative procedures. This will markedly increase the exposure and greatly facilitate careful component removal and reinsertion. Resorting to trochanteric osteotomy "only when necessary" may severely compromise reattachment. Surgical exposure also requires resection of the very thick pseudocapsule around the proximal femur. In essence, the proximal femur must be completely mobilized, often to the point of even skeletonizing it so that damage to the femur can be avoided and accurate prosthetic positioning can be accomplished.

Prosthesis and cement removal. The loose standard femoral component is usually removed with relative ease. Special stems with fenestrations, dimples, extra length, double curves, or bony ingrowth surfaces may present very special problems. For the standard component, once the cement laying over the lateral curved shoulder of the prosthesis is removed, extraction is easily accomplished by applying force directed in line with the stem.

The special problem of removing the distal end of a broken prosthesis can be solved in one of four ways: (1) loosening the entire mass of cement around the prosthesis, (2) making a window in the cortex of the femur, (3) drilling into the broken surface of the distal stem and attaching an extractor, or (4) cutting between the broken stem and the femoral cortex with a large trephine.

Removal of a broken stem by loosening the cement around the entire distal broken tip is not usually the method of choice, because loosening that cement creates a serious risk of damage to the femoral cortex. Making a controlled window in the femur is safer and can be accomplished with standard osteotomes and power saws. It requires carefully making a template of the window over the broken stem and carefully sculpting so that the piece of bone can be replaced to fill the defect. Placing this cortical window anteriorly significantly diminishes the resultant weakening of the femur.

One special technique for extracting the distal broken stem involves carefully drilling into the broken surface of the distal stem with a high-speed drill, placing a special distraction device into the hole, and using an extraction hammer to remove the stem.[2] This method does require special equipment and laboratory practice so that the specific protocol is followed carefully to avoid damaging the femur.

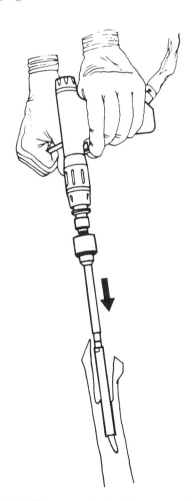

Fig. 17-2. Drilling over the broken stem with a specially designed large trephine allowing the stem to act as a drill guide. (From Collis, D., and Dubrul, W.: Contemp. Orthop., **8:**62, May 1984.)

Recently, another method for removing the broken stem from within the canal of the femur has been developed.[1] In this method, the cement surrounding the stem tip is cut by frictional sawing, using a large trephine with specially designed teeth. Placing the appropriately sized circular saw over the broken stem allows the stem to act as a guide (Fig. 17-2). Although very effective, this method also requires special equipment and operative techniques that demand the procedure be tried in the laboratory before being used in the operating room. This method does have the potential advantage that it can be used to remove bony ingrowth or other prostheses with uneven surfaces.

Special equipment is essential for the safe and effective removal of cement retained within the femoral canal. Many surgeons have proposed high-speed power equipment as the solution to this taxing problem. These expensive pieces of equipment operate at very high speed, and it should be remembered that potentially they can remove the bone more easily than the cement. Some surgeons have suggested using image intensification to avoid bone damage by these high-speed instruments, but this introduces the risks of contamination and irradiation.

My preference is to remove as much of the cement as possible under direct vision by the slow, careful, and often tedious use of hand instruments. These specially designed instruments greatly facilitate this removal (Fig. 17-3). The cement is split into relatively large fragments (Fig. 17-4), which then can be removed readily using special chisels (Fig. 17-5). The internal aspect of the femoral canal can be cleaned of cement, bone chips, and fibrous tissue with a reverse cutting curette (Fig. 17-6).

Removal of a distal cement plug can be accomplished using a special guide placed in the femoral canal that directs a small drill through the center of the cement plug (Fig. 17-7). Then, this hole is enlarged by 1 mm increments by using a series of drill bits that are specially designed for cement removal (Fig. 17-8). Visualization in the distal canal is enhanced by appropriate lighting. Very often, simply an adjustment of the operating table or overhead lights will accomplish this. Other aids include fiberoptic lights, head lamps, and a specially designed, battery-powered disposable light source. Adequate irrigation and suction equipment must be available, and a special suc-

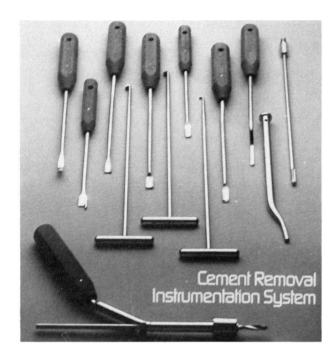

Fig. 17-3. Numerous special hand instruments helpful in removal of cement without using high-speed power equipment. (Courtesy The Depuy Co., Warsaw, Ind.)

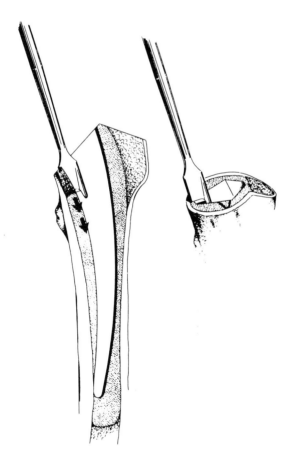

Fig. 17-4. Splitting the proximal cement into large fragments for easy removal. (Courtesy The Depuy Co., Warsaw, Ind.)

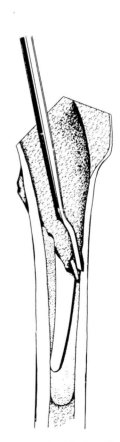

Fig. 17-5. Using curved chisels of various angles to remove cement. (Courtesy The Depuy Co., Warsaw, Ind.)

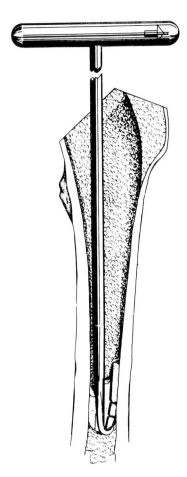

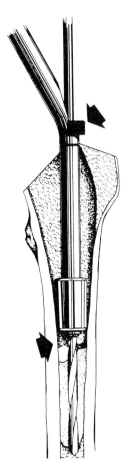

Fig. 17-6. Long-handled reverse cutting curette for canal cleaning. (Courtesy The Depuy Co., Warsaw, Ind.)

Fig. 17-7. Drill guide to allow making a hole in the center of a large retained distal cement plug. (Courtesy The Depuy Co., Warsaw, Ind.)

Fig. 17-8. Special design of drill point on the right compared with a standard drill point on the left. These cutting edges on a series of drill bits enlarging in 1 mm increments allow removal of cement by "chipping" it out from the interior of a permanently drilled hole in the cement mass. (Courtesy The Depuy Co., Warsaw, Ind.)

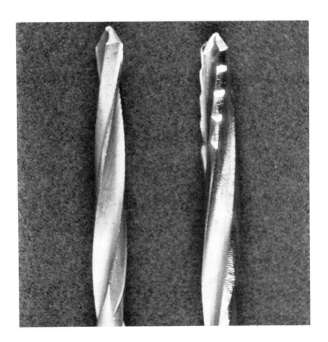

tion apparatus called the Super Sucker is helpful to avoid repetitive clogging of the suction equipment by the chips of cement. Pulsatile lavage facilitates final debridement of the canal.

Reinsertion of the new prosthesis. In most hips when a loose, uninfected prosthesis has been removed, revision surgery is possible. A rare exception may exist when very massive bone destruction is present. Recently there has been significant interest in doing revision hip reconstruction with press-fit or bony ingrowth prostheses with or without bone grafting. This interest stems from the frequently reported fact that the results from revision of cemented total hip arthroplasty using cement the second time are markedly inferior to those of primary hip replacements. I do not believe that the results need be as bad as suggested and that carefully done revision surgery, using cement, can produce quite reasonable results. My opinion is supported by a follow-up of 70 aseptically loose or broken femoral components that I have revised between 1974 and 1984. Only one of these hips has required re-revision, and that was for loosening after 8 years in a patient who weighed 330 pounds. Another hip required surgical drainage of an acute infection 2 years after the original revision surgery. There was one death from pulmonary embolus 3 weeks after surgery. There have been no repetitive dislocations or permanent nerve injuries in this group. The average length of follow-up was 43 months with an average Iowa rating of 91 points. Prostheses with extra neck lengths usually were used. No custom-made prostheses were needed. The stem lengths varied from 120 to 300 mm.

Some surgeons have proposed that all revision surgeries should be done with long stems. I do not believe this to be essential. What is essential is that a reasonably good-quality cortical bone be reached for recementing somewhere between 4 and 10 cm. Certainly, any cortical defect should be bypassed by a length of stem at least one and a half times the diameter of the femur. Large defects warrant greater length of bypass (Fig. 17-9).

Cement technique for reinsertion is even more critical than in primary total hip replacement. A large body of orthopaedic literature has evolved outlining and stressing these techniques. First, a proper bed must be obtained. This includes removal of all fibrous tissue or loose bony or cement

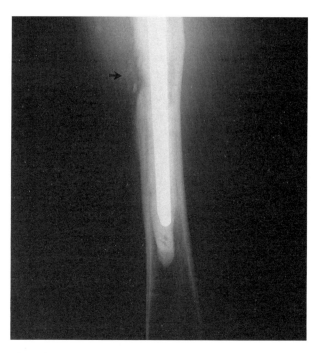

Fig. 17-9. Large cortical defect with generous stem bypass. Effective cement containment without formal plugging.

fragments. Careful drying of the endosteal surface is important. (Frequently hypotensive anesthesia will aid in this effort.) If possible, plugging of the distal femoral canal with bone, plastic, or a separate cement plug is helpful. Occasionally the stem required is so long that placing a special plug in the expanding medullary canal of the metaphyseal region of the distal femur is neither practical nor effective (see Fig. 17-9). Centrifugation of the cement seems to be a helpful aid in increasing its fatigue life. Injection of the cement with some form of injection system is definitely beneficial. Because of the large area to be filled (this may be the entire canal), several mixes of cement started at slightly different times can be helpful.

The question of whether to add antibiotics to the cement is still an unanswered one. Good results are reported with treating infections with antibiotic-loaded cement. However, the FDA has not approved any commercially prepared cement with antibiotics added. My preference is to mix approximately 300 mg of tobramycin to each 40 g of methacrylate powder before adding the liquid monomer. I have not used antibiotics in the cement on all revision cases. Since most revision series report infection rates considerably higher than primary total hip replacement, a good case could be made for that practice.

A number of surgeons are proposing that all revision of cemented total hip arthroplasties should be done with press-fit or bony ingrowth prostheses. The advisability of that practice certainly will have to await the scrutiny of long term follow-up of those cases before it is enthusiastically endorsed. Documented evidence also has not been presented to support the practice of either autografting or allografting in order to improve immediate and permanent fixation of the prosthesis. No evidence has been presented that new bone actually will replace the bone graft placed between an artificial implant and the femoral cortex.

Postoperative protocol. The postoperative protocol for a revised total hip replacement in which cement is used is usually very similar to that of a primary total hip arthroplasty. The patient is often out of bed in a day or so, on crutches for 6 to 8 weeks, and using a cane for another 6 to 8 weeks. In patients who have hips where the bone stock is significantly compromised, a longer period of external support may be required, and in very rare instances, lifetime use of a cane may be recommended.

When prosthetic instability is present at the conclusion of surgery, because of either bony anatomic deficits or weak soft tissue repair, a period of 1 to 3 weeks of bedrest after surgery may be advisable. In very rare instances, a pantaloon, single hip spica, from above the waist to above the knee, may be appropriate.

It is even more important than with total primary hip replacement that these patients be aware of the need to avoid significant lifting or impact loading. However, since they already have had one failure of an artificial joint, making that need understood usually is not difficult.

In conclusion, careful attention to preoperative planning and skillful application of special surgical techniques can result in the successful revision of most failed femoral components.

REFERENCES

1. Collis, D., and Dubrul, W.: The removal of fractured prosthetic components from medullary cavities: A new technique, Contemp. Orthop. **8**(5):61-63, 1984.
2. Harris, W.H., White, R.E., Mitchell, S., and Barber, F.: A new technique for removal of broken femoral stems in total hip replacement: A technical note, J Bone Joint Surg. **63A:**843-845, 1981.

Part D

Revision of total hip arthroplasty for aseptic loosening: the acetabulum

RICHARD C. JOHNSTON

This portion of the instructional course will cover revision of the aseptically loose acetabular prosthesis. Diagnosis, incidence, and results of aseptic revision have been covered previously. I will discuss indications, objectives, and results briefly and then concentrate on technique with emphasis on the rationale of technique.

My indications for aseptic revision are disabling symptoms or bone destruction of sufficient degree that additional bone destruction will make the performance of revision surgery much less predictable or impossible. The overall objective of revision surgery is to provide the patient with a hip that will function as normally as possible and be least likely to loosen again. The steps to reaching this objective are: first, the hip must be taken apart completely so that the surgeon has direct visual and instrumental access to the acetabulum circumferentially. Second, a bed of bone of adequate strength that is completely devoid of soft tissue and debris must be prepared. Third, a new prosthesis should be selected that distributes the applied load as evenly as possible and thus minimizes peak stresses on bone and/or cement. This prosthesis must be inserted in such a manner as to create a new anatomic geometry that, during function, will place as little load on the hip as possible. Finally, the prosthesis must be solidly fixed to bone. If these objectives are reached, the results of total hip revision will be quite satisfactory and rather durable.

My personal experience is indicated in Table 17-1. Through 1983, I have done 143 revisions; 81 of these were for a loose acetabulum or loose femoral and acetabular components. Thirty-five had positive cultures and are considered septic, and 46 were aseptic. The bulk of those in the last column of Table 17-1 had aseptic femoral component loosening without acetabular loosening. Follow-up is current in all but three. Cement fixation has been used in all; none has been bone grafted. The Charnley prostheses were used until I began using Iowa prostheses a few years ago. Since 1974 antibiotic powder has been used in the cement, and systemic antibiotics for 2 to 6 months

Table 17-1. Total hip revisions performed from 1971 to 1983

	Loose acetabulum		
	Septic	*Aseptic*	*Other*
1971	1	—	—
1972	1	1	—
1973	—	2	—
1974	—	2	1
1975	1	1	4
1976	6	1	3
1977	3	5	7
1978	1	2	3
1979	3	1	6
1980	3	6	9
1981	2	8	9
1982	5	7	10
1983	9	10	10
TOTAL	35	46	62/143

have been used. Those operations done in 1971, 1972, and 1973 all failed, and further surgery has been necessary. In the remaining group, except for one hip infected with *Pseudomonas* organisms and converted with a Girdlestone procedure, no revisions because of component loosening have been necessary. There are abundant thin radiolucent lines, but there are none 2 mm in width and no implant migration.

Even though the numbers are not huge and the length of follow-up is relatively short, I have been rather reluctant to change what I am doing for new and unproved procedures. Revisions are being done today that use bone ingrowth fixation. These are experimental procedures, and follow-up of 1 to 2 years of small numbers of patients makes it impossible to know results at this time. It is difficult, if not impossible, to fill the space about the acetabulum previously occupied by bone, which is now destroyed, with prosthesis. Therefore some surgeons are filling this space with bone graft, usually allograft, in conjunction with prostheses designed for bony ingrowth fixation. Although it is too early to know results, it is difficult to imagine bone growing from dead allograft into porous prosthesis to produce fixation. The remainder of this presentation will concern cement fixation only.

Exposure. The exposure method I have used includes trochanteric osteotomy and capsulectomy for complete mobilization of the proximal femur and wide exposure of the acetabulum.

Preparation of bone. A hip gouge may be slipped in the cement–bone interval, and the acetabular prosthesis can be removed, revealing the granulation tissue membrane and bits of cement in the acetabular bed. I have not found a need to cut the implant into pieces before removal. The membrane should be grossly removed with hip gouges and a rongeur. It is this membrane that appeared radiolucent on x-ray study. The membrane, microscopically, is a mass of histiocytes. Remaining membrane and flimsy bone are removed with an acetabular reamer. Extreme care is taken to remove no more bone than absolutely necessary. I believe it is impossible to remove the cells immediately adjacent to the bone with a curette, therefore this final bit of membrane is removed most efficiently and with the least bone destruction by the use of a high-speed, rather large, burr, which finally prepares a bed of acetabular bone of adequate strength. The acetabular cavity at this point is very irregular in shape and has usually been enlarged considerably, but much more superiorly than anteroposteriorly.

A decision must now be made whether to proceed with joint replacement or to settle for pseudoarthrosis or possibly a very large bipolar femoral prosthesis with or without bone graft. The integrity of the posterior and anterior columns is very important in this decision. If the posterior column is not intact, there is no way a joint replacement will be successful. If the anterior column is not intact, the prognosis is certainly guarded. Defects in the bone centrally are less important. The usual case is that, even in situations of significant medial migration of the old, loosened acetabular prosthesis, a layer of new bone about 2 mm thick has been formed ahead of the migrating prosthesis, and there is no significant central defect.

However, central defects of varying sizes can occur. Small central defects are not too important and certainly do not contraindicate joint replacement or, by themselves, require grafting. Large central defects of more than 2 or 3 cm may require grafting but do not contraindicate joint replacement.

Selection of prosthesis. Everyone seems to

agree that polyethylene is a quite adequate bearing material and should be left alone. We became concerned with potential acetabular component loosening a number of years ago when we saw loosening of two general types. One was radiolucency at the cement–bone junction circumferentially that is caused by fatigue failure of trabeculae of either bone or cement or both at that junction. The other mode of failure appears with a crack in the cement near the center of the acetabulum. This is rather clearly fatigue failure of methyl methacrylate.

We reasoned, and I think that most now agree, that reduction of the peak stress in cement or bone would result in a lower incidence of fatigue failure and therefore a lower incidence of prosthetic loosening. We used a computer to study this problem with a mathematic, three-dimensional axisymmetric model. It was found that the peak stresses in compression were at the site of the crack in the cement and that stresses in compression, tension, and shear could be reduced rather significantly by stiffening the prosthesis. The most effective way to stiffen the prosthesis is to give it a metal back. This profoundly reduces the peak stress in both cement and bone by distributing the load much more evenly.[5] Carter and associates subsequently found similar results with a two-dimensional model.[2] Therefore, it is apparent that it is quite desirable to use a metal-backed acetabular prosthesis.

Although adding a ring helps a little, it does not help enough to justify significant dissection to make the ring fit. The effect of mesh is so minimal compared to the metal shell that it no longer deserves a place in our armamentarium. Just a small increase in the external diameter of the prosthesis from 40 to 48 mm results in a rather dramatic increase in the volume and surface area of the hemisphere. The greater the surface area, the greater the area through which the load is transferred from prosthesis to cement and presumably the lower the stresses in the cement. Therefore the largest prosthesis that will fit in the AP diameter in the inferior aspect of the cavity should be used. The internal socket diameter is irrelevant.

Reconstruction of the geometry of the hip. The acetabular prosthesis should not be placed medial to the floor of the original acetabular notch so that the load is distributed to the dense bone in the iliac bar. Within this constraint, the acetabular prosthesis should be placed as far medially, inferiorly, and anteriorly as possible. This placement results in the lowest possible total load across the hip joint. This is the most important point of all the variables in acetabular reconstruction. If the center of rotation of the prosthetic acetabulum is much more than 1 cm superolateral to its normal location, the total load on the joint will be increased considerably with resultant increase in the incidence of recurrent loosening. In addition, the force needed in the abductor muscles to prevent limping is so high that a significant limp is almost inevitable.[1,4] Therefore it is very important that the acetabular prosthesis be placed in the same location. This usually results in the creation of a gap previously occupied by bone now destroyed. This gap may be predominantly medial, as in Fig. 17-10, or predominantly superior, as in Fig. 17-11. In either case the gap must be filled with something, either prosthesis, bone graft, or cement.

An inventory of prostheses would need to be unrealistically large to fill the gap with prosthesis. Use of bone allografts can be accomplished tech-

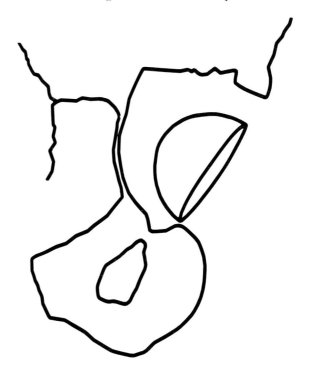

Fig. 17-10. Line drawing of postoperative x-ray film demonstrating gap between prosthesis and bone, which is predominantly medial.

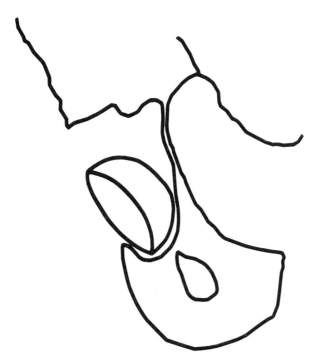

Fig. 17-11. Line drawing of postoperative x-ray film demonstrating gap between prosthesis and bone, which is predominantly superior.

nically and is currently popular, but it results in short term (3- to 5-year) failure rates in the 20% range.[3,6] However, cement can be used to fill the gap quite nicely. As long as cement is used for fixation there is no reason not to use it to fill the gap. The results have been predictably good.

Cement fixation. There has been much controversy through the years concerning whether low viscosity cement or doughy cement is more advantageous. The less viscous the cement, the easier it is to get the cement to penetrate trabecular bone. In my judgment, it is necessary that the cement penetrate the bone probably 1 mm or less, only so far as to produce just enough interdigitation to create a strong bond. If the bone is bleeding—and in my experience it is always bleeding, even with hypotensive anesthesia—it is necessary that the cement be viscous enough to displace the blood, or the blood will mix with the cement. It is well known that the mixing of cement and blood or fat profoundly weakens the cement. Therefore using cement in a rather doughy state is desirable.

Putting pressure on acetabular cement makes it more likely to fill the cavity and probably more likely to penetrate bone. The question is, how do you put pressure on acetabular cement? I try to do so with a flat plunger-type apparatus, most of the time with at least partial success. However, the acetabulum has a rather wide and sometimes irregular mouth, therefore it is not really practical to put a lot of pressure on acetabular cement, as desirable as it may be. I certainly find the argument for centrifuging cement sensible and convincing, and I have been centrifuging cement for the last couple of years. However, even though centrifugation removes the small voids in the cement, if in handling the cement the surgeon permits larger voids to develop, the cement will be just as weak.

SUMMARY

Very predictable results can be obtained from revision of the aseptically loose acetabular prosthesis by using cement fixation if: (1) the hip is taken apart completely so that complete access to the acetabulum is obtained, (2) a bed of bone of adequate strength completely devoid of soft tissue is prepared, (3) a new prosthesis, backed with a metal shell, is selected to distribute the applied load as evenly as possible and thus minimize peak stresses in cement or bone, and (4) this prosthesis is inserted as far medially, inferiorly, and anteriorly as possible to create a new anatomic geometry that, during function, will place as little load on the hip as possible.

REFERENCES

1. Callaghan, J.J., Salvati, E.A., Pellicci, P.M., Wilson, P.D., Jr., and Ranawat, C.S.: Two to five year results of revision total hip replacement: Have we improved? J. Bone Joint Surg. **67A**(7):1074-1085, 1985.
2. Carter, D., Vasu, R., and Harris, W.: Stress distributions in the acetabular region—II: Effects of cement thickness and metal backing of the total hip acetabular component, J. Biomech. **15**(3):165-171, 1982.
3. Conn, R., Peterson, L., Stauffer, R., and Ilstrup, D.: Management of acetabular deficiency: Long-term results of bone grafting the acetabulum in total hip arthroplasty, scientific program, American Academy of Orthopaedic Surgeons, Jan. 1985.
4. Johnston, R., Brand, R., and Crownshield, R.: Reconstruction of the hip, J. Bone Joint Surg. **61A**(5):639-652, 1979.
5. Peterson, D., Crownshield, R., Brand, R., and Johnston, R.: An axisymmetric model of acetabular components in total hip arthroplasty, J. Biomech. **15**(4):305-315, 1982.
6. Trancik, T., Stulberg, B., Wilde, A., and Feiglin, D.: Allografting of severely deficient acetabulae in revision total hip arthroplasty, scientific program, American Academy of Orthopaedic Surgeons, Jan. 1985.

Part E

Revision of femoral component loosening with titanium ingrowth prosthesis and bone grafting

RAMON B. GUSTILO

The current standard practice in the United States is for the orthopaedic surgeon to revise a failed cemented primary total hip arthroplasty with another cemented total hip. However, accumulating reports[1-5,7-11] strongly suggest that the expected failure rate associated with such revision is unacceptably high.

The basic problems on removal of a loose cemented femoral component are:

1. There is a large proximal canal with thin cortices and often bone loss medially. Good cementing even with two or more packages of cement is difficult to achieve (Fig. 17-12, *A*).
2. A longer stem is needed for stability. Sometimes a window is made for cement removal, or with use of power reamers, a hole is inadvertently made and a longer stem is needed to go beyond the defect to provide stability and protection from fracture at the defect area.
3. Instability leads to high incidence of dislocation.

During the last 4 years, we started a treatment program for nonseptic loosening of femoral component with a press-fit anatomic design prosthesis (BIAS) and primary cancellous bone grafting proximally in an attempt to solve the problem of increased failure of revision with a cemented femoral component.[6] The concept is based on:

1. Proximal biologic ingrowth, located anteriorly and posteriorly (Figs. 17-12, *B* and 17-13)
2. Long curved stem and AP dimensions to fit the intramedullary canal
3. Anteverted head and neck of 12 degrees and carefully measured neck length to provide stability and prevent dislocation. New prosthesis design provides variable, interchangeable head neck length
4. Proximal bone grafting proximally with autogenous iliac cancellous bone

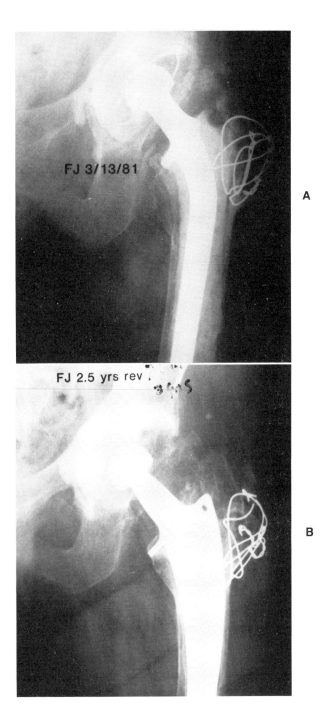

Fig. 17-12. A, F.J., 76 years old, 1 year after third revision with long stem and two packages of bone cement had severe pain and used two crutches for ambulation. AP x-ray films showed loosening at cement–bone interface and marked thinning of the cortices. **B,** F.J., 2½ years after ingrowth revision prosthesis with bone graft; patient is doing well without pain, and x-ray film showed increased cortical thickness.

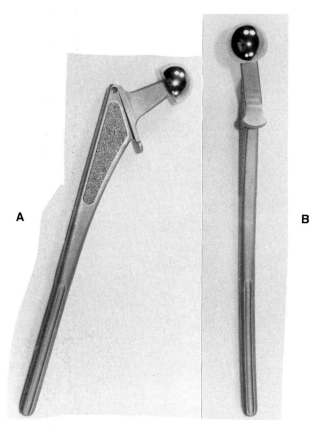

Fig. 17-13. A, Front view of titanium porous ingrowth prosthesis. **B,** Lateral view of titanium porous ingrowth prosthesis.

SURGICAL TECHNIQUE

We take large AP and lateral x-ray films in 3- or 6-foot projections and make a template of these x-ray films with 20% or 10% distortion magnification. The intramedullary canal then is measured using the x-ray template with correct magnification.

Two sizes of the intramedullary stem are recommended for every revision procedure to achieve intramedullary stability by proper selection of stem size. Hip revision surgery is to be done with trochanteric removal. The surgeon should have a straight view of the intramedullary canal from above. Bone cement is removed with specialized osteotomes and powered reamers, which seldom have been used over the last 2 years. A window rarely is made on the shaft to remove cement. The canal is irrigated copiously with jet lavage, which is followed by flexible reaming until the isthmus is passed. I usually ream 2 mm or more than the actual size of the stem to accommodate the long curved stem. A proximal rasp usually is not needed because of

the wide canal. The prosthesis is inserted slowly. As the stem passes through the isthmus and fills up the canal, the proximal canal is filled with cancellous bone anteriorly and posteriorly. Cancellous iliac strips are routinely removed through the same incision but extended proximally to the iliac crest. It is not uncommon, however, to supplement autogenous bone with bank bone femoral head. Occasionally a large flexible reamer up to 25 mm in size is needed to accommodate the large-stem prosthesis. The average size that I use now is 15 mm (11 to 21 mm).

The average blood loss was 2021 ml, and average replacement was 2 units of packed red blood cells and 1 unit of whole blood. I have routinely used a cell saver in all revision total hip arthroplasty in the last 2 years and have given back an average of 400 to 500 red blood cells during surgery from the cell saver. Routinely, x-ray films are taken in the operating room on insertion of the femoral component prosthesis before wound closure.

POSTOPERATIVE PROGRAM

The patient is advised to stay on partial weight bearing for the first 6 weeks and full weight bearing after 6 weeks. On the average the patient uses crutches for 3.1 months.

Results. This is a preliminary report of 24 cases of revision total hip arthroplasty for nonseptic loosening with titanium ingrowth prosthesis and cancellous bone grafting proximally. All surgeries were performed by me. The average age of the patient was 55.4 years (range 37 to 74). Mean follow-up after insertion of the ingrowth prosthesis was 23.3 months (range 12 to 44). The results are shown in Table 17-2 using the Harris functional hip scoring system. All patients have done well and improved their functional hip score from 45 preoperatively to 84 postoperatively.

COMPLICATIONS

Postoperative complications consisted of two dislocations, treated successfully with cast immobilization for 6 weeks in one patient, and in another with replacement of acetabular component with a bipolar prosthesis. One acute hematogenous infection occurred following a dental procedure; this was treated successfully with an incision and drainage, leaving the prosthesis in place, and 6 weeks of antibiotic therapy. This patient has been followed for 2 years after sur-

Table 17-2. Hip score of 24 revision hip arthroplasties with ingrowth prosthesis and bone grafting

Maximum points	Preoperative	6 months	1 year	2 years	3 years
Total score (100)	48.0	80.2	83.0	88.3	88.2
Pain (44)	17.9	38.1	41.7	41.6	42.0
Limp (11)	2.5	7.8	8.4	9.2	9.5
Support (11)	6.8	7.8	7.9	10.2	11.0
Distance (11)	4.7	7.8	6.3	8.6	8.0
Function (14)	9.1	10.5	10.0	10.8	9.0
Deformity (4)	3.0	4.0	4.0	3.2	4.0
ROM (5)	4.5	4.6	4.7	4.7	4.7

gery without recurrence of sepsis and with a normal sedimentation rate. None has been revised so far for loosening of the femoral component.

SUMMARY

Preliminary results of 24 cementless revision hips are very encouraging and show no evidence of loosening at 12 to 45 months follow-up. With the problem inherent in femoral component loosening and the high incidence of failure from cemented revision total hip arthroplasty, the use of a porous ingrowth long stem prosthesis fitted to the canal with bone grafting proximally offers a logical solution to a very difficult problem.

REFERENCES

1. Amstutz, H.D., Ma, S.M., Jinnah, R.H., and Mai, L.: Revision of aseptic loose total hip arthroplasties, Clin. Orthop. **170:**21, 1982.
2. Broughton, N.S., and Rushton, N.: Revision hip arthroplasty, Acta Orthop. Scand. **53:**923, 1982.
3. Cavanaugh, B.F., and Fitzgerald, R.: Analysis of 219 revisions of total hip replacements. Papers presented at the Mid-American Association Meeting, Mayo Clinic, Rochester, Minnesota, 1982.
4. Dandy, D.J., and Theodorou, B.C.: The management of local complications of total hip replacement by the McKee-Farrar technique, J. Bone Joint Surg. **57B:**30, 1975.
5. Esses, S., Hastings, D., and Schatzker, J.: Revision of total hip arthroplasty, Can. J. Surg. **4:**345-347, 1983.
6. Gustilo, R.B., and Kyle, R.F.: Revision of femoral component loosening with titanium ingrowth prosthesis and bone grafting, Symposium on revision of failed total hip arthroplasty. In Welch, R.B., editor: The hip: Proceedings of the twelfth open scientific meeting of The Hip Society, St. Louis, 1984, C.V. Mosby Co.
7. Hoogland, T., Razzano, C.D., Marks, K.E., and Wilde, A.H.: Revision of hip Mueller total hip arthroplasties, Clin. Orthop. **161:**180-185, 1981.
8. Hunter, G.A., Welsh, R.P., Cameron, H.U., and Bailey, W.H.: The results of revision of total hip arthroplasty, J. Bone Joint Surg. **61B:**419, 1979.
9. Pellicci, P.M., Wilson, P.D., Sledge, C.M., Salvati, E., Ranawat, C.S., Callaghan, J., and Poss, R.: Long term results of revision total hip replacements, Orthop. Trans. J. Bone Joint Surg. **8:**202, 1984.
10. Pellicci, P.M., Wilson, P.D., Sledge, C.M., Salvati, E., Ranawat, C.S., Callaghan, J., and Poss, R.: Revision total hip arthroplasty, Clin. Orthop. **170:**34, 1982.
11. Reigstad, A., and Hetland, K.R.: Rearthroplasty after conventional total hip prosthesis and double-cup prosthesis, Arch. Orthop. Trauma Surg. **103:**152-155, 1984.

Part F

Salvage of acetabular insufficiency with cementless components

WILLIAM R. MURRAY

Acetabular insufficiency resulting from failed total arthroplasty, trauma, or tumor leaves few alternatives with which to salvage a functional hip. When, in the surgeon's judgment, the use of bone cement is not indicated (for example, inadequate bone stock, fracture nonunion, sensitivity to cement, infection), the alternatives include bipolar devices, press-fit cementless acetabular components with porous outer surfaces, threaded metallic outer shells with polyethylene inserts, and threaded ceramic acetabular components. This report will not discuss our experience with nonthreaded, porous-surfaced devices (for example, A.M.L.*, P.C.A.†, H.G.‡, APR§) used for acetabular revision.

---

*Richards Medical Co., Memphis, Tenn.
†Howmedica, Rutherford, N.J.
‡Zimmer, Warsaw, Ind.
§Intermedics Orthopedics, Austin, Tex.

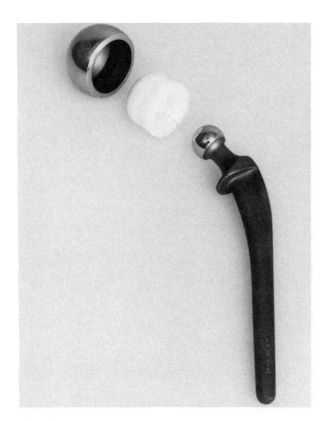

Fig. 17-14. Photo of a disassembled bipolar prosthesis.

BIPOLAR PROSTHESIS SALVAGE FOR ACETABULAR INSUFFICIENCY

Bipolar prostheses (Fig. 17-14), usually with supplemental bone graft, were used in 79 patients (81 hips) between November 1977 and December 1985 as salvage procedures for bone-deficient acetabula or nonunited acetabular fractures at the University of California, San Francisco (UCSF). Seventy-three patients (75 hips) had failed total arthroplasties; five, nonunited acetabular fractures; and one, metastatic carcinoma to the right ilium.

The femoral component was removed for cause only, for example, loosening, malposition, malrotation, or leg-length discrepancy. Therefore it is necessary to have bipolar prostheses available whose inside diameter is consistent with the diameter of the head of the femoral component in place (22, 26, 28, or 32 mm) and whose outside diameter fills the acetabulum.

Technique. A transtrochanteric lateral approach is our standard approach: it was used in all revision arthroplasties and in two of the nonunited acetabular fractures. The patient is placed routinely in the lateral decubitus position, and the extremity is draped free, with the iliac crest included in the operative field. No scrubbing or washing of the skin is done in the operating room. All patients shower with pHisoHex the night before and the morning of surgery; the skin preparation in the operating room is 1% tincture of iodine. A total capsulectomy is performed routinely. Intravenous antibiotics are started at the time of induction of anesthesia in those who have not been operated on before and after representative tissue specimens are obtained for microscopic and bacteriologic analysis in patients who have had surgery. In the patients who have not had prior surgery, the intravenous antibiotics are discontinued on the third to fifth postoperative day, whereas in the revision group, antibiotics are continued intravenously until the final bacteriologic report is submitted (usually 5 to 7 days postoperatively). Our routine is to initially administer 1 g of cefazolin sodium intravenously as a push dose over 3 to 5 minutes and then to add 1 g to the intravenous solution to be run in slowly during the remainder of the operation. Postoperatively, 1 g of cefazolin sodium is given intravenously every 6 hours during the postoperative period.

The acetabular component and all cement and scar are removed while preserving as much acetabular bone stock as possible. In all cases the fit between the remaining acetabular bone and the acetabular component is as tight as possible consistent with optimal seating or containment of the prosthesis in the acetabulum. To produce a tight equatorial, or rim, fit of the prosthesis, the acetabulum is reamed with reamers whose cutting diameters are 1 to 2 mm less than the outside diameter of the selected prosthesis. Standard, readily available components range from 44 to 62 mm in outside diameter. Custom or special order prostheses of 64 to 75 mm can be obtained.

Acetabular defects, irregularities, cement fixation holes, penetrations, and nonunited fractures are filled with bone grafts as necessary. Although allografts are frequently used, the patient's own bone is the preferred source of graft. If the femoral head is available, it serves as the bone graft; if not, the ipsilateral iliac crest and outer table of the adjacent ilium may be used. Large defects are filled with solid sections of bone. The remaining bone then is morselized or ground into a "slurry" with a burr. The selected acetabular component then is snapped onto the femoral head and the hip is reduced. The acetabular component with its tight rim fit holds and molds the bone graft (Figs. 17-15 and 17-16).

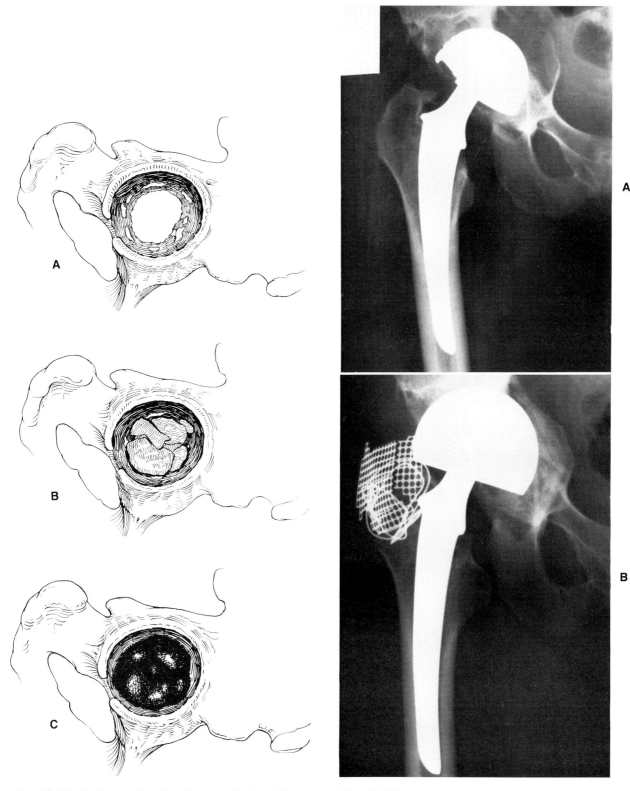

Fig. 17-15. A, Illustration showing acetabular defects. **B,** Major defect filled in with solid sections of bone. **C,** Remaining spaces filled in with morselized bone, or "slurry".

Fig. 17-16. A, Preoperative roentgenogram showing deficiency of medial acetabular wall. **B,** Roentgenogram 11 months after revision shows incorporation of bone graft.

THREADED ACETABULAR DEVICES

The threaded ceramic acetabular device has limited application in revision total hip surgery, since it must be used only against a ceramic head. (Ceramic acetabular devices are no longer used at UCSF.) Recently, three types of threaded metallic shells with polyethylene inserts have become available: two are hemispheric, and the other is a truncated cone (Bio-Met) identical in size and shape to the ceramic devices (Fig. 17-17). They all accept high-density polyethylene (HDP) inserts of 22, 26, 28, and 32 mm inside diameters. The hemispheric devices are of two types: the Mecron ring, in which the HDP insert is fitted flush to the rim of the ring; and the Anderson ring, with 10-degree and 20-degree offset inserts that can be "dialed" into position to produce maximal stability, resulting in the offset portion of the insert being proud of the rim of the ring (see Fig. 17-17).

Technique. All cement and scar are removed, defects are grafted, and the acetabulum is reamed to the inner-thread diameter. The self-

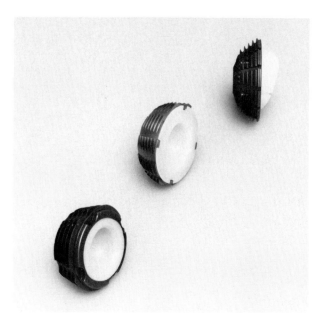

Fig. 17-17. Photograph of the three types of metal threaded shells. *From left to right:* the Bio-Met, the Mecron, and the Anderson. The Anderson device illustrates the 20-degree offset insert.

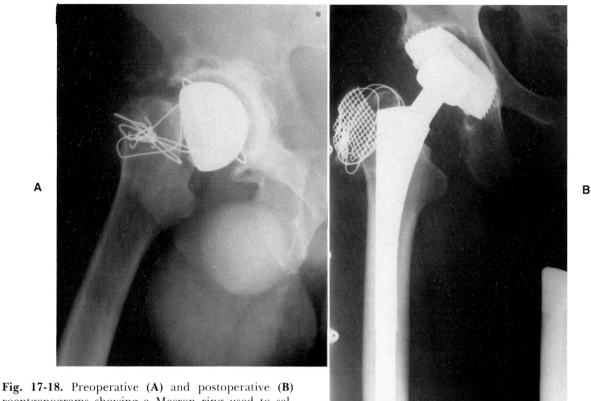

Fig. 17-18. Preoperative **(A)** and postoperative **(B)** roentgenograms showing a Mecron ring used to salvage a failed surface replacement with a cementless femoral component.

tapping rings are inserted to the base of the acetabulum. The HDP inserts are then fixed in position.

Indications. The threaded devices have been used at UCSF to salvage acetabular deficiency following total hip arthroplasties when inadequate bone stock would not permit the use of either cemented devices or nonthreaded porous surface devices, or, when there was insufficient coverage to result in a stable hip joint with a bipolar device (Fig. 17-18). In addition, five patients with five bipolar prostheses that had been inserted following failed standard total hip arthroplasty experienced chronic or repeated dislocations or subluxations because of inadequate bone containment of the bipolar device. Use of the threaded Anderson ring with 20-degree offset inserts resulted in stable, pain-free, functional hip joints (Fig. 17-19).

POSTOPERATIVE CARE

Postoperative care is essentially the same for the bipolar and threaded devices. Postoperatively, the patients are placed in either balanced suspension or a continuous passive motion machine. Out-of-bed activity is started when the suction drains are removed, usually by the third day. Weight-bearing with two crutches (with 25% body weight on the affected side) is continued for 8 weeks. If at that time there is no evidence of component migration, the grafts appear to be incorporating or are incorporated, and the trochanteric repair is stable, weight-bearing is increased to 50% of body weight with one or two walking aids. However, if pain or limp is present, the patient is advised to continue using two crutches. All patients are advised that these are salvage procedures, and permanent external support is prescribed (but the prescription is not universally followed).

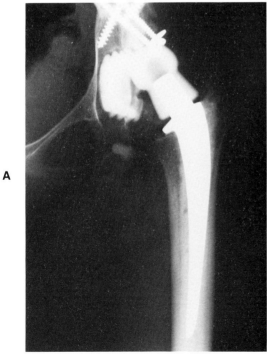
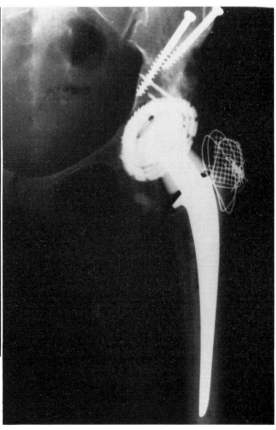

A **B**

Fig. 17-19. Preoperative (**A**) and postoperative (**B**) roentgenograms of an Anderson ring used to salvage an unstable and fractured ceramic total hip replacement.

SUMMARY

In conclusion, it appears that large outside-diameter bipolar devices or threaded, cement-free acetabular components (with or without porous surfaces) provide excellent hip stability when used to salvage hips with acetabular insufficiency. The bipolar or threaded devices can maintain or restore normal or nearly normal hip mechanics, minimize pain by preventing motion between the cup and the bone, and permit fill-in of bony defects and healing of nonunited fractures. Bone grafting should be used whenever possible, since it may prevent medial migration and allow for replacement with a cemented or cementless porous-surfaced cup in the future should pain occur. A cane or crutch should be used to minimize stress across the joint and thereby prolong the life of the reconstruction. All patients must realize that these are salvage procedures.

Chapter 18

Principles, techniques, results, and complications with a porous-coated sintered metal system

CHARLES A. ENGH

J. DENNIS BOBYN

In response to the overall dissatisfaction with the long-term results associated with cemented hip arthroplasty, particularly in younger and more active patients, a variety of porous-coated implants designed for biologic fixation by tissue ingrowth are being evaluated.[1,9] The goal with the concept of biologic fixation is to establish a more natural and enduring interface between artificial and living materials and hence overcome the problem of aseptic late loosening that is so prevalent in joint replacement surgery. Since the early 1970s the sintered type of metallic porous surface has been shown experimentally to be extremely efficacious for bone ingrowth.[11] Clinical use of a modified Moore-type femoral stem incorporating the sintered porous coating began cautiously in a few North American centers in the middle to late 1970s and has grown rapidly and widely since FDA approval in 1983. Our clinical follow-up currently encompasses over 1000 noncemented primary cases since 1977, and the success that has been obtained to date has resulted in optimism for the future and continued advocation of the use of this new technique.

Throughout the past 8 years a learning curve has naturally been experienced. Surgical principles and implant designs have been refined and modified to respect the different and sometimes demanding nature of noncemented fixation. Some of the problems unique to biologic fixation

arthroplasty have been recognized and solved; expanding knowledge and improving technology no doubt will result in further change. This chapter will discuss the most important principles related to surgery and implant design, the clinical results for primary cases, and the problems that are unique to bone ingrowth implant systems and some of their solutions. Emphasis will be placed on the femoral side of arthroplasty because of greater experience with porous-coated femoral prostheses.

PRINCIPLES OF IMPLANT DESIGN
Femoral component

The most difficult problems with implant fixation in total hip arthroplasty exist on the femoral side. The high loads acting on the femoral head in combination with the complex loading configuration and the eccentric nature of the neck and shaft are the cause. The use of a porous surface to enhance press-fit fixation is therefore more important on the femoral side than on the acetabular side. Bone growth into a porous metal surface is an extremely effective tool—cortical bone ingrowth can result in shear fixation strength on the order of 1 ton per square inch.[2] In order to maximize the potential for this type of fixation strength, it is important that the stem be of a design that will be inherently stable within the femur upon implantation. It is also important to achieve uniform contact of the porous surface of the implant with host bone, particularly cortical bone in view of its high inherent strength and ability to fully withstand weight-bearing loads. Adherence to these principles will result not only in good immediate implant stability by a frictional fit but also in the optimal conditions for the fastest rate of development of additional implant stability by bone ingrowth.[3,4]

There are two general approaches to femoral implant design. One is to design "anatomic" stems with shapes that reflect the internal geometry of the femur. The anatomic shape is typically derived by averaging contour information obtained by image analysis (such as CT scanning) of a large number of femurs and is chosen to conform closely to the inner, most cortical, shape of the femur. The advantage of this approach is that a tight fit can be achieved with extensive cortical bone–implant contact area. Anatomic stems are generally slightly curved, and this helps to render the implanted stem stable against rotational forces. A problem with this approach is that the "averaged" stem shape does not conform well in cases with pathologic distortion of anatomy in the femoral neck region. Also, preparation of the

channel for an anatomic stem is not as easily or as accurately performed as it is for a stem with more regular or symmetric geometry. Finally, anatomic stems leave the surgeon little or no scope for slight adjustment in stem position to optimize the degree of head anteversion for maximum stability against dislocation.

The second approach to femoral implant design, which we prefer, is to use a more symmetric straight stem geometry as depicted in Fig. 18-1. This allows the inner shape of the proximal femur to be simply but precisely modified to a regular implant configuration. A round straight stem facilitates modification of the femur by drilling to obtain a tight press fit in the isthmus region of the femur well away from the area of common pathologic distortion and nonanatomic geometry. It also allows rotation within the pre-drilled intramedullary canal to a position approximating the patient's degree of femoral head anteversion. Finally, a symmetric implant design eliminates the need for right and left versions, thus reducing inventory.

The prosthesis in use is fabricated from surgical grade cobalt-based alloy (ASTM F-75). The implant is initially cast and subsequently porous

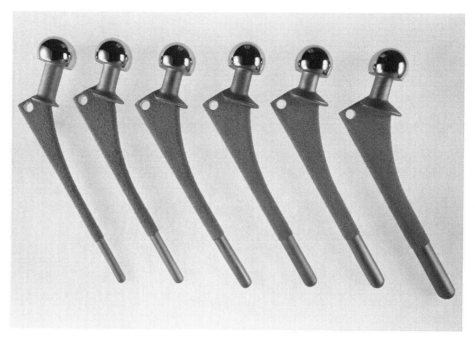

Fig. 18-1. Photograph of the partially porous-coated femoral stem design in a range of stem diameters. (From Engh, C.A., and Bobyn, J.D.: Biological fixation in total hip arthroplasty, Thorofare, N.J., 1985, Slack, Inc.)

coated using powder metallurgy and sintering techniques previously described in the literature.[10,11] Computerized image analysis of the porous surface structure has indicated a volume porosity of 35% to 40% and an average pore size of approximately 250 micrometers.[6] More than 80% of the pores fall within the size range of 45 to 410 micrometers, a range demonstrated under controlled experimental conditions to be optimal for the development of the greatest fixation strength in the shortest time period.[2] From 1977 to 1982 the femoral component was available in fully porous-coated design with a diameter of 10.5 mm. Since 1982 the porous coating was removed from the distal 5.0 cm of the stem, and a range of stem diameters from 9.0 mm to 18.0 mm in 1.5 mm increments has been available. In 1984 clinical trials began with the same stem design but with the porous coating confined to the proximal two fifths of the stem length. These changes in the level of the porous coating were made in response to the concerns about stress shielding and implant removal.

Acetabular component

Component fixation on the acetabular side is not as much of a problem because of the simpler geometry and loading configuration. It is generally accepted that a hemispheric component design is preferable, because it simplifies surgical preparation of the implant site and minimizes bone resection. Immediate implant stability can be achieved by using spikes or screws in the case of porous-coated implants or self-tapping threads for threaded cup designs. Because of the inherently stable shape of the acetabulum, it may not be necessary to use micromechanical interlock such as achieved by bone growth into a porous surface to ensure enduring fixation. Increasing evidence exists that the macromechanical interlock achieved with self-tapping threaded cup designs may prove to suffice in the long term.[9] It is also generally agreed that a noncemented cup should be designed to be modular, with an outer reinforcing metal shell and an inner polyethylene liner (Fig. 18-2). This two-part system is versatile, allowing for replacement or interchanging of the liner should it ever be necessary. The use of a liner with an eccentric extended bearing surface is helpful in preventing dislocation.

Noncemented porous-coated or threaded acetabular components have been used since 1982. Before then conventional cemented acetabular components or bipolar-type components were

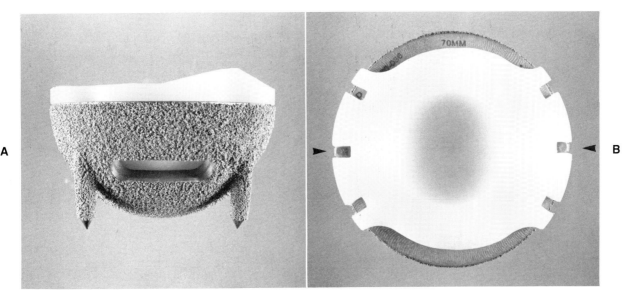

Fig. 18-2. A and **B,** Photographs of a porous-coated modular acetabular cup design. Initial stability is achieved with three spikes. The metal shell has slots to enable positive determination of complete seating during impaction. The polyethylene liner has an eccentric lip that can be adjusted to one of three positions for maximal stability against dislocation (see *arrow,* **B**). (From Engh, C.A., and Bobyn, J.D.: Biological fixation in total hip arthroplasty, Thorofare, N.J., 1985, Slack, Inc.)

used in conjunction with the porous-coated femoral components.

SURGICAL PRINCIPLES
Femur

To simplify understanding of the principles underlying preparation of the femur and insertion of the prosthesis, the femoral implant can be divided into three parts: a straight rod portion to fit the hollow femoral tube or intramedullary canal, a proximal triangular portion to fit the intertrochanteric region, and a head and neck portion adjustable to accommodate leg length and hip stability considerations (Fig. 18-3). As illustrated in Fig. 18-4, the rod section of the prosthesis is inserted down the canal and positioned so that the triangular section fits the intertrochanteric region, accepting when possible the pathologic degree of anteversion or retroversion already present. The channel for the rod portion is prepared by intramedullary reaming, and all subsequent surgery is oriented to that channel.[6]

Acetabulum

Because it can be difficult or impossible to adjust the rotation of the femoral component to the perfect amount of anteversion, the acetabulum should be prepared bearing in mind the predetermined degree of femoral implant rotation. For instance, if a pathologic process such as hip dysplasia forces the neck of the implant to lie in forward rotation of 45 degrees or more, the acetabulum must be placed in a subnormal forward placement to prevent anterior hip subluxation. Since it is not always possible to fix mechan-

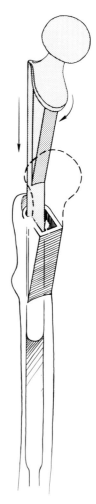

Fig. 18-4. Schematic illustration of the rod portion of the prosthesis being inserted down the drilled intramedullary canal and rotated to a position filling the intertrochanteric region corresponding to the degree of head anteversion. (From Engh, C.A., and Bobyn, J.D.: Biological fixation in total hip arthroplasty, Thorofare, N.J., 1985, Slack, Inc.)

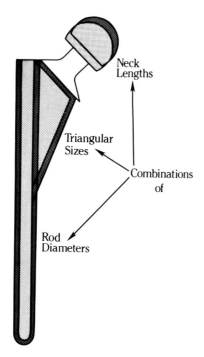

Fig. 18-3. The femoral stem inventory consists of combinations of different rod diameters, triangular sizes, and neck lengths. (From Engh, C.A., and Bobyn, J.D.: Biological fixation in total hip arthroplasty, Thorofare, N.J., 1985, Slack, Inc.)

ically a porous-coated or threaded acetabular component with the optimal orientation to match the femoral rotation, an eccentric polyethylene liner can be used to compensate for such a deficiency and thus enhance hip stability.

Preoperative planning and templates

Because the noncemented implants generally fill the prepared implant site and leave little or no room for further adjustment during the final implantation step, the procedure should be planned preoperatively using true AP and lateral radiographs and implant template overlays. The preoperative planning sequence should take place in a stepwise fashion similar to the surgical implantation of the components. The femur must be assessed for implant fit in terms of rod diameter, rod length, proximal triangular width, and neck length. The lateral x-ray films of the femur should be used to determine the best location for drilling the pilot hole (usually anterior to the intertrochanteric fossa) for the path down the intramedullary canal to compensate for variations in the amount of anterior and forward flexion of the femoral neck and the extent of the curve of the femoral shaft. The lateral x-ray films are also very important in determining the maximum diameter of the implant, since this is dictated largely by the size of the double bow or S shape of the femur, a geometry not appreciated on AP inspection alone. The acetabulum must be assessed for implant size, sphericity of shape, and overall orientation. The exact position of the acetabular component within the pelvis must be determined before selection of the head and neck length segment for the femoral component in order to accurately plan restoration of leg length equality.

Surgery

The surgical procedure has been detailed and illustrated in a prior publication.[6] The five sequential steps should include:

1. Intramedullary drilling
2. Evaluation of femoral head and neck rotation and preparation of the recess for the triangular portion of the implant to match this rotation
3. Insertion of the porous-coated or threaded acetabular shell in a matching position of rotation
4. Insertion of the trial femoral component to check for femoral leg length and hip stability
5. Selection of the proper rotation for the acetabular liner to maximize hip stability

Certain aspects of this sequence need to be emphasized.

1. The channel for the femoral stem is prepared before resection and preparation of the femoral neck to ensure that the neck preparation is precisely oriented to the intramedullary pathway.
2. The pilot hole for the intramedullary channel must be started well back in the trochanter to ensure a straight path down the femoral shaft. The pilot hole must be selected to allow for the S shaped femoral curve.
3. The channel is prepared with a series of progressively larger rigid reamers with cutting flutes extending for a length equivalent to the stem length. Use of a flexible reamer or reamer with only a small length of cutting edge and a narrower shank will prevent reaming of a perfectly straight channel and result in problems with stem impaction. The diameter of the final reamer must match that of the prosthesis.
4. Preparation of the acetabulum for a noncemented acetabular component generally requires greater exposure than with cemented arthroplasty, particularly for threaded components, since the capsule must be stripped away from the rim around its entire circumference to prevent soft tissue impingement during screw insertion.
5. The final implant sites are prepared with exacting tolerances, and changes in implant position cannot be made during final implant insertion. Thus the use of trial components for establishing tightness of fit, leg length equality, and hip stability is particularly important before implantation.
6. The components are inserted with an extremely tight frictional fit. They should not easily "drop in" to the implant site. The femoral component, for example, should only advance several millimeters at a time with each mallet blow until final seating. Implant removal after this type of forceful impaction would be difficult, emphasizing the importance of the use of trial components.

Postoperative management

If the components are inserted with a tight press fit and the postoperative x-ray films demonstrate good canal filling on the femoral side and complete seating on the acetabular side, the patient is kept on crutches for 6 weeks after surgery. If otherwise, it may be necessary to restrict weight bearing for longer postoperative intervals (up to 12 weeks) to give more time for biologic fixation by bone ingrowth. It should be strictly emphasized, however, that the process of bone ingrowth cannot be relied on routinely for stabilization of a poorly inserted or fitting component.

FOLLOW-UP

The cases have been assessed clinically in terms of a modified D'Aubigne 6-point pain and walking scale (Table 18-1). This modification was made in order to render the scales more applicable to the study of bone ingrowth prostheses. Variables such as patient age, disease process, and implant design were examined for influence on the clinical results. The cases were divided according to stem fit based on study of a postoperative AP radiograph, category 1 representing those in which there was a press fit at the isthmus and category 2 representing those in which there was an obvious mismatch in stem and canal diameter. The influence of this parameter on the clinical results was also evaluated. In addition to the clinical assessment, AP and lateral radiographs of comparable orientation and exposure were taken at regular intervals and studied for evidence of bone ingrowth and adaptive bone modeling adjacent to the implants. For these purposes the femur was divided into 4 levels. Level 1 corresponds to the proximal triangular portion of the stem, level 2 to the straight portion of the stem above the isthmus that does not contact the endosteal cortex, level 3 to the isthmus region where the stem fits tightest, and level 4 to the region below the region of tightest fit (Fig. 18-5). The anterior, posterior, medial, and lateral aspects of the femur in each level (a total of 16 sites) were examined at each time interval for evidence of bone formation or resorption. In order to assess the validity of the concept of biologic fixation, several femora intact with the prosthesis have been retrieved at autopsy and processed for undecalcified thin-section histology to permit light microscopic examination of the bone-implant interface.[6]

Patient evaluation currently extends to 8 years. The total number of consecutive primary cases at each yearly interval is listed in Table 18-2 (as of January, 1985). Also included is the number of cases followed at each yearly interval. The difference in the yearly numbers represents those cases lost to follow-up because of patient death or the inability to obtain records. A total of 341 of the 400 cases performed before 1985 have both an adequate 1-year clinical assessment and a complete series of comparable x-ray films. The prevalent diagnosis in these 341 cases was osteoarthritis (228 of 341), followed by rheumatoid arthritis (47 of 341) and avascular necrosis (47 of 341). There were 189 females and 148 males. One hundred and eleven cases were in patients 50 years or younger and the remaining 230 were in patients over 50 years of age. In 179 cases the

Table 18-1. Description of the D'Aubigne 6-point pain and walking scores*

Pain	Points	Walking
No pain	6	No cane

No pain
  tires easily
	5	No cane
		  limps intermittently

Pain on weight bearing
  only a start up hesitancy
	4	Cane
		  outdoors, only for distance

Pain on weight bearing
  upon start up and with use
	3	Cane
		  always outdoors

Pain—restricted activity
  not at rest
	2	Cane—restricted activity
		  severe limp

Continuous pain	1	Housebound

*Modified to be more applicable to bone ingrowth fixation prostheses. Modified from D'Aubigné, R.M., and Postel, M.: J. Bone Joint Surg. **36A:**451, 1954.

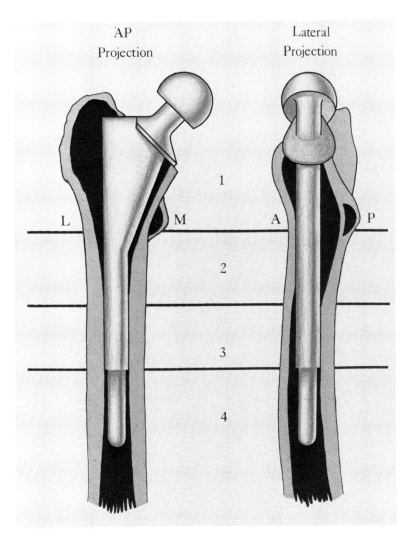

AP
Projection

Lateral
Projection

Fig. 18-5. Schematic illustration of AP and lateral views of an implanted partially porous-coated stem with the femur divided into 4 levels (see text). These are the 4 levels referred to in Tables 3 and 4. (From Engh, C.A., and Bobyn, J.D.: Biological fixation in total hip arthroplasty, Thorofare, N.J., 1985, Slack, Inc.)

Table 18-2. Cases followed by yearly intervals/mean D'Aubigne pain and walking scores

| | *Years since surgery* | | | | | | |
	1	*2*	*3*	*4*	*5*	*6*	*7*
Total number of cases	400	214	124	57	26	14	6
Cases with complete follow-up	341	178	103	50	20	4	2
Average pain score	5.8	5.7	5.7	5.8	5.8	5.5	5.5
Average walking score	5.6	5.5	5.6	5.7	5.6	5.5	5.5

femoral stems were fully porous coated, in 145 they were coated to within 5.0 cm of the stem tip, and in the remaining 17 they were coated only on the proximal two fifths of the stem.

RESULTS
Clinical evaluation

The average D'Aubigne pain and walking scores at yearly intervals are listed in Table 18-2. The scores are all excellent, averaging 5.5 out of 6.0 or better. As a group, patients 50 years and younger have an average score 0.1 or 0.2 point higher at all time intervals compared with patients over 50 years of age. A similar result has been found for patients with a category 1 stem fit as compared with a category 2 stem fit. No difference in clinical ratings has yet been demonstrable with the cases divided according to disease process or stem design (in terms of extent of porous coating). No difference has been observed between cases with cemented and noncemented acetabular components, although the follow-up time for the porous-coated and threaded cups is much shorter than for the cemented cups. One femoral component has been removed for loosening. There have been no infections. Complications not related to the implant design itself have been no different from those of cemented arthroplasty.

Radiographic and histologic evaluation: bone modeling

The details of adaptive bone modeling have been discussed in previous publications.[5-8] Evidence of both bone resorption and formation has been observed radiographically, and for the most part this occurs within the first year after surgery. There is a general trend for bone resorption to

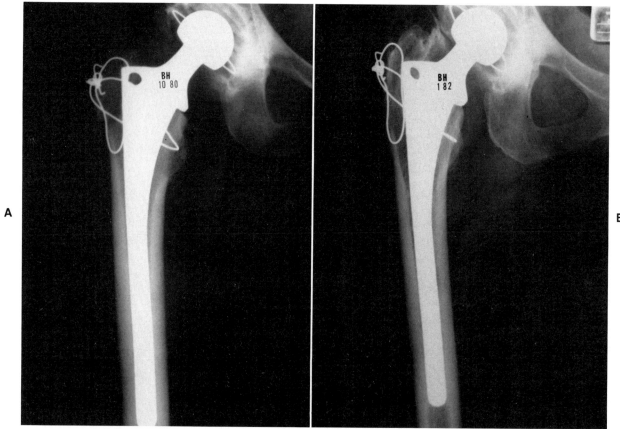

Fig. 18-6. Postoperative **(A)** and 18-month **(B)** radiographs of an implanted 10.5 mm fully porous-coated stem. Rounding off and slight loss of density in the proximal medial cortex (level 1) has occurred. The remainder of the femur appears unchanged. (From Engh, C.A., and Bobyn, J.D.: Biological fixation in total hip arthroplasty, Thorofare, N.J., 1985, Slack, Inc.)

occur proximally and bone formation to occur distally, indicating that the femoral stem funnels load away from the intertrochanteric region to the region of tight fit in the shaft. In the vast majority of cases the resorption has not been serious, remaining confined to the proximal medial cortex as illustrated in Fig. 18-6. This is particularly true with cases in which 9.0, 10.5, 12.0, 13.5, or 15.0 mm stem diameters were used. More recently the use of larger and more flexurally rigid stems has increased, and the degree of bone loss has been noticeably more extensive and serious (Fig. 18-7). As a means of illustrating this general trend, the incidence of bone resorption (either thinning or darkening of the cortex on x-ray films) at 1 year as a function of level in the femur and stem diameter is listed in tabular form in Table 18-3. It is clear (from Table 18-3) that the incidence of bone resorption is greatest

with stem diameters above 12.0 mm and in levels 1 and 2 (as highlighted by the bold type). The incidence of bone formation (either thickening or whitening of the cortex on x-ray film) at 1 year as a function of level in the femur and stem diameter is listed in Table 18-4. There is a tendency for bone to form primarily adjacent to the distal portion of the stem, in levels 3 and 4, regardless of stem diameter (in bold type).

Another common manifestation of adaptive bone modeling is that of radiopaque line formation. The typical radiopaque line is about 1.0 mm in thickness and develops adjacent to the stem but separated from it by a radiolucent space varying from about 0.5 to 1.0 mm. These radiopaque lines are almost exclusively limited to the areas of the uncoated portions of the femoral stem and generally develop only adjacent to small regions of the stem, although the rest of the bone-implant

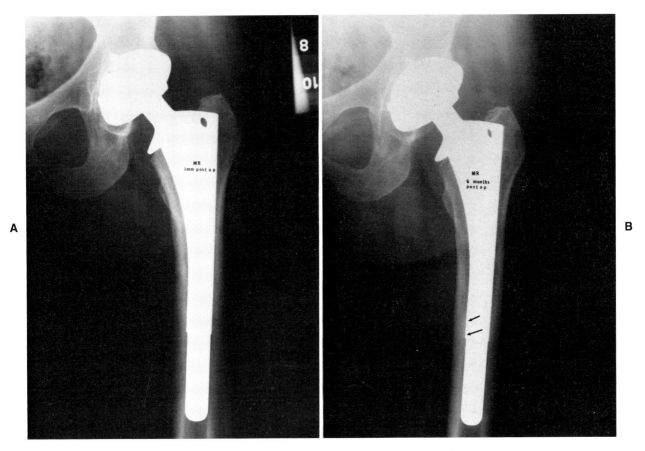

Fig. 18-7. Postoperative **(A)** and 6-month **(B)** AP radiographs of an implanted 16.5 mm partially porous-coated stem. A rapid loss of density in the medial cortex occurred throughout levels 1 and 2. (From Engh, C.A., and Bobyn, J.D.: Biological fixation in total hip arthroplasty, Thorofare, N.J., 1985, Slack, Inc.)

Table 18-3. Incidence of bone resorption as a function of stem diameter and region in the femur at 1 year*

	Stem diameter (mm)							
	9.0	10.5	12.0	13.5	15.0	16.5	18.0	22.5
Level 1 triangular section of stem	17%	30%	23%	67%	44%	94%	50%	100%
Level 2 rod section above press fit	0%	4%	3%	39%	28%	45%	75%	100%
Level 3 press fit at isthmus	0%	1%	0%	5%	11%	12%	50%	100%
Level 4 below press fit	0%	1%	0%	0%	0%	0%	0%	0%
Number of cases	6	133	74	18	71	33	4	1

*See Fig. 18-5.

Table 18-4. Incidence of bone formation as a function of stem diameter and region in the femur at 1 year*

	Stem diameter (mm)							
	9.0	10.5	12.0	13.5	15.0	16.5	18.0	22.5
Level 1 Triangular section of stem	0%	4%	5%	5%	1%	3%	0%	0%
Level 2 Rod section above press fit	17%	1%	0%	0%	0%	3%	0%	0%
Level 3 Press fit at isthmus	17%	5%	5%	28%	18%	27%	0%	100%
Level 4 Below press fit	33%	10%	13%	33%	28%	39%	25%	100%
Number of cases	6	133	74	18	71	33	4	1

*See Fig. 18-5.

interface is stable and has an appearance suggestive of bone ingrowth. The lines are believed to represent localized regions of relative motion between the implant and the femur, which in the case of the proximally porous-coated femoral implants, implies that the implant is well fixed proximally and that there is flexure of the femur relative to the smooth and rigid distal stem. In a few of the early cases in which small diameter stems were used in large intramedullary canals (for example, at 1 year 12 of 341 or 3.5%) the radiopaque lines develop more extensively, in 2 or more of the 4 levels and 6 or more of the 16 sites. This more extensive line formation suggests that the stem is fixed entirely by fibrous and not osseous tissue ingrowth (Fig. 18-8).

Histologic study of the bone-implant interface has demonstrated unequivocally that the powder-made sintered porous surface with an average pore size of 250 micrometers is efficacious for biologic fixation by bone ingrowth (Fig. 18-9).[6] From extensive study of both animal and human specimens, both radiographically and histologically, it has become possible to interpret certain radiographic features as indicative of bone ingrowth. These features include proximal stress shielding, endosteal hypertrophy and cortical thickening at the junction of porous and smooth implant surfaces, and absence of radiopaque lines except around the smooth uncoated portion of the stem. Features not compatible with adequate bone ingrowth fixation include subsidence, the presence of radiopaque lines at more than one level or five sites around the porous-coated part of the prostheses, absence of calcar atrophy and localized hypertrophy along the lateral cortex (indicative of a lack of uniform stress transfer along the stem and high compressive contact

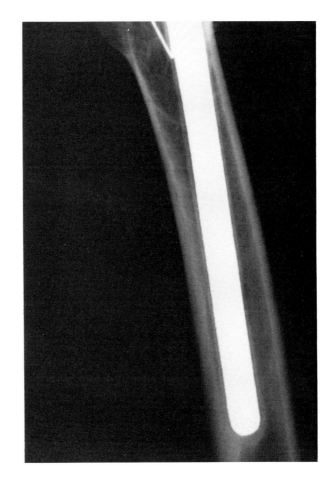

Fig. 18-8. Five-year lateral radiograph of a case with a fully coated 10.5 mm stem in which extensive radiopaque lines developed around the entire implant, indicating fibrous tissue fixation. (From Engh, C.A., and Bobyn, J.D.: Biological fixation in total hip arthroplasty, Thorofare, N.J., 1985, Slack, Inc.)

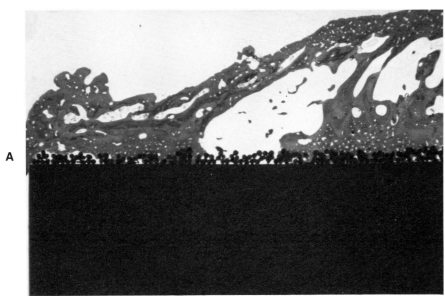

Fig. 18-9. Photomicrographs of an undecalcified histologic section prepared from a specimen retrieved at autopsy 3 years after surgery (stained with paragon). **A,** ×2, posterior bone-implant interface just under the implant collar. Extensive bone growth is evident within the surface porosity. From Engh, C.A., and Bobyn, J.D.: Biological fixation in total hip arthroplasty, Thorofare, N.J., Slack, Inc.

Continued.

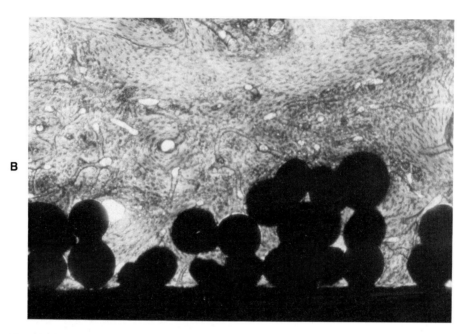

Fig. 18-9, cont'd. B, ×20, higher magnification of a region in **A** illustrating the cellularity and vascularity of the ingrown osseous tissue. (From Engh, C.A., and Bobyn, J.D.: Biological fixation in total hip arthroplasty, Thorofare, N.J., 1985, Slack, Inc.)

loading at these sites), and progressive intramedullary enlargement indicating disuse osteoporosis and lack of stress to the endosteal surfaces by the stem.

PROBLEMS UNIQUE TO POROUS IMPLANTS AND BIOLOGIC FIXATION ARTHROPLASTY

The learning curve associated with any new technique has resulted in the recognition of several problems or complications that are unique to bone ingrowth arthroplasty.

Immediate (perioperative) problems

Shaft fractures. Because of the need to achieve a tight fit of the stem within the intramedullary canal at the time of surgery, the most obvious immediate problem relates to fracture either of the neck or shaft. Shaft fractures are caused by improperly sizing the canal with the intramedullary reamers so that the implant is either too large or too long. They are prevented by proper preoperative planning using template overlays on lateral x-ray films of the femur and by the proper use of rigid intramedullary drills marked for appropriate drilling length. The side cutting flutes must extend the entire length of the

reamers to ensure that the prepared channel is the same diameter as the cylindric rod over its entire length. The prosthesis must be no longer or no larger than the predrilled channel. When shaft fractures occur, it must be determined if the fracture is either incomplete and therefore stable or complete and unstable. Most of the fractures are incomplete and consist only of a splitting and slight spreading of the anterior femoral cortex where the excessively long stem contacts the bow of the femur. These anterior cracks are treated by a longer interval of protected weight bearing, and, if more extensive, by the use of a one leg spica fiberglass cast. Unstable fractures must be treated by surgical stabilization of the fracture, which sometimes requires temporary removal of the implant. Longer periods of protected activity are required in these instances.

Neck fractures. Femoral neck fractures occur either if the triangular channel through the femoral neck is too small or if the prosthetic stem has not been oriented to account for the amount of forward flexion and rotation of the femoral neck. These problems can be prevented by the use of proper preoperative templates, proper placement of the pilot hole considering orientation both to the neck and the shaft, and the use of trial components of different rod and triangular sizes to ensure proper seating of the rod, collar, and triangular portion of the prosthesis before insertion of the final porous-coated component. If these steps are not carried out and a femoral neck fracture occurs, the extent of the fracture must be determined. If the neck fracture does not extend below the level of the lesser trochanter and if there is a tight implant fit at the isthmus, the fractured femoral neck can be stabilized with a circumferential wire through the lesser trochanter. The patient's postoperative rehabilitation will not change.

Excessive leg lengthening. Excessive leg lengthening is apt to occur in patients with hip dysplasia and protrusio acetabuli; it may occur also in smaller patients in whom the intertrochanteric triangular region of the femur is proportionally small with reference to the intramedullary canal diameter. In these situations the use of the standard triangular-sized femoral implant can prevent collar seating, and when the shortest neck length prosthesis is inserted to its fullest and the femoral head is brought down to the level of the new acetabulum excessive leg lengthening still occurs. The problem is prevented by preoperative planning with accurate x-ray studies of the femur in the proper rotation. These steps allow the surgeon to recognize the need for a prosthesis with a proportionally smaller triangular size and arrange to have it available on a custom basis.

Posterior dislocations. The posterior surgical approach to the hip has been associated historically with a higher incidence of dislocation. The need to excise the capsule and labrum to insert the threaded acetabular components requires more extensive exposure, which compounds the problem. Most hip dislocations are caused by impingement and a levering of the femoral head out of the acetabulum. Removing osteophytes from the rim of the acetabulum and the anterior femoral neck, the use of modular femoral and acetabular components to adjust leg length and maximize stability, and the careful use of trial implants before final implant insertion will lessen this problem.

Postoperative (delayed) problems

Stress shielding. The most serious problem with porous-coated implants, at least on the femoral side, is the tendency for stress shielding and disuse osteoporosis of bone. This is a function of several factors that include the stiffness of the implant material relative to bone, the moment of inertia of the stem (a geometric factor related to the 4th power of the stem diameter), and the integrity of the bond between the implant and host bone. On a theoretical basis, the worst possible situation is to have a femoral stem of high stiffness and large diameter well bonded to the femur along its entire length. Apart from the tendency for axial load to be borne preferentially by the metal stem, bending and torsional stresses in the femoral shaft are also reduced as a result of the presence of the implant. These concepts have been discussed in some detail in a prior publication.[6]

It must be recognized and accepted that any stem is going to cause stress redistribution that results in some regions of resorption and other regions of hypertrophy. The use of small diameter stems (<13.5 mm) has not caused radiographically demonstrable resorption that is of serious concern. As explained earlier, there is a definite tendency for larger stem diameters to cause proximal resorption in a higher percentage of cases. Even in most of these cases, however, the resorption is localized to the calcar and is relatively minor. It is only in about 5% of all cases with stems 13.5 mm and larger that more worrisome (greater resorption over a greater area) proximal resorption occurs to an extent that is detectable radiographically.

The current proposed solution to this problem is to confine the implant porosity to more proximal regions of the stem. In theory, this will force stress transfer in the proximal region of good bonding and help maintain bone stock. Clinical trials with a stem that is 40% coated are promising in this regard, although the number of cases with longer than 1 year follow-up is still few. In addition to this design modification, it may be necessary to render the rod portion of the stem more "isoelastic" with the femoral shaft through modification of materials or design.

Thigh pain. About 10% of the patients experience some form of thigh pain with activity within the first postoperative year. This thigh pain has been of two general types. One occurs immediately at onset of load bearing such as typically occurs with a symptomatically loose cemented prosthesis. Patients with this type of thigh pain tend to have a category 2 (poor canal filling) type of implant fit and extensive radiopaque line formation around the stems. This does not mean that all patients with small stems in large canals and extensive radiopaque lines experience thigh pain. In fact many of these patients score 5 or 6 on both pain and walking scales indicating that fibrous ingrowth can effectively stabilize the implant. The results, however, are not consistent or predictable. The second type of thigh pain is not "start up" in nature but is felt in the midthigh region after extended activity and typically occurs with a well-fitting partially coated stem that shows evidence of bone ingrowth fixation proximally and evidence of flexure of the endosteal cortex against the distal stem tip. This feature is manifested on x-ray studies by radiopaque line formation around the tip of the stem and by endosteal or periosteal hypertrophy of the cortex at the site of high point contact compressive loading. This pain may arise from the stress concentration at the level where the stem tip contacts the endosteum and is generally present during the first and second postoperative years. This problem may be preventable by tapering the stem tip so that point contact cannot occur or by using a lower modulus material that is more effective in distributing load.

Materials problems. Concern has been expressed about the fatigue strength of the materials that undergo sintering heat treatment. While sintering does reduce fatigue strength (about 10% for cobalt-based alloy compared with cast material) the material still retains high strength characteristics, and the use of larger stems (compared with conventional cemented designs) increases fatigue strength considerably. No problems have been encountered with the porous-coated Moore design with follow-up extending now to 8 years.

Concern has also been expressed about the quality of the bond between the porous coating and the implant substrate. In about 3% of the early cases, postoperative radiographs indicated small localized regions where several sintered particles had loosened from the implant as a result of tight impaction. More recently, with improved metallurgy and sintering techniques, this has not been a problem. The cases with loosened particles can develop into a problem if the implant is not stabilized by bone ingrowth, and cyclic loading results in fretting wear and corrosion of the implant against the loosened particles. Excessive implant loosening and production of fretting debris may result in the need for revision.

Implant removal. The bond that can develop between porous metal and ingrown bone is so strong that it renders implant removal a potential problem. Certainly this problem is aggravated with stems that are porous-coated along their entire length. Thin osteotomes can be used effectively to progressively divide the bone-implant interface and allow removal. The reduction in the level of porous coating is a design modification that renders the entire bone-porous implant interface more accessible and facilitates extraction without serious loss of bone stock.

Metal ion release. The higher surface area–metallic porous systems can release greater amounts of constituent elements through corrosion mechanisms compared with smooth-surfaced implants.[12] Concern has been expressed about the possible toxic or even carcinogenic effects of systemic overload of these elements. This is a potentially serious problem that is under widespread investigation. The reality of this concern has yet to be documented clinically with porous systems either in North America or Europe, where experience dates back to the early 1970s.

SUMMARY

Experience with biologic fixation hip arthroplasty using the powder-made sintered porous system has been very encouraging over the past 8 years. With simple implant design, accurate instrumentation, and careful attention to surgical technique, the results of surgery can be made equal to those obtained with conventional cemented arthroplasty (using the current improved implant designs and cementing techniques). Most of the problems associated with this new technology have been recognized and solved. The most serious problem is probably that of stress shielding and disuse osteoporosis, and this may well be overcome through judicious design modification. It is the next decade that will determine whether the incidence of late aseptic loosening is reduced through design for a "living" interface between implant and bone.

REFERENCES

1. Bobyn, J.D., and Engh, C.A.: Biologic fixation of hip prostheses: Review of the clinical status and current concepts, Adv. Orthop. **7:**137, 1983.
2. Bobyn, J.D., Pilliar, R.M., Cameron, H.U., and Weatherly, G.C.: The optimum pore size for the fixation of porous-surfaced metal implants by the ingrowth of bone, Clin. Orthop. **150:**263, 1980.
3. Cameron, H.U., Pilliar, R.M., and Macnab, I.: The effect of movement on the bonding of porous metal to bone, J. Biomed. Mater. Res. **7:**301, 1973.
4. Cameron, H.U., Pilliar, R.M., and Macnab, I.: The rate of bone ingrowth into porous metal, J. Biomed. Mater. Res. **10:**295, 1976.
5. Engh, C.A.: Hip arthroplasty with a Moore prosthesis with porous coating—a five year study, Clin. Orthop. **176:**52, 1983.
6. Engh, C.A., and Bobyn, J.D.: Biological fixation in total hip arthroplasty, Thorofare, N.J., 1985, Slack Inc.
7. Engh, C.A., Bobyn, J.D., and Gorski, J.M.: Biological fixation of a modified Moore prosthesis, Orthopaedics **7:**285, 1984.
8. Engh, C.A., and Bobyn, J.D.: Biological fixation of a modified Moore prosthesis—II: Evaluation of adaptive femoral bone modeling. In Welch, R.B., editor: The hip: Proceedings of the twelfth open scientific meeting of the Hip Society, St. Louis, 1984, The C.V. Mosby Co.
9. Morscher, E., editor: The cementless fixation of hip endoprostheses, New York, 1983, Springer-Verlag.
10. Pilliar, R.M.: Powder metal-made orthopaedic implants with porous surface for fixation by tissue ingrowth, Clin. Orthop. **176:**42, 1983.
11. Pilliar, R.M., Cameron, H.U., and Macnab, I.: Porous-surfaced layered prosthetic devices, J. Biomed. Eng. **10:**126, 1975.
12. Woodman, J.L.: Nickel and titanium release in a carcinogenesis study of orthopaedic implant materials, Proceedings of the 29th Annual Orthopaedic Research Society meeting, Anaheim, Calif., March 8-10, 1983.

Chapter 19

Factors controlling optimal bone ingrowth of total hip replacement components

WILLIAM H. HARRIS

Investigations of the past 15 years have identified 10 key factors that dominate the optimization of bony ingrowth for fixation of total hip replacements. It is clear that the biology of this process is analogous in its early phases to fracture healing and that this biologic response depends on blood supply, limited motion, and the absence of sepsis. Since only meager human data are available dealing with the study of optimization of bony ingrowth in joint replacement, the bulk of this experimental data dealing with bony ingrowth has been derived from animal studies.

The 10 key factors are the following:
1. Apposition
2. Pore size
3. Rigid initial fixation
4. Type of bone
5. Weight bearing
6. Biocompatibility
7. Remodeling
8. Bone grafting
9. Other stimuli
10. Distinction between the human and the animal experience

Since bony ingrowth in its simplest form is the osseous biologic response to fill a gap, apposition is important. The smaller the gap between the host material and the porous surface, the easier it is for bony ingrowth to take place. The problem until now has been the lack of knowledge about the magnitude of gap that can be bridged successfully and the absence of any quantification of the magnitude of the deleterious effect of having substantial gaps.

The study of these questions has been impossible because of the inability to quantify the fit of the implant against bone, the magnitude of the gap, and most basically, the amount of bony ingrowth. It is now possible to quantify the accuracy of the fit quite precisely using the pressure-sensitive film called Prescal manufactured by Fuji in Japan. The insertion of a thin layer of this film at the time of trial insertion of a bony ingrowth implant makes it possible to identify quite precisely the exact areas and points of contact between the implant and the host bone.

Far more difficult has been the problem of quantification of bony ingrowth. In the past this has been possible only in crude terms. But now with the development of the Jasty system of image analysis,* it is possible for the first time to quantify with high accuracy and great rapidity the exact amount of bone present in microradiographic or histologic sections of porous layers using sophisticated computer analytic techniques. Thus it has been possible to quantify the effect of apposition.

In a series of adult dogs studied in our laboratory we have shown that in the canine the presence of a gap of 0.5 to 1.0 mm reduces the amount of bony ingrowth by 50%.[7] The total amount of bone formed in the porous layer in these experiments has averaged 13% and thus the average figure for bony ingrowth in comparable

---

*Murali Jasty, M.D., Orthopaedic Biomechanical Laboratory, Massachusetts General Hospital, Boston, MA 02114.

cases in which intimate apposition was not achieved but a gap of 0.5 to 1.0 mm was present was only 6.5%.

In terms of pore size it has long been recognized that a pore size below 75 micrometers and even below 100 micrometers resulted in fibrous ingrowth rather than bony ingrowth. Substantial debate exists about the effect of pore sizes above 100 micrometers. We have recently completed a canine study that also showed that, even in the presence of excellent apposition and rigid immediate fixation, the pore sizes of 125 micrometers were distinctly inferior in terms of total bone ingrowth compared to those at 250 or 450 micrometers. The data, again using the Jasty quantification system, showed that bony ingrowth fills 13% of the total porous layer if the pore size is 250 or 450 micrometers but only 6% if the average pore size if 125 micrometers, an important and statistically significant reduction.

RIGID FIXATION

Rigid fixation clearly is essential. If motion occurs, fibrous tissue goes in rather than bone. However, it is not known *how* rigid the fixation has to be. Clearly some motion always exists between a press-fit implant and the adjacent bone, and as yet no one has quantified the lower end of this scale.

In terms of implant design it is clear that the acetabular component is best designed as a hemisphere because of its intimate apposition, adaptability, positioning, and minimization of the destruction of host bone to provide optimal fit.[4] However, the hemisphere is the least stable configuration and thus requires some augmentation of fixation to provide the rigid immediate stability. Experimental studies in dogs have shown that the optimal way to do this is to use screws, either periacetabular screws or screws that penetrate through the base of the acetabular component.[4]

For rigid fixation on the femoral side the optimal circumstances are (1) a component designed with a cylindric stem that is driven into the isthmus of the femur after it has been reamed with a cylindric reamer of identical size, (2) a body or metaphyseal portion that occupies the bulk of the metaphyseal region of the proximal femur and flares in its proximal portion so that a wedge press fit is created both medial-lateral and anteroposterior in the cancellous bone of the metaphysis, and (3) a collar that fits precisely on an accurately reamed calcar and medial femoral neck region to further substantially reduce micromotion and eliminate subsidence.

In the postoperative management of patients with bony ingrowth devices, most authors agree that crutches should be used for a period of time to support muscular rehabilitation and to reduce load across the hip joint to decrease the inevitable, minimal micromotion.

However, some weight bearing plays an important role. Although it has long been recognized that decreased stress leads to bone resorption, the question of the positive or negative effect of weight bearing in stimulating bony ingrowth has never been resolved. We have just completed an experiment in which a series of total hip replacements that were done in dogs provided excellent fixation and excellent apposition.[7] However, half of the animals had the hip dislocated and left dislocated; thus the only difference between the groups was load bearing. Using the Jasty computer technique for quantification of new bone formation, we showed that the bony ingrowth was reduced by 50% in those dogs which had the hip dislocated. It is clear that some weight bearing is a distinct advantage to stimulating new bone formation.

Experimental studies have shown clearly that bony ingrowth can occur well from either cancellous or cortical bone. The rate is faster with cancellous bone, but the ultimate resistance to shear is greater when the bony ingrowth has occurred adjacent to cortical bone. The explanation of this strength difference is quite simple. In pull-out push-out tests the failure occurs through the adjacent bone and not through the porous material; thus it is easier to break the surrounding cancellous bone than it is to break the surrounding cortical bone. Therefore shear strength of bony ingrowth from cortical bone is greater than from cancellous bone.

The next major concern is that of biocompatibility. Because of the increased surface area of all porous implants, there is a substantial increase in metal ion release from metallic porous surfaces. This can have an adverse effect locally in the early or late period and in remote parts of the body in the late period.

In humans the long term biocompatibility issues both locally and remotely remain unresolved. However, the strongest long term scientific information on biocompatibility and toxicity comes from extensive studies by Galante and his group using titanium tivanium porous implants in rats, dogs, and subhuman primates.[1,9,11,12] These studies cover a decade and include complete autopsy studies in primates after 10 years. No such data exist for chrome cobalt. No deleterious effects were seen of the titanium-tivanium implants.

LATE REMODELING

In the long run the success or failure of most porous implants will hinge not so much on the initial bony ingrowth but rather on the late remodeling. It has been shown that, using proper techniques, it is possible to obtain bony ingrowth in most instances. Maintaining it is the key issue. Excessive stress can lead to bone resorption. The stress within normal limits will lead to bone formation. Decreased stress will lead to bone resorption, and striking examples of this have been clearly demonstrated both experimentally and in humans. Studies by Hedley and associates[5] and Pilliar[10] have shown extraordinary disuse osteoporosis and focal bone resorption in areas of major reduction in stress secondary to a variety of porous implants. A few striking examples of this also have been seen in human cases as, for example, reported by Lord.[8]

Thus it becomes extremely important to avoid major stress shielding. This is most likely to occur in the proximal femur. Consequently every effort should be made to transfer stress as much as possible proximally and as far proximally as possible. It is widely held now that the porous system surface should be confined to the metaphyseal area, and a collar is of major advantage. Major stress transfer from the tip of the prosthesis to the isthmus of the femur represents a significant potential long term hazard.

Bone grafting plays a very important role in bony ingrowth implants. It is often necessary to bone graft cysts or defects on the acetabular side. This is particularly true in case of revision surgery. On the femoral side bone grafting also plays an important role. Based on general experience autogenous cancellous bone is probably the optimal tissue. A great deal of particulate allografting has been done in humans with reports of early radiographic success. It is doubtful that massive single pieces of allograft material will provide a satisfactory stimulus to bony ingrowth.

Major investigative work is now being done in other forms of stimulation of bony ingrowth. Although the potential for this approach is high, nothing as yet has been shown to be significant in a major way. The leading candidates for success in this area are hydroxyapatite, electrical stimulation, bone morphogenic protein, and other similar compounds. This is an area of intense interest and should be watched carefully, but at the moment it is an unproved area.

Finally, since so much of the data on the subject are derived from animals, we must keep in mind the potential difference between humans and the other, experimental, animals. In general the human behavior has followed what would be predicted from the animal experiments, but it must be reemphasized that extremely limited human data are available. For example, with the AML femoral component the first design that was inserted was available in a single size that was relatively small and had a porous layer that had an average pore size of 125 micrometers. Eleven such components have been retrieved, and virtually no bony ingrowth was present.[2] Equally important, virtually none of these patients showed extensive osteoporosis at least over a period of 2 to 4 years.

However, as larger AML stems were introduced with a pore size averaging about 250 micrometers and the fit became substantially better, certain patients showed distinct abnormalities. The radiographic evidence of bony ingrowth was substantially better, and simultaneously the evidence of disuse osteoporosis was substantially greater.[3]

It is reasonable to speculate that the first version was used primarily as a press fit, did not involve significant bony ingrowth, and was not subjected to the major problems of disuse. All of these things were reversed with a larger implant with a better porous coat. However, without the histologic data from the retrieved specimens none of these differences would have been intelligible. Thus much more data will need to be analyzed with great care to fully establish the behavior of bony ingrowth implants in humans and the differences between humans and animals in the responses of bony ingrowth.

One distinction that does appear to be clear is that, at least judged by radiographic evidence, the human will fill in larger gaps than the dog. Gaps of 2.0 mm and more have been shown radiographically to fill in the human acetabulum after the introduction of bony ingrowth components.

Equally important, in the human experience with a variety of femoral components, it has been clear that major changes take place in the stress distribution and that these are reflected by substantial alterations in the trabecular bone pattern and major osteoporosis in the proximal-femoral cortical areas. These changes can occur in relative short time intervals.[3,6,8] The full extent and the full importance of these remain to be shown.

SUMMARY

The major factors dealing with optimization of bony ingrowth for total hip replacement have been shown by experimental and limited clinical experience to be apposition, pore size, rigid initial fixation, the type of bone surface, weight bearing, biocompatibility, remodeling, bone grafting, other forms of stimuli, and the distinctions between the human response and the response of the experimental animals.

REFERENCES

1. Andersson, G.B.J., Gaechter, A., Galante, J.O., and Rostoker, W.: Segmental replacement of long bones in baboons using a fiber titanium implant, J. Bone Joint Surg. **60A:**31-40, 1978.
2. Collier, J.P., Mayor, M., Engh, C., and Brooker, A.: Bone ingrowth of porous-coated Moore prostheses, Second World Congress of Biomaterials, 10th annual meeting of the Society of Biomaterials, Washington, D.C., April 27-May 1, 1984.
3. Engh, C.: Personal communications, April 5, 1986.
4. Harris, W.H., White, R.E., Jr., McCarthy, J.C., Walker, P.S., and Weinberg, E.H.: Bony ingrowth fixation of the acetabular component in canine hip joint arthroplasty, Clin. Orthop. **176:**7-11, 1983.
5. Hedley, A.K., Clark, I.C., Bloebaum, R.D., Moreland, J., Gruen, T., Coster, I., and Amstutz, H.: Viability and cement fixation of the femoral head in canine hip surface replacement. In Sledge, C.B., editor: The hip: Proceedings of the seventh open scientific meeting of The Hip Society, St. Louis, 1979, The C. V. Mosby Co.
6. Hungerford, D.: Current status of the PCA hip, paper presented to the twelfth open scientific meeting of The Hip Society, Rochester, N.Y., Sept. 1984.
7. Jasty, M., Weinberg, E.H., Rogers, S., and Harris, W.H.: Factors influencing bone ingrowth into porous coated canine acetabular replacements, paper presented at the annual meeting of the American Academy of Orthopaedic Surgeons, Feb. 9-14, 1984, Atlanta, Ga.
8. Lord, G.: Personal communication, March 21, 1986.
9. Memoli, V.A., Woodman, J.L., and Galante, J.O.: Long term biocompatibility of porous titanium fiber metal composites, paper presented at the 29th Annual Orthopaedic Research Society meeting, Anaheim, Calif., March 8-10, 1983.
10. Pilliar, R.M., Cameron, H.U., Welsh, R.P., and Binnington, A.G.: Radiographic and morphologic studies of load bearing porous surfaces structured implants, Clin. Orthop. **156:**249-258, 1981.
11. Woodman, J.L., Jacobs, J.J., Galante, J.O., and Urban, R.M.: Titanium release from fiber metal composites in baboons—a long term study, paper presented at the 28th Annual Orthopaedic Research Society meeting, New Orleans, La., Jan. 19-21, 1982.
12. Woodman, J.L., Jacobs, J.J., Urban, R.M., and Galante, J.O.: Vanadium and aluminum release from fiber metal composites in baboons—a long term study, paper presented at the 29th Annual Orthopaedic Research Society meeting, Anaheim, Calif., March 8-10, 1983.

Chapter 20

Self-bearing, uncemented, ceramic total hip replacement arthroplasty

EDWARD H. MILLER

ROBERT S. HEIDT

MICHAEL C. WELCH

WARREN G. HARDING

ROBERT S. HEIDT, JR.

S. MICHAEL LAWHON

For various reasons, orthopaedic surgeons are searching for alternatives to conventional cemented total hip replacement. The conventional method, however, is difficult to surpass; it has been a standard for many years and gives predictable results. Newer types of arthroplasty must be compared to the cemented type. From this, two basic questions must be answered. First, in primary total hip replacement in older patients, is the new type as effective, as safe, and as durable as the cemented type? Second, do the indications for the new type extend to patient groups who are not candidates for the cemented type?

The search for alternatives is stimulated by problems such as aseptic loosening, or metal-on-metal bearing of conventional hip replacement, or by problems resulting from the extension of operative indications to patients who were inappropriately chosen. One must remember, however, that we are facing primarily the poor results of the *earliest* types of cementation. Finger packing with less than meticulous debridement and cleansing still provided satisfactory results in most cases. With current cementation techniques the results may be even better. We must keep this in mind as we review the results of newer, uncemented methods.

The implants addressed in this review were developed by Professor Dr. Heinz Mittelmeier at the University of Saar Medical School in Homburg, Germany. Late in the 1950s Dr. Mittelmeier began to investigate alternatives to methylmethacrylate fixation. By 1974 he had developed the prototype of the acetabular and femoral head components that are currently in use. He changed the femoral stem in 1976; results reported here pertain to the improved design that resulted from that change.

DEVELOPMENT AND CONCEPT OF THE CERAMIC TOTAL HIP REPLACEMENT

Cement fragmentation and the accumulation of polyethylene wear debris at the cement-bone interface are among the problems with cemented prostheses. Samples of the cement-bone interface characteristically contain large fragments of polyethylene wear debris and polymethylmethacrylate surrounded by histiocytes and giant cells. These fragments are too large to be ingested by histiocytes and cannot be removed from the area by these cells (Fig. 20-1).

Mittelmeier searched for a material that would not produce so much wear debris and that need not require methylmethacrylate fixation. He

188

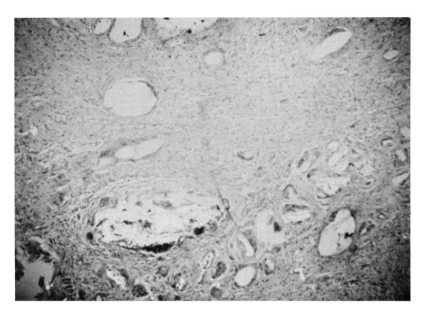

Fig. 20-1. Wear debris from conventional metal-polyethylene total hip replacement.

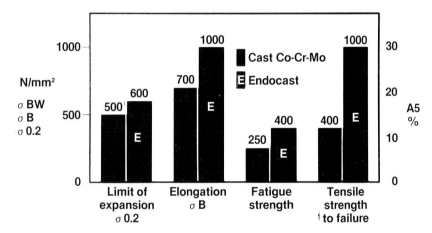

Fig. 20-2. Characteristics of cobalt-chrome alloy and Endocast (Richards Medical Co.).

chose an aluminum oxide ceramic for the acetabular and femoral head components and a cobalt-chrome-molybdenum super alloy for the femoral stem (Table 20-1 and Fig. 20-2). The friction and wear characteristics of the ceramic-on-ceramic bearing were excellent (Fig. 20-3). Compared to metal on plastic, the ceramic on plastic was also superior (Fig. 20-4).

The extreme smoothness that can be achieved on the ceramic surface made this material an excellent bearing for a ball-and-socket joint. The tremendous reduction of friction and wear in vitro is primarily a result of the extreme lubricity or slipperiness of the ceramic in water-based lubricant, which is comparable to joint fluid. One measure of lubricity is the angle subtended by a drop of lubricant on a lubricating surface. Because water molecules are polarized and attracted to the crystal aluminum oxide surface, the surface is very wettable (Fig. 20-5). The lubricity of alumina ceramic is one factor that encouraged the development of a comprehensive ceramic hip system (Fig. 20-6) for cementless (or cemented) application.

Table 20-1. Mechanical properties of German biomaterials

	Glass	Calcium-ceramic	Hydroxylapatite	Aluminum oxide
Compressive strength (N/sq mm)	500	120-190*	300	4000
Bending strength (N/sq mm)	150	Unknown	Unknown	500
Microhardness	1000	Unknown	Unknown	2000

*Depends on porosity.

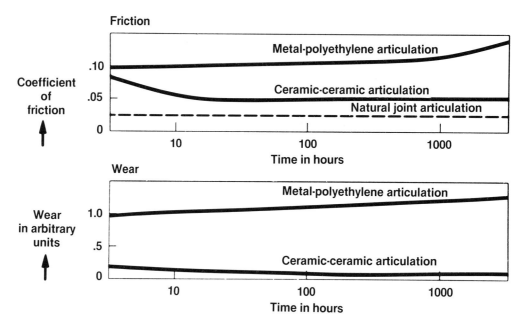

Fig. 20-3. Friction and wear characteristics of ceramic-ceramic and metal-polyethylene articulation.

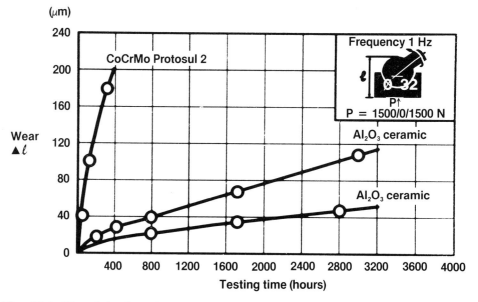

Fig. 20-4. Wear behavior of material combinations for hip joint endoprostheses in water.

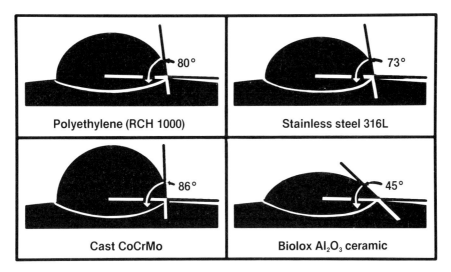

Fig. 20-5. Lubricity as measured by the angle subtended by a drop of water on various biomaterials.

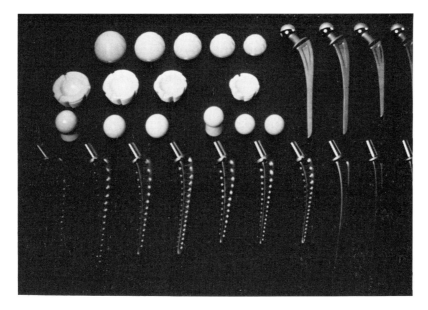

Fig. 20-6. Comprehensive cementless hip system for ceramic-ceramic articulation *(all but top row)* or metal-polyethylene articulation *(top row)*.

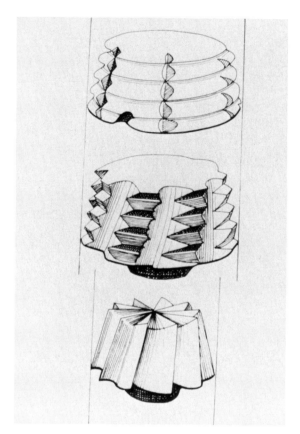

Fig. 20-7. Acetabular cup, threadcutter, and reamer for cementless cup implantation.

CEMENTLESS OPERATIVE TECHNIQUE

Mittelmeier initially used the Watson-Jones incision and recommends appropriate instrumentation for acetabular (Fig. 20-7) and femoral preparation (Fig. 20-8). The aim is minimal removal of acetabular bone and resection of the femoral neck so that the central and perpendicular axes of each subtend a 50-degree angle from the horizontal (Fig. 20-9). The femur is broached until the femoral component can be inserted with finger pressure so that there is 10 to 15 mm between the cut femoral neck and the prosthesis collar (Fig.

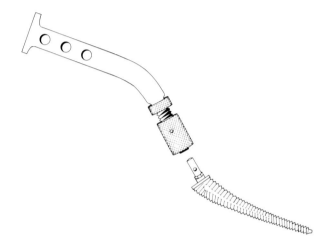

Fig. 20-8. Femoral broach-trial and handle for cementless stem implantation.

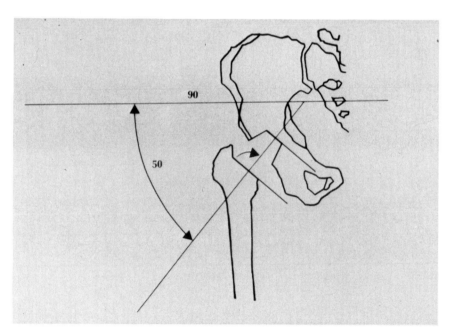

Fig. 20-9. Correct resection and reaming angles for femoral and acetabular preparation.

20-10). Morselized bone graft is inserted with the femoral stem. The femoral component is press fitted, and the acetabular component, which is threaded on the outside, is screwed in for immediate firm fixation.

PATIENTS AND METHODS

This report is of 231 total hip replacements in 212 patients; 100 underwent surgery between June 1982 and February 1983, and the others underwent surgery between February 1983 and February 1984. The minimum follow-up periods were 2 years for the first group and 1 year for the second. The distribution of diagnoses (Table 20-2) differed from that of most groups undergoing primary total hip replacement. Because the procedure is more appropriate for younger individuals, posttraumatic arthritis and osteonecrosis were more prevalent, and the average age at surgery was lower (Fig. 20-11; range, 17 to 82

Table 20-2. Distribution of diagnoses

Disease	Percentage of patients
Osteoarthritis	33
Posttraumatic arthritis	30
Osteonecrosis	21
Rheumatoid arthritis	11
Other	5

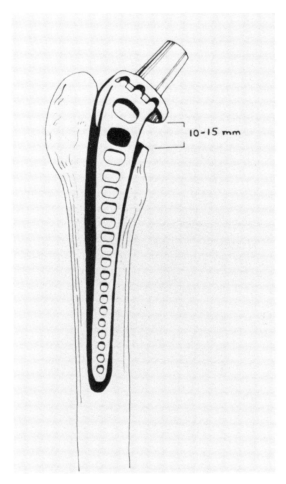

Fig. 20-10. Depth of femoral stem in femur after insertion with finger pressure.

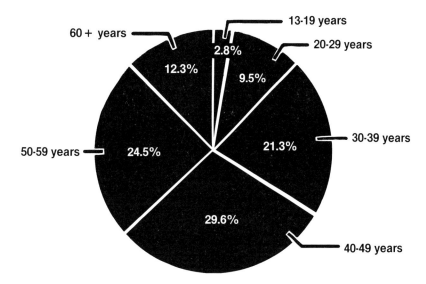

Fig. 20-11. Age at time of surgery.

years). (Typical examples of primary osteoarthritis, posttraumatic arthritis and osteonecrosis are depicted in the clinical illustrations.)

RESULTS

Complications. Table 20-3 shows the complications in each group. The first group had one infection, but the second group had none. The two dislocations in the first 100 patients were associated with hip revision—both done through the posterior approach with trochanteric osteotomy. The second group had one transient femoral nerve and sciatic nerve palsy. There was one femoral fracture in each group. One death due to aspiration pneumonia occurred in the first group.

Prosthesis failure. There was a difference in the characteristics of clinical failure of uncemented hips compared to conventional cemented ones. With cemented hips there is a "grace period" even when the prosthesis has been poorly implanted. With uncemented hips, by contrast, the grace period is absent—a hip system that is not going to work *never* works; immediate postoperative symptoms do not abate and revision comes early. This has been the European experience, in which about 4.8% of patients required revision, all within 18 months after surgery. From 18 months to 10 years after surgery there were no revisions for late loosening.

In the current study, five patients had femoral loosening that required revision of the uncemented prostheses to cemented ones. In one case a 68-year-old wife of a hospital administrator had intractable thigh pain from primary osteoarthritis (Fig. 20-12, *A* and *B*); the uncemented hip was therefore revised (Fig. 20-12, *C*). Another case involved a 19-year-old man, the youngest patient in the first group. He underwent surgery for osteonecrosis (Fig. 20-13, *A*), then developed activity-related pain due to femoral stem loosening (Fig. 20-13, *B*), underwent revision to a larger femoral stem (Fig. 20-13, *C*), and continued to have pain that prompted a second revision to a conventional cemented total hip.

Revision of failed cemented hips. It may be that a main indication for the uncemented hip is failed cemented arthroplasty. We have done 44 revisions of this type, including two for a 70-year-old retired executive with classic aseptic loosening with osteolysis (Fig. 20-14, *A*). Bilateral revisions were to uncemented, self-bearing, ceramic total hip replacements (Fig. 20-14, *B*). A year later,

Table 20-3. Complications

	First group N = 100	Second group N = 100
Dislocations	2	0
Femoral nerve palsy	0	1
Sciatic nerve palsy	0	1
Femoral fracture	1	1
Phlebitis	2	1
Death	1*	0
Heterotopic ossification	4	2
Femoral loosening	4	1
Vascular injury	0	0

*Aspiration pneumonia.

despite an ununited trochanter (Fig. 20-14, *C*), he has excellent regeneration of bone in both proximal femora, walks unaided, plays golf 3 times a week (with a golf cart), and is quite satisfied with the results.

The uncemented acetabular cup is also satisfactory for revision cup arthroplasty (Fig. 20-15), double cup arthroplasty (Fig. 20-16), and arthroplasty after sepsis (Fig. 20-17, in this case, with an interval of resection arthroplasty because of the gram-negative nature of the pathogen).

The same principles of complete cement removal and reestablishment of a viable prosthesis-bone interface apply when cementation is used in revision. Partial revision of the total hip system may involve a new metal-backed polyethylene-lined acetabular component when the conventional metallic femoral component is to be left in place. However, a ceramic acetabular component cannot be combined with a metallic femoral head; the extreme hardness of the ceramic cup will cause severe, destructive wear of the metallic femoral head. Alternatively, partial revision may involve a new uncemented femoral component with a ceramic femoral head when the intact polyethylene acetabular component is to be left in place. This is possible because of the excellent tribology of the ceramic femoral head and the polyethylene cup.

There are two other important warnings. Never heat-sterilize a ceramic femoral head mounted on the metallic stem. The difference in the coefficients of expansion of these two materials will cause inappropriate stresses in the ce-

Text continued on p. 200.

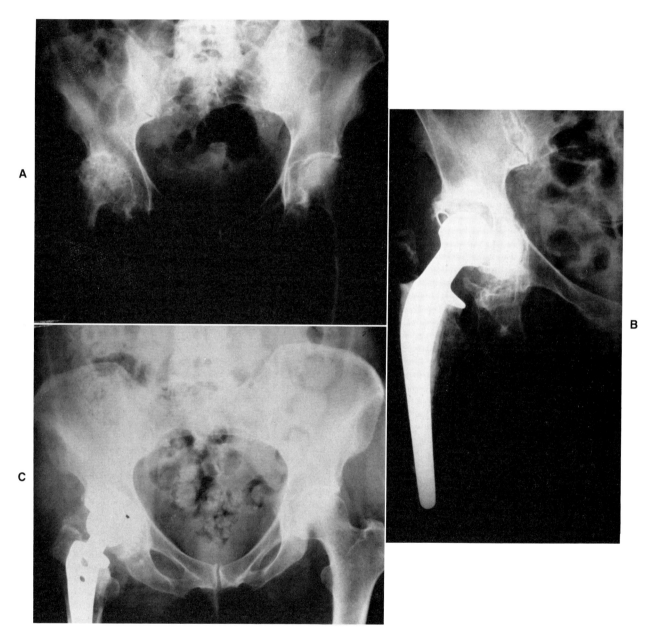

Fig. 20-12. Case A; 68-year-old woman with osteoarthritis of the right hip. **A,** preoperative. **B,** Postoperative—cementless ceramic total hip associated with thigh pain. **C,** Postoperative—hip revised to a cemented total hip.

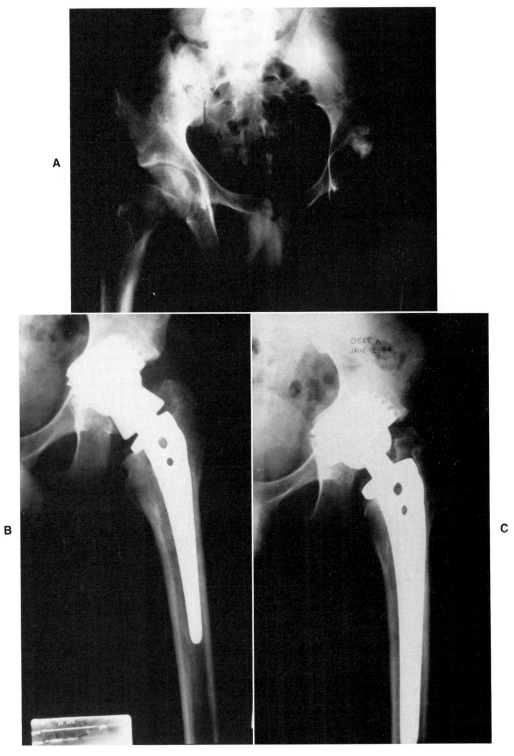

Fig. 20-13. Case B: 19-year-old man with osteonecrosis of the left femoral head. **A,** Preoperative. **B,** Postoperative—cementless ceramic total hip with stem loosening. **C,** Postoperative—hip revised to a larger femoral stem (still cementless).

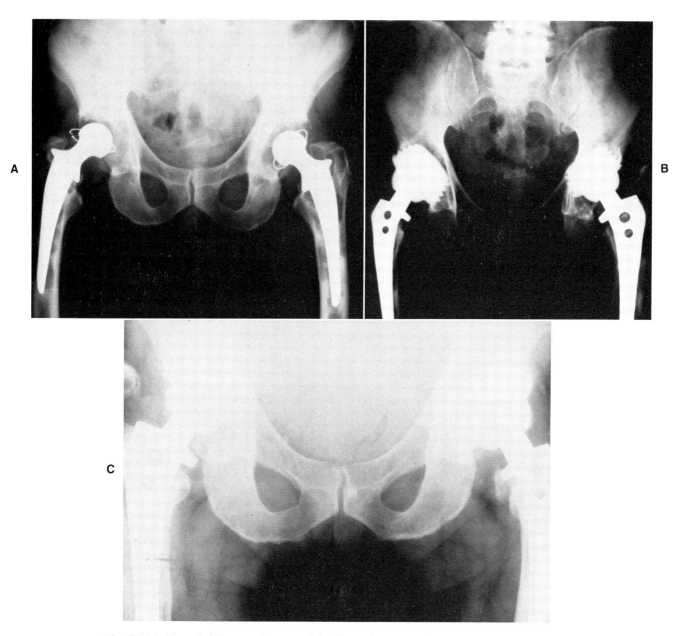

Fig. 20-14. Case C: 70-year-old man with bilateral cemented total hip replacements. **A,** Preoperative—classic aseptic loosening with osteolysis. **B,** Postoperative—bilateral revision to cementless ceramic total hips. **C,** 1 year postoperative—normal function despite ununited trochanter.

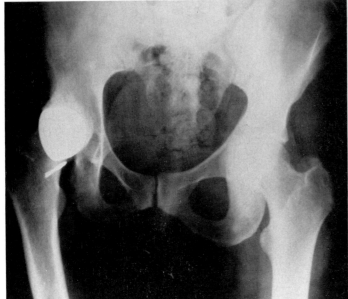

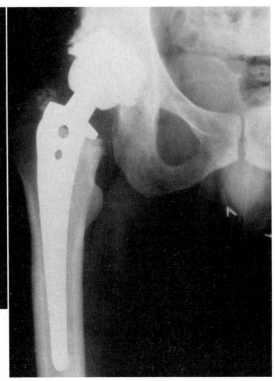

Fig. 20-15. Revision-cup arthroplasty.

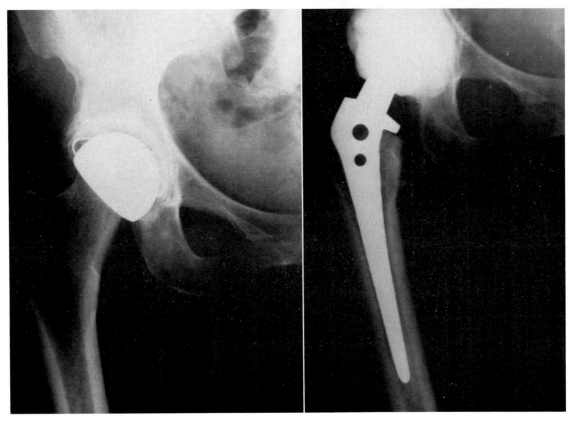

Fig. 20-16. Double-cup arthroplasty.

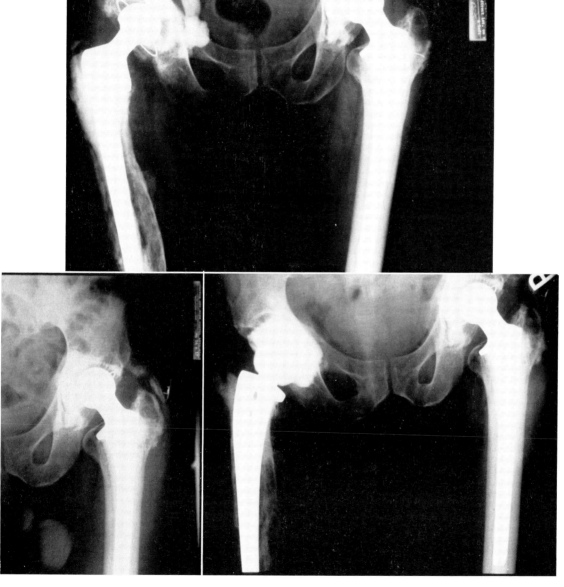

Fig. 20-17. Cup arthroplasty after sepsis and total hip replacement.

ramic component, leading to failure. For the same reason never quench a ceramic component in cold water immediately after autoclaving.

Now under way is a clinical evaluation of an uncemented bipolar femoral component having a ceramic head that articulates with a polyethylene-lined metal outer shell. This prosthesis is used when the acetabulum is undamaged (Fig. 20-18) and in revision.

Difficult cases. The frequency of using the uncemented ceramic system in extraordinarily difficult cases has been noted. An illustrative case, represented in Fig. 20-19, is of advanced destruction of the acetabulum (*Panel A*) that resulted from sepsis in childhood. The uncemented ceramic total hip was implanted with facility (*Panel B*) by applying a bone graft with a malleolar screw after acetabular component insertion.

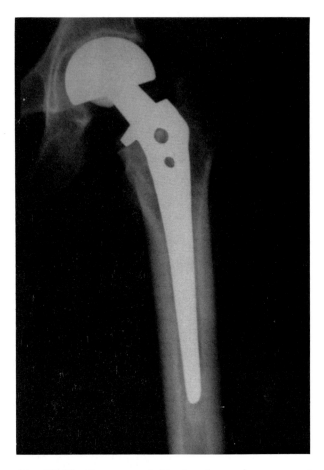

Fig. 20-18. Uncemented bipolar femoral component with ceramic head.

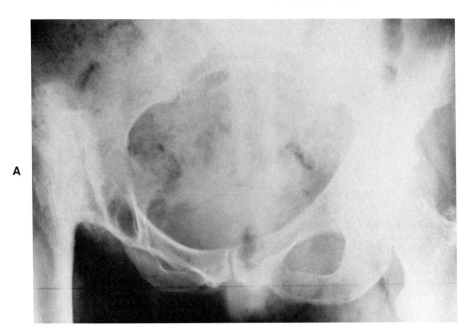

Fig. 20-19. A, Advanced destruction of the acetabulum.

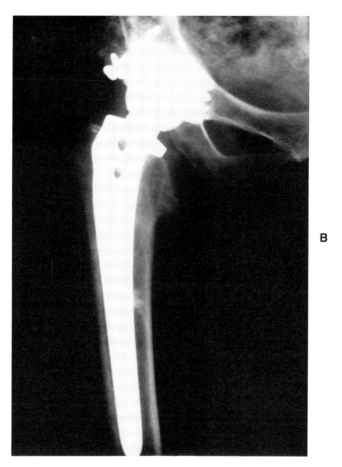

Fig. 20-19, cont'd. B, Cementless ceramic total hip replacement with bone grafting on the acetabular side.

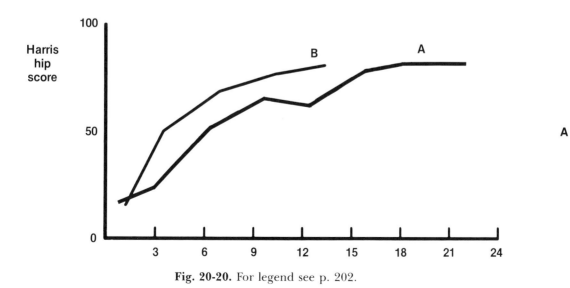

Fig. 20-20. For legend see p. 202.

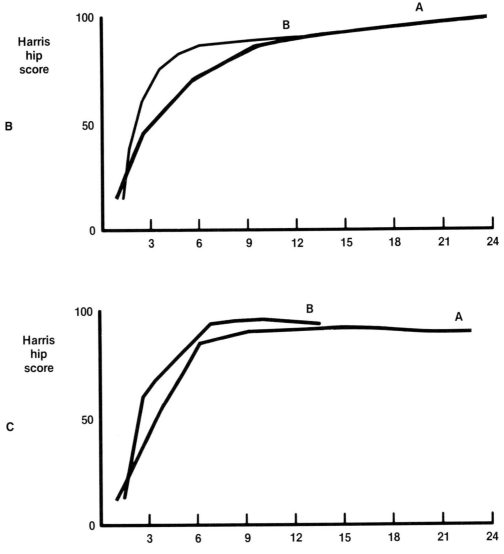

Fig. 20-20, cont'd. Harris hip scores for uncemented (**A**) and cemented (**B**) total hips. Panel **A,** patients with osteoarthritis; Panel **B,** patients with posttraumatic arthritis, Panel **C,** patients with osteonecrosis.

SUMMARY

The results for young patients in three diagnostic groups—osteoarthritis, posttraumatic arthritis, and osteonecrosis—show clearly that the uncemented procedure requires longer a recovery time than the cemented procedure (Fig. 20-20). A more aggressive physical therapy program has resulted in an earlier return to function, as shown in these graphs.

In conclusion, our experience with this operative procedure includes excellent patient acceptance, a failure rate comparable to that in Europe, a longer period of recovery than that for cemented arthroplasty, excellent results in revision of failed cemented arthroplasty, and an encouraging facility in the difficult case.

Chapter 21

A cementless titanium hip endoprosthesis system based on press-fit fixation: basic research and clinical results

KARL ZWEYMÜLLER

The anchorage of implants serving as a replacement for hip joints has been the subject of increasing discussion in the last few years. However, this only proves that a best standard method has not been found so far. Some authors attribute the failures experienced with cement prostheses over the past years to operative errors and in particular to the deficiencies of the cementing technique. They also hold the opinion that the improved handling of the acrylate must go hand-in-hand with the optimization of these techniques. Others believe that the cement aging processes lead to its destruction solely because of the changed physical properties[13,18,33] and the associated atrophy of the osseous bed.[22]

It is said that toxic admixtures to the cements can be identified for many years and, in combination with the ossification disturbance of the bony bed, ultimately lead—as a long-term-consequence—to loosening of the implant.[6,25]

From the problematic alone, and it is only barely outlined here, it is no wonder that the cementless anchorage is attracting more and more attention. About a decade ago, solutions to problems of cementless anchorage were proposed by pioneers like Ring, Judet, and Siwash.[20,36,40] In the ceramics sector Boutin, Griss, Mittelmeier, and Salzer reported on the first clinical results.[8,16,29,37] A great deal of knowledge, particularly about the anchorage of the stem, was taken over from the era of Moore and Thompson, when there was no cement for the fixation of implants.[31,43] Their knowledge really triggered the modern development of cementless systems.

It is interesting to note that the difficulties experienced with the anchorage of the stem apparently are much greater than those associated with the cup. The number of possible solutions is large, ranging from the "anatomical design," in the sense of a right-left variant,[17,21] to straight cylindrical stems,[12,27,35] and also to models with quadratic or rectangular cross-sections.[29,46]

Even more attention is being paid to the stem surfaces. With the cast alloy stems of Lord,[27] Hungerford,[21] and Engh,[12] for example, the surface area has been enlarged by means of a porous coating. Others[14,15] prefer titanium wires instead. Mittelmeier[29] favors large holes and recently an implant with a finer structure.[30] Homsy, for his part, prefers a metal prosthesis with a plastic coating.[19] He believes in a tissue-ingrowth implant fixation by way of a soft porous coating. Morscher uses a plastic prosthesis with a metal core.[32] In the sense of a biologic isoelasticity in relation to the bone this material combination should favor the anchorage of the implant. Nearly all of these authors assume that a permanent anchorage ultimately will result through the ingrowth of newly developed bone tissue in the coarse- or fine-structured, or "madreporous," or "porous-coated" surfaces specially provided for this purpose. Although a primary "press fit" is not ruled out, most of the authors feel that it contributes too little to the permanent anchorage.

Since no standard best solution has been elaborated so far for cementless implants (and it appears that there is still a long way to go), various questions may be posed.

1. In the light of current technologic knowledge, which material constitutes the optimal basis for hip implants?
2. Which surface commends itself for a primary stable implantation and also for a secondary stable permanent anchorage?
3. Is there any possibility of removing the stem again once it has been implanted?
4. What are the clinical findings, and how do the fine tissues react to the implant?
5. Can such implants replace cemented prostheses, and, if so, under which indications?

The following answers, based on my personal results, are confined to the stem.

MATERIALS AND METHODS
Concept of the modular system and anchorage principle

The hot-forged straight prosthetic stem made of titanium alloy is available in 10 different sizes (Fig. 21-1). There are also two undersized versions for extremely small femora and an over-sized model for the upper range. The individual anatomic variances of the femur, such as the size of the medullary cavity, anteversion-anteflexion, and antecurvature, thus are fully considered. The experience gained to date shows that all femora, except for extremely narrow or curved bones, allow satisfactory implantation of the prosthesis. The length of the anchorage stem ranges from 145 to 185 mm. Three ceramic ball heads with three different neck lengths are available. The present modular system therefore comprises 13 components and the possibility of 30 variations.

The design of the stem provides for a firm seating over a large area on the cortical bone. With a taper of 3 degrees the distal portion of the conical stem resembles the head of an arrow; that is, the medial and lateral conicities increase and it ends in a rounded tip (Fig. 21-1). Sagittally, the lower end of the stem also tapers off gradually to a rounded tip. In the proximal region the stem broadens out leaflike in the frontal plane. Consequently, good rotational stability is assured. This part of the stem has a number of holes. The cranial-most hole is designed for holding the extracting hook. Two holes are located in the axis of the neck, which is located at an angle of 49 degrees (or 131 degrees) to the axis of the prosthesis. These holes facilitate radiographic measurement. The other ones enable the surgeon to monitor the healing process, because the ingrowth of the regenerated osseous tissue can be

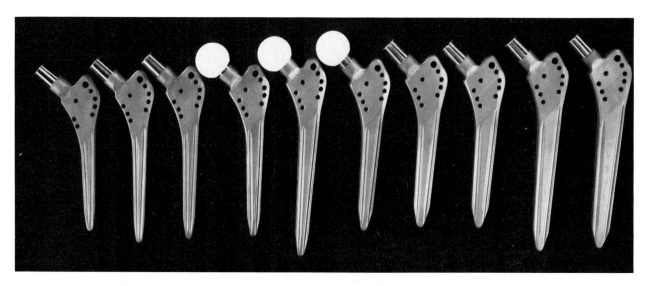

Fig. 21-1. Modular hip prosthesis, System Zweymüller, comprising 10 stems of different sizes made of wrought Ti-6Al-4V alloy Protasul-64 WF and three Biolox ceramic ball heads with three different neck lengths.

followed readily on radiographs (Fig. 21-1).

Torsional forces, however, also are taken up by the cross-sectional shape of the stem. Since the cross section of the prosthesis is rectangular, the four rounded edges can be fixed in the corticalis of the femur in the sense of a four-point anchorage. The full length of the prosthesis achieves area contact (Fig. 21-2). Depending on the preparation of the preexistent bone during the operation, the narrow and wide sides of the stem also contribute to the anchorage. Consequently the cardinal objective of the new design is to achieve maximal stable primary fixation of the stem in the metadiaphyseal region. Accordingly, the anchorage is effected as a press fit in a precisely prepared osseous bed corresponding in size to that of the prosthesis. No doubt exists that the cross section and the surface structure of the stem contribute to subsequent stabilization through the growth of newly developed bony tissue. Here again the extremely biocompatible titanium alloy offers optimal preconditions for this process too.

The acetabular socket that has proved itself with this femoral component is the polyethylene screw-type socket designed by Endler[10,11] (Fig. 21-3). This socket, which is also implanted without the use of acrylic bone cement, is available in seven different sizes. Any other cementable type

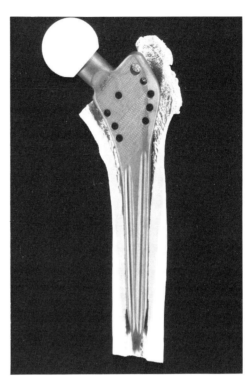

Fig. 21-2. Specimen femur after preparation of the bone and implantation of a prosthesis of corresponding size. Pronounced metadiaphyseal contact of the implant with the surrounding bone. Macerated after the preparation.

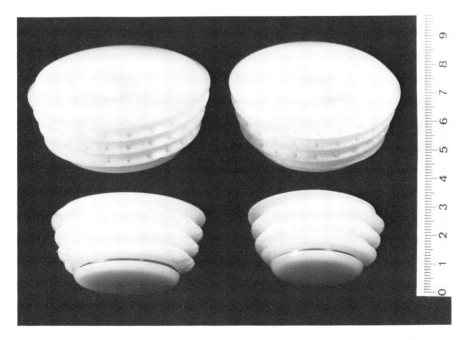

Fig. 21-3. Various-sized conical screw-type cups (Endler) made of ultrahigh molecular weight polyethylene Chirulen.

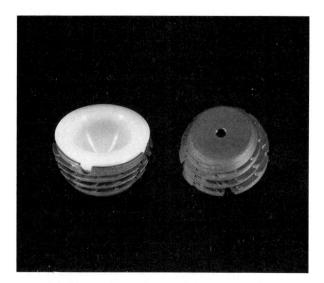

Fig. 21-4. Conical self-tapping metal cup made of pure titanium with and without polyethylene insert (Zweymüller).

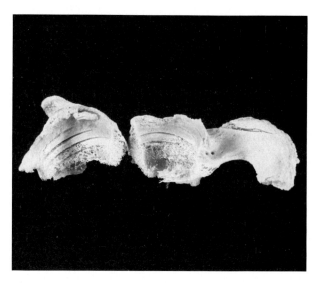

Fig. 21-5. Osseous acetabulum cut into two pieces after implantation of the self-tapping titanium cup shell. The flanks of the threads are clearly visible. Macerated after the preparation.

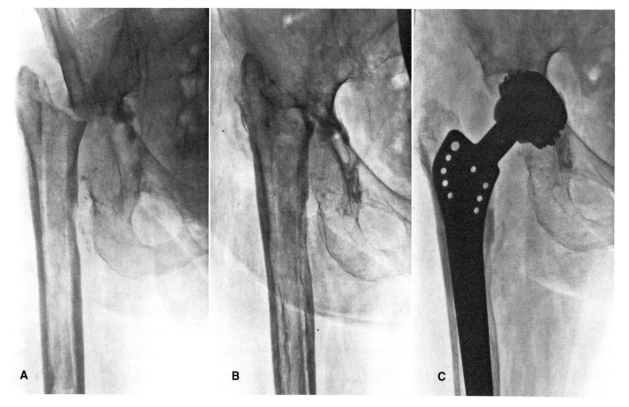

A   B   C

Fig. 21-6. P.C., female, 61 years old. **A,** After removal of a Lord stem and a cemented cup. Massive loss of the surrounding bone stock. The ventral area of the diaphysis had to be fenestrated to permit removal of the prosthesis. **B,** Preoperative state. **C,** Good fit of the self-tapping titanium cup and stem. The conical cup showed good primary stability during surgery even though there had been a massive dystrophy of the acetabular bone. This stability was possible because of sufficient medialization. Inconspicuous postoperative development.

Table 21-1. Standardized implant materials

Component	Implant material	DIN	Standard ASTM	ISO
Cup shell	Pure titanium Protasul* Ti		F 67	5832-2
Cup and cup insert	Ultra-high molecular weight polyethylene Chirulen‡	58834	F 648	5834-1
		58836		5834-2
Ball head	Aluminium oxide ceramic Biolox†	58835	F 603	6474
Stem	Ti-6Al-4V wrought alloy Protasul-64 WF*		F 136	5832-3

*Sulzer Brothers Ltd., Winterthur, Switzerland.
†Feldmühle AG, Plochingen, Federal Republic of Germany.
‡Ruhrchemie AG, Oberhausen, Federal Republic of Germany.

of polyethylene cup also may be used, provided that it matches the 32 mm ceramic ball head.

In addition there is also a self-tapping conical metal shell made of forged pure titanium with a polyethylene insert (Figs. 21-4 and 21-5 and Table 21-1). The sizes correspond to those of the Endler cup. The experience gained with this cup system over a period of more than 1 year is very promising, because the possibilities for anchoring the cup even under difficult conditions are good, for example, in connection with replacement operations associated with cemented cups that have become loose (Fig. 21-6).

Materials and design safety

In developing this hip prosthesis system, consisting of stem, ball head, and socket, clinically proved implant materials used in human implantation for many years have been deliberately chosen to preclude any risks on the part of the material. The material combination of hot-forged titanium (cup shell), ultra-high molecular polyethylene (cups), aluminium oxide ceramic (ball heads) and hot-forged titanium alloy (femoral stems) fulfills the requirements of both national and international standards (Table 21-1).

The slip-on connection developed in Winterthur at the beginning of the 1970s, which permits Biolox ceramic ball heads to be attached to the specially structured metal spigots of hip prosthesis stems, has been employed clinically in more than 40,000 cases (of which over 10,000 are Zweymüller femoral stems made of titanium alloy) since 1975. There has not been one single report of loosening or damage to the extremely hard, mirror-finish ceramic ball head. The extremely scratch-resistant ceramic surface, which is

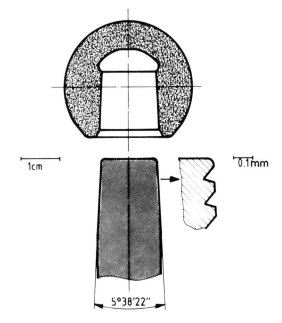

Fig. 21-7. Cross-section through the Biolox ceramic ball head for slip-on connection by means of a metal spigot with a specially structured surface. The conical spigot is made of hot-forged Protasul-64 WF.

readily wettable with body fluid, contributes markedly to the reduced polyethylene abrasion on the synthetic cup (Fig. 21-7).

In the case of all stem models detailed investigation of the nondeformability under static (Fig. 21-8) and dynamic (Fig. 21-9) load allows us to expect a long service life without the risk of fracture for the hip prostheses that are anchored directly to the bone and subject to million-fold loads in the body.[38,39] The results of these time-consuming pulsating tests entered in a Woehler stress-cycle diagram (Fig. 21-9) reveal that under these extremely stringent test conditions (most severe loosening for several years) the smallest prosthesis model 8 (representing the smallest undersized version) still can be pulsated with a load of 6000 N (corresponding to about six times the body weight of 100 kg) without fracturing. This corresponds to a safety factor of 2.1 against fracture when the critical limit is set at 2800 N under the same test conditions. This is based on long-term clinical experience with other femoral prosthesis models. With a sustainable pulsating loadability of 7500 to 10,000 N, the safety factor against fracture of the larger models 10 and 12.5 is even higher, namely 2.7 to 3.6.

Biolox ceramic ball heads with completely fixed prosthetic stems, joined by means of the special slip-on conical spigot connection featuring a specially structured surface, have been subjected to 50 million pulsating load cycles between 300 and 8,300 N (corresponding to eight times the body weight of 100 kg) both in air-fluxed Ringer's solution and in blood serum. No signs of cracking or fracture have been observed, however, even under these most severe conditions.

The high safety factor against fracture of the wrought Protasul-64 WF stem and the Biolox ceramic ball head of the modular Zweymüller total hip prosthesis system designed for cementless fixation has been corroborated by the results of extensive static and dynamic strength tests and investigations so far conducted.

Operative technique

In the planning of a cementless hip prosthesis system, it must be realized from the very outset that the success of the operation depends on the precision with which it is performed. Conse-

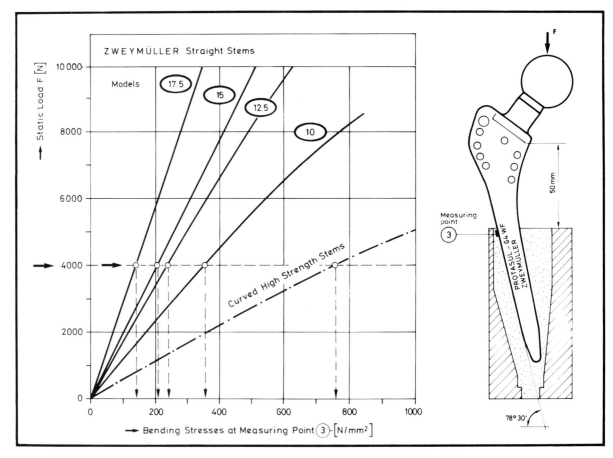

Fig. 21-8. Bending stresses at measuring point 3 at the lateral aspects of four Zweymüller hip prosthesis stems (10 to 17.5) and a curved stem of high strength as a function of the static load *F* applied to the 50 mm simulation-loosened hip prostheses.

quently it is absolutely essential to determine the size of the prosthesis to be used with the aid of the femoral templates before the operation. This measuring will conform with the operative situation in about 80% of the cases. Nevertheless, deviations to the extent of one size are possible, in some cases because of the different enlargements of the radiographs resulting from the individual circumstances. With adipose patients, for example, the medullary cavities of the femora appear to be larger, because they are positioned farther away from the plates. With slender patients exactly the opposite can be expected.

The operation is performed with the patient in the supine position. A modified Watson-Jones approach is used.[5] It is obvious, however, that the operation also may be performed via a dorsolateral access. After resection of the neck of the femur and detachment of the femoral head, the joint capsule is removed and the osseous acetabulum prepared accordingly. This part of the operation may be considered completed as soon as the osseous acetabulum is of such conical shape over the major part of its circumference that it matches the corresponding curvatures of the implant. If a polyethylene cup is selected, the thread must be cut before the socket is screwed in. If the newly developed titanium shell is preferred, there is no need to cut a thread. In other words, surgery is reduced by one working operation. The advantage of a conical cup is that such implants have large anchoring surfaces on the lateral portions of the cone and thus also can be medialized to an optimal degree. This is particularly important in the case of patients suffering from dysplasia arthrosis. In addition, the conical shape offers an optimal safeguard against tilting (Fig. 21-4).

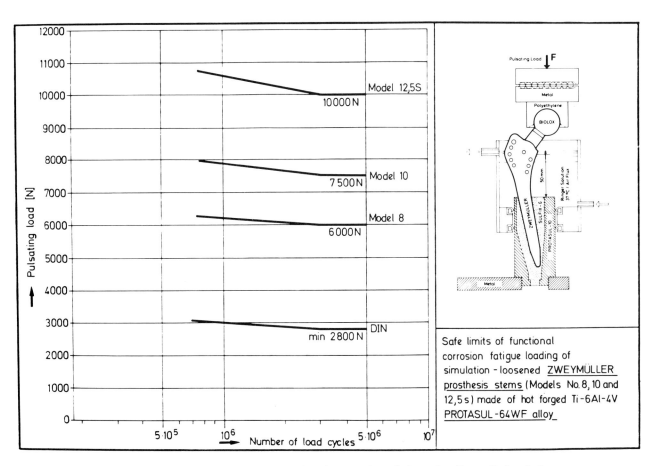

Fig. 21-9. Safety limits of the functional corrosion fatigue loading of simulation-loosened Zweymüller hip prostheses: Model 8, 6000 N; Model 10, 7500 N; Model 12.5 S, 10,000 N; all with stems of hot-forged Ti-6Al-4V titanium alloy Protasul-64 WF under the specified test conditions.

The next task is to prepare the medullary cavity of the femur. This is effected with the femoral rasps, which are applied to the medullary cavity in increasing sizes (Fig. 21-10). Their conical shape also conforms with that of the prosthesis. The rasping operation is complete as soon as the rasp is in tight contact with the corticalis of the medullary cavity. The relatively small differences in the sizes of the femoral rasps facilitate a step-by-step procedure and thus an exact preparation. The required neck length is determined as soon as the femoral component has been implanted. The medullary cavity then is closed off at the proximal end of the prosthesis with cancellous bone. The appropriate ball head is selected, and the protective cap removed immediately before its attachment to the structured surface of the spigot, whereupon it is turned slightly and given a slight tap. Particular care has to be exercised here with regard to the cleanliness of the two conical surfaces.

After repositioning and a check to determine movement of the joint, the wound is irrigated in a thorough manner to reduce the possibility of postoperative periarticular ossifications to a minimum and then closed in accordance with the operative access.

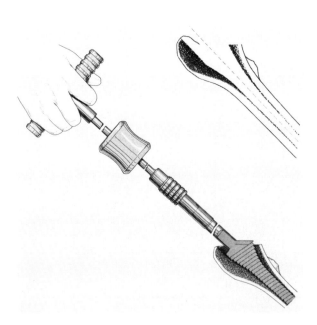

Fig. 21-10. Scheme of the preparation of the femur in the longitudinal axis with the femoral rasp.

CLINICAL RESULTS
Patient evaluation

During the period from October 1979 to June 1985, 1225 cementless implants were inserted at the Orthopaedic University Clinic in Vienna. Ten reoperations have been necessary up to now. It was considered of particular interest to follow up the earlier operations in order to obtain information on the clinical and radiographic results (Tables 21-2 through 21-11).

Table 21-2. Cementless implantations: Follow-up more than three years (N = 154)

Patients not included in statistics

Deceased patients	8
No follow-up possible	8
Infections (Girdlestone)	1
Cemented stem	1
TOTAL	18
Patients remaining	*136*

Table 21-3. Cementless implantations (N = 136)

Minimum follow-up period	28.0 months*
Maximum follow-up period	60.0 months
Average follow-up period	44.9 months
Male patients	58
Female patients	78
Age distribution	22-77 years
Average	56.8 years

*Only one case less than 36 months included because of radiologic interest (settlement of the prosthesis).

Table 21-4. Diagnosis (N = 136)

Idiopathic arthritis	75
Rheumatoid arthritis	9
Dysplasia	31
Avascular necrosis	13
Status posttrauma	3
Status postepiphysiolysis	3
Status post-Perthes	1
Others	1
TOTAL	136

Table 21-5. Walking capacity (preoperative)

Unable to walk	1	(0.7%)
At home	37	(27.2%)
>100 m	44	(32.4%)
>500 m	30	(22.1%)
>1 km	24	(17.7%)

Table 21-6. Walking capacity (postoperative)

Unable to walk	2	(1.5%)
>100 m	8	(5.9%)
>500 m	11	(8.0%)
>1 km	51	(37.5%)
Unlimited	64	(47.1%)

Table 21-7. Supports (preoperative)

None	53	(38.9%)
Cane, occasionally	6	(4.5%)
Cane, permanently	58	(42.7%)
Crutches	19	(14.0%)

Table 21-8. Supports (postoperative)

None	94	(69.1%)
Cane, occasionally	25	(18.4%)
Cane, permanently	11	(8.0%)
Crutches	6	(4.4%)

Table 21-9. Complaints (postoperative)

None	102	(75%)
Minor, without any impairment of daily life	30	(22.1%)
Serious, with impairment	4	(2.9%) (in two cases, trochanteric pain)

Table 21-10. Localization of the complaints at clinical examination

Bursitis trochanterica or scar pain	18
Soft tissue pain in inguine	4
Pain in the cup region	2
Soft tissue pain in the thigh	4
Femoral pain during inward rotation	8

An early infection *(Staphylococcus aureus)* was experienced with one patient. The prosthesis was removed, and the hip was left as a Girdlestone hip. The patient still has not made a decision with regard to a reoperation. In another case a lesion of the inguinal nerve and vessels occurred during the cutting of the thread for the cup. The vessels were reconstructed successfully, but a cable transplant of the nervus femoralis proved negative. In this particular case the stem had been anchored with cement and was therefore excluded from the follow-up statistics. Additional complications involved the tearing off of two trochanters and two fissures of the femur. These occurred in the region of the prosthesis tip and were treated in a conservative manner, that is, with a plaster cast. To a certain extent these fractures may be attributed to the instrumentarium that had not been optimized at that time. However, fractures of this kind also can be caused by nonoptimal operative technique. This can occur if the rasp is tilted when the osseous bed is prepared or if the prosthesis is implanted despite the fact that it does not conform with the prerasped osseous bed. The frequency of fracture can be rated now at 1%.

The walking capacity and the aids needed for walking preoperatively and postoperatively are specified in Tables 21-5 to 21-8.

The postoperative complaints and the localization of the complaints found at clinical examination are shown in Tables 21-9 and 21-10.

When we consider the assessment of the result by the patients themselves, the especially large percentage of patients who were (very or largely) satisfied with the operation is particularly interesting (Table 21-11).

At the same time we should realize that the operation was performed on average some 45 months before, that is, a period that already allows us to make an objective statement as well.

As is the case with every operative technique,

Table 21-11. Assessment of the result by the patients

Very satisfied	123	(90.4%)
Largely satisfied	12	(8.8%)
Unsatisfied	1	(0.7%)

failures were experienced. These will be described in detail, because such cases yield particularly valuable knowledge.

Reoperations

Reoperations proved to be necessary on three occasions with this first series of 136 stems. In the first case new bone formations had to be removed 7 months after the initial operation because of massive periarticular ossifications and functional ankylosis of the hip. Only slight recurrence was experienced, and the mobility improved significantly. On the other hip the patient was suffering from an osseous ankylosis following massive ossifications after a double cup arthroplasty. An individual reaction was certainly evident here. The distribution of the periarticular ossifications is shown in Table 21-12.

This table shows only two cases of ossification that had reached such a state that mobility was badly impaired, i.e. Stage III according to Arcq.[4] Stages I and II do not involve any functional restrictions. In addition to the individual factors, the occurrence of periarticular ossifications depends on the operative approach and the traumatization of the tissue. This statement is generally applicable to any hip operation. With the cementless implantation there is also the possibility of postoperative bleeding from the medullary cavity. This can be more or less stopped by closing off the proximal end of the femur by compression of the cancellous bone or through the insertion of cancellous bone from the head of the femur along the proximal end of the implant.

It was necessary to reoperate the stem in one case and on the stem and cup in another. These two cases will serve as an aid to answer the following questions at the same time.

1. How easy or difficult is it to remove a cementless prosthesis on the basis of a press-fit anchorage?
2. Can a loosened cementless prosthesis be replaced by a cementless model?

Table 21-12. Periarticular ossifications

None	71	(52.2%)
Arcq I*	32	(23.5%)
Arcq II	31	(23.0%)
Arcq III	2	(1.4%)

*See Arcq, M.: Arch. Orthop. Unfall - Chir. **77:**108, 1973.

3. What is the condition of the osseous bed around such a loosened implant?

The first case involved a 59-year-old female patient weighing about 95 kg. She had been provided with an implant that was too small and that had a small prosthesis collar, which was used at that time. It soon led postoperatively to the formation of a pronounced radiolucent line around the implanted stem (Fig. 21-11). Nevertheless, the patient had no complaints and was satisfied until she had an accident 4 years after the implantation. From then on, she suffered severe and, above all, load-dependent pain, which undoubtedly was attributable to the stem. The latter was changed by means of a reoperation. The prosthesis was removed without difficulty and the medullary cavity prepared with a curette. A model, two sizes larger, was implanted—again without the use of cement. Since the osseous bed was largely intact, it was easy to establish a stable anchorage in the cortical bone. Up to now, 14 months after the reoperation, the patient is well, and no new radiolucent lines have formed around the implant.

The second case concerned a 42-year-old woman whose pelvis had undergone osteotomy according to Chiari because of a severe dysplasia arthrosis 4 years before the implantation of the cementless hip. A titanium stem was implanted in combination with an Endler polyethylene cup in February 1980. As a result of a technical operative error, the implanted stem was too small (Fig. 21-12). Furthermore, the prosthetic component was anchored proximally and not diaphyseally because of a coxa valga. As a consequence of this, the medial curvature of the proximal portion of the stem jammed on the extremely valgus calcar portion of the femur. Through settling, the stem tried to establish osseous contact, which was not possible in this case because of the parallel cortical shape of the diaphyses (Fig. 21-12, *C*). A radiolucent line formed encircling the complete stem.

It is interesting to note that this patient was also free of complaints until she was involved in a motoring accident 3 years after the operation. From then on she suffered severe pain, and the prosthesis had to be replaced. It was found that the stem and the cup were loose. The two components were able to be removed without difficulty. The granulation tissue was removed with great care and found to be thicker in the region

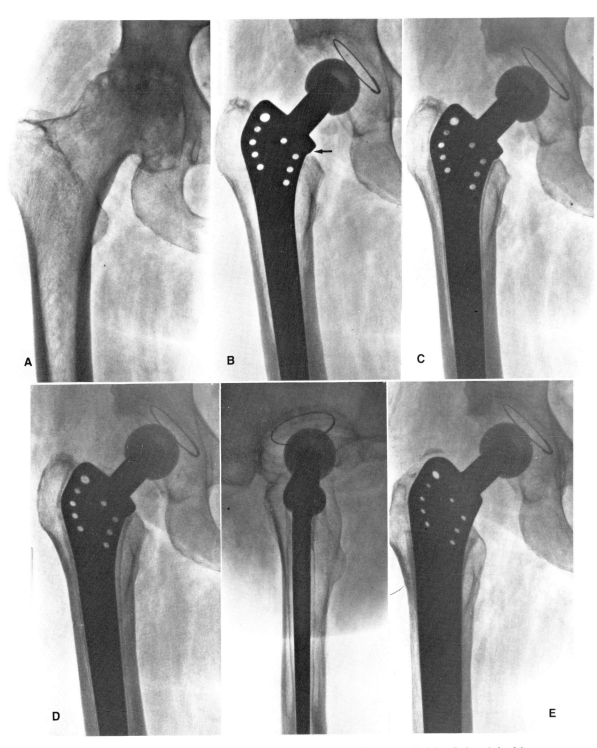

Fig. 21-11. S.K., female, 59 years old. **A,** Pronounced osteoarthritis of the right hip. Wide medullary canal. **B,** 4 months after surgery. Comparatively little contact of the implant with the diaphysis. The collar has been placed upon the resection line of the femoral neck *(arrow).* **C,** 15 months after surgery. Wide radiolucent line around the proximal and the intermediate thirds of the stem. **D,** 39 months after surgery. Increase of the radiolucent lines around all of the stem in the AP and the axial x-ray film. **E,** 59 months after primary surgery and 14 months after replacement surgery with a larger model. Good diaphyseal cortical contact. Except for a trochanter bursitis, there are no complaints.

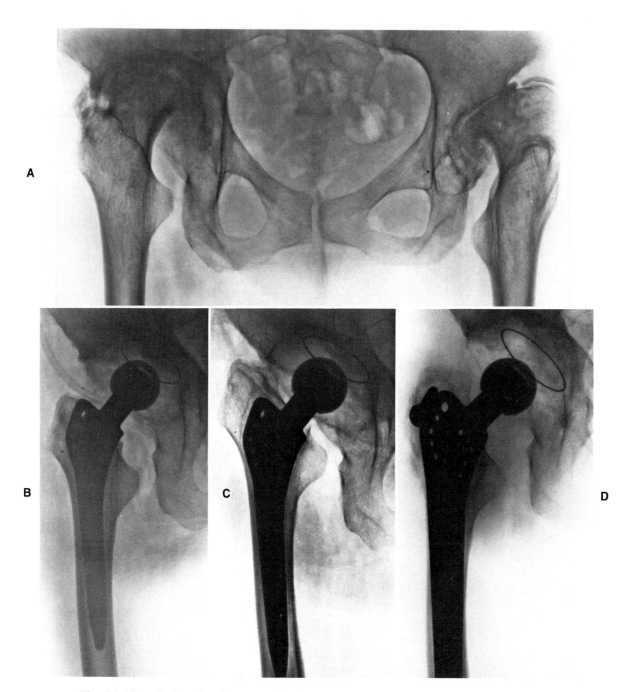

Fig. 21-12. L.J., female, 42 years old. **A,** Massive bilateral dysplasia arthrosis, after Chiari's pelvic osteotomy on the right side. Pronounced coxa valga. **B,** Operation site: implantation of the stem in a valgic position as a result of the contact of its medial curvature with the calcar. Insufficient diaphyseal contact. **C,** 39 months following surgery. Distinct settling of the prosthesis. Radiolucent lines around its proximal parts as well as around the tip. **D,** After exchange operation of both components with larger implants. Additional fixation of the major trochanter with a cortical screw.

of the stem than the cup. A larger cementless model was implanted in each case. The bone around the stem was partly resorbed and thinner than the original. Nevertheless, it was possible to establish a primary stable anchorage (Fig. 21-12, *D*). The patient's condition may be rated as "good" 8 months after the operation.

Investigation of the inner polyethylene faces of the Endler screw cup (implantation time 45 months) revealed a total wear extending to a depth of only 0.35 mm, which corresponds to an annual rate of 0.09 mm. This low value for a polyethylene screw-type cup has been confirmed by the measurement results published by Weber[44] for the polyethylene wear (0.09 mm per year) for Weber-Stühmer total hip prostheses with polyethylene cups and 32 mm Biolox ceramic ball heads.

These two cases allow us to answer the questions asked at the beginning in the following manner.

1. In cases of loosening, a prosthesis anchored with a press fit can be removed quite easily. No great operative effort is needed.
2. A loosened cementless prosthesis also can be replaced by a cementless implant.
3. Depending on the duration and extent of loosening, the osseous bed can be resorbed to a major or minor degree. The earlier assumed hypothesis that a loosened cementless prosthesis does not cause any, or only very slight, rarefication of bone is true only in some cases. Nevertheless, it would be unwise to implant a cement prosthesis in such an already damaged osseous bed, because it would rob the bone of any recovery possibility.

As to the further knowledge gained from these two cases, it should be stated that clinically manifested signs of loosening still can occur after complaint-free implantation of some years duration. Admittedly, the follow-up of radiographs leaves open the question as to why pain did not occur before.

Radiograph evaluation

The radiograph constitutes a valuable aid for the assessment of the postoperative development. However, the radiographs must be made accurately in both planes, and regular follow-ups are a necessity. Possible changes in the position of the prosthesis, radiolucent line formations, and osseous changes are of particular interest, providing they indicate an increasing incorporation of the implant or signs of loosening.

Tables 21-13 and 21-14 indicate the position of the implants postoperatively and at the time of the follow-up. Even the slightest but just determinable radiologic dislocation also was rated. It was now considered of particular interest to examine the patients exhibiting changes in the position of the implant with regard to their complaints. It was established that there was a significant percentage of patients with complaints in the case of positional changes in varus and in the longitudinal axis, combined with a varus dislocation. With the exception of one patient, however, the mere settlement in the longitudinal axis did not have any clinical relevance. Apart from one patient the complaints were so slight that they did not interfere with the daily activities (Table 21-15). On the other hand, changes in the position of the implant can take place without being expressed clinically.

The evaluation of radiolucent lines (double contours) located around the implant is much more difficult. Here again, every minimal line was rated. They were found around the implant in a large percentage of cases and chiefly located in the region of the proximal end of the prosthesis. Clinically, these lines proved to be completely insignificant (Fig. 21-13). Double contours around the whole implant were observed only in 7% of the cases. In the majority of those they were only 1 mm or less.

Table 21-13. Stem position (postoperative)

Exactly in the longitudinal axis of the femur	100	(73.5%)
<5-degree varus	22	(16.2%)
>5-degree varus	8	(5.8%)
Slightly in valgus	6	(4.4%)

Table 21-14. Stem position (follow-up)

Unchanged	106	(78.0%)
Migration into varus position	9	(6.6%)
Migration into valgus position	1	(0.7%)
Settlement in the longitudinal axis	7	(5.1%)
Settlement + varus	13	(9.6%)

Table 21-15. Stem position: postoperative complaints

	No complaints	*Minor complaints*	*Major complaints*
No change	86	17	3
Migration into varus	4	5	0
Migration into valgus	0	1	0
Settlement in the longitudinal axis	6	1	0
Settlement + varus	6	6	1

The follow-up based on the series of radiographs showed that these radiolucent line formations were already pronounced after about 6 months. In the subsequent years, however, neither their appearance nor, above all, their thickness was altered. Accordingly, these cases were rated as "indifferent" in the assessment of the incorporation of the prostheses; that is, on the basis of the unchanged radiologic situation over the last few years there was no change. Although no increasing incorporation could be established here, there was no degradation of the surrounding bone structure either. (Table 21-16). In cases with an increase in the bone structure immediately adjacent to and around the implant, the result was classified as "increasing incorporation" (see Table 21-16).

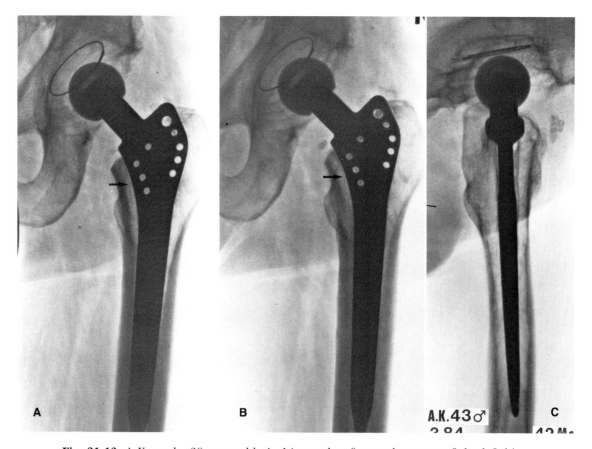

Fig. 21-13. A.K., male, 39 years old. **A,** 14 months after replacement of the left hip. Slight radiolucent line in the proximal region of the prosthesis *(arrow)*. **B,** 42 months after surgery. The AP picture shows increasing incorporation of the prosthesis. No increase of the radiolucent line *(arrow)*. **C,** The axial picture shows a radiolucent line in the proximal part of the prosthesis too. No increase of this line in the last years. Excellent clinical result.

An implant was rated "loose" if pronounced radiolucent lines were observed around the whole prosthesis. As previously stated, the radiologic changes do not correspond with the clinical findings. In four of these five cases the patients had only minor complaints. One of them had a double-sided implantation, and so both hips must be subject to pronounced loads here (Fig. 21-14).

The cause of the clearly evident radiolucent line formations is primarily implantation-

technical errors. Should, for example, the implanted prosthesis be too small, that is, no ideal cortical contact is realized with the implant as a result of the operation, we must expect loosening later. Because of its straight conical stem, this prosthesis still can settle and thus achieve a secondary stabilization. However, the evaluation of these cases shows that this leads only to complete freedom from complaints in a certain percentage of cases. On the other hand, patients whose implants were absolutely stable also had complaints. Such complaints are not related to the implantation of a cementless prosthesis, but they are the consequences of the operative approach and related problems (see also Table 21-10).

However, we should not forget that here we are concerned with the first cases to be treated with a new method, for which neither the implantation

Table 21-16. Assessment of the incorporation

Prosthesis exhibits increasing incorporation	93	(68.3%)
Bone reacts indifferently	37	(25.7%)
Prosthesis becoming loose	5	(5.1%)
Radiograph not assessable	1	(0.7%)

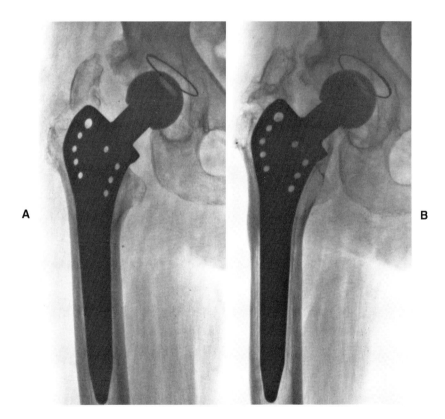

Fig. 21-14. K.H., female, 66 years old. **A,** After total replacement of the right hip. Partial avulsion of the major trochanter. The implant used is too small. **B,** 30 months after surgery. The stem is almost completely surrounded by a radiolucent line. Slight migration toward the varus position.

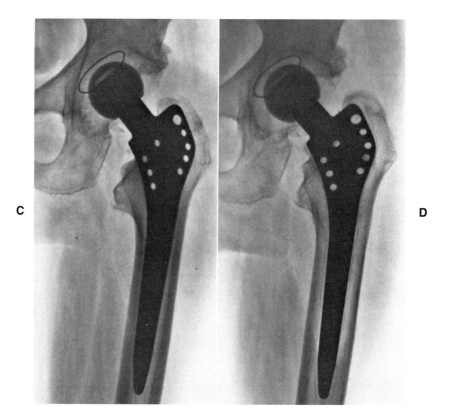

Fig. 21-14, cont'd. C, After total replacement of the left hip. The implant used is much too small. **D,** 33 months after surgery. Radiolucent lines of constant width around the implant. Distinct spongiosation of the cortex. Patient walks a couple of miles daily without the aid of a cane. She has no complaints.

technique nor the instruments were perfected to the extent they are today. It can be assumed therefore that the results also will improve as more and more experience is gained with this operation. Undoubtedly this method places greater demands on the surgeon than is the case with the implantation of a cemented prosthesis. Cemented implants are most stable immediately after the operation. However, the cement is able to conceal, at least for some time, technical errors in implantation.

SPECIAL INDICATIONS

A further point of discussion is the ongoing question of possible contraindication for the cementless implantation with regard to the preoperative bone quality and the age of the patient. The cementless anchorage of course should be encouraged in the case of younger patients with good bone structure. However, sur-

geons also encounter old (and very old) patients with a bone quality that one would expect with an appreciably younger patient; therefore individual factors must be considered. It has not been proved so far that the results realized with older patients are inferior to those achieved with younger persons. Nevertheless, caution has to be exercised in cases where the patient to be operated on will probably never learn to walk with crutches; thus partial weight-bearing, at least, cannot be expected postoperatively.

Osteoporosis is also no contraindication for the cementless anchorage, providing the implant is anchored exactly cortically. As to polyarthritis, the changes taking place in the bone do not constitute any contraindication for the cementless implantation either. According to my own findings, there is no difference between the results achieved with patients suffering from idiopathic arthrosis and rheumatoid arthritis (Fig. 21-15).

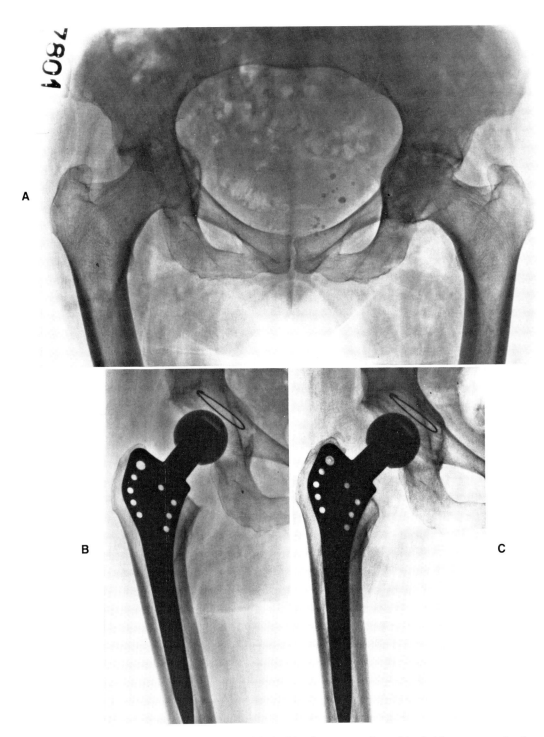

Fig. 21-15. L.H., female, 58 years old. **A,** Massive protrusion of both hips as a result of rheumatoid arthritis. The acetabular floor of the right side shows infractions already. **B,** 2 months following surgery. Good fit of cup and stem. Slight threads in the conical area of the cup. A spongioplasty has been done in the acetabular floor. **C,** 37 months following surgery. Good incorporation of the cup. No tendency to protrude. The position of the stem remains unchanged. No radiolucent lines. Distinct increase of the trabecular structure in the medullary cavity. Excellent clinical result. The other hip has been replaced meanwhile.

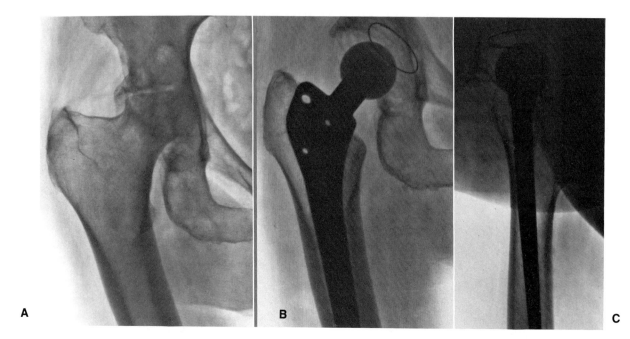

A   B   C

Fig. 21-16. F.M., female, 53 years old. **A,** Massive destruction of the right hip caused by rheumatoid arthritis. **B,** 8 months after total replacement of the right hip. Inconspicuous postoperative development. **C,** Good position of the stem in the axial x-ray film as well.

Particularly in the case of patients with rheumatoid arthritis the radiologic follow-ups reveal increasing incorporation of the implant resulting from newly formed bone, especially in the cancellous bone region. This radiologic impression was verified histologically in a patient with severe destructive inflammation (Fig. 21-16). As a complication of a cervical fusion, this female patient died 10 months after implantation of the right hip joint and 3 months after surgery on the left hip joint. Up to that time she was quite mobile at home. The microsection showed increased incorporation of the implant through newly formed bone tissue. The bone extended—without any intermediate layers of connective tissue—to the metal and followed every surface roughness (Figs. 21-16, *E* and *F*). This increasing ingrowth was still not completed after 10 months (see Fig. 21-16). The cross-section of the titanium stem as shown in Fig. 21-16, *G*, with the directly neighboring bone substance was analyzed for calcium (29 ± 1%) and phosphorus (10 ± 1%) in the electron beam microprobe. These values conform well with the calcium/phosphorus content of the

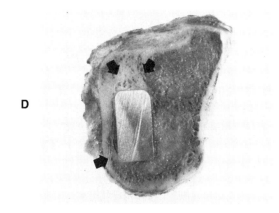

D

Fig. 21-16, cont'd. D, Macroscopic cross-section of the metaphysis 10 months after surgery. The arrows show sclerosis zones of the cortex in close contact with the metal surface.

load-bearing calcium hydroxide apatite of the compact femoral bone. The good degree of mineralization exhibited by the bone material that had grown onto the titanium surface of the stem was substantiated by means of x-ray studies of fine structural analysis.

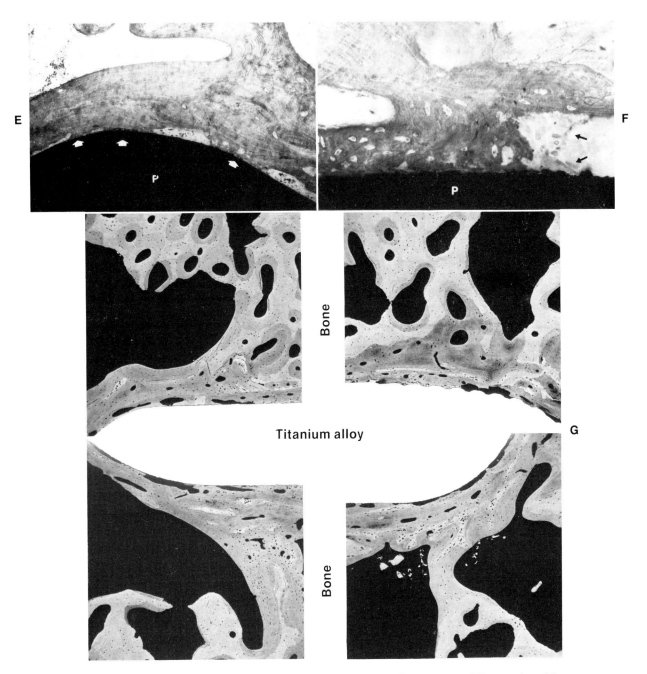

Fig. 21-16, cont'd. E, Edge of the prosthesis, 10 months after surgery. (Microsection, 10 μ, toluidin blue, undecalcified, ×160.) Direct contact of lamellar newly built bone *(arrow)* with the metal. *P,* prosthesis. **F,** Direct area of contact of the newly built lamellar bone with the metal. No interposed connective tissue, no foreign body giant cells. Vital osteoblasts. Wide osteoid seam *(arrows)* with immediate contact to the metal. (Microsection, 10 μ, toluidin blue, ×400.) **G,** Backscatter electronic-current images (magnification ×40) of the cross-section of the titanium stem with good bone contact after an implantation duration of 10 months.

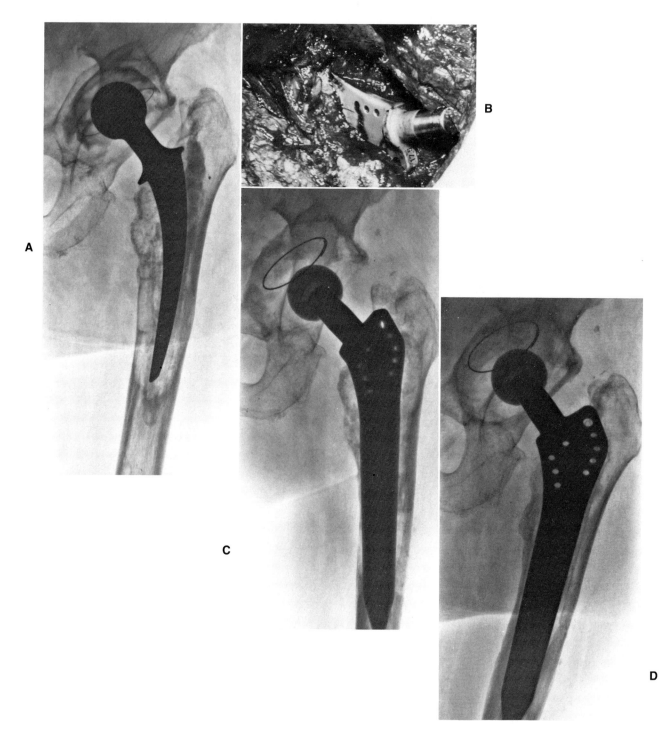

Fig. 21-17. R.H., female, 75 years old. **A,** Massively loosened cemented total hip prosthesis, 7 years after implantation. Almost complete resorption of preexisting bone, especially in the region of the calcar and the medial diaphysis, as well as in the acetabulum. **B,** Operation site: stem already implanted. Large defect of the calcar. The hollow areas around the proximal part of the prosthesis have been filled up with homologous spongy bone. **C,** 2 months after surgery. **D,** 29 months after surgery. Significant enlargement of the diaphyseal bone. The spongious graft has healed around the calcar. Excellent clinical result.

A further indication area, which I believe will become increasingly important in the future, is the replacement of a loosened cemented implant. One has to consider the following.

1. The osseous bed around the loosened endoprosthesis is massively impaired by the broken cement and wear particles. Should cement be reintroduced into this frequently, although partly, destroyed bone stock?
2. Does bone react differently and more positively to a cementless implant than to a cemented one?
3. Therefore does the cementless implantation of an exchange prosthesis offer a real advantage?

The answer to the first question is that we must avoid the use of cement in such cases wherever possible. One of the many arguments here is that a replacement cemented prosthesis must be anchored in healthy bone. This usually begins, however, distal of the original stem tip. In case of repeated loosening the size of the defect usually rules out a sufficient therapy.

With the cementless reoperation the bone has the chance to react again, in the sense of increased bone substance. As an example, I cite the case of a 75-year-old female patient who was admitted to our clinic with massively loosened cemented joints on both sides. The bone exhibited distinct signs of recovery following the replacement of the left hip (Fig. 21-17). The patient now uses this leg as the weight-bearing leg 29 months after the operation. A review of the first series of 50 replacement operations shows that this trend may be observed generally among numerous patients.[45] This, in turn, answers the second question: in the absence of bone cement the bone apparently is given the chance of entering a regeneration phase.

In my opinion these results show that the cementless implantation is a real alternative to the conservative reoperation methods. As with every technique, especially in such problem areas, the results depend largely on patient selection, operative skill, and postoperative care. Taking these factors into consideration, this method should be appraised for the larger number of cases that we shall surely encounter in the future.

SUMMARY

The follow-up of the first 136 cases operated on 3 to 5 years ago revealed a high percentage of excellent and good results. They certainly compare favorably with the early results realized with cementable prostheses. At the same time we should remember that these results have been achieved with a new method embodying a number of uncertainties and weaknesses at the beginning. As a result of the initial experience, intensive efforts were made to realize improvements without at all changing the principle of a primary stable metadiaphysary cortical anchorage on the basis of a press fit. The improvements are found in the improved accuracy of the operative planning and the refinement of the surgical procedure. This includes selection of the optimal prosthesis size, compression of cancellous bone, which thus also reduces the bleeding from the medullary cavity, and thorough irrigation of the wound area. The range of available stems was extended with a view to reducing the size graduations between the individual implants. Furthermore, it was decided to do away with the small prosthesis collars that were used in the initial phase. The mounting of the collar on the resection face of the neck of the femur could give the false impression of a stable metadiaphysary cortical anchorage. The collar has proved to be disadvantageous in these cases (Fig. 21-11). The development of a metal cup made of pure titanium constitutes a further step forward. Taking these facts into account, we can expect a further improvement in future results.

The questions posed at the outset have been partly answered by the presentation of the results and the possibility of employing this system for special indications. There is no doubt that the cementless implant can be employed instead of a cementable model. Even osteoporotic bone substance frequently reacts to the biocompatible cementless implant with an enlargement of bone substance and remineralization. The conventional bone cement on the other hand leads to demineralization at the bone cement–bone interface and should therefore not be used in cases of major osteoporosis.[24]

From the theoretic standpoint of bone healing, in the sense of an osseointegration according to Albrektsson,[1] the patient should not subject the involved joint to any weight for 3 months—an unrealistic requirement. I believe that, even though this prosthesis system is primarily stable and permits immediate weight bearing, it should be protected in the first 6 weeks following surgery. With patients suffering from rheumatoid arthritis, we should use the advantages provided by the cementless anchorage even when the polytopic localizations associated with the disease render weight-relieved mobilization impossible or restrict the same to an extensive degree.

As far as the material is concerned, the employed titanium stem definitely offers optimal preconditions. In contrast to the cast implants it is almost impossible for even the smallest implant to break in the postoperative period (Fig. 21-9). Should a reoperation prove necessary because of loosening or infection, the prosthesis can be removed without any further destruction of the surrounding bone stock, because a large area of the stem surface is provided only with a fine structure that facilitates the explantation of the stem.

The histologic examination of stems removed from deceased patients showed that the employed titanium alloy is extremely biocompatible.[26] Otherwise the newly formed bone would not have grown so close to the metal surface (Fig. 21-16). In the sense of Albrektsson,[2,3] we can truly speak here of an osseointegration. Electronic spectroscopic investigations[28,41] showed that a layer of titanium oxide (TiO_2), serving as an active passivator of the metal surface, forms continuously on the surface of the titanium alloy in the body environment. This layer favors the chemisorption of superoxide O_2^- and hydroxide OH^-. Up to now, no reports exist in the literature on any negative effects of implants made of the titanium alloy Ti-6Al-4V on the neighboring bone, even though this material has been employed clinically since the 1960s. The excellent compatibility of titanium—in the sense of biocompatibility—was substantiated by the investigations made by Bothe that established the tendency of the bones to make contact with titanium.[7] These characteristics were used particularly in the area of oral and dental implants, where excellent long-term results have been achieved.[2,3,9]

In comparison with conventional bone cements and with the aid of a so-called bone growth chamber, Albrektsson[1] was able to show that the use of polymethylmethacrylate (PMMA) cements leads to the formation of connective tissue and less new bone formation, whereas with titanium there was direct bone contact and a significant increase in the formation of new bone. This reflects the low biocompatibility of the PMMA bone cement and the excellent compatibility of titanium.

The primary stability and mechanical quiescence that are achieved by the primary stabilization of the prosthetic stem in the corticalis through the press fit are prerequisite for primary ingrowth. In combination with the bioinertness of the titanium, it is first the primary stabilization that facilitates the osseointegration of the stem. In the stems investigated, this osseointegration occurred mainly in the medial and lateral press-fit regions and spread from there to the dorsal and ventral sides.[24] Like Swanson and Freeman,[42] and also Linder,[23] we believe that a porous-coated surface is not necessary for osseointegration.

REFERENCES

1. Albrektsson, T.: Osseus penetration rate into implants pretreated with bone cement, Arch. Orthop. Trauma Surg. **102:**141, 1984.
2. Albrektsson, T., Branemark, P.J., Hannsson, H.A., Kasemo, B., Larsson, K., Lundström, I., McQueen, D.H., and Skalak, R.: The interface zone of interorganic implants in vivo: Titanium implants in bone Ann. Biomed. Eng. **11:**1, 1983.
3. Albrektsson, T., Branemark, P.J.; Hansson, H.A., and Lindström, J.: Osseointegrated titanium implants, Acta Orthop. Scand. **52:**155, 1981.
4. Arcq, M.: Die periartikulären Ossifikationen—eine Komplikation der Totalendoprothese des Hüftgelenkes, Arch. Orthop. Unfall-Chir. **77:**108, 1973.
5. Bauer, R., Kerschbaumer, S., Poisel, S., and Oberthaler, W.: The transgluteal approach to the hip, Arch. Orthop. Trauma Surg. **95:**47, 1979.
6. Bösch, P., Harms, H., and Lintner, F.: The proof of dimetylparatoluidine in bone cement even after long-time implantation, Arch. Toxicol. **51:**157, 1982.
7. Bothe, R.T., Beaton, K.E., and Davenport, H.A.: Reaction of bone to multiple metallic implants, Surg. Gynecol. Obstet. **71:**598, 1940.
8. Boutin, P.: L'arthroplastie totale de la hanche par prothèse en alumine. Résultats de 150 cas d'ancrage direct de la pièce acétabulaire, Internat. Orthopaedics (SICOT) **1:**87, 1977.
9. Branemark, P.J., Hansson, B.O., Adell, R., Breine, U., Lindström, J., Hallen, O., and Öhman, A.: Osseointegrated implants in the treatment of the edentulous jaw, Scand. J. Plast. Reconstr. Surg. **11**(suppl. 16) 1977.
10. Endler, M.: Theoretisch-experimentelle Grundlagen und erste klinische Erfahrungen mit einer neuen, zementfreien Polyäthylenschraubpfanne beim Hüftgelenkersatz. Acta Chir . Austriaca, Suppl. **45:**3, 1982.
11. Endler, M., Endler, F., and Plenk, H., Jr.: Experimental and early clinical experience with an uncemented UHMW polyethylene acetabular prosthesis. In Morscher, E., editor: The cementless fixation of hip endoprostheses, New York, 1984, Springer-Verlag.

12. Engh, C.A., and Bobyn, J.D.: Biological fixation in total hip arthroplasty, Thorofare, N.J., 1985, Slack, Inc.
13. Gächter, A.: The bone cement cuff in hip endoprostheses: Results of 80 postmortem studies. In Morscher, E., editor: The cementless fixation of hip endoprostheses, New York, 1984, Springer-Verlag.
14. Galante, J.H., Harris, W.H.: Paper presented at the fifty-second annual meeting of the American Academy of Orthopaedic Surgeons, Las Vegas, 1985.
15. Galante, J.H., Rostoker, W., Lueck R., and Ray, R.D.: Sintered fiber metal composites as a basis for attachment of implants to bone, J. Bone Joint Surg. **53A**:101, 1971.
16. Griss, P., and Heimke, G.: Five years experience with ceramic-metal-composite hip endoprostheses. I. Clinical evaluation. Arch. Orthop. Trauma Surg. **98**:157, 1981.
17. Henssge, E.J.: Gegossene spongiös-metallische Implantate, Paper presented at the twenty-sixth annual meeting of the Austrian Society of Surgery, Vienna, 1985.
18. Holz, Z., Hemminger, W., and Gasse, H.: Mechanische Untersuchungen an explantierten und frischen Knochenzementen, Arch. Orthop. Trauma Surg. **91**:121, 1978.
19. Homsy, C.A.: Biocompatibility of perfluorinated polymers and composites of these polymers. In Williams, D.F., editor: Biocompatibility of clinical implant materials, vol. 2, Boca Raton, Fla., 1982, CRC Press.
20. Judet, R.: Total-Hüftendoprothesen aus Porometall ohne Zementverankerung, Z. Orthop. **113**:828, 1975.
21. Hungerford, D.S., and Kenna, R.V.: Preliminary experience with a total knee prosthesis with porous coating used without cement, Clin. Orthop. **146**:95, 1983.
22. Küsswetter, H., Gabriel, E., Stuhler, T., and Töpfer, L.: Remodelling of the femur in conventionally-implanted hip prostheses. In Morscher, E., editor: The cementless fixation of hip endoprostheses, New York, 1984, Springer-Verlag.
23. Linder, L., Albrektsson, T., Branemark, P.J., Hansson, H.A., Invarsson, B., Jönsson, U., and Lundstrm, I.: Electron microscopic analysis of bone-titanium interface, Acta Orthop. Scand. **54**:45-52, 1983.
24. Lintner, F.: Die Ossifikationsstörung an der Knochenzement-Knochengrenze. Acta Chir. Austr. Suppl. **48**: 1983.
25. Lintner, F., Bösch, P., and Brand, G.: Histological examinations of remodelling proceedings on the cement-bone surface of endoprostheses after implantation from 3-10 years, Pathol. Res. Pract. **173**:376, 1982.
26. Lintner, F., Zweymüller, K., and Brand, G.: Tissue reactions to titanium endoprostheses: Autopsy studies in four cases, J. Arthroplasty, 1986. (In press.)
27. Lord, G., Hardy, J.J., and Kummer, F.J.: An uncemented total hip replacement, Experimental study and review of 300 madreporique arthroplasties, Clin. Orthop. **141**:2, 1979.
28. Maeusli, P.A., Bloch, P., Burri, C., Moosmann, A., and Gerret, V.: Oberflächenprozesse an Titan und Titanlegierungen, 5, Berlin, 1984, Vortragsreihe DVM-Arbeitskreis Implantate.
29. Mittelmeier, H.: Total hip replacement with the autophor cementfree ceramic prosthesis. In Morscher E., editor: The cementless fixation of hip endoprosthesis, New York, 1984, Springer-Verlag.
30. Mittelmeier, H.: Paper presented at the meeting of the Austrian Society of Orthopaedic Surgeons, Vienna, 1985.
31. Moore, A.: A metal hip joint, a new selflocking vitallium prosthesis, South. Med. J. **45**:1015, 1952.
32. Morscher, E., Bombelli, R., Schenk, R., and Mathys, R.: The treatment of femoral neck fractures with an isoelastic endoprosthesis implanted without bone cement, Arch. Orthop. Trauma Surg. **98**:93, 1981.
33. Oest, O., Müller, K., and Hupfauer, W.: Die Knochenzemente, Stuttgart, 1985, Ferdinand Enke, Verlag.
34. Pflüger, G., and Zweymüller, K.: Austauschoperationen gelockerter Hüftendoprothesen mit zementfreien Implantaten: Operations, technik und Frühergebnisse. In Bauer, R., and Kerschbaumer, F. editors: Die Koxarthrose, Uelzen, 1984, ML Verlag, West Germany.
35. Reichelt, A., and Bläsius, K.: First experience with PM prosthesis. In Morscher, E., editor: The cementless fixation of hip endoprostheses, New York, 1984, Springer-Verlag.
36. Ring, P.A.: Total replacement of the hip joint: A review of a thousand operations, J. Bone Joint Surg. **56B**:44, 1974.
37. Salzer, M., Zweymüller, K., Locke, H., Zeibig, A., Stärk, N., Plenk, H., and Punzet, G.: Further experimental and clinical experience with aluminium oxide endoprostheses, J. Biomed. Mater. Res. **10**:847, 1976.
38. Semlitsch, M.: Metallic implant materials for hip joint endoprostheses designed for cemented and cementless fixation. In Morscher, E., editor: The cementless fixation of hip endoprostheses, New York, 1984, Springer-Verlag.
39. Semlitsch, M., and Panic, B.: 10 years of experience with test criteria for fracture-proof anchorage stems of artificial hip joints, Eng. Med. **12**:185, 1983.
40. Siwash, K.M.: The development of a total metal prosthesis for the hip joint from a partial joint replacement, Reconstr. Surg. Traumatol. **11**:53, 1969.
41. Steinemann, S.G., and Perren, S.M.: Titanlegierungen für Implantate-physikochemische Fragen, 5, Vortragsreihe DVM-Arbeitskreis Implantate, Berlin, 1984.
42. Swanson, A.B., and Freeman, M.A.R.: The tissue response to total joint replacement prostheses. In: The scientific basis of joint replacement, Tunbridge Wells, England, 1977, Pitman Medical Publishing Co., Ltd.
43. Thompson, F.R.: Two and a half year's experience with a vitallium intramedullary hip prosthesis, J. Bone Joint Surg. **36A**:489, 1959.
44. Weber, B.G., Semlitsch, M., Sieber, H.P., and Egli, A: Wear of the components of the trunion bearing total hip and its varieties, In: Fourth meeting of the European Society of Biomechanics, Davos & Switzerland, 308, 1984.
45. Zweymüller, K.: Austauschoperationen gelockerter Zementprothesen. In: Das zementfreie Hüftendoprothesensystem Zweymüller-Endler, Vienna, 1986, Facultas Verlag. (In press.)
46. Zweymüller, K., and Semlitsch, M: Concept and material properties of a cementless hip prosthesis system with Al_2O_3 ceramic ball heads and wrought Ti-6Al-4V stems, Arch. Orthop. Trauma Surg. **100**:229, 1982.

Chapter 22

One-staged exchange arthroplasty for septic total hip replacement

WILLIAM H. HARRIS

PREOPERATIVE CONSIDERATIONS

The three major options in the management of a septic total hip replacement are:

1. Resection arthroplasty
2. Immediate replantation
3. Resection arthroplasty followed by delayed replantation

The advantages of immediate replantation are great. If successful, it means only one operative procedure rather than two operative procedures as in the delayed replantation, or it means substantially better functional results than a resection arthroplasty. Either way this represents significant advantages to the patient in terms of hospital time, operative time, the apprehensions and risks of having two operations, and the major improvement in pain relief and function.

Conversely, the risks involved are high compared to the other two options, since a major foreign body is implanted in the face of infection.

The resolution of these two divergent positions requires three key elements:

1. Highly specific selection of the patient
2. Reconstructive surgery of high technical ability
3. Excellent management of the antimicrobial therapy

Without the coordination of these three elements, the risks are prohibitive, and immediate replantation should not be undertaken. However, in the presence of these three elements, immedi-

ate replantation can be carried out with a high degree of success, at major reduction in morbidity to the patient, and major reduction in cost to the community.

What are the key issues in patient selection? First, the patient must be healthy. If sepsis recurs, the patient will become moderately or severely ill again and may die. Consequently, such immediate replantation should not be undertaken unless the patient is otherwise generally quite healthy.

The second key issue is the presence of only a single organism of infection. In addition, that organism should be a gram-positive organism. The experience with multiple organism infections and gram-negative infections in terms of immediate replantation is significantly worse than in single organism gram-positive infections. In my judgment immediate replantation should not be undertaken if there are multiple organisms or gram-negative organisms.

Next, the infection should be one in which the patient has already demonstrated a substantial symbiosis with the organism. In other words, immediate replantation should not be done in the face of active, aggressive sepsis but rather should be limited to those patients in which the process of infection is slow, smoldering, and relatively nonvirulent.

Finally, there should be no evidence of extensive osteomyelitis.

It is clear, then, that only a small portion of patients who have a septic total hip replacement will be candidates for immediate replantation. On the other hand, in this selected group of patients

Supported in part by The William H. Harris Foundation.

the results of immediate replantation are very gratifying indeed.

What about antibiotic management in immediate replantation? Three approaches to the delivery of antibiotics in these circumstances have been advocated: triple systemic antibiotics, single systemic antibiotics, and antibiotic cement. The experience of those advocating triple systemic antibiotics has shown no advantage in terms of the clinical success of the procedure, and the toxicity associated with this approach is prohibitive. Single systemic antibiotics should be used in high doses, based on the sensitivity of the demonstrated organism involved. The evidence in favor of the capacity of antibiotic cement to deliver high concentrations of antibiotics locally and safely is overwhelming. Therefore, in immediate replantation I strongly urge the use of antibiotic cement.

What then are the prerequisites for immediate replantation? It is essential not only to establish that sepsis is present but also to establish the identity and sensitivity of the organisms. This requires an aspiration. I rarely, if ever, use a bone scan in these circumstances, because bone scans are inaccurate and insensitive. Even if a bone scan provided information that suggested strongly that sepsis was present, this information would be insufficient. Bone scans cannot identify the organism or allow you to determine the sensitivity of the organism. Aspiration can do both.

This clinical setting is one instance in which it is neither necessary nor worthwhile to carry out an arthrogram at the time of the aspiration. In the presence of sepsis both components should be exchanged whether they are loose or not. Therefore, if sepsis is known to be present, no arthrogram is needed.

RESULTS

What results can be expected in such surgery? Obviously, the results of this surgery will depend very heavily on whether infection is actually present, and in some cases the definition of the presence of sepsis can be difficult. In our work[4] we have required a positive culture in addition to the other conventional means of identifying sepsis. It is important to appreciate that sepsis in the hip joint may be very subtle indeed and that the common parameters indicating a septic process may be completely lacking. For example, erythema and swelling may be totally absent. The

white blood-cell count may be normal in total and devoid of a shift to the left. The sedimentation rate may be completely normal. There may be nothing specific about the radiographic appearance, and thus the clinical setting may be one that appears extremely benign. Usually the patients in this group are afebrile.

We studied a group of 18 patients in whom definite sepsis has been established by the determination of positive cultures, growing the same organisms on multiple occasions, and testing multiple sites at the wound.[4] The mean age of these patients was 61.3 years with a range from 28 to 74 years. They had had 30 previous hip procedures. The mean follow-up period was 42 months with a range from 24 to 84 months. In this group, 11 patients had single drug therapy and 7 had combined therapy, generally two antibiotics and occasionally three. In only two instances in this series was gentamicin cement used. We would currently recommend antibiotic cement in all cases.

The antibiotic treatment was continued parenterally for 6 weeks in most cases and orally for 12 months in most cases.

The organisms involved were *Staphylococcus epidermidus* in ten patients and *Staphylococcus aureus* in two. One case was infected with *Pepticoccus* organisms and one with *Proprionibacterium acnes.*

In four cases, the organisms were gram-negative or mixed organisms, namely: one case of *Proteus mirabilis,* one of *Salmonella-B,* and one case with both alpha hemalytic streptococcus plus *Enterococcus* and one case with *Staphylococcus epidermidus* plus *Proprionibacterium.*

This approach has led to a 78% success rate in terms of freedon of sepsis and excellent functional results at 4 years average follow-up.

In a much larger series reported from Buchholz's group, in which the use of antibiotic cement was employed, similar results have been obtained in direct exchange.[1]

It is of special interest that the four failures with recurrent sepsis in this series were the four patients with gram-negative or mixed infections. All other patients were free of infection.

SURGICAL CONSIDERATIONS

The essential feature of the surgery is a radical debridement, including all of the bone cement. Generally, this can best be accomplished by the wide exposure afforded by trochanteric osteotomy, despite the disadvantages of trochanteric osteotomy under these circumstances. Those disadvantages are predominantly the presence of the wires and the risk of nonunion. Nevertheless, more effective debridement with a lower incidence of technical complications can be produced by the improved exposure afforded by trochanteric osteotomy. In our experience the addition of the wires for reattaching the greater trochanter is but a small part of the total foreign material that is implanted, and the use of trochanteric wires for reattachment of the greater trochanter has not been a disadvantage.

Crucial to these successful replantations is the use of contemporary cementing techniques.[3] This means that the medullary canal must be plugged with a bone cement plug,[2] which is distinctly preferable to any silastic plug or to a bone plug itself. The cement must be centrifuged,[2] introduced through a cement gun, and pressurized. That is true on both the femoral side and the acetabular side.[5-7]

Extensive studies have been done of the advantages of centrifugation. It more than doubles the fatigue life of the bone cement and is strongly recommended in all instances. The preferred bone cement is Simplex P containing erythromycin and colistin. Its antibiotic activity is excellent, and the strength of centrifuged Simplex is substantially greater in fatigue than Palacos. In addition, the penetration of Simplex P into the bone is substantially better than Palacos.

For the cementing on the femoral side, the viscosity of the centrifuged Simplex P containing erythromycin and colistin (AKZ bone cement) can be improved (lowered) by chilling the monomer.

On the acetabular side this is unwise because the viscosity is so low that it is difficult to control the cement.

This approach has led to a 78% success rate in terms of freedom of sepsis and excellent functional results at 4 years average follow-up.

In a much larger series reported from Buchholz's group, similar results have been obtained in direct exchange.[1]

Clearly, it is a high-risk operative procedure, but it is an operative procedure whose risk does not exceed that of the indirect exchange if patient selection is done carefully.

REFERENCES

1. Buchholz, H.W., Engelbrecht, E., Lodenkamper, H., Rottger, J., Siegel, A., and Elson, R.A.: Management of deep infection of total hip replacement, J. Bone Joint Surg. **63B:**342, 1981.
2. Burke, D.W., Gates, E.I., and Harris, W.H.: Centrifugation as a method of improving tensile and fatigue properties of acrylic bone cement, J. Bone Joint Surg. **66A:**1265, 1984.
3. Harris, W.H., McCarthy, J.C., Jr., and O'Neill, D.A.: Loosening of the femoral component of total hip replacement after plugging the femoral canal. In The hip: Proceedings of the tenth open scientific meeting of The Hip Society, St. Louis, 1982, The C.V. Mosby Co.
4. Jupiter, J.B., Karchmer, A.W., Lowell, J.D., and Harris, W.H.: Total hip arthroplasty in the treatment of adult hips with current or quiescent sepsis, J. Bone Joint Surg. **63A:**194, 1981.
5. Oh, I., Bourne, R.B., and Harris, W.H.: The femoral cement compactor: An improvement in cementing technique in total hip replacement, J. Bone Joint Surg. **65A:**1335, 1983.
6. Oh, I., and Harris, W.H.: A cement fixation system for total hip arthroplasty, Clin. Orthop. **164:**221-229, 1982.
7. Oh, I., Merckx, D.B., and Harris, W.H.: Acetabular cement compactor: An experimental study of pressurization of cement in the acetabulum in total hip arthroplasty, Clin. Orthop. **177:**289, 1983.

Chapter 23

Treatment of the infected total hip arthroplasty

WILLIAM R. MURRAY

DEFINITION AND TREATMENT

Deep-wound infection is an infection in the periprosthetic space. Factors to be considered in treatment are (1) early or late infection, (2) virulence of the organism of infection, and (3) component loosening.

Treatment modalities available are (1) incision and debridement, plus local and systemic antibiotic treatment; (2) debridement and direct-exchange arthroplasty, plus local and systemic antibiotic treatment; (3) removal of both components, debridement of all scar tissue, cement, and devitalized tissue, plus local and systemic antibiotic treatment; and (4) removal and debridement as described, plus local and systemic antibiotic treatment, and delayed reinsertion.

Antibiotics in the cement. Although the FDA has not approved the addition of antibiotic to bone cement by the manufacturer of the cement, interpretation of the FDA regulations indicates that combining of bone cement with an appropriate antibiotic by a physician does not contravene any law or regulation if, in the physician's judgment, it is medically advisable; that is, if the antibiotic either reduces the chances of infection or treats an infection and does not alter the strength or character of the cement below acceptable standards.

The antibiotic added to the cement must be eluted (or leached out) from the cement in bactericidal or bacteriostatic concentration and must not be inactivated by the polymerization process. Antibiotics that have shown sustained release in tests are gentamicin, penicillin, erythromycin, oxacillin, cloxacillin, methicillin, lincomycin, clindamycin, cephalosporins, colistin, fucidin, neomycin, kanamycin, and ampicillin. Chloramphenicol and tetracycline appear to be inactivated by the polymerization process and should not be used in bone cement. The usual method at the University of California at San Francisco (UCSF) has been to mix 1 g of erythromycin and 300 mg of colistin with 40 g of polymethylmethacrylate (PMMA) (Simplex P) or 60 g of PMMA (Zimmer LVC). Thorough mixing is accomplished by adding PMMA powder to the antibiotic powder in 2-tablespoon doses (Fig. 23-1) and mixing after each addition. The mixing bowl then is covered with another bowl and shaken like an old-fashioned cocktail shaker (Fig. 23-2) for not less than 2 minutes to ensure even distribution of the finely powdered antibiotic throughout the PMMA powder.

Wound irrigation at surgery. Copious quantities of a solution containing kanamycin (one g per 500 ml of saline or Ringer's solution) are used routinely at UCSF for wound irrigation during surgery.

Postoperative wound instillation. Postoperative instillation of antibiotics into the wound with a suction–irrigation system has been successful in controlling or preventing infection. We have used Jergesen's and Jawetz's high-concentration, low-volume system, in contrast to the high-volume, low-concentration system popularized by Compere. Superinfection with *Pseudomonas* or other organisms has not occurred (or if it has, we are not aware of any such case). Two or more K-10 tubes are left in the depths of the wound at the time of surgery and are connected to a sterile trap

229

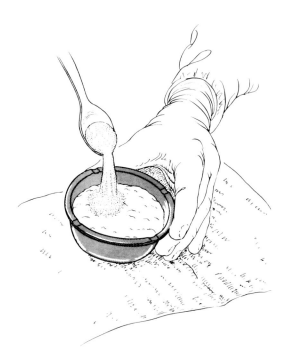

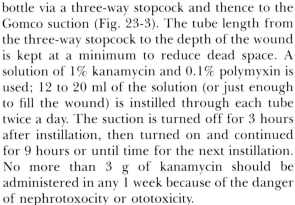

Fig. 23-1. Polymethylmethacrylate powder (PMMA) is added to antibiotic powder in 2-tablespoon doses.

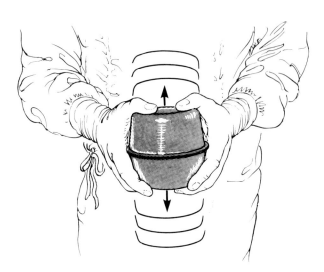

Fig. 23-2. Antibiotic powder and PMMA powder are shaken in two bowls placed one on top of another.

bottle via a three-way stopcock and thence to the Gomco suction (Fig. 23-3). The tube length from the three-way stopcock to the depth of the wound is kept at a minimum to reduce dead space. A solution of 1% kanamycin and 0.1% polymyxin is used; 12 to 20 ml of the solution (or just enough to fill the wound) is instilled through each tube twice a day. The suction is turned off for 3 hours after instillation, then turned on and continued for 9 hours or until time for the next instillation. No more than 3 g of kanamycin should be administered in any 1 week because of the danger of nephrotoxocity or ototoxicity.

The patient's renal and auditory status should be monitored with tests of serum creatinine every other day and audiograms twice a week. Treatment is stopped if the creatinine is rising or hearing acuity is falling. The instillations are stopped routinely after 1 week. Suction is continued, however, and cultures are obtained 24 and 48 hours after the last tube instillation. The regimen of tube instillation and alternate suction is then resumed for another 72 hours. If the cultures are negative, the tubes are removed after the 72 hours. If the cultures are positive, the program is continued for another 5 days, at which time cultures are obtained once again.

Intravenous and oral antibiotics. The intravenous antibiotics used must be the most appropriate to treat the infection based on sensitivity studies, and preferably should be continued for 6 weeks after surgery. At the present time at UCSF, the most frequently used intravenous antibiotic is cefazolin (Ancef) in a dosage of 1 g every 6 hours. Following this 6-week period of intravenous antibiotic use, one or more oral antibiotics, once again appropriate to the bacteria cultured and its (or their) antibiotic sensitivities, are continued for 6 more weeks. Most frequently we have used cephradine (Velosef) in a dosage of 500 mg 4 times per day.

Surgical treatment

Incision and debridement, plus local and systemic antibiotic treatment. The decision to limit the surgical treatment to drainage, debridement, and closure over suction-irrigation tubes rests with the surgeon. At UCSF this modality of treatment is used only for those patients whose infection is detected early, that is, less than 3 months after surgery, or in whom the bacterial strain recovered is of relatively low virulence, for example, *Staphylococcus epidermidis, Micrococcus,* or *Streptococcus* organisms. We have been unsuccess-

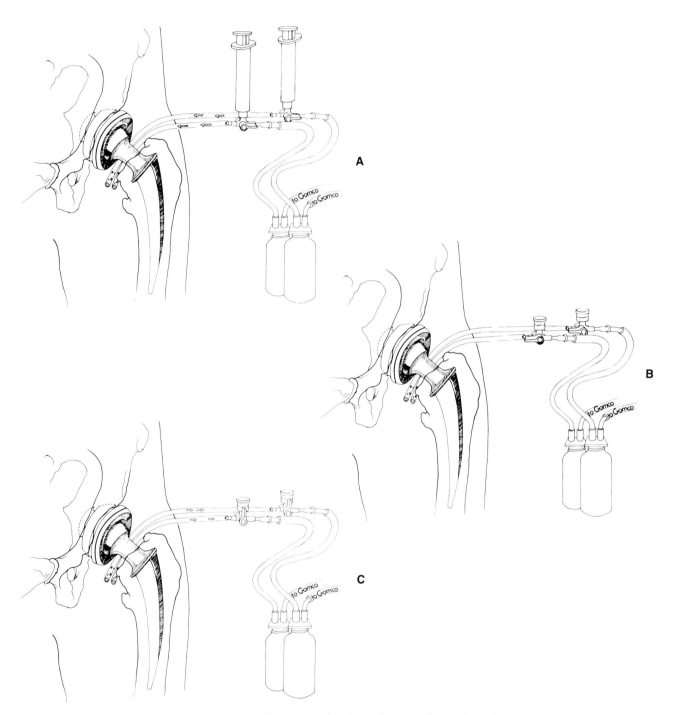

Fig. 23-3. The Jergesen-Jawetz Gomco suction-irrigation. **A,** Illustration of the tubes in place and direction of antibiotic-solution flow during instillation. **B,** The suction is stopped for 3 hours. **C,** Illustration of the tubes and direction of flow during the 9-hour suction. (From Leach, R.E., Hoaglund, F.T., and Riseborough, E.J., editors: Controversies in orthopaedic surgery, Philadelphia, 1982, W.B. Saunders Co.

ful in using this modality of treatment to manage infection with high-virulence organisms such as *Staphylococcus aureus* or any of the gram-negative bacteria. When used, there must be adequate debridement of all devitalized tissue from the wound; excessive granulations are "debulked" to allow optimal antibiotic penetration into the soft tissues and the periprosthetic space. Suction and irrigation (the Jergesen-Jawetz technique described earlier) are preceded by copious irrigation of antibiotic-containing solution at the time of surgery. This is followed by the intravenous antibiotic routine for not less than 4 and preferably for 6 weeks, and then by oral antibiotics as previously described. This combined surgical–antibiotic treatment has been successful in controlling infection in only 21.2% of the patients in whom it has been used.

Debridement, direct exchange, plus local and systemic antibiotic treatment. For direct-exchange arthroplasty, antibiotic-containing cement is used routinely. If the organism is known, the most appropriate antibiotic is administered. As noted earlier, our usual routine at UCSF has been to add 1 g of erythromycin and 300 mg of colistin to 40 or 60 g of PMMA powder. On occasion, at the discretion of the surgeon, the antibiotic dose has been doubled, to 2 g of erythromycin and 600 mg of colistin per 40 or 60 g of PMMA. This amount of antibiotic stays well within the limits set by the ASTM F-4 Committee, which has determined that the minimum compressive strength level for PMMA is 70 megapascals (MPa). The addition of over 4.5 g of powdered antibiotic to 40 g of powdered PMMA would be required to reduce the compressive strength below 70 MPa; it would also reduce the diametral tensile strength below acceptable levels. Compressive and diametral tensile strengths also are reduced below acceptable levels if the antibiotic is added as a liquid or if powdered antibiotic is added to the liquid monomer before it is mixed with the powdered polymer.

Although direct-exchange arthroplasty admittedly is less morbidity-producing than the Girdlestone resection, we restrict its use to instances where the organisms of infection are of low virulence, because we have been unable to control infections with *Staphylococcus aureus* or gram–negative organisms with this method. Our original routine was to remove only the loosened component. For the past year both components have been removed even if only one was loose.

The patients are treated with local antibiotics via tube instillation and aspiration and with intravenous and oral antibiotics as described earlier.

Removal of both components, debridement, plus local and systemic antibiotic treatment. Removal of both components and all cement, devitalized tissue, and scar tissue, supplemented by skeletal traction and local and systemic antibiotics, has been successful in controlling infection in over 86% of the patients in whom it has been used regardless of the infectious organism involved. Copious quantities of kanamycin irrigating solution are used during surgery. The local tube instillation and aspiration techniques are followed, as are the intravenous antibiotic and oral antibiotic programs previously outlined. The patients are kept at bedrest in balanced suspension and tibial tubercle skeletal traction for not less than 4 weeks and usually for 6 weeks postoperatively in order to maintain limb length, prevent deformity, and rest the operative area. When out-of-bed activities are permitted, a shoe lift of 50% to 75% of the measurable shortening is applied, and patients are permitted weight-bearing as tolerated.

Removal of both components, debridement, plus local and systemic antibiotic treatment and delayed reinsertion. The technique for removal and the antibiotic program are the same as outlined previously. After completion of their 4- to 6-week skeletal traction plus intravenous antibiotic course and 6 weeks of oral antibiotics, the patients are evaluated and a decision is made to attempt to reinsert the prosthetic device. In most cases we have elected to wait for a minimum of 3 months after all antibiotics have been stopped before reinserting another total hip prosthesis. If delayed reinsertion is to be performed, it should not be done until there is clear clinical and laboratory evidence of absence of infection. The pertinent tests include, but are not limited to, wound inspection, normal sedimentation rate and white blood cell count, culture–negative aspiration arthrogram, normal indium granulocyte, or gallium radionuclide scans. No antibiotics are administered at the time of delayed reinsertion until after tissue specimens have been obtained for culture; appropriate intravenous antibiotics then are started, based on previous culture and sensitivities and continued for at least 7 days postoperatively. If at that time the operative specimen cultures are negative, the antibiotics are discontinued. If the cultures are positive, the

Table 23-1. UCSF experience with 174 deep-wound infections

Patient signs and symptoms	Percentage of patients	Results of treatment	Control or eradication of infection achieved (% of hips)
Pain	75.3	Incision and debridement	21.2
Drainage or cellulitis	21.3	Direct exchange	50.0*
Sepsis	3.4		85.2†
Elevated erythrocyte sedimentation rate	57.4	Primary removal	86.8
Positive preoperative culture	57.0	Removal and reinsertion	90.4
Negative preoperative culture— positive intraoperative culture	43.0		

*All had positive preoperative cultures.
†Includes those who had only positive surgical cultures.

most appropriate antibiotic or antibiotics are continued for 6 weeks intravenously and then 6 more weeks orally at the discretion of the surgeon.

Experience in treatment of deep-wound infection. At UCSF we have treated 174 deep-wound infections after total hip arthroplasty. The 174 comprised those referred with a deep-wound infection (43), our own 51 cases (which included nine deep-wound infections in 1756 index or virgin total hip arthroplasties, an incidence of 0.5%), and another 80 patients who had only a positive intraoperative culture. Our experience indicates that excisional arthroplasty is probably the treatment of choice.

Table 23-1 depicts the signs and symptoms of these 174 patients and the results of treatment. Of those patients treated only by incision and drainage, debridement, and local and systemic antibiotics, only 21.2% emerged free of infection. The results of direct-exchange arthroplasty are difficult to interpret; direct exchange controlled or eradicated the infection in 50% of those patients who had positive preoperative cultures at the time of their aspiration arthrogram. However, if one adds to this group 72 patients who had a negative preoperative culture but a positive intraoperative culture (in most instances probably a contaminant), then the success rate in direct exchange goes up to 85.2%. Removal of the prosthesis (Girdlestone resection) successfully combatted infection in 86.8% of patients when used as the final procedure, and removal and delayed reinsertion of the prosthesis in patients was successful in 90.4%.

SUMMARY

Based on our present experience, excisional arthroplasty is the most reliable option. Infections caused by organisms of significant virulence are best treated with excisional arthroplasty or Girdlestone resection followed by delayed reinsertion after adequate antibiotic treatment has controlled the sepsis, as determined by clinical and laboratory criteria. In patients with infections caused by organisms of relatively low virulence, for example, *Staphylococcus epidermidis* or anaerobic diphtheroids, the surgeon should seriously consider either incision and drainage, debridement, and local and systemic antibiotics if there is no component loosening, or direct exchange (removing both components and reinserting them with antibiotic cement) if there is loosening of one or both components. However, if incision and debridement or direct exchange fails, then excisional arthroplasty as a definitive procedure or as a first stage of a removal and reinsertion should be carried out.

While we have not been successful in treating even early infections caused by *Staphylococcus aureus* with incision, drainage, and antibiotics, the morbidity associated with this procedure is extremely low compared with that of the other procedures; therefore it seems reasonable to use this modality as an emergency treatment for acute infections, with the full realization that it probably will not succeed as the definitive procedure, and the surgeon should prepare for early, more definitive surgical intervention.

Chapter 24

Prosthetic reimplantation for salvage of the infected hip

EDUARDO A. SALVATI

JOHN J. CALLAGHAN

BARRY D. BRAUSE

The Hospital for Special Surgery in New York has been committed since 1967 to the study of infection following total hip replacement (Figs. 24-1 and 24-2). Since that time approximately 150 infected hip arthroplasties have been reimplanted. The earlier experience included cases reimplanted primarily in one stage, with antibiotic therapy selected by the treating orthopaedic surgeon.[8,19]

Since 1976, a standardized 6-week intravenous regimen was instituted.[13] Antimicrobial therapy, based on tube dilution studies, was administered parenterally for 6 weeks in doses sufficient to attain a peak bactericidal serum titer of at least 1:8. Determination of these titers required bacteriologic isolation of the patient's organism from a clinical specimen. The choice of drug and dosage was dependent on the sensitivities of the organism, with consideration given to the ability of the drug to penetrate and kill, as opposed to inhibit. The test was terminated at the point of highest dilution of serum that caused 99% destruction of a standard inoculum of the infecting organism. A serum bactericidal level of 1:8 or greater was set arbitrarily as the adequate antibiotic level to resolve the infection on the basis of the accepted effectiveness of similar titers in the treatment of bacterial endocarditis.[6] These studies were performed under the supervision of a single consultant in infectious disease (B.B.).

Patients undergoing reimplantation had to meet the following criteria: a minimum 1:8 bactericidal serum level, adequate medical health including no immunodeficiency or immunosuppression, adequate bone quality and soft tissue for reconstruction, and good potential for rehabilitation.

MATERIALS AND METHODS

Between January 1976 and March 1982, 32 hips in 31 patients were reimplanted with total hip arthroplasties to salvage infected joints. All of these patients were studied prospectively.

Mean age at reimplantation was 64.7 years (range 28 to 85 years). Mean age at follow-up was 68.8 years (range 35 to 88 years). Mean follow-up was 4.1 years (range 2 to 8 years).

Organisms grew on both broth and agar plate mediums in all cases at the time of one-stage reimplantation or at the first stage in two-stage reimplantation. The organisms cultured are listed in Table 24-1. Cultures were negative in the second stage of all two-stage reimplantations.

The index procedures that became infected are listed in Table 24-2. Nineteen patients had a preoperative hip aspirate. Fifteen of these had a positive culture from an aspirate where fluid was obtained. In the four "dry" taps, where no fluid was obtained until saline was injected into the hip joint, only one grew out a positive culture. All cultures were the same as those obtained at the time of surgery. Thirteen hips were not aspirated

234

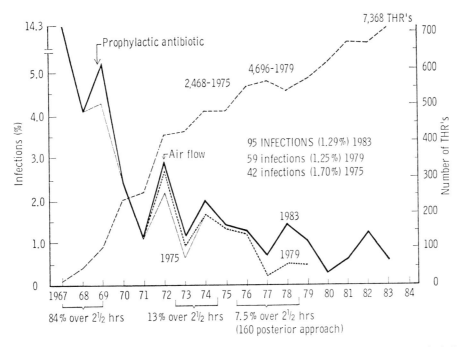

Fig. 24-1. Annual deep infection rate in total hip replacement at The Hospital for Special Surgery from August 1967 to December 1983, inclusive. The dotted lines below the solid line show the annual deep infection rate up to 1975 and up to 1979. The other dotted line shows the number of total hip replacements performed per year. The decreasing duration of surgery through the years is shown below.

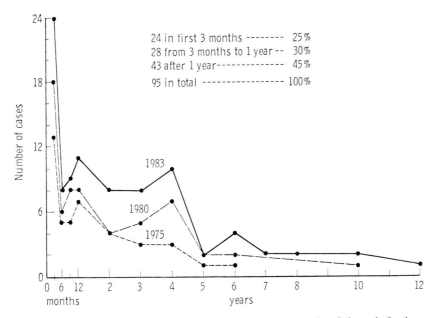

Fig. 24-2. Graph showing the postoperative time of diagnosis of deep infection as of December 1975, December 1980, and December 1983.

Table 24-1. Organisms cultured

Staphylococcus epidermidis	17*
Staphylococcus aureus	5*
Pseudomonas aeruginosa	2
Enterobacter	2
Microaerophilic streptococcus	2
Escherichia coli	1
Propionibacterium acnes	1
Bacteroides fragilis	1*
Staphylococcus epidermidis and enterococcus	1

*Recurrence.

Table 24-2. Infections

Total hip replacement	20
Uncemented endoprosthesis	5
Cemented endoprosthesis	4
McLaughlin nail	1
Hematogenous infection	2

Table 24-3. Antibiotic dilution titers

Bactericidal titers achieved	Number
1 : 8	3
1 : 16	8*
1 : 32	4†
1 : 64	4
1 : 128	4‡
1 : 256	3
1 : 512	3
1 : 1024	2
1 : 2048	1

*Recurrence of *Staphylococcus aureus*.
†Recurrence of *Bacteroides fragilis*.
‡Recurrence of *Staphylococcus epidermidis*.

because either the diagnosis of infection had been made elsewhere (six hips) or infection was not suspected before surgery (seven hips).

SURGICAL MANAGEMENT OF INFECTION

A transtrochanteric approach was used in 29 cases (which includes all 20 infected total hip replacements), and a posterior approach in three. Fourteen cases were performed in one stage. A one-stage reimplantation was limited to those infections caused by very sensitive bacteria with negative Gram stain and benign tissues by macroscopic and frozen section observation at the time of surgery. In addition, the seven infections not suspected at surgery had a one-stage reimplantation. Eighteen hips were performed in two stages with the second stage done 2 weeks to 11 months after the first stage (mean 4.3 months) and during the same hospitalization in nine cases (50%).

At the time of debridement a careful and meticulous effort was made to remove all necrotic, devitalized tissue, sinus tract, prosthetic components, wires, other foreign bodies, and acrylic cement. In several cases this required windows in the femur (these were performed on the anterior surface and right angle corners were avoided. One surgeon used a Cloward drill to make round windows). If there was uncertainty concerning complete acrylic removal, an intraoperative radiograph was performed. No patient received preoperative antibiotics, which were administered only after all cultures were obtained.

In all 32 hips, intraoperative Gram stains were performed, aerobic, anaerobic fungal, and TB cultures were taken of the intraarticular fluid, and multiple tissue samples were sent from the acetabulum and femur for frozen and permanent section and culture. In all 32 hips intraoperative cultures grew infecting organisms in both broth and agar. Acute inflammation was seen on histopathology in 25 cases. In the other seven cases only chronic inflammation or reactive tissue was demonstrated.

In all 18 hips, at the second stage, cultures of the fluid and tissue were again sent for microbiologic and pathologic examination. None of these cultures was positive.

In two-stage reimplantation, after the first stage, closed-tube suction irrigation was instituted for 2 to 4 days. Most patients were placed in proximal tibial skeletal traction for 3 to 4 weeks. In five cases long-stem femoral components were required to bypass previous defects in the femur (windows or perforations). No intraoperative femoral fractures occurred. No antibiotic was mixed into the new acrylic cement. The antibiotic dilution titers obtained are listed in Table 24-3, including the three recurrences.

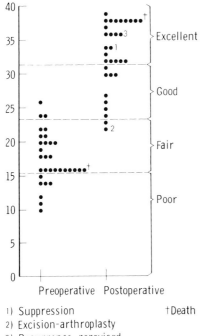

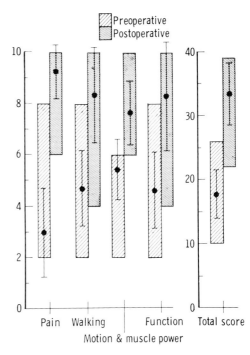

1) Suppression   †Death
2) Excision-arthroplasty
3) Recurrence, rerevised

Fig. 24-3. Preoperative and last postoperative rating of each hip.

Fig. 24-4. Preoperative and postoperative rating of all hips, including mean and standard deviation for pain, walking, motion and muscle power, function, and total score.

RESULTS

All 31 patients with 32 hips were followed a mean of 4.1 years (range 2 to 8 years). Both clinical and radiographic results were obtained at last follow-up. Twenty-two hips were rated excellent, eight good, and two fair (Figs. 24-3 and 24-4). There were three recurrences of infection, and their clinical rating included is at last follow-up.

RADIOGRAPHIC EVALUATION

Radiographs were analyzed comparing the first good-quality postoperative anteroposterior radiograph with the last follow-up radiograph. Initial postoperative and follow-up radiolucencies on the acetabular and femoral sides are pictured in Fig. 24-5 and 24-6. There was progression of acetabular radiolucencies in four hips (13%) and of femoral radiolucencies in five hips (16%).

DISCUSSION

Use of a standardized intravenous antibiotic regimen, sufficient to obtain a peak bactericidal serum titer of at least 1:8, has been highly effective in the treatment of infected hips by

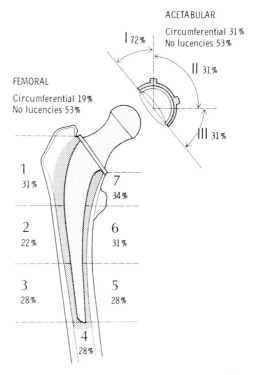

Fig. 24-5. Initial postoperative acetabular and femoral radiolucencies.

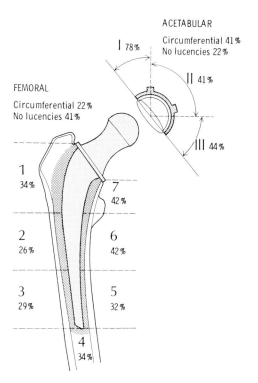

ACETABULAR
Circumferential 41%
No lucencies 22%

| 78%

|| 41%

||| 44%

FEMORAL
Circumferential 22%
No lucencies 41%

1 34%

7 42%

2 26%

6 42%

3 29%

5 32%

4 34%

Fig. 24-6. Last follow-up acetabular and femoral radiolucencies.

reimplantation with total hip arthroplasty (see Table 24-3). The regimen appears to have erradicated infection and allowed good function in 29 of 32 hips (90.6%). It was effective in all 12 cases of infected hardware, infected endoprostheses (cemented and uncemented), and hematogenous infections (100%). It was also effective in 17 of 20 infected total hip replacements (85%). Finally, 12 of 14 one-stage (86%) and 17 of 18 two-stage reimplantations (94.5%) demonstrated no recurrence.

We recognize the limited number of cases studied and the innumerable variables involved. However, we believe that these cases probably represent the best results that we can obtain by careful selection, meticulous surgery, and strictly controlled intravenous antibiotic therapy. Thus far, no study reveals better success in eradicating infection and restoring hip function by reimplantation, unless it includes antibiotic-impregnated cement (Table 24-4). Future studies with antibiotic-impregnated cement will have to be judged against these results.

RATIONALE FOR THE USE OF ANTIBIOTIC IMPREGNATED CEMENT

In the hope of improving the success rate and decreasing the contraindication to reimplantation of total hip replacement following infection, since mid-1982 the use of Palacos-Gentamicin antibiotic-impregnated cement (PG) was included,

Table 24-4. Results of reimplantation

	One-stage		Two-stage	
With antibiotic-impregnated cement	*Number*	*Percent*	*Number*	*Percent*
Buchholz et al., 1981[1]	667	77.00	—	—
Lindberg, 1981[11]	59	90.00	18	78.00
Murray, 1981[12]	13	38.50	22	95.50
Turner et al., 1982[16]	101	86.00	—	—
TOTAL	840	72.90	40	86.75
Without antibiotic-impregnated cement				
Hunter, 1979[9]	55	18.00	10	60.00
Talbott et al., 1980[14]	—	—	25	80.00
Cherney and Amstutz, 1981[3]	5	80.00	28	64.00
Fitzgerald, 1981[4]	—	—	111	90.00
Jupiter et al., 1981[10]	18	78.10	—	—
Present study	14	86.00	18	94.5
TOTAL	110	65.52	202	77.7

based on European experiences that reported 77% to 90% success with one-stage reimplantation using PG, despite extending the indications to all infections.[1,2,11] In addition, we used PG in patients undergoing joint replacement who were at higher risk of infection, that is, complicated revision surgery, multiple previous operations, suspicion of sepsis, infections in other body sites, previously irradiated joints, and immunodeficient or immunosuppressed patients.

Beads of antibiotic impregnated cement (Palacos-Gentamicin Septopal)[7,17] were also incorporated in the treatment of infected joints. The beads were introduced after thorough debridement and removal of prosthetic components and acrylic cement. To maintain the local gentamicin levels, no irrigation was used in these cases (only suction for 24 hours).

PG was selected based on previous reports confirming that the elution rates of antibiotics were higher with Palacos cement,[15,18] the demonstration of bactericidal concentrations throughout the cortex, including the endosteal surface, for 7 months after implantation,[5] and confirmation that the fracture properties were not significantly affected by the addition of 0.5 g of gentamicin.[20]

Gentamicin was preferred because of the following favorable properties: broad spectrum and bactericidal activity, rare resistance, thermostabilility, non-allergenic drug, free solubility in water, and ample experience in Europe using this combination.

A prospective study was performed to evaluate the joint fluid, serum, and urine antibiotic levels in 38 patients implanted with PG (0.5 g of gentamicin per 40 g of cement) and in 18 patients with gentamicin-impregnated beads. Each bead is 7 mm in diameter and contains a 4.5 mg gentamicin base. The beads are strung on a chromium-nickel multistranded thread with 30 beads to a chain.

Radioimmune assays were performed on joint fluid, serum, and urine samples at various times after surgery. On day one high joint fluid levels of gentamicin were eluted from PG implanted patients (mean 14.9 µg/ml, range 2.7 to 38.9) and bead implanted patients (mean 36.9 µg/ml, range 19.6 to 69.5) with very low serum and urine levels (Figs. 24-7 and 24-8).

The joint levels of gentamicin obtained in PG implanted patients on day one were seven times higher and in bead implanted patients 17 times

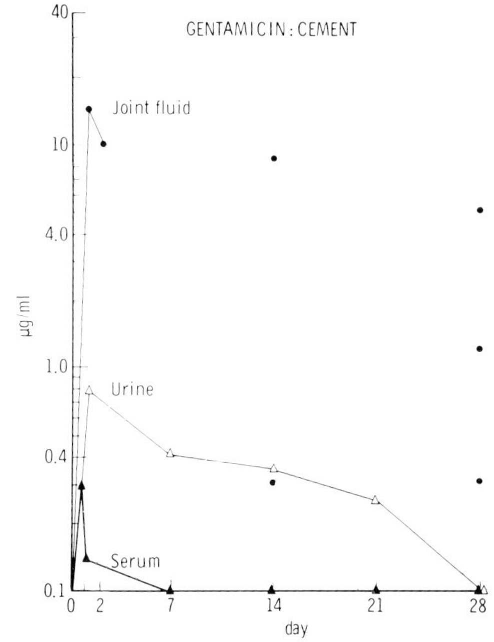

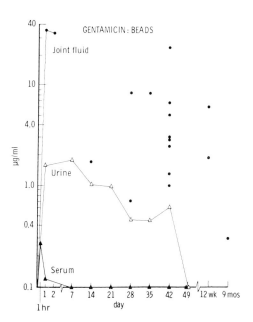

Fig. 24-7. Joint fluid, urine, and serum levels obtained in patients implanted with gentamicin cement (logarithmic scale). Dots represent single joint aspirates.

Fig. 24-8. Joint fluid, urine, and serum levels obtained in patients implanted with gentamicin impregnated beads (logarithmic scale). Dots represent single joint aspirates.

higher than those obtained in the joint with intravenous administration of gentamicin. The serum and urine levels were about 10 to 20 times less in patients with PG or beads compared to those levels obtained in controls after intravenous administration of gentamicin. These very low systemic levels should preclude nephrotoxic and ototoxic effects; in fact, no toxicity was observed in our patients.

Bioactivity of gentamicin in the specimens was confirmed. Staphylococci were exquisitely sensitive, whereas streptococci were less sensitive to gentamicin (Fig. 24-9). Gentamicin's potency against gram-negative organisms is well docu-

mented. Both gentamicin-impregnated beads and cement appear safe and effective in the treatment of infected joints and in reimplantation of prosthetic joints.

The addition of antibiotic was not detrimental to the fracture properties and, in fact, was beneficial, possibly as a result of a plasticizing effect of the antibiotic. Centrifugation did not improve the resistance to fracture, a result consistent with fracture mechanics concepts. The intrusion of PG was found to be inferior to that for either Zimmer or Simplex, although volume contraction on setting was indistinguishable for the three cements.

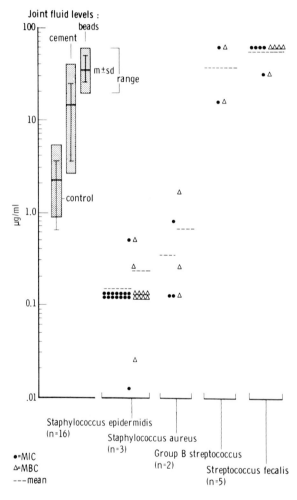

Fig. 24-9. MICs and MBCs to gentamicin, of gram–positive aerobic organisms retrieved from infected hip replacements. Mean, standard deviation, and range of gentamicin joint fluid levels are represented at the left. Control represents joint fluid levels obtained after intravenous gentamicin administration.

REFERENCES

1. Buchholz, H.W., Elson, R.A., Engelbrecht, E., Lodenkamper, H., Rottger, J., and Siegel, A.: Management of deep infection of total hip replacement, J. Bone Joint Surg. **63B:**342-353, 1981.
2. Carlsson, A.S., Josefsson, G., and Lindberg, L.: Revision with gentamicin-impregnated cement for deep infections in total hip arthroplasties, J. Bone Joint Surg. **60A:**1059-1064, 1978.
3. Cherney, D.L., and Amstutz, H.C.: Total hip replacement in the previously septic hip, J. Bone Joint Surg. **65A:** 1256, 1983.
4. Fitzgerald, R.H., Jr.: Indirect exchange of the infected hip implant, Orthop. Trans. **5**(3):372, 1981.
5. Hoff, S.F., Fitzgerald, R.H., Jr., and Kelly, P.J.: The depot administration of penicillin G and gentamicin in acrylic bone cement, J. Bone Joint Surg. **63A:**798, 1981.
6. Hook, E.W., and Guerrant, R.L.: Therapy of infectious endocarditis. In Kaye, D., editor: Infective endocarditis, Baltimore, 1976. University Park Press.
7. Hovelius, L., and Josefsson, G.: An alternative method for exchange operation of infected arthroplasty, Acta Orthop. Scand. **50:**93-96, 1979.
8. Hughes, P.W., Salvati, E.A., and Wilson, P.D., Jr., et al.: Treatment of subacute sepsis of the hip by antibiotics and joint replacement: Criteria for diagnosis with evaluation of twenty-six cases, Clin. Orthop. **141:**143, 1979.
9. Hunter, G.A.: The results of reinsertion of a total hip prosthesis after sepsis, J. Bone Joint Surg. **61B:**422, 1979.
10. Jupiter, J.B., Karchmer, A.W., Lowell, J.D., and Harris, W.H.: Total hip arthroplasty in the treatment of adult hips with current or quiescent sepsis, J. Bone Joint Surg. **63A:**194, 1981.
11. Lindberg, L.T.: The experience with antibiotic cement in Sweden (abstract), The Second American Orthopaedic Association Symposium, Boston, 1981.
12. Murray, W.R.: Treatment of established deep wound infection after total hip arthroplasty: A report of 65 cases. In Leach, R.E., Hoaglund, F.T., and Riseborough, E.J., editors: Controversies in orthopaedic surgery, Philadelphia, 1981, W.B. Saunders Co.
13. Salvati, E.A., Chekofsky, K.M., Brause, B.D., and Wilson, P.D., Jr.: Reimplantation in infection: A 12-year experience, Clin. Orthop. **170:**62-75, 1982.
14. Talbott, R.D., Glassburn, A.R., Jr., Nelson, J.P., McElhinney, J.P., and Greenberg, R.L.: Implantation of total hip arthroplasty after known deep infection, Orthop. Trans. **4**(1):97, 1980.
15. Torholm, C., Lidgren, L., Lindberg, L., and Kahlmeter, G.: Total hip joint arthroplasty with gentamicin-impregnated cement: A clinical study of gentamicin excretion kinetics, Clin. Orthop. **181:**99-106, 1983.
16. Turner, R.H., Miley, G.B., and Fremont-Smith, P.: Septic total hip replacement and revision arthroplasty. In Turner, R.H., and Scheller, A.D. Jr. editors: Revision total hip arthroplasty, New York, 1982, Grune & Stratton, Inc.
17. Wahlig, H., Dingeldein, E., Bergmann, R., and Reuss, K.: The release of gentamicin from polymethylmethacrylate beads: An experimental and pharmocokinetic study, J. Bone Joint Surg. **60B:**270-275, 1978.
18. Wahlig, H., Dingeldein, E., Buchholtz, H.W., and Bachmann, F.: Pharmacokinetic study of gentamicin-loaded cement in total hip replacements: Comparative effects of varying dosage, J. Bone Joint Surg. **66B:**175-179, 1984.
19. Wilson, P.D., Jr., Aglietti, P., and Salvati, E.A.: Subacute sepsis of the hip treated by antibiotics and cemented prosthesis, J. Bone Joint Surg. **56A:**879, 1974.
20. Wright, T.M., Sullivan, D.J., and Arnoczky, S.P.: Report on an investigation of the effect of antibiotic additions on the fracture properties of polymethylmethacrylate bone cements, Acta Orthop. Scand. **55:**414-418, 1984.

Chapter 25

Treatment concepts and lessons learned in the treatment of infected implants

CARL L. NELSON

Treatment of surgical sepsis in orthopaedic surgery must be based on the principles of treatment of any surgical sepsis and the factors influencing the chronicity of infection. In addition, the difficulty in understanding the surgery of bone infection is a frustration to both the student and the expert. As in any neglected field, it has retained the methods of previous eras without a sharp focus on the principles and pathophysiologies. It is therefore a field in which patterns, rather than principles, are recommended. The absolute answers are still not available, but I will try to synthesize and condense the principles and the developing concepts into an organized approach. These concepts are not unequivocally mine, and I have borrowed heavily from historic information and newer recommendations. I believe that the application of these principles, based on pathophysiology, is most important. As Whitehead has said, "knowledge should be useful."

SUSCEPTIBLE CHARACTERISTICS OF BONE

Bone has peculiar characteristics that make it susceptible to chronic infection: a limitation of soft tissue space, a blood supply that favors necrosis, and an inadequate mechanism to resorb necrotic bone.[12] If infection occurs in the medullary canal, it is forced into the relatively small volume of soft tissue space that is encompassed by the rigid cortical walls. As it passes down the canal, it enters the Haversian system and further deprives the area of its blood supply. Once necrotic, bone is slow to revascularize. When the

bone is reamed, there is immediate death around the reamed area—very similar to the death that takes place when a projectile enters tissue. If adequate space exists, as in cancellous bone, vessels can penetrate the area and revascularize the bone or anneal it; thus antibiotics and antibodies can enter this area. Where reaming is eccentric and methylmethacrylate is directly against cortical bone, devascularization occurs, and dead bone may be present for at least a year following surgery.[21] Patients with orthopaedic implants may have large amounts of dead bone for prolonged periods with little vascular supply to combat infection. Consequently, they are at risk to develop an infection and may require extensive debridement.

ENVIRONMENT AND FOREIGN BODIES

A relationship exists between the number of bacteria deposited and the status of the environment. A markedly compromised environment requires small numbers of bacteria to produce infection; conversely, in a noncompromised host, relatively large numbers of bacteria are required before the body's defense mechanisms are overcome and an infection is produced.

Foreign bodies play a significant role in relation to bacterial dose; Elek showed an increased incidence of infection when a foreign body was introduced. A subcutaneous injection of up to 1 million *staphylococcus aureus* organisms will not produce an infection; however, when 2 to 8 million inoculums are injected, the host is overcome and an infection develops. However if a foreign body was present (in this study a skin

242

suture was examined), only 100 *Staphylococcus aureus* organisms produced an infection.[5]

Furthermore, orthopaedic implants have been shown to be a suitable substratum for microbiologic growth, suggesting that phagocytes are unable to phagocytize glycocalyx-enclosed microcolonies.[8]

PATHOPHYSIOLOGY OF INFECTION

When infection is superimposed on avascular bone and foreign bodies, more dead bone is produced. In infection, bacteria proliferate, producing local edema, inflammation, and necrosis; within 72 hours the blood supply and the local tissue circulation are compromised, causing a reduction of local antibodies, leukocytes, oxygen, and tissue nutrients. Waste products accumulate, as well as bacterial toxins, while phagocytes die, releasing cytologic enzymes that cause suppuration, which causes further granulation-tissue and local-tissue destruction. It has been taught that the pressure from purulent material causes the increasing bone necrosis. Experimental work suggests that toxins produced by the bacteria necrotize bone immediately near the bacteria much as hunters kill their prey before feeding.

Furthermore, the toxins inhibit osteoblasts and bone formation in the immediate area.[9] Infection around implants produces granulation tissue and then fibrous tissue to wall off the infection (Fig. 25-1). In 2 weeks increasing fibrous formation and new bone formation exist; the fibrous membrane is an attempt to wall off the infection and results in an abcess formation that contains both products of the infectious process and necrotic,

sequestrated bone. By 6 weeks there is continued osteoclastic removal of dead bone and increasing new bone formation. The infection further stimulates new reactive bone involucrum around the infection, which may occur in the medullary canal or periosteum. At 12 weeks in the normal host, thick dense membranes with the cancellous bone become dense to form involucrum (Fig. 25-2).

After the sequestrum and involucrum have formed, the body attempts to resorb the sequestra by granulation tissue. A contest then occurs between the host and the microorganisms. As best stated by Enneking, if the body wins, the process is absorbed and may leave no bony scar.[6] If the infection wins, it will break through the membranous tissue and involucrum and burrow through the soft tissue and erupt, forming a sinus (Fig. 25-3). The necrotic bone and abscess may be

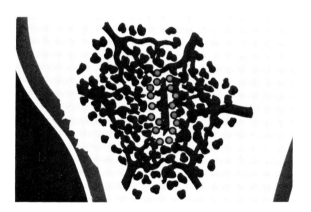

Fig. 25-2. The "walling-off" and attempt to eradicate bacteria and the locally compromised tissue.

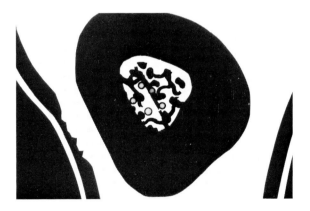

Fig. 25-1. Inflammatory response to devitalized bone and bacteria.

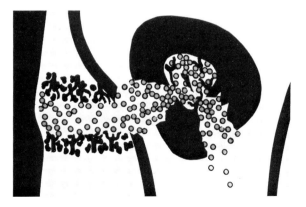

Fig. 25-3. Failure to eradicate the infection, breaking through the involucrum and sinus tract formation.

evacuated and healing may occur, or the sequestrum may be retained producing intermittent drainage. Clinically, in humans a similar process takes place, but the intensity of the new bone formation is usually not clinically observed. That is not to say that significant involucrum is not seen; in fact, if infections are allowed to continue for significant periods, this does occur.

In general, however, the patient with a surgical implant sepsis is diagnosed before marked new formation is usually encountered, and more often the pathophysiology is reflected as lysis. The sequelae then are bacterial growth, toxin formation, bone death, granulation tissue formation, fibrous membrane development, and bone absorption without new bone formation, producing bone erosion that is reflected as decreased radiodensity on x-ray studies.

The bacterial toxins then produce a continuing favorable environment, and the necrotic bone establishes an environment ideal for bacterial growth; that is, nutrients are present without an adequate blood supply.

Necrotic bone. Excision of necrotic bone is as important as the eradication of the bacteria, and to paraphrase Pasteur, "The environment is everything—the bacteria is nothing." Without an environment that allows bacteria to grow, infection may not persist.

The limited capacity to then resorb mineralized tissue is another related problem. There appears to be no biologic enzyme that digests mineralized bone in one stage, and necrotic bone must have contact with granulation tissue.

Necrotic trabecular bone is not as much of a problem as is cortical bone, since cancellous bone has a larger peripheral surface area compared to its mass. The surface area of cortical bone is small, and resorption is slow; therefore a large amount of necrotic cortical bone seriously impedes the attempts to heal the patient and is often the cause for failure.[12]

Hematoma. Soft tissue hematoma is a problem related to early surgical sepsis. Hematoma is not only a nidus for infection; if it becomes tense and taut, it devascularizes the surrounding soft tissue, impedes the natural defense mechanisms of the patient, and prevents antibiotics and antibodies from penetrating the hematoma. In our studies of delaying administration of antibiotics in patients with total hips arthroplasties, we found that, with one patient in which a hematoma developed, the hematoma was not penetrated by

antibiotic.[18] That patient had a very large, tense, taut hematoma.[18] Tense, taut hematoma in orthopaedic surgery is to be avoided to prevent infection and eradicated in treatment.

ANTIBIOTICS

Antibiotic therapy that is based on suppression or eradication should be directed by the surgeon and by the infectious disease consultant. The most commonly used regimen is to give a precise antibiotic aimed at the specific organism, to give it intravenously for a minimum of 2 weeks (preferably 6 weeks), and then to place the patient on oral antibiotics with the belief that this regimen will eradicate the bacteria.[10] Although supressive antibiotic therapy has been used, it has not gained popularity because of the amount of drug suggested, as well as the duration of therapy.

One hopes to achieve eight to ten times the minimal inhibitory concentration at the site of infection. Do antibiotics get to the area where the bacteria are? Bacteria in infection exist in the marrow space and in the Haversian canals but not in the canaliculi—they are simply too large; Fig. 25-4 demonstrates the relative size of the bacteria. Therefore antibiotics will reach the area of infection unless the area is encapsulated or the bone is dead. The duration of antibiotic use is a personal preference without hard data to substantiate an end point. Many believe that the physician should treat the patient as long as areas of sequestration

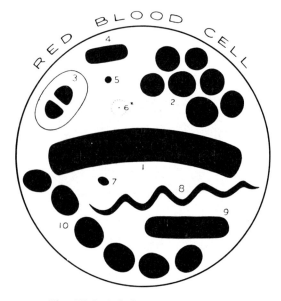

Fig. 25-4. Relative size of bacteria.

and avascularity may be present and therefore have recommended 6 months to a year of therapy.[16]

PATIENTS TREATED

Once antibiotic therapy is agreed on, surgery for acute infections is started. My experience using these principles in the treatment of infected total hips is divided into long-term, follow-up case reports to emphasize certain lessons learned.

In 13 patients who had infected total hips, we have followed the patients for an average of 10 years. It is interesting that nine of the patients ended with resection arthroplasties, whereas four have retained their prostheses.[19]

Acute infections

Our experience in treatment of an acutely infected total hip suggests it should be treated as any surgical infection—debridement of the soft tissue, leaving the stable prosthesis intact, and appropriate antibiotic treatment. Of three patients with acute infections followed for 11 years who were treated in this manner, two are successful. One had a streptococcal infection, and the other a *Staphylacoccus epidermidis*. Both remain uninfected at 10 years.

PRINCIPLES OF TREATMENT

Based on these pathophysiologic concepts, the principles of treatment are clear: diagnosis, evaluation, antibiotics, debridement, and rehabilitation. Debridement may need to be repetitive, involves sequestrectomy, can be considered a method of decontamination, and produces dead space.

Before surgery, several practical points should be kept in mind. First, an infectious disease consultation is mandatory. Second, some important factors should be assessed before surgery: the degree and extent of bone necrosis and the condition of the host. The immunologic status of the patient must be assessed before surgery and enhanced, if possible. Many patients are depleted nutritionally and must be replenished before surgery and maintained during the postoperative period so that they are capable of adequate metabolic activity.

Hickman catheter

Long-term antibiotic therapy and laboratory blood sampling become major problems in finding venous access to the patient. It is our recommendation that a Hickman catheter be used before any surgical procedure in which long-term intravenous antibiotic therapy is anticipated, not only for humanitarian reasons but to reduce the complications associated with long-term intravenous treatment. Furthermore, the Hickman catheter can be used for outpatient intravenous treatment and the concomitant administration of hyperalimentation through a secondary lumen.[1]

NUTRITIONAL ASSESSMENT

One of the least-recognized aberrations that may lead to the development of surgical sepsis or create a host environment conducive to chronic infection is a state of malnutrition and secondary loss of immunocompetence. If any one lesson has been learned, it is to prove that any patient who has an infected implant is not malnourished. The incidence of malnourishment is surprisingly high[13]; certainly the debilitation associated with chronic sepsis must increase the rate of malnutrition. Without question surgical procedures designed to eradicate chronic sepsis will not be successful if the patient is significantly malnourished.

Simple screening tests, serum albumin, transferrin, total lymphocyte count, triceps skin fold, arm muscle circumference, and skin antigen tests can be used to calculate a prognostic level of risks and the state of malnutrition.[4,15,20] If the patient is malnourished, he or she should be restored nutritionally before any definitive surgery.

BACTERIOLOGIC DIAGNOSIS

A precise bacteriologic diagnosis must be made, and joint aspirations should be done, realizing that cultures from sinus tracts are considered by many as inaccurate.[14] Cierny has stated an average of 80% accuracy after identifying the infected organism by biopsy, whereas Patzakis found near 50% accuracy by culturing the sinus tract.[3,22] Plain x-ray films and tomograms are the best method of assessing the extent of the disease, although CT scans are best for determining soft tissue extension. Bone scans are not usually helpful but can identify skip lesions.[3]

The third patient constituted a failure. This patient had a colostomy, and developed a *Pseudomonas* infection that was debrided with the prosthesis left in place. The patient developed an osteomyelitis of the entire femur; she was followed for many months, too ill to have further surgery, and eventually died. The lesson learned:

patients with nonvirulent organisms who are healthy and have an acute infection can be managed successfully in this way. The very ill patients who are immunosuppressed and nutritionally depleted, who have virulent difficult organisms, and who can tolerate only one operative procedure probably should have complete debridement of the prosthesis and cement, as well as appropriate antibiotic therapy. It was also found with these patients that closed-suction irrigation became secondarily contaminated, and on occasion superinfected if used longer than 48 hours.[19]

LATE INFECTIONS

The choice of antibiotics should be determined before surgery and based on the organism found in the preoperative hip aspiration. If there is any question whether the organism cultured is contaminant or if the aspiration cultures show no growth, the antibiotic should not be started prior to surgery. Multiple cultures, aerobic as well as anaerobic, and biopsy material should be sent to the laboratory, after which the antibiotic should be started. If the surgeon is not sure at the time of surgery whether infection is present, Gram stains may be helpful; however, antibiotics should be given until all culture reports return proving or disproving that the patient has an infection.

After 3 months the infection is insidious. As long as the component parts are not loose, the principles of treatment remain the same. If the parts are loose, there are three surgical choices: complete debridement, complete debridement with the delayed reimplantation, or a complete debridement with an acute reimplantation. Some of the factors that may help in deciding what to do are:

1. *The degree of debility.* If the patient can only tolerate one operation, do the one most likely to cure.
2. *The quality of the tissue.* A patient with massively scarred fibrous tissue is a poor candidate for acute or delayed reimplantation.
3. *The organism.* Infections caused by highly virulent organisms, resistant organisms, or gram-negative organisms appear less likely to respond to treatment.

A disabled patient who is immunosuppressed and nutritionally depleted and who has a massively scarred hip and highly virulent gram-negative organism will probably never respond to reimplantation, whether acute or delayed.

A 69-year-old male had a total hip replacement arthroplasty done in 1974, following which he developed an *Escherickia coli* and *Proteus vulgaris* infection and was treated with multiple debridements and then long-term antibiotics. This therapy took place over 3 years; the infectious organisms became resistant, his prosthesis became loose, and the bone and soft tissue became badly scarred. The patient was extremely debilitated, since he was both anemic and bedfast.

He underwent complete debridement, appropriate antibiotics were administered, and the wound was left open for 3 months. His wound closed, and he is now asymtomatic. He uses crutches and is pain-free and mobile.

Debridement in these instances must be considered debridement of the prosthesis, bone, and soft tissue. The wound needs to be left open because of the immense amount of dead space. A frequently recurring mistake is to close a wound in a patient such as this too early or without muscle transplantation, thus producing dead space and a cloaca in which bacteria may thrive. Should the surgeon remove all the cement? If there is infected avascular bone around it, which is almost always the case, it should be removed.

DIRECT EXCHANGE VS. DELAYED EXCHANGE

What about acute reimplantation (direct exchange)? One patient who underwent a total hip replacement in 1972 developed an infection 3 months postoperatively. His aspiration grew enterococcus and alpha streptococcus organisms that were sensitive to ampicillin. His total hip was acutely replaced, ampicillin was used in the acrylic cement, and he was also given 6 weeks of antibiotic therapy. He was last seen 12 years after total hip replacement, and his hip score was 97. This healthy individual, with nonresistant, relatively insensitive organisms and without bone or soft tissue scar, had a successful reimplantation. Should you use direct reimplantation? What are the criteria? Data from Buchholtz show a high rate of cure with the antibiotic-ladened acrylic cement.[2,17] However, Hunter, in reviewing the Canadian series, found that the occasional use of direct reimplantation was successful only in 10 of 33 patients treated in this manner.[11]

Another patient underwent a total hip replacement in August 1973 and did well until 8 months postoperatively, when he developed an *E. coli* urinary tract infection that required 3 weeks of hospitalization. Following release from the hospital, he developed hip pain and was again admitted; aspiration and culture grew *E. coli.* Two months later, his total hip was removed and replaced after debridement with the antibiotic, acrylic-ladened cement. By 1975 he had recurrent pain in the hip and was admitted. Aspiration of the hip revealed purulent material, and resistant *E. coli* were cultured. He was taken to surgery, and the prosthesis was removed and packed open. At the present time he is having some discomfort as a result of soft tissue ossification but functions as a city controller. This individual, who is young, robust and healthy and does not have severe bone or soft tissue scarring but rather a virulent organism, would have been better-served by an acute debridement and a consideration of delayed reimplantation.

RESECTION ARTHROPLASTY

What about the resection arthroplasty or the so-called Girdlestone procedure? Girdlestone popularized the procedure in another era with different types of patients. Now, although the procedure is lifesaving, it has not produced routinely good clinical results. Our results have not been as good. In an 11 year follow-up of nine resection arthroplasties, two patients became bedfast, five can only get about on crutches, two can do light work; persistent drainage of the wound has been a problem in some of these patients. For an older patient who is debilitated and ill, the operation will not necessarily improve the patient's function, but it may be lifesaving. Of 13 infected patients followed for seven years, six eventually died. The relatives believed that all the patients deaths were related to the infections.[19]

Muscle transplantation

One of the formidable frustrations is the overwhelming, cavernous dead space occasionally produced by resection arthroplasty. Attempts to deal with this problem often meet with failure: the patient is debrided, closed over tubes, breaks down, and the pattern is repeated. The other alternative, long-term open drainage, is physiologically and aesthetically displeasing to many, whereas disarticulation may be unacceptable. We believe that a decision to use muscle flaps to fill the dead space should be made early in treatment and will reduce repeated attempts at

closure and prolonged hospitalization.

As a rule the local soft tissue and osseous blood supply are diminished by previous procedures and chronic infection. Dead space, necrotic tissue, and low oxygen tension create an environment conducive to chronic drainage. Well-vascularized flaps have the ability to survive in spite of significant bacterial challenge, and they have the capacity to delivery oxygen, leukocytes, and immunologic humeral factors. Our choice has been the use of the vastus lateralis muscle transposition, because it usually has been spared disruption by previous surgery, it is anatomically consistent, it has sufficient bulk to fill the defect, and the remaining quadriceps appear sufficient to compensate for any deficiency from the vastus lateralis transfer.[7]

SUMMARY

In summary, if the pathophysiology of surgical infection is understood and the principles of treatment are followed, dealing with the complex problems of infected transplants should be less formidable.

REFERENCES

1. Berman, A.T., and Miers, D.J.: The use of the Hickman catheter in orthopaedic infections: Brief note, J. Bone Joint Surg. **67A:**650-651, 1985.
2. Buchholz, H.W., Elson, R.A., Englebrecht, E., et al.: Management of deep infection of total hip replacement, J. Bone Joint Surg. **63B:**342, 1981.
3. Cierny, G., and Mader, J.T.: Management of adult osteomyelitis. In Evarts, C.M., editor: Surgery of the musculoskeletal system, vol. 10, New York, 1983, Churchill Livingstone, Inc.
4. Dreblow, et al.: Nutritional assessment of orthopaedic patients, Mayo Clin. Proc. **56:**51-54, 1981.
5. Elek, S.D., and Conen, P.E.: The virulence of Staph. pyogenes for man: A study of problems of wound infection, Br. J. Exp. Pathol. **38:**573, 1957.
6. Enneking, W.F.: Infections. In: Clinical musculoskeletal pathology, 1977. Lithoprinted by Storter Printing Co., Gainesville, Fla.
7. Garvin, K.L., Collins, D., and Nelson, C.L. Infected resection arthroplasties: Natural history and treatment with vastus lateralis transfer. (Submitted for publication.)
8. Gristina, A.G., and Costerton, J.W.: Bacteria-laden Biofilms: A hazard to orthopedic prostheses, Infections in Surg. **3:**655-662, 1984.
9. Haynes, D.W., Morrissy, R.T., and Nelson, C.L.: Systemic cellular changes with osteomyelitis, Transactions of the twenty-eighth Annual Orthopaedics Research Meeting, New Orleans, Jan. 19-21, 1982.
10. Hughes, P.W., Salvati, E.A., and Wilson, P.O., Jr.: Treatment of subacute sepsis of the hip by antibiotics and joint replacement: Criteria for diagnosis with evaluation of twenty-six cases, Clin. Orthop. **141:**143-157, 1979.

11. Hunter, G., and Dandy, D.: The natural history of the patient with an infected total hip replacement, J. Bone Joint Surg. **59B:**293, 1977

12. Kahn, D.S., and Pritzker, K.P.H.: The pathophysiology of bone infection, Clin. Orthop. **96:**12-19, Oct. 1973.

13. Jensen, Jack E., Jensen, Terri G., and Smith, Taylor K., Nutrition in orthopaedic surgery, J. Bone Joint Surg. **64A:**1263-1272, 1982.

14. Mackowiak, P.A., Jones, S.R., and Smith, J.W.: Diagnostic value of sinus tract cultures in chronic osteomyelitis, JAMA **239:**2772-2775, 1978.

15. Mullen, J.L., Buzby, G.P., Matthews, D.C., Smale, B.F., and Rosato, E.F.: Reduction of operative morbidity and mortality by combined preoperative and postoperative nutritional support, Ann. Surg. pp. 604-613, Nov., 1980.

16. Nelson C.L.: Antibiotics in bone, joints, and hematoma. In: Instructional course lectures: American Academy of Orthopaedic Surgeons, vol. 26, St. Louis, 1977, The C.V. Mosby Co.

17. Nelson, C.L., and Bergman, B.R.: Antibiotic-impregnated acrylic composites. In Eftekhar, N.S., editor: Infection in joint replacement surgery: Prevention and management, St. Louis, 1984, The C.V. Mosby Co.

18. Nelson, C.L., Bergfeld, J., Schwartz, J., and Kolcqun, M.: Antibiotic levels in hematoma and wound fluid, Clin. Orthop. **108:**138-144, 1975.

19. Nelson, C.L., Evarts, C.M., Marks, K.E., and Andrish, J.: Infected total hip replacement arthroplasty: Results and complications, Clin. Orthop. Rel. Res. **147:**258-262, 1980.

20. Pratt, W.B., Veitch, J.M., and McRoberts, R.L.: Nutritional status of orthopaedic patients with surgical complications, Clin. Orthop. Rel. Res. **155:**81-84, 1981.

21. Rhinelauder, F.W., Nelson, C.L., Stewart, R.D., and Stewart, C.L.: Experimental reaming of the proximal femur and acrylic cement implantation: Vascular and histologic effects. In: The hip: Proceedings of the seventh open scientific meeting of The Hip Society, St. Louis, 1979, The C.V. Mosby Co.

22. Symposium on Infections in Orthopaedic Surgery, San Diego, May 31 to June 1, 1985.

Chapter 26

Preoperative planning of total hip arthroplasty

WILLIAM N. CAPELLO

The value of preoperative planning of total hip surgery has been recognized for many years. Deyerle published an article in 1972 on the preoperative planning of unipolar prostheses[1] and called the planning "shadow surgery." Müller included preoperative planning as an exercise in his course on total hip arthroplasty in 1977. Although accurate, his method was time-consuming and, probably for this reason and others, never achieved wide acceptance. Another reason was that the dimensions of prostheses then available were very limited. There were some variations in neck length, but, at most, three sizes were available. Stem length varied little, and the AP dimension remained essentially bladelike until very recently. The only major variations in stems at that time were some incremental increases in the medial-lateral dimension. Therefore even if the surgeon wished to fit the prosthesis to the patient's anatomy, the fitting could not be accomplished because of the limited prosthetic sizes available.

Recently the proportionality of the human femur has been appreciated, and prosthetic hip systems have been designed to accommodate these anatomic variations. This has resulted in a major increase of prosthetic inventory. Current stem designs include considerable variation in all three dimensions and offer many more neck lengths. The introduction by a variety of manufacturers of hip prostheses for uncemented implantation has added to the size variability. Presently most hip systems offer from five to nine sizes, each varying in length, medial-lateral, and anteroposterior dimensions. The use of modular head and neck segments allows the surgeon to adjust neck length over a wide spectrum of sizes that range from 25 to 55 mm.

Furthermore, the advent of uncemented prostheses brings with it the need for firm, immediate fixation of the implant. This can be accomplished only by accurate fitting of the stem to the femur, using an implant system that has a large spectrum of prosthetic sizes and accompanying instruments that allow surgical precision.

Even with cemented arthroplasty the need for precision has increased. It is now recognized that an uninterrupted cement mantle around the implanted stem is beneficial. Precise preoperative planning can ensure the presence of this mantle.

Thus the combination of new, highly variable implants with precision instrumentation and the awareness by the surgeon of the need for precise fitting of the prosthesis demands careful and accurate preoperative planning. This type of planning is necessary, particularly in uncemented arthroplasties, if the goals of arthroplasty of the hip are to be met routinely.

GOALS OF PREOPERATIVE PLANNING

The goals of preoperative planning are manyfold. The prime objective is to shorten the learning curve that is a necessary aspect of using any new implant system. In this regard selection of the appropriate size of the implant is essential. An undersized uncemented stem can lead to early loosening, whereas over estimating the actual size may result in a significant intraoperative fracture of the femur. Reliance solely on the instruments for sizing can be misleading. The "feel" of the instruments is dependent on a number of factors, including the quality of the available bone and the surgeon's prior experience with similar systems. Proper preoperative planning can provide accurate predetermination of prosthetic size and give the surgeon immediate feedback regarding the correct feel of the instruments in various clinical settings, thereby shorting the learning curve.

Proper preoperative planning also allows the surgeon to consider the equalization of leg-length discrepancies in total hip arthroplasty. The surgeon can accurately measure the discrepancy and plan precisely how it will be corrected during the procedure. In addition, preoperative planning allows the surgeon to formulate alternative plans if the procedure of choice cannot be performed. It allows the surgeon to identify the need for special equipment, such as custom prostheses, and AO fixation equipment, high speed burrs, and autograft or allograft.

Overall, preoperative planning minimizes intraoperative guesswork. It is valuable in this regard, not only to the surgeon, but to the entire operative team. It permits the nursing staff to better prepare for the procedure by having available the correct implants and any additional equipment that is required. Finally, proficient preoperative planning is rewarded by a significant reduction in surgical time. It minimizes or eliminates the need for repeating steps in the procedure—a major cause of prolonged surgical time.

METHOD OF PLANNING

Before planning can be accomplished, two items are essential. First, radiograms of good quality must be available, and, second, magnification of the radiograms must be known. Assuming that all are identical in magnification is erroneous. Because of the variations in body build, camera position, and film cassette position, uniform magnification is impossible in the clinical setting. Some type of marker must be included in the radiogram to permit precise determination of the magnification factor. This is critical because, as will be shown later, overlay templates that have built-in magnification are needed to complete the plan. One method of determining magnification is to use a plexiglas rod with lead spheres exactly 100 mm apart embedded in either end. If the rod is positioned at the level of the proximal femur and parallel to the x-ray film, the distance between these spheres can be measured from the film and the magnification calculated.

Good quality radiograms in the anteroposterior and lateral projections are needed for accurate planning. Fig. 26-1 is an AP view of the pelvis that is not suitable for preoperative planning of total hip replacement. It does not include a sufficient amount of the proximal femur to allow for accurate templating nor does it provide any way to assess the magnification of this film. Finally, the rotation of the hip, which will be discussed later, is not correct. Fig. 26-2 is an orthopaedic pelvis film that is ideal for preoperative planning of hip arthroplasties. An ample amount of the upper femur is seen, as is the entire hip joint. In addition, a marker is included that allows for calculation of the magnification of this film. Finally, rotation of the femur is more correct.

Proper use of overlay templates requires a true, AP projection of the upper femur. When the patient is positioned so that the knee is pointing straight up, the head, neck, and proximal femur are rotated secondary to the anteversion of these structures. A radiograph taken with this positioning gives an oblique projection of the head, neck, and upper femur, not a true AP projection. Therefore internal rotation of the hip until the head and neck are parallel with the cassette is necessary if a true AP projection is to be obtained. Obviously, this is difficult to accomplish in a clinical setting with hips that are diseased. However, the closer the surgeon gets to this ideal AP projection, the less error there is in templating. The degree of error in sizing is a function of the rotational distortion. Table 26-1 relates the rotational distortion to the sizing error. If a true AP projection is not possible, two things can be done to compensate. The x-ray technologist can tilt or rotate the pelvis to compensate for the lack of internal rotation, or the angular error introduced into the x-ray can be measured (assuming 15-degree anteversion) and the sizing adjusted accordingly (see Table 26-1).

Rotation influences lateral radiograms in a similar fashion. Thus, if true cross-table surgical lateral films are being used, rotation must be taken into consideration. One method of taking this radiogram so that the resultant film is magnified 15% to 20%, with gradation of density uniform, is described later. An alternative is the Lowenstein view (Fig. 26-3), which is easier tech-

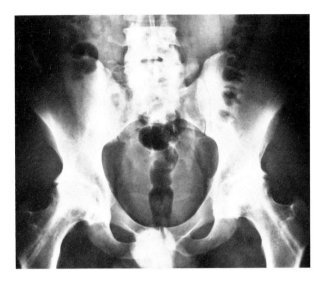

Fig. 26-1. AP view of the pelvis: an x-ray film view not suitable for preoperative planning.

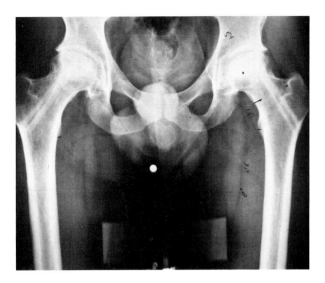

Fig. 26-2. AP view of the pelvis (orthopaedic pelvis) suitable for preoperative planning of total hip replacement.

Table 26-1. Effect of rotation in an AP radiogram on dimension sizing error

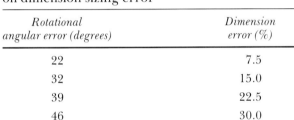

Rotational angular error (degrees)	Dimension error (%)
22	7.5
32	15.0
39	22.5
46	30.0
51	37.5

nically and also provides another view of the acetabulum.

Once the appropriate views are in hand and magnification is known, planning can begin. Most of the planning involves the AP view. First, a line is drawn at the level of, and parallel to, the ischial tuberosities. The relationship between this line and the lesser trochanter of the femur allows for accurate assesment of leg length discrepancies. Any discrepancy is measured and recorded (Fig. 26-4).

Next the acetabular overlay templates are used to determine the position and size of the prosthetic acetabulum (Figs. 26-5, 26-6, and 26-7). They must be positioned so that the center of the prosthesis reproduces the center of rotation of the head. Often this position is one where the inferior margin of the acetabulum lies at the level

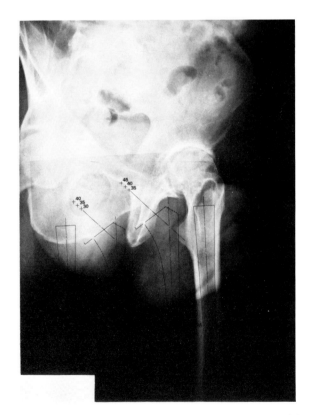

Fig. 26-3. Lowenstein lateral view of femur (with overlay template in place).

Fig. 26-4. Diagram of x-ray film showing line drawn parallel to ischial tuberoscities (*B* to *C*, Determination of leg-length discrepancies). *A*, Distance between x-ray film marker spheres.

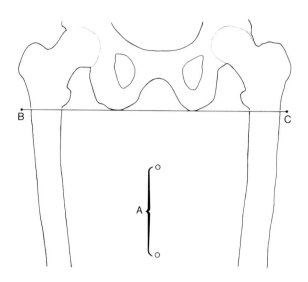

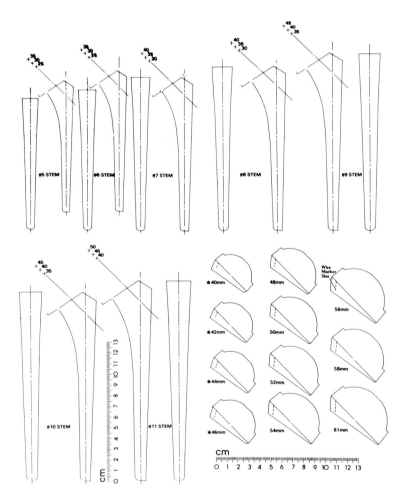

Fig. 26-5. Overlay templates used in preoperative planning showing AP and lateral projection of the stem, acetabular component, and magnified rulers.

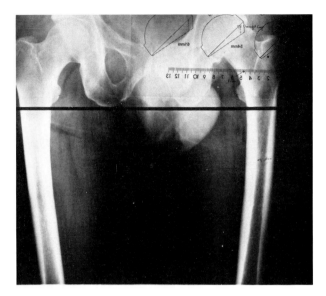

Fig. 26-6. AP x-ray film with acetabular template in proper position.

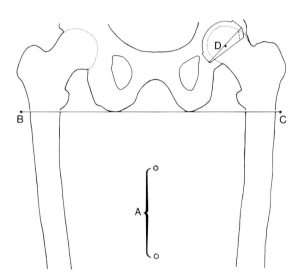

Fig. 26-7. Diagram of correct position of acetabular template with center of rotation marked.

of the obturator foramen. Sizing should be such that the implant will contact as much of the acetabular bone as possible without excessive removal of the strong subchondral bone. The medial position should be at the level of the tear drop. Major eccentricities in the acetabulum can be managed by eccentric cement mantles or, if uncemented components are planned, by bone grafting. Thus identifying the need for acetabular bone grafting is done at this time.

Making a template of the femur is the next step. In cemented arthroplasties, allowances are needed for a cement mantle. The size and location of this mantle are left to the discretion of the surgeon. In uncemented systems filling of the proximal canal is frequently necessary. Therefore a template that best fits the upper femur will indicate the stem size to be used. Once the stem size is determined, the appropriate head and neck segment can be chosen. If no leg-length discrepancies exist, exact superimposition of the center of the prosthetic head and femoral head to the previously identified acetabular center of the hip will maintain the existing leg length (Figs. 26-8 and 26-9). If a discrepancy is present, then the distance from the acetabular center to the femoral center should equal the previously measured discrepancy and subsequent superimposition will reestablish leg lengths. Once this determination has been made, the template will indicate the neck resection level. This is measured easily from

the proximal aspect of the lesser trochanter and can be accurately reproduced at surgery, providing the lesser trochanter is exposed during the procedure.

An alternative method is to note the relationship between the tip of the greater trochanter and the prosthetic femoral head. This relationship can be assessed during surgery, using trial prostheses and the neck cut accordingly. I prefer exposing the lesser trochanter and measuring from it at the time of surgery. Any measurements that are made during the planning, such as the distance from the lesser trochanter to the intended neck resection level, must be done with a ruler whose scale is magnified the same amount as the x-ray film. Most templates include such a scale. If one is not available, a standard ruler can be used and the magnification factor subtracted from the reading. Figs. 26-10 and 26-11 show the complete plan an AP x-ray film.

A lateral x-ray template is done in a similar manner. Because the intended neck resection level already has been determined, it can be taken into account on the lateral film. Occasionally, the surgeon will encounter a discrepancy between sizes on the AP film and the lateral film because some femurs are oval-shaped proximally. The surgeon then will have to decide if excessive bone can be reamed to accommodate the larger of the two sizes or if it is prudent to use the smaller one.

If a medullary plug is planned in a cemented

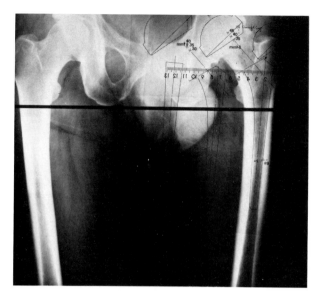

Fig. 26-8. AP x-ray films of femoral template in place matching contour of canal and the appropriate neck length (plus 40) matching acetabular center of rotation.

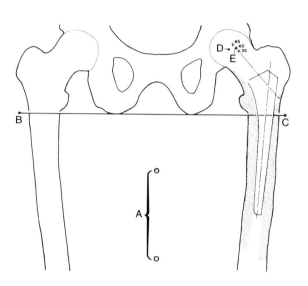

Fig. 26-9. Diagrams of femoral template and matching centers of rotation, acetabular and femoral.

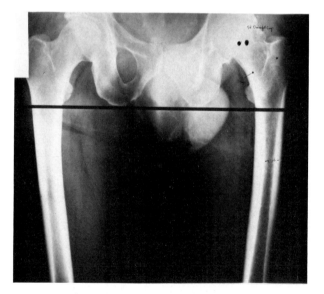

Fig. 26-10. AP x-ray films showing completed plan with leg length discrepancies measured, neck cut indicated, and centers of rotation marked for femoral and acetabular component.

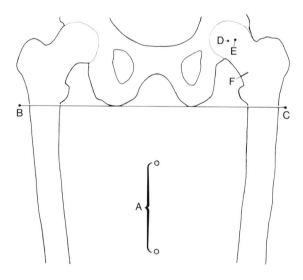

Fig. 26-11. Diagram showing completed templating with line *B* to *C*, any leg length discrepancy. Point *D*, Center of acetabulum. Point *E*, Center of femoral head. Line *F*, Intended neck resection level from lesser trochanter.

arthroplasty, its size can be determined at this time by measuring the canal diameter at the level of the prosthetic stem. As mentioned, alternative plans also can be drawn at this point, and the need for special equipment can be assessed.

In complicated cases such as revision arthroplasty, it is sometimes necessary to make a template of the opposite unoperated hip to assess component size and determine the need for special equipment or bone graft.

CHECKING THE PLAN

There are at least three methods of checking the preoperative plan. First, the instruments, including the trial prostheses, improve the surgeon's "feel" and permit the identification of major discrepancies in this predetermined size by how the instruments and trial prostheses are fitting the bone.

Second, in uncemented hip arthroplasties, the development of an intraoperative criteria for tightness of the prosthetic stem gives the surgeon some assurance that the implanted stem is firmly fixed. I suggest that surgeons develop some means of applying predetermined rotation and extraction forces to the implanted stem. Should the stem move during this test, an error has been made in sizing, and either a larger size should be used or the implant should be cemented.

Finally, good quality postoperative x-ray films are essential and provide another method of checking the preoperative plan (Figs. 26-12 and 26-13). Should the implanted prosthesis differ in size from that determined preoperatively, the surgeon can return to the preoperative plan and search for reasons why the plan was either not followed or proved inaccurate. Leg-length discrepancy also can be measured postoperatively and compared to the preoperative plan. In addition, acetabular placement and orientation are checked.

TECHNIQUE FOR TAKING SURGICAL LATERAL X-RAY FILMS

The modified surgical lateral x-ray film is used to view the lateral aspect of the femur.

The patient is supine with the femur of interest fully extended. The patella should be rotated 10 to 20 degrees inward. The opposite leg should be suspended above the patient. The 10 cm marker is placed on the anterior surface of the patient's leg (see Fig. 26-15) parallel with the film and halfway between the medial and lateral borders of the thigh. The superior-most end of the marker should lie at the level of the crease of the leg. The patient then is adjusted so the marker is 17 cm from the film. (See Fig. 26-14.) A linear grid is employed to decrease cutoff but still allow

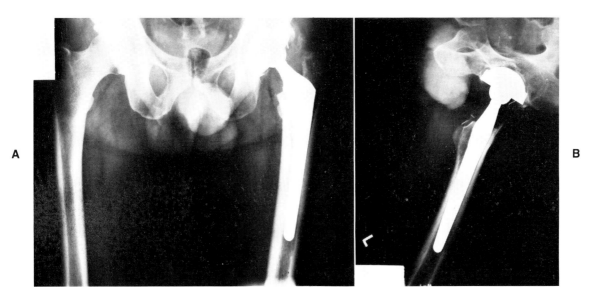

Fig. 26-12. A, AP x-ray film showing postoperative appearance of implant corresponding to previously described preoperative plan. **B,** Lateral view of patient.

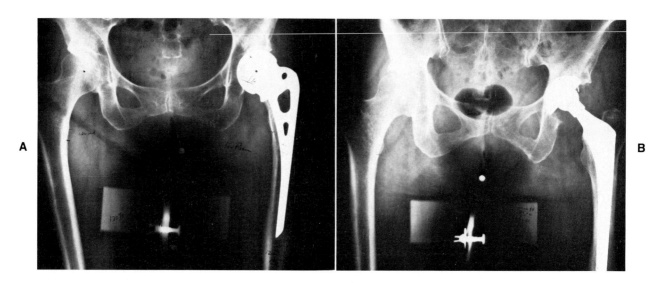

Fig. 26-13. A, Preoperative x-ray film of patient undergoing revision surgery for painful Austin-Moore prosthesis. **B,** Postoperative AP x-ray film of patient showing revision arthroplasty conforming to preoperative plan and restoration of leg lengths.

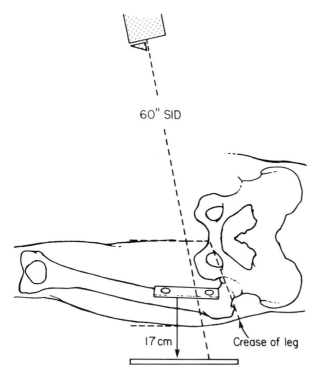

Fig. 26-14. Relationship of femur film cassette and camera for lateral x-ray resulting in film magnification of 15% to 20%.

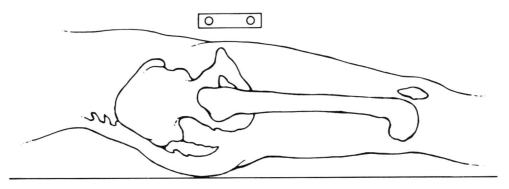

Fig. 26-15. Positioning of patient for lateral x-ray with x-ray marker on anterior thigh.

for some angulation. The marker will not be distorted. The grid is placed next to the hip of interest with a 14-inch square or 14-inch-by-17-inch cassette placed behind it.

There should be a 60-inch target film distance, with no more than a 10- to 20-degree tube angulation from the perpendicular. The tube is centered to the lesser trochanter or the crease of the leg. Careful collimation to include the marker is important in the final visualization. An aluminum filter wedge approximately 3 inches long, 4 inches wide, and ¾ inch at its thickest edge is needed. This filter is placed with the thick end at the midline of the collimator box. With this positioning of the wedge, the radiogram should demonstrate an even density from hip to femur. This allows for absorption of unwanted radiation in the femoral area.

Positioning by these methods should create a 15% to 20% magnification of the radiographic image. This can be confirmed by measuring the distance between the centers of the two radiopaque balls. A reading of 11.5 cm is ideal; however, an error margin of ±0.5 cm is acceptable (11.0 cm to 12.0 cm).

SUMMARY

Preoperative planning of a total hip replacement is a necessary first step in arthroplasty. If properly done, it can shorten the learning curve for new prosthetic systems, minimize intraoperative guesswork, and decrease surgical time. It also will allow the surgeon to fulfill one of the universal goals of reconstructive surgery—precision with reproduceability.

REFERENCES

1. Deyerle, W.M.: Complications of hip prostheses: An atlas of new preventive technical aids, Clin. Orthop. **53:**61-79, 1967.

Chapter 27

Corrosion and ion transfer from porous metallic alloys to tissues

J.E. LEMONS

L.C. LUCAS

Metals and alloys have extensive and long-term applications for reconstructive surgery procedures. In general the biocompatibility profiles for most systems have demonstrated very few limitations for established classes of biomaterials.[9] The evaluations of metallurgic properties have always emphasized corrosion studies for correlation with *in vivo* tissue responses.[1] Interfacial interactions with the nonporous alloys have shown clearly that minimal amounts of biocorrosion products can be tolerated by human patient populations, and in general the dose-response-time relationships have not exceeded normal tissue limits within the local or systemic environments. However, with the recent introduction of porous metals and alloys for biologic tissue ingrowth for the mechanical stabilization of many different types of prostheses, new questions have been raised about the specific types and amounts of metallic constituents that would be transferred to the *in vivo* environment, especially over the long term.[8,10] Pressing questions about dose-response-time relationships not previously established and the very long-term influences of specific elements that may be accumulated in organs have caused expanded interest in this area of biocompatibility research.

This paper will address questions about (1) surface and metallurgic microstructural features for currently available systems, (2) *in vitro* corrosion and the influence of porosity on susceptibility and rate of corrosion, (3) the elements preferentially released during corrosion and biocorrosion, and (4) biologic responses to metallic ions in tissue culture and at implant interfaces.

MATERIALS AND METHODS
Materials

The metallic systems investigated in our laboratories and the types of porous surfaces provided for biologic fixation are summarized in Table 27-1. The metallic systems include single composition alloys and combinations of titanium (Ti), titanium-aluminum-vanadium (Ti-6A1-4V), and cobalt-chromium-molybdenum (Co-Cr-Mo). The porous surfaces range from sintered wire compacts of Ti on Ti-6A1-4V to sintered and plasma-sprayed Ti, Ti-6A1-4V, and Co-Cr-Mo. The microstructures of the substrate and porous regions include the fine-grain size alpha-beta Ti-6A1-4V, cast Ti-6A1-4V with an acicular microstructure, medium grain–size titanium wire, cast Co-Cr-Mo with a large grain size, and the polyphase regions of the plasma-sprayed surfaces. More detailed metallurgic studies of these alloys have already been presented.[6]

Corrosion

The various alloys in porous and nonporous surface conditions were analyzed using potentiostatic polarization methods. The test conditions included an oxygenated phosphate–buffered water solution with 0.9% sodium chloride maintained at pH 7.00 ± 0.05 and $37 \pm 1C$. Triplicate anodic and cathodic polarization curves were generated for each alloy. Methods for generating

Table 27-1. Summary of porous metallic systems

Material	Fabrication method	Surface type
Co-Cr-Mo	Sintered, cast	Regular spherical
Ti-Al-V	Sintered, VMC	Regular and irregular
	Plasma sprayed	Irregular
Ti	Sintered	Wire, regular or irregular spherical Irregular
	Plasma sprayed	Irregular
Ti/Ti-Al-V	Sintered	Wire, irregular
	Plasma sprayed	Irregular
Ti-Al-V/Co-Cr-Mo	Sintered	Irregular
	Plasma sprayed	Irregular
Ti-Al-V/C	Sintered and coated	Irregular

these curves have been described in previous publications.[3,4] Data were averaged, and the corrosion rate (i_c) for each alloy system was obtained by extrapolating (Tafel extrapolation) the cathodic curves to the measured corrosion potential. The anodic curves were generated to include a reverse scan after entering the transpassive (higher potential range) region to evaluate the reverse scan–hysteresis behavior and the possibilities for pitting and crevice corrosion.

To determine the preferential release of elemental constituents, accelerated corrosion tests also were conducted. For these tests, a potential greater than the breakdown potential was applied to the test alloy specimens for a series of time periods. After each test the corrosion solutions were analyzed for the type and amount of metallic elements present. These chemical analyses then could be correlated with prior microstructural studies of the corrosion specimens. Specimen surfaces were examined by optical and scanning-electron microscopy techniques including metallurgic metallographic sections. These data were generated from solid specimens, and complete data have not been collected for the various porous metallic materials.

Tissue interactions

Tissue culture studies included the addition of the primary elements from the alloys and combinations of the elements at concentration ranges from 0.4 to 100 parts per million (ppm). Cell morphologies and numbers were compared to controls as a measure of fibroblast-type cellular responses to metallic-corrosion product environments.[2] Implants of the alloys and implants where corrosion products were provided along the soft tissue to biomaterial interface also were studied for establishing correlations between the cell culture and *in vivo* implantation conditions. These evaluations also were correlated, when possible, with human clinical information about tissue responses to metallic corrosion products.

RESULTS
Materials and microstructural features

Titanium (Ti) wire on titanium alloy (Ti-6Al-4V) showed the substrate to be of two different types. The specimens for higher strength applications showed an alpha-beta type microstructure for the alloy, whereas other specimens showed a cast microstructure. The cast Ti-6Al-4V microstructure showed the acicular-type features with large dimensions at the sintered contact points between the titanium wire and the substrate. Standard powder metallurgy–porous surfaces (sintered) from Ti-6Al-4V showed a midrange grain size of primarily alpha phase, alpha-beta type microstructure. The cobalt-base alloys were castings and always showed a large grain structure. Regions of localized multiphase structures were located at many of the contact points between the spherical particulate surface regions and the alloy substrate. These regions could influence mechanical and corrosion-property characteristics.

The plasma sprayed–alloy surface regions showed mixed polyphase mirostructures with multiple internal interfacial boundaries. Some specimens showed a second phase–type boundary between the substrate and the porous surface coating. The microstructural features were quite irregular for the plasma-sprayed materials.

Measurements of surface area relationships showed an increase from 1.2 to 7.2 times the nominal surface area compared to the nonporous systems. In general these surfaces showed a depth not exceeding about 3 times the average dimensions of the porosity openings (approximately 150 to 300 micrometer-size porosity).

Corrosion

The results of the potentiostatic polarization analyses for corrosion potential (E_c) and rate (i_c) are summarized in Table 27-2. In general the corrosion potentials of these alloys were not significantly altered by the addition of a porous surface region. This was true for similar alloy combinations (Ti-6Al-4V and Co-Cr-Mo). The corrosion-rate increases were somewhat proportional to the relative increases in surface area associated with the porosities. The relative increases in corrosion rate at the corrosion potential ranged from $\times 1.2$ to $\times 5.2$ as compared to overall increases of surface area of $\times 1.2$ to $\times 7.2$. At potentials greater than the corrosion potential for each porous system, the corrosion current magnitudes continue to be greater than those of

the solid forms of the alloys. Thus porous alloy systems would release increased quantities of metallic ions to the adjacent systemic tissues.

The comparisons of cyclic anodic–corrosion cycles showed limited hysteresis behavior for the Co-Cr-Mo alloys, indicating that these porous alloys should not be susceptible to pitting or crevice corrosion. The titanium alloys did not show hysteresis behavior.

The analyses of elemental distributions within selected corrosion solutions showed that the relative quantities of released ions were not the same as the nominal composition of the alloy. This is not surprising, since these alloys were subjected to potentiostatically driven anodic corrosion conditions. However, since in vivo implants have shown localized regions of corrosion, the elemental distributions of elements provided to the in vivo environment also should be specific to the region of the alloy undergoing corrosion.

Tissue interactions

The implant interface studies showed the titanium- and cobalt-base alloys to be biocompatible materials when evaluated by standard histologic methods. The surfaces resulted in passive fibrous tissue capsules, which have been demonstrated in previous studies.[7] In general clinicians believe that increases in the quantity of localized corrosion products result in increased amounts of tissue reaction, with a general trend of more reaction with more corrosion products. Detailed histologic studies demonstrate that this may not always be true, because reaction magnitudes also depend on the type and relative amounts of the constituents available to the tissues at the implant site.

The tissue culture studies to which metallic salt solutions (simulated corrosion products) were added showed reactions that were dependent on both the type and the amount of elemental constituents present. Selected elements such as vanadium and chromium (Cr^{+6}) displayed toxic responses at significantly lower concentrations than the other elements investigated. A general trend for titanium alloy showed that mixtures of elements caused cellular changes at lower concentrations, thereby supporting a theoretic concept of synergistic interactions being associated with multiple ionic constituents. Extended studies of cell culture systems and the role of metallic constituents on cells also have shown the value of

Table 27-2. Corrosion potentials (E_c) and rates (i_c) for porous alloys

Material and condition	$E_c(mV)$	$i_c(\mu A/cm^2 \times 10^{-2})$
Ti-solid	−14	1.3
Ti-Al-V-solid	−50	0.3
Ti-Al-V-porous	−75	1.4
Ti/Ti-Al-V (fiber)	−10	4.4
Co-Cr-Mo-solid	−10	1.1
Co-Cr-Mo-porous	−35	2.8
Co-Cr-Mo/Ti-Al-V	−72	2.0

E_c, corrosion potential; i_c, corrosion rate.
E_c and i_c from Tafel extrapolations taken from potentiostatic polarization relationships.

transmission electron microscopy for the detailed descriptions of cellular morphologies. Correlations between the quantities of elemental constituents for iron, chromium, and nickel (316L) combinations have been evaluated for tissue culture and surgical implant conditions, showing quantitative interrelationships between these types of samples.[5] These types of studies are continuing in several research laboratories.

SUMMARY

Investigations on porous and nonporous alloys currently available for surgical implant device stabilization through tissue ingrowth have shown (1) microstructures that are characteristic of the thermal processing history of the device and alloy with differences between the nonporous and porous devices of the same nominal chemical analysis, (2) in vitro corrosion potentials that are similar for porous and nonporous alloys and corrosion rates that are approximately proportional to the increases in relative surface areas ($\times 2$ to $\times 10$); (3) local tissue interactions at the cellular level that are specific to the type and amount of elemental constituents present at the interface; and (4) no direct correlations between the local cellular responses (fibroblasts) and the potential for hypersensitivity and other systemically mediated responses.

Evaluations of the available published literature and available information on device retrievals and analyses support the opinion that no quantitative, statistically based epidemiologic studies have yet established significant correlations between se-lected metallic ions and major types of tissue lesions. However, with the changes in surface area and basic surface chemistry for existing alloy systems, research on the long-term tissue responses should be emphasized. In our opinion, biomaterial surface modifications are possible, whereby the relative quantities of released ions available to the environment could be significantly reduced.

REFERENCES

1. Annual book of ASTM standards, Medical devices, ASTM, Philadelphia, 1984.
2. Lucas, L.C.: Biocompatibility investigations of surgical implant alloys, doctoral dissertation, Birmingham, Ala., 1982, University of Alabama at Birmingham.
3. Lucas, L.C., Buchanan, R.A., and Lemons, J.E.: Investigations on the galvanic corrosion of multi-alloy total hip prostheses, J. Biomed. Mater. Res. **15:**731-747, 1981.
4. Lucas, L.C., Buchanan, R.A., Lemons, J.E., and Griffin, C.D.: Susceptibility of surgical cobalt-base alloy to pitting corrosion, J. Biomed. Mater. Res. **16:**799-810, 1982.
5. Lucas, L.C., Lemons, J.E., Lee, J., and Dale, P.: *In vitro* corrosion characteristics of Co-Cr-Mo/Ti/6Al-4V/Ti alloys, ASTM Special Publication, 1986.
6. Luckey, H.A., and Kubil, F., Jr., editors: Titanium alloys in surgical implants, ASTM special technical publication 796, Philadelphia, 1983 ASTM.
7. Meers, D.C.: Materials and orthopaedic surgery, Baltimore, 1979, Williams & Wilkins Co.
8. Williams, D.F., editor: Biocompatibility of orthopaedic implants, vol. 1, Boca Raton, Fla., 1982, CRC Press.
9. Williams, D.F., and Roaf, R.: Implants in surgery, London, 1973, W.B. Saunders, Ltd.
10. Woodman, J.L., Black, J., and Jiminez, S.A.: Isolation of serum protein organometallic corrosion products from 316SS and HS-21 *in-vitro* and *in vivo*, J. Biomed. Mater. Res. **18:**99-115, 1984.

TOTAL KNEE

Chapter 28

General considerations in total knee arthroplasty

DAVID A. HECK

DONALD B. KETTELKAMP

The primary indication for total knee arthroplasty is pain with weight bearing. Night pain may be present, but it is more common in inflammatory arthritides such as rheumatoid arthritis. These pain patterns are associated with the primary structural abnormality of loss of articular cartilage. Synovitis and intraosseous hypertension also contribute to clinically significant pain. Pain usually is significant enough that walking is reduced to a distance of less than three blocks. Varying degrees of deformity and ligamentous insufficiency may be associated with the articular cartilage loss.

Infection generally contraindicates total knee arthroplasty. Recent experience has indicated that under some circumstances, particularly with gram-positive infections, implantation may be carried out after the infection has cleared. In addition, neurotrophic arthritis contraindicates total joint replacement. Patients with vascular compromise should be treated with caution. If the vascular insufficiency is severe, total joint replacement should not be performed. Relative youth, particularly with combined ligamentous instability, remains a contraindication at this time.

A surprising number of patients can be improved significantly by nonoperative intervention. Nonoperative treatment includes the use of a cane, activity modification, weight reduction when appropriate, and the use of nonsteroidal antiinflammatory agents. If this proves unsatisfactory, nonreplacement surgical alternatives, especially with the very young, should be explored.

Severe tricompartmental disease, particularly when combined with ligamentous insufficiency, is a prime indication for knee fusion. In unicompartmental degenerative arthritis the orthopaedic surgeon should consider other alternatives, such as osteotomy, in addition to unicompartmental total knee replacement. The relative roles of abrasion arthroplasty, joint debridement, and osteochondral grafts require further delineation in the future.

The operative procedure, anticipated results, potential complications, and alternate modes of treatment should be discussed in detail with the patient. The decision to have or not to have a surgical procedure and the choice of the specific procedure reside with the patient. The final decision as to type of implant resides with the surgeon. Many years ago Larson recommended that elective surgery not be scheduled for a patient at the first office visit. This allows the patient to consider the procedure and the risks over a 24-hour period before scheduling. This is excellent advice when considering reconstructive surgery.

The patients' expectation from a total knee arthroplasty should be less pain. Younger and heavier patients in particular should expect to have continued restriction in their activity level. At the present state of the art, eventual loosening of the implant should be anticipated, although the exact frequency, longevity of implants, and the optimal conditions for implant survival are not yet well defined. The clinical risks of infection, phlebitis, pulmonary embolus, peroneal nerve palsy, vascular compromise, transfusion reaction, allergies to medications, anesthesia, and implant complications (loosening, fracture, wear), should be discussed with the patient.

Because medicine is an inexact science, each orthopaedic surgeon should develop a philosophy concerning the application of total joint arthroplasty. We believe the surgeon should approach the arthroplasty with the goal of replacing only the nonfunctioning structures and to retain as many secondary options as are compatible with obtaining pain relief and improved ambulatory ability.

APPLIED KINEMATICS

The orthopaedic surgeon will find that basic knowledge of knee kinematics is necessary to understand the functioning of the knee in its varied normal and abnormal conditions. Furthermore, this basic knowledge can help the surgeon select appropriate prosthesis and instrument systems to allow for maximal restoration of function and implant longevity.

To fully describe the relative motions of two rigid bodies in space, information on six independent motions must be defined. These motions can be described as three rotations and three translations. In order to describe motions at the knee joint, Grood and Suntay[16] have proposed the use of two linked coordinate systems that are related by six clinically relevant independent motions. In the sagittal plane, rotation corresponds to flexion/extension and translation to anterior/ posterior drawer. In the transverse plane, rotation is internal or external in direction and translation is either medial or lateral. To fully specify the final location, the coronal plane rotation is abduction or adduction, and translation is axial compression or distraction.

LaFortune[24] has measured these motions by using pins rigidly fixed to the femur and tibia in five normal adult subjects. Her data can be summarized as follows:

1. In the sagittal plane during level gait, rotation (sagittal flexion) at heel strike averages 2 degrees. In early stance phase, the knee flexes to 20 degrees. It then extends and finally flexes reaching a maximum of 60 degrees during swing phase. Anteroposterior translation is approximately 5 mm during stance phase. Posterior translation of the tibia with respect to the femur increases to approximately 15 mm in swing phase. Overall translation closely parallels the sagittal flexion.

2. Rotation in the transverse plane closely parallels sagittal flexion of the knee. The tibia is in relative external rotation at heel strike. The tibia then proceeds into internal rotation with flexion during early stance to an average of 4 degrees. In swing phase extension, the tibia again goes into external rotation relative to the femur. The average total motion is 9 degrees. Medial to lateral translation occurs from an initial neutral position at heel strike proceeding to medial displacement, oscillating toward lateral displacement, and returning in a medial direction just before toe off. Stance phase translation averages 4 mm. During swing phase, maximal medial translation of 6mm occurs.

3. Rotation in the coronal plane is limited. The knee is in slight abduction at heel strike, which then generally increases to 6 degrees in swing phase. Overall coronal rotation averages only approximately 5 degrees. Axial translation (compression/distraction) also closely parallels sagittal rotation. This translation predominately represents the varying radii of curvatures of the femoral condyles and averages 3 mm.

According to other authors using external monitoring systems, other activities such as stair climbing require a mean 87 degrees of sagittal flexion. Descending stairs requires an average of 91 degrees.[2] Activities such as getting out of a chair require approximately 105 degrees of sagittal plane rotation. Lifting objects requires 117 degrees of flexion.[25,37]

To fully reproduce these normal motions, a delicate balance must be achieved between articular surface design and the supporting ligamentous structures. If the articular surfaces are highly constraining and minimal disruption has occurred in the surrounding ligamentous and capsular envelope, marked increases in both residual ligament tensions and bone prosthesis interface stresses will be seen. This constellation of events probably is represented best by early attempts at total knee arthroplasty in which a single-axis, single-degree-of-freedom prosthesis such as the Herbert prosthesis was used. Clinical experiences with loosening, premature device failure, and restricted range of motion were all evident. This is not to say, however, that the prosthesis should be designed without constraint. The ICLH prosthesis, as originally conceived, had no constraint to medially or laterally directed forces. This resulted in translational instability in the transverse plane.[14] Excessive unconstrained tibial rotation also may be associated with patello-femoral disorders.[7,20,31]

IMPLANT SELECTION

Selection of an individual implant is therefore dependent on the initial patient status. The patients with relatively minimal degrees of deformity and generally intact supporting ligamentous structures will be served best through the use of a minimally constrained prosthesis. Preservation of the cruciate ligaments, especially the posterior cruciate, will assist in deceleration functions such as descending stairs.[2,10,38]

One must, however, be wary of the preservation of the posterior cruciate ligament when using prostheses with higher levels of femorotibial constraint. This combination of restraints can cause rocking of the femorotibial articulation, increased wear, increased bone prosthesis interface stresses, and excessive ligamentous stresses. These phenomena are particularly associated with a constraining elevated flange along the posterior aspect of the tibial surface.[26]

In patients who have greater degrees of deformity, especially those with flexion contractures of greater than 30 degrees, it is frequently necessary to resect the posterior cruciate ligament in order to obtain full extension. In these cases and in those with greater than 25 degrees of varus or valgus deformity, a more constrained prosthesis will be required. In cases of maximal ligament and bone deficiency, as in tumor surgery or certain revision procedures, it is necessary to proceed to more highly constrained prostheses such as the Total Condylar III,[6] or a rotating hinge design, or even to a custom prosthesis.[8] Prostheses with such increased articular constraint require greater degrees of activity reduction to minimize loosening and device failure.

FEMORAL COMPONENT DESIGN

Femoral component design should incorporate a central patellar groove with lateral condylar buttressing to prevent patellar subluxation. The condylar radii should vary anatomically in the

sagittal plane to duplicate normal kinematics. However, the exact curvature of the runners in the frontal plane is open to question. Relatively flat condylar surfaces result in improved surface load distribution on unconstrained polyethylene tibial surfaces. This design feature also improves stability to varus and valgus forces through the maximization of the contact moment arm.[1] However, flattening of these surfaces can, especially when ligament insufficiency exists, increase the potential for loading at the prosthetic edges. This flattening, through a "teetering" effect, will result in increased interface bony stresses and surface wear. The use of a central stem in a primary femoral arthroplasty is generally not necessary for load transmission but may assist in establishing the proper alignment.

TIBIAL COMPONENT DESIGN

Because total knee replacement failures have occurred most commonly on the tibial side,[17] special attention must be directed at this component in order to reduce failure.[11] The tibial component must offer a low-friction surface to articulate with the femoral component. The most satisfactory materials to date for this low-friction surface have been high-molecular-weight polyethylene contacting cobalt chrome molybdenum. In addition, the tibial component surface should be capable of being contoured to present variable degrees of constraint to accommodate the existing ligamentous status. Relatively thin layers of polyethylene, which are not metal backed, should not be used because they have been associated with cold flow, breakage, loosening, and tibial subsidence.[5] Thick layers of polyethylene or a metal backing can distribute the load over a broad area. To minimize bony resection, metal backing appears to be the most rational approach at present. Furthermore, because of its thermal conductivity metal backing can decrease peak temperatures during the insertion of components with methyl methacrylate cement.[30]

Adding carbon fibers to high molecular–weight polyethylene in an attempt to reinforce it has been investigated extensively. Indeed, the ultimate strength and stiffness of this composite structure is increased. However, fatigue resistance is decreased.[9] Furthermore, the increased stiffness results in a decreased contact area and increased surface stress. Since most failures begin at the surface, it seems unlikely that this approach will help address the concerns of wear in total knee arthroplasty.[5,32] The use of other composite types of polyethylene, however, may reduce surface contact stress while allowing for anatomic bone-strain distribution.[22,34]

The use of a single central tibial stem is the best way to obtain satisfactory bony fixation.[27] This requires resection of only the relatively weak intercondylar bone and decreases peak interface stresses.[15] It is quite clear, however, that none of the currently available prostheses or prosthetic approaches is capable of anatomically redistributing the load across the proximal tibial surface.[32,33] Optimization of load transfer requires maximization of proximal tibial contact.[4] However, achieving this exact contact is difficult with the variability in tibial bone resection and the presence of tibial anthropometric differences, even if performed on a custom basis.

The role of cemented porous-backed tibial components is controversial. The predominant mode of loosening does not occur at the prosthesis cement interface but rather at the bone cement interface. Relatively rough surfaces indeed allow improvement in cement strength because of a local reinforcement effect. The technology used to apply the porous surface is still in evolution. Fatigue failure of the underlying tibial component resulting from the alteration in grain size as a function of sintering is a major concern. In addition, the introduction of numerous notches at every point of application of the bead or wire is alarming because of its deleterious effect on fatigue performance.[29] Finally, problems of surface delamination and breakage (loose beads and wires) need to be resolved.[17]

Optimal parameters for tibial component design in the biologic ingrowth mode are currently ill-defined. It may be likely that a combination of smooth stems and porous plateaus will prove satisfactory.[19] Whether the use of a single central stem or the use of multiple stems is the most satisfactory will require further investigation. Finally, it is unclear what the optimal type of biologic tissue ingrowth is, either fibrous or bony, and which will produce a lasting painless arthroplasty.[18]

PATELLAR COMPONENT DESIGN

Relatively little information is available on the ideal patellar component design. Currently three shapes are available. A trapezoidal component is used in some knee designs to prevent dislocation of the patella. However, this design constrains the femoral component runners to a nonanatomic, grooved design. It appears that, with appropriate lateral soft tissue release and adequate femorotibial rotational constraint, this high degree of patellar articular constraint is unnecessary.

A dome-shaped component is the most commonly used configuration. Technically, it is easy to insert because no attention need be given to rotational alignment. It is axisymmetric and therefore can be used in the right or left knee, reducing inventory. However, it has the theoretic disadvantage of concentrating load in relatively small areas of articulation, which may predispose to polyethylene failure.[36]

An anatomically designed prosthesis that is metal backed may minimize the problems of polyethylene failure and give adequate levels of constraint to patellar subluxation or dislocation. Surgical precision is necessary during insertion to be certain that proper rotational alignment is present, because improper alignment will result in increased surface and interface stresses. Patellar fixation is probably best accomplished through the use of multiple small stems rather than a single central stem. This allows for greater rotational stability at the bone-prosthesis interface and minimizes problems with patellar fracture associated with single large central posts.

EX-VIVO MACHINE TESTING

Murray and coworkers tested the Variable Axis, Total Condylar, Stabilo-condylar, Spherocentric, and Noiles implants to failure in a knee simulator. The variable axis with no constraint to rotation and the Noiles Hinge Prosthesis survived 10 million cycles without failure. The total condylar sustained plastic cold-flow at 8 million cycles. The tibial component of the stabilo-condylar became loose at 4.8 million cycles. Data are not currently available for the commonly used resurfacing implants.

The wear characteristics of implants are relatively poorly understood as they relate to changes in stiffness and area of contact over time. Hillberry and coworkers at Purdue tested the Insall-Burnstein, multi radius, geopatellar/geometric, RMC, cruciate condylar, and anametric knees in a knee simulator. The stiffness varied with the number of simulated steps, and the area of contact gradually increased between zero and 100,000 steps. Misalignment was found to result in altered wear, increased shear stress at the bone cement interface, and instability at the articulating surfaces.[1]

SURGICAL PRINCIPLES

The surgical principles for total knee arthroplasty require careful preoperative planning, intraoperative precision, and sensible postoperative management.

1. Preoperative planning is necessary to determine the appropriate design and size of the prosthesis. Alternatives must be available in the operating room.
2. Accurate alignment of the limb and all prosthetic components (including the normal or resurfaced patella) should be determined and restored to normal.
3. The minimum in bone resection should be performed.
4. Ligamentous stability must be assessed and maximally restored.
5. Accurate instrumentation to ensure optimal prosthetic-bony interface fit must be available. Good cement technique should be used.

Implant selection is based on the preoperative evaluation of deformity, bone loss, and ligamentous integrity, but the final decision is made in the operating room. The soft tissue releases necessary to obtain limb alignment will also allow for minimization of bone resection. The implant design chosen should have the minimum in surface-design constraint compatible with restoring knee stability. It should be of a resurfacing design if possible. Poorer results are associated with more constrained implants. Subsequent salvage is easier after initial use of resurfacing implants.

When a revision implant is necessary, it should be chosen to meet the deficits present. It should minimize bone resection and restore the three planes of motion. The primary consideration is to save bone. The problems associated with excessive bone loss or bone resection are those of loss of orientation, inability to use jigs and instrumentation to restore alignment, anatomic limitations to further resection, compromised implant fixation, increased instability, and the difficulty in subsequent salvage arthrodesis.[21]

A number of authors associate prosthetic or limb malalignment with subsequent loosening.[3,14,28,35] To restore alignment in varus deformity, all osteophytes must be removed, the capsule sectioned, the medial collateral ligament stripped from the tibia, and occasionally the semimembranosus tendon lengthened. After each of these steps, alignment should be checked and only those releases performed that are necessary to obtain limb alignment.

The steps for correction of valgus deformity include lateral retinacular release, section of the iliotibial band, release of the lateral collateral ligament and popliteus tendon from the femur, posterolateral capsular section, and lengthening of the biceps tendon. Again only those steps necessary to correct alignment are carried out.

Correction of flexion contracture may include soft tissue release, bone resection, and occasionally quadriceps reefing for restoration of quadriceps length where significant bone has been resected. When possible, preservation of the posterior cruciate ligament is desirable.

Tibial or femoral bone loss may be managed by use of cement with or without reinforcement, bone grafting, or custom prostheses. Close attention should be given to cement technique to improve interdigitation with cancellous bone, minimize laminations, and avoid contamination.

In general, patellar resurfacing should be carried out in all rheumatoid arthritic patients but may be applied selectively in the osteoarthritic patient depending on the patellar cartilage status. No more than 1 cm of bone should be resected. At least 1 cm of patella should remain to minimize the risk of fracture. The combined prosthesis and remaining patella should be of normal height. When necessary, an oblique lateral retinacular release will permit patellar realignment with minimal sacrifice to the patellar blood supply.

CLINICAL RESULTS

With close attention to detail and proper patient selection, resurfacing implants including the total condylar, duopatellar, PC retaining kinematic, Townley, posterior stabilized total condylar, PCA, Eftekar, and variable axis. All give about 85% good or satisfactory results with 2 years and longer follow-up. This rivals or exceeds current results with total hip replacement. Constrained implants, including the spherocentric, rotating hinge and total condylar III, are less satisfactory and provide 2 years or longer satisfactory results, from 65% to 93%. However, the overall results tend to deteriorate with time.[12,13,23,31]

SUMMARY

1. Total knee replacement is a powerful but complex surgical procedure.
2. Recognizing and addressing all planes of motion at the knee is mandatory for good results.
3. Accurate alignment of the prosthetic component and the limb is crucial.
4. Close attention to surgical detail and prosthetic interaction is necessary.
5. Current prosthetic replacement fails to return the bone to its normal strain environment.
6. Clinical results with current resurfacing components rival or exceed those obtained with conventional total hip replacement in properly selected patients.

ACKNOWLEDGEMENT

We would like to thank Dr. William Capello for his constructive editorial comments and our secretary, Charlotte Kerkhoff, for her cheerful attitude during preparation.

REFERENCES

1. Abarotin, V.A.: In vitro measurement of forces in prosthetic knees, master's thesis, Lafayette, Indiana, 1984, Purdue University.
2. Andriacchi, T.P., Galante, J.O., and Fermier, R.W.: The influence of total knee-replacement design on walking and stair-climbing, J. Bone Joint Surg. **64A**(9):1328-1335, 1982.
3. Bargren, J.H., Blaha, J.D., and Freeman, M.A.R.: Alignment in total knee arthroplasty: Correlated biomechanical and clinical observations, Clin. Orthop. **173**:178-233, 1983.
4. Bargren, J.H., Day, W.H., Freeman, M.A.R., and Swanson, S.A.V.: Mechanical tests on the tibial components of non-hinged knee prostheses, J. Bone Joint Surg., **60B**(2):256-261, 1978.
5. Bartel, D.L., Bicknell, V.L., and Wright, T.M.: Analysis of stresses causing surface damage in metal-backed plastic components for total knee replacement, Transactions of the thirtieth annual meeting of the Orthopaedic Research Society, vol. 9, 1984.
6. Bartel, D.L., Burstein, A.H., Santavicca, E.A., and Insall, J.N.: Performance of the tibial component in total knee replacement, J. Bone Joint Surg. **64A**(7):1026-1033, 1982.
7. Buchanan, J.R., Bowman, L.S., Shearer, A., Gallaher, B.A., and Greer III, R.B.: Clinical evaluation of the variable axis total knee replacement, Final program, forty-ninth annual meeting of the American Academy of Orthopaedic Surgeons, Jan. 21-26, 1982.
8. Chao, E.Y.S., and Sim, F.H.: Tumor prosthesis design: A system approach. In Chao, E.Y.S., and Ivins, J.C., editors: Tumor prostheses for bone and joint reconstruction, New York, 1983, Thieme-Strotton, Inc.
9. Connelly, G.M., Rimnac, C.M., Wright, T.M., Hertzberg, R.W., and Manson, J.A.: Fatigue crack propagation behavior of ultrahigh molecular weight polyethylene, J. Orthop. Res. **2**(2):119-125, 1984.
10. Draganich, L.F., Anderson, G.B.J., Andriacchi, T.P., and Galante, J.O.: The influence of the cruciate ligaments on femoral-tibial contact movement during knee flexion, Transactions of the thirtieth annual meeting of the Orthopaedic Research Society, vol. 9, 1984.
11. Ducheyne, P., Kagan II, A., and Lacey, J.A.: Failure of total knee arthroplasty due to loosening and deformation of the tibial component, J. Bone Joint Surg. **60A**(3):384-391, 1978.
12. Eftekhar, N.S.: Total knee-replacement arthroplasty, J. Bone Joint Surg. **65A**(3):293-309, 1983.
13. Ewald, F.C., Jacobs, M.A., Miegel, R.E., Walker, P.S., Poss, R., and Sledge, C.B.: Kinematic total knee replacement, J. Bone Joint Surg. **66A**(7):1032-1040, 1984.
14. Goldberg, V.M., and Henderson, B.T.: The Freeman-Swanson ICLH total knee arthroplasty, J. Bone Joint Surg. **62A**(8):1338-1344, 1980.
15. Goldstein, S.A., Wilson, D.L., Sonstegard, D.A., and Matthews, L.S.: The mechanical properties of human tibial trabecular bone as a function of metaphyseal location, J. Biomech. **16**:965-969, 1983.
16. Grood, E.S., and Suntay, W.J.: A joint coordinate system for the clinical description of three-dimensional motions: Application to the knee, J. Biomech. Eng. **105**:136-144, 1983.
17. Heck, D.A., Chao, E.Y., and Kelly, P.J.: The biomechanical performance of a conical coupling in porous-coated modular prosthesis design, Transactions of the thirtieth annual meeting of the Orthopaedic Research Society, vol. 9, 1984.
18. Heck, D.A., Nakajima, I., Chao, E.Y., and Kelly, P.J.: The effect of immolization on biologic ingrowth into porous titanium fibermetal prostheses, Transactions of the thirtieth annual meeting of the Orthopaedic Research Society, vol. 9, 1984.
19. Hedley, A.K., Clarke, I.C., Cozinn, S.C., Coster, I., Gruen, T., and Amstutz, H.C.: Porous ingrowth fixation of the femoral component in a canine surface replacement of the hip, Clin. Orthop. **163**:300-311, 1982.
20. Kettelkamp, D.A.: Personal communication, March 1985.
21. King, T.V., and Scott, R.D.: Femoral component loosening in total knee arthroplasty, Clin. Orthop. **194**:285-290, 1985.
22. Knee Replacement Surgery, American Academy of Orthopaedic Surgeons continuing education course, Chairman S. Ranawat, New York, N.Y., Nov. 5-7, 1984.
23. Knets, I.C., Kalnberz, V.K., Yanson, K.A., and Saulgozis, J.Z.: Material for making bone endoprosthesis and endoprosthesis of said material. Patent specification filed with patent office, London, Sept. 16, 1976.

24. LaFortune, M.A.: The use of intra-cortical pins to measure the motion of the knee joint during walking, doctoral dissertation, University Park, Pa., 1984, Pennsylvania State University.

25. Laubenthal, K.N., Smidt, G.L., and Kettelkamp, D.B.: A quantitative analysis of knee motion during activities of daily living, Phys. Ther. **52:**32-42, 1972.

26. Lew, W.D., and Lewis, J.L.: The effect of knee-prosthesis geometry on cruciate ligament mechanics during flexion, J. Bone Joint Surg. **64A**(5):734-739, 1982.

27. Lewis, J.L., Askew, M.J., and Jaycos, D.P.: A comparative evaluation of tibial component designs of total knee prosthesis, J. Bone Joint Surg. **64A**(1):129-135, 1982.

28. Lotke, P.A., and Ecker, M.L.: Influence of positioning of prosthesis in total knee replacement, J. Bone Joint Surg. **59A:**77-79, 1977.

29. Mooz, A.: Mechanical properties of a surgical grade titanium alloy, master's thesis, Toronto, Ontario, 1980, University of Toronto.

30. Mjoberg, B., Pettersson, H., Rosenqvist, R., and Rydholm, A.: Bone cement: Thermal injury and the radiolucent zone, Acta Orthop. Scand. **55:**597-600, 1984.

31. Murray, D.G., and Webster, D.A.: The variable-axis knee prosthesis, J. Bone Joint Surg. **63A**(5):687-693, 1981.

32. Murrish, D.E.: Finite element analysis of the tibia with and without knee prostheses, master's thesis, Lafayette, Indiana, 1984, Purdue University.

33. Murrish, E.E., Hillbery, B.M., and Heck, D.A.: Strain distribution in the proximal tibia with and without tibial prostheses: A fem study, Transactions of the thirty-first annual meeting of the Orthopaedic Research Society, **10:**122, Jan. 21-24, 1985.

34. Parsons, J.R., Alexander, H., and Weiss, A.B.: Absorbable polymer—filamentous carbon composites: A new concept in orthopaedic biomaterials. In Szycher, M., editor: Biocompatible polymers, metals, and composites, Lancaster, Pa., 1983, Technomic Publishing Co., Inc.

35. Rand, J.A., and Coventry, M.B.: Stress fractures after total knee arthroplasty, J. Bone Joint Surg. **62A**(2):226-233, 1980.

36. Schaff, J.A.: Stability tests and clinical correlation of laboratory tested knee prostheses, master's thesis, Lafayette, Indiana, 1983, Purdue University.

37. Sledge, C.B., and Walker, P.S.: Total knee replacement in rheumatoid arthritis. In Insall, J.N., editor: Surgery of the knee, New York, 1984, Churchill Livingstone, Inc.

38. Soudry, M.J., Walker, P.S., Reilly, D., and Sledge, C.B.: Interface forces of tibial component: The effect of PCL sacrifice and conformity. Transactions of the twenty-ninth annual meeting of the Orthopaedic Research Society, vol. 8, 1983.

Chapter 29

Total knee arthroplasty: technical planning and surgical aspects

KENNETH A. KRACKOW

This chapter addresses details of the technical aspects of total knee arthroplasty, including preoperative planning and intraoperative execution. The material is presented without strong reference to particular prostheses or instrumentation systems. The points covered represent factors—some of which are certainly very obvious, some of which may not be so—that are important to the successful performance of total knee arthroplasty.

PREOPERATIVE PLANNING
Basic technical goals

The technical, as contrasted with clinical, goals of total knee arthroplasty involve several basic factors: (1) accurate prosthetic seating on optimal quality bone, especially in cases of press-fit, uncemented arthroplasties, (2) proper axial alignment, (3) adequate ligament balance throughout the range of motion, and (4) maximum range of motion. At the same time the surgeon must respect tissue via careful handling, while still achieving adequate exposure for high-quality cementing techniques and clearing of extraneous cement.

Assessment of difficulty

The relative difficulty of an individual case should be determined early in the preoperative phase. Factors that relate heavily to this consideration are: (1) the patient's preoperative range of motion, (2) the degree of deformity, (3) the nature of that deformity, (4) the amount of bone loss present, and (5) the general bone quality.

Preoperative motion, especially limited flexion, can pose major technical difficulties. This is more obvious in cases of failed fusion and suspected ankylosis than in such cases as shown in Fig. 29-1. Removal of osteophytes, as well as mobilization of collateral and posterior capsular-ligamentous structures, is usually required in such cases and can be technically very challenging.

Major preoperative deformity increases the surgical difficulty of a given case. Such situations necessitate complex ligament balancing techniques and also may present special problems with bone loss and primary bone deformity (Fig. 29-2). The basic principles of deformity management are addressed later in this chapter.

Bone quality deserves some preliminary attention. Hard, sclerotic bone may present some difficulties for accurate, effective bone sawing techniques. However, extreme osteoporosis is likely to pose even more significant problems. Heavy bone instruments of a total knee instrumentation system have to be handled extremely carefully to avoid turning a *primary* total knee arthroplasty into something that looks more like a *revision* as a result of inadvertent bone damage.

The surgeon is especially cautioned regarding the occurrence of asymmetric bone density seen with long-standing severe varus or valgus deformity (Fig. 29-2). On the lateral side in the case of varus or the medial side of a valgus knee, the surgeon may find pathologically soft bone that requires special attention. Also, any soft tissue reattachment to bone may be complicated by such osteoporosis.

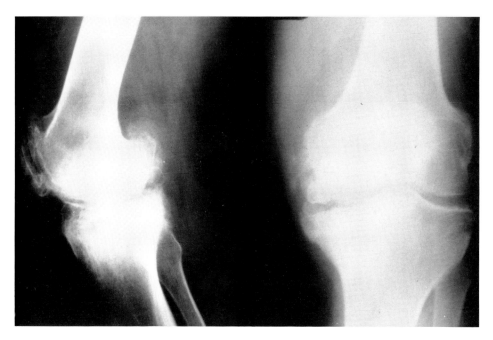

Fig. 29-1. Lateral and AP radiographs of a patient with inability to flex the knee beyond 40 degrees. Interlocking osteophytes at the posterior margins of the femur and tibia necessitated a posteromedial exposure for their removal before the knee could be flexed beyond 45 degrees.

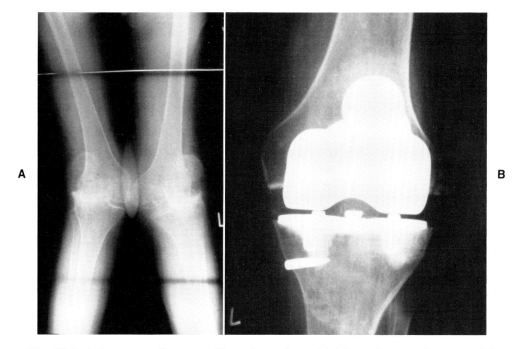

Fig. 29-2. A, Long-standing x-ray films of a patient with bilateral genu valgum. Medial soft tissues have stretched so that the medial joint spaces gap open with weight bearing. Close inspection indicates relative osteoporosis medially with normal to slightly sclerotic bone laterally. **B,** Short postoperative AP x-ray film shows horizontal joint line and staple used to reattach medial capsular ligamentous structures after concurrent medial ligamentous reconstruction.

Continued.

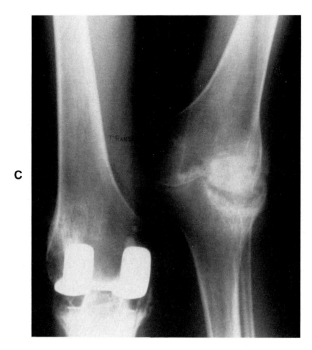

C

Fig. 29-2, cont'd. C, AP view of left knee shows major valgus deformity. The level of the joint line and the magnified size of the knee suggest a flexion contracture. There is major bone loss at the lateral tibial plateau.

Selection of prosthesis

Even without considerations of cement vs. uncemented arthroplasty techniques, prosthesis selection involves several general choices in terms of prosthetic constraint, prosthetic replacement for bone loss, and prosthesis size. The issue of appropriate prosthesis constraint can be a very lengthy topic in which such factors as patient age, deformity, and surgeon's expertise weigh heavily. Minimal constraint with maximal reliance on natural or reconstructed soft tissue stabilizers is preferred, and the overwhelming majority of cases can be managed satisfactorily with minimally constrained, even posterior cruciate–sparing condylar-type, implants.

In cases of major, especially asymmetric, bone loss, custom implants, metal wedges, and bone grafting techniques are available. To determine proper prosthetic size, manufacturers' templates and specific x-ray film magnification determinations may be used. Determination of the x-ray tube-to-knee distance and tube-to-film distance for both AP and lateral x-ray films provides ratios that allow the surgeon to obtain the true dimen-

sions of the knee outline from the magnified appearance on the finished x-ray film.

$$\frac{\text{Tube to knee distance}}{\text{Tube to film distance}} = \frac{\text{Actual size}}{\text{X-ray film size}}$$

ALIGNMENT AND INSTRUMENTATION

The following discussion, dealing with axial alignment, rotational alignment, and instrumentation, addresses points that must be understood at the preoperative phase. These are general considerations that are relevant to all cases as opposed to preoperative planning considerations for an individual case.

Axial alignment

The past 10 to 12 years of experience with total knee arthroplasty have shown that poor axial alignment represents one of the most significant factors in premature loosening. There is little disagreement on surgeons' basic goals for proper alignment that are summarized in these two considerations:

1. The prosthetic knee joint should be centered on the mechanical axis of the lower extremity
2. There should be "proper" orientation of the joint line

Diagrams in Fig. 29-3 depict a knee joint centered on the mechanical axis, the mechanical axis being defined as a line connecting the center of the femoral head to the center of the ankle. The condition of the knee being centered in this manner is independent of the position of the entire lower extremity in space, under the assumption that the knee is extended. That is, a knee properly centered remains so whether the extremity is relatively adducted or relatively abducted.

The second condition of proper orientation of the joint line is a generally accepted goal; however, what constitutes "proper" may not be universally defined. Surgeons speak of a joint line that is parallel to the ground, perpendicular to the "vertical," perpendicular to the joint reaction force, or perpendicular to the mechanical axis. These are not all equivalent states.

Although the condition of the prosthesis as being *centered* on the mechanical axis is invariant, not depending on the relative position of the lower extremity in space, the orientation of the joint line *does* depend on the extremity's position in space. As the lower extremity, extended at the

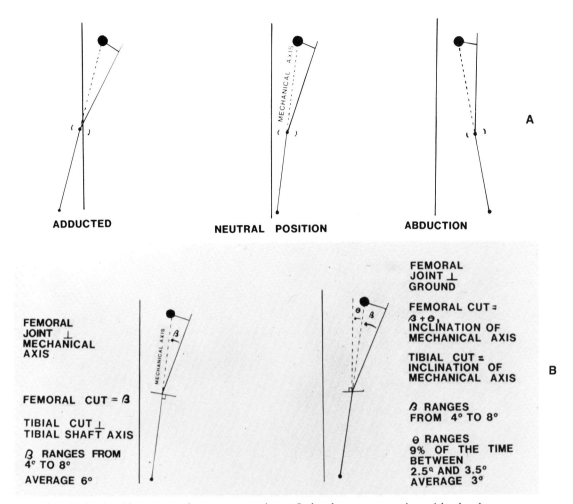

ADDUCTED   **NEUTRAL POSITION**   **ABDUCTION**

A

FEMORAL
JOINT ⊥
MECHANICAL
AXIS

FEMORAL CUT = β

TIBIAL CUT ⊥
TIBIAL SHAFT AXIS

β RANGES FROM
4° TO 8°

AVERAGE 6°

FEMORAL
JOINT ⊥
GROUND

FEMORAL CUT =
β + θ,
INCLINATION OF
MECHANICAL AXIS

TIBIAL CUT =
INCLINATION OF
MECHANICAL AXIS

β RANGES
FROM 4° TO 8°

θ RANGES
9% OF THE TIME
BETWEEN
2.5° AND 3.5°
AVERAGE 3°

B

Fig. 29-3. A, Diagrammatic representation of the lower extremity with the knee centered on the mechanical axis. Although this condition holds as the extremity is moved from adduction to abduction at the hip, the orientation of the joint line with respect to the ground changes with this movement. **B,** Diagrammatic representation of two different alignment setups. *Left,* Knee centered on the mechanical axis with the prosthetic joint line perpendicular to the mechanical axis. *Right,* Knee centered on the mechanical axis; the joint line is parallel to the ground with the ankle positioned adjacent to the midline as it would be during gait.

knee, is moved from a position of adduction to abduction, the joint line rotates relative to the ground. For this reason the relationship of the joint line to the ground requires some specification as to the relative position of the lower extremity at the time this alignment is being judged.

Essentially two joint-line orientation schemes are in current vogue. The overall differences between them are minimal; however, for the sake of clearer understanding and terminology, an analysis follows.

The first and most traditional joint orientation is one in which the joint line is perpendicular to the mechanical axis (Fig. 29-3). Here the tibial cut is perpendicular to the tibial shaft axis, and the femoral cut is made at a valgus angle β, typically between 5 and 8 degrees, where β represents the actual angle between the femoral shaft axis and the femoral portion of the mechanical axis, that is, a line from the center of the femoral head to the center of the knee. The proper angle of the distal femoral cut is not fixed absolutely but depends on the structure of the femur itself. However, it is usually quite close to 6 degrees.

A second scheme that has assumed significant popularity could be described as the "anatomic" joint-line orientation where the joint line is not perpendicular to the tibial shaft axis but is actually, or closer to, perpendicular to the vertical (parallel to the ground) during gait (Fig. 29-3). During normal gait the foot strikes the ground adjacent to a center line near the midpoint of the body. As a result the mechanical axis from the femoral head to the ankle has an inward inclination, θ (between 1.5 and 3.5 degrees). In order for the joint line to be parallel to the ground (perpendicular to the vertical) during gait, its relationship to the tibial shaft axis must be different from perpendicular by the small angle, θ. Furthermore, its relationship to the femoral shaft must be at a greater "valgus" angle by the amount of the angle, θ, also. Therefore, in this second joint-line orientation scheme the femoral cut is made at $\beta + \theta$ or approximately 7 to 11 degrees valgus, and the tibial cut is made at θ or approximately 1 degree to 3 degrees varus.

The resulting tibiofemoral angle in both schemes is β, approximately 6 degrees, and the orientation of the joint line is either perpendicular to the mechanical axis in the first case or approximately parallel to the ground during gait in the second.

Rotational alignment

Several points are important to establish proper prosthetic rotational alignment. Beyond a thorough knowledge of the anatomic landmarks that are useful for reestablishing alignment, it is appropriate to recognize the limitations of correcting preexisting malrotation. To a large extent total knee arthroplasty involves modification of bone and joint surfaces within or between most of the major soft tissue attachments spanning the distal femur and proximal tibia. Significant rotational malalignment, which exists after appropriate soft tissue releases and bone excision for the distal femur and proximal tibia, cannot be totally corrected by placing (typically) the tibial component in strictly normal anatomic position. For example, the patient with persistent external tibial rotation of 20 degrees cannot effectively be

"derotated" simply by turning the tibial component into 20 degrees of external rotation with respect to the femur (that is, normal rotation with respect to the tibia) and hoping that the joint surfaces will then track normally. A minimally constrained prosthesis so implanted will simply tend to rotate outward at the tibia, a situation that may even invite subluxation. The surgeon would rather err on the side of correcting such a deformity than of accentuating it; therefore in this example the tibial component would be placed perhaps 5 to 10 degrees toward the proper anatomic orientation. However, the full 20-degree correction may lead to problems. Certainly the surgeon must not err in the opposite direction.

The point to appreciate is that "anatomic" landmarks of rotation must be assessed in terms of patient rotation immediately before surgery and in terms of positions achievable after bone cutting and soft tissue releases. At this stage, however, persisting malrotation may need to be accepted to some extent; the positions of normal rotational landmarks have to be appreciated in the context of the case at hand in addition to "textbook normal standards."

Femur

Several anatomic references available in assessing femoral component rotation are available. When relatively minimal or symmetric degeneration is present, gross inspection at the end of the femur will reveal proper alignment. Beyond this the anatomic references available are the axis (medial to lateral) formed by the posterior femoral condyles, the axis formed by the medial and lateral femoral epicondyles, and the position and appearance of the trochlear groove (Fig. 29-4).

The primary reference for femoral component position usually can be taken as the axis of the posterior femoral condyles, even if slight dif-

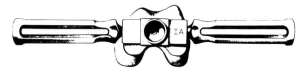

Fig. 29-4. Diagrammatic end-on view of a distal femur. A total knee instrument has been aligned parallel to the imaginary axis formed by the posterior femoral condyles.

ferential wear of one condyle necessitates some "eyeball" correction. This axis actually defines neutral femoral rotation, and the anterior and posterior cuts are made parallel to this line.

The axis of the femoral epicondyles may be used as a secondary rotational reference, keeping in mind that this axis is approximately 10 degrees rotated with respect to neutral—the medial epicondyle being more anterior than the lateral.

Although proper femoral rotation is most important for the positioning of the anterior and posterior femoral cuts, it is also fairly important in performing the distal femoral cut, because this cut is not perpendicular to the femoral shaft axis.

Tibia

The importance of establishing proper rotation may be viewed as it impacts on setting up and performing bone cuts and as it relates to rotational placement of the tibial component. In the alignment scheme where the tibial cut is made perpendicular to the tibia shaft axis, alterations of rotation will not affect anything at the time of bone resection, but only at the time of the component orientation. If the tibia is to be cut in slight inclination to yield a joint line parallel to the ground during gait, then the "setup" for this cut needs to be done with the tibia in neutral rotation.

The anatomic landmarks available for establishing tibial rotation include the tibial tubercle, the intermalleolar axis, the appearance of the top of the tibial surface, and the axis defined roughly by the posterior cortical margins of the tibia at the joint line. Assessment of the relative positions of each of these anatomic aspects with regard to "textbook normal" and to the preexisting position for a given patient is very important.

Tibial tubercle position that is anatomically lateral to the midline may be quite variable. The intermalleolar axis is typically at a position of 25 degrees to 30 degrees external rotation *with the knee in extension,* and the axis of the posterior margin of the tibia is at neutral to slightly internally rotated, that is, farther posterior on the medial side compared to the lateral.

Alignment pitfalls

The surgeon must be aware of several pitfalls and avoid them. Some relate to features of anatomy and deformity, whereas others relate to individual instrumentation systems.

In patients with major varus or valgus deformity, such deformity persists when the knee is flexed, causing a corresponding rotation of the femur when the tibia is held "vertical" during the surgical exposure. Fig. 29-5 shows how a varus knee brought into flexion undergoes internal rotation at the femur as the tibia is brought to a vertical orientation. The opposite is seen in some valgus cases where the femur externally rotates. This is an observation that I have neither read of nor heard in an oral presentation but that is nevertheless quite real and consistent. The rotation of the femur becomes apparent only if close attention is given to anatomic indicators of rotation—namely, the posterior femoral condyles. The importance of this observation is that the surgeon must align the instruments accurately to the anatomy of the femur and not according to the operating room table or to the "horizon."

On the tibial side, in addition to appreciating individual variations of preexisting rotation and rotational landmarks, it is important to be aware of changes in tibial rotation that can accompany knee flexion. These changes are of two types. In many knees the well-known screw-home rotation persists even after removal of joint surfaces and cruciate ligaments. In these cases the tibia passively rotates internally as the knee is flexed to 90 degrees or more. In other cases, however, the tibia may be seen to rotate externally with flexion caused by a tethering effect imparted by the everted patella and tight extensor mechanism. For these reasons it may be safest to establish "neutral" tibial rotation while the knee is in extension or to establish it relative to a bony landmark or axis whose position has been first checked with the knee in extension.

Axial alignment pitfalls generally relate to individual characteristics of knee instrumentation systems. Short intramedullary femoral rods offer obvious sources of error. Extramedullary femoral shaft pins can present problems of parallax error and problems in the presence of bowed femurs. Alignment relative to the femoral head also invites uncertainty, since the position of that structure under the drapes and deep within the body is not directly known.

Simple trigonometry reveals that 1 inch of error in the positioning of a femoral indicating rod at the level of the hip introduces a 3 to 4 degree varus/valgus error—an amount that may certainly prove significant.

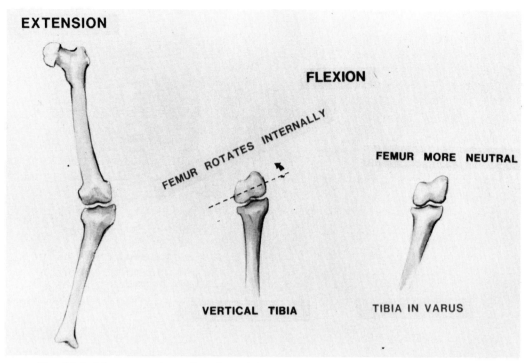

EXTENSION

FLEXION

FEMUR ROTATES INTERNALLY

FEMUR MORE NEUTRAL

VERTICAL TIBIA

TIBIA IN VARUS

Fig. 29-5. Diagrammatic explanation of femoral rotational artifact seen in varus knee deformities. The varus deformity persists in flexion and leads to internal rotation of the femur if the tibia is positioned vertically.

On the tibial side, the surgeon must be alert for bowing of the tibia in both the frontal and sagittal planes. For this reason it is probably safest to align according to the overall tibial shaft axis, that is, the imaginary line connecting the center of the knee to the center of the ankle.

INSTRUMENTATION

Whatever knee prosthesis and accompanying instrumentation system may be chosen, it is absolutely essential that the surgeon understand the alignment assumptions inherent in that instrumentation and the landmarks that will be used in trying to follow these assumptions. It is important to understand the joint-line orientation sought and the femoral alignment reference(s) to be used, that is, the femoral shaft or femoral head. In the case of the femoral shaft whether the surgeon will be aligning with the entire axis of the femur or just the distal aspect must be known.

For these reasons when tibial alignment is considered, it may be best to use the entire tibial shaft axis and assess the instrumentation in these terms.

Femoral component positioning

It is next important to appreciate how the instrumentation will guide femoral component positioning other than its varus/valgus orientation, that is, how the relative anteroposterior and medial/lateral positions of the component are to be determined.

Instrumentation systems characteristically have used three approaches for this positioning. Many systems such as those used for some total condylar type prostheses have relied on the position of a drill hole in the intercondylar region. This is generally placed in relationship to the position of the origin of the posterior cruciate ligament or the general appearance of the intercondylar notch. There are other instrumentation systems that key from the anterior femoral cortex.

The third anteroposterior alignment reference is the level of the posterior femoral condyles.

Whichever reference technique is used to determine anteroposterior position of the femoral component, a worthy goal is to place the new femoral component in proper relationship to the ligament attachments on the femur. In this way proper ligament balance in flexion and extension and a proper kinematic pattern of motion can be achieved.

Flexion-extension ligament balance

Intimately related to femoral component positioning is the question of flexion-extension ligament balance. It is absolutely essential to understand how the instrumentation system seeks to lead to proper ligament balance in a flexion vs. extension sense.

Early knee systems, especially the geometric technique, did not address this question as explicitly as more recent instrumentation. Currently, the most common way of achieving flexion-extension ligament balance is to attempt to create equal bone gaps in flexion and extension. Generally, a gap is created with the knee in 90 degrees of flexion between the posterior femoral cut and the proximal tibial transverse cut. The knee is brought into full extension, and the distal femur is resected so that the gap in extension matches that in flexion. A second approach gaining some popularity today is introduced by the Universal Knee Instrument System, wherein specifically measured thicknesses of posterior and distal femur are removed because they will be replaced by appropriately matching thicknesses of femoral component. Following this, a minimum thickness of tibial bone is removed to allow seating of the tibial component, and the thickness of the tibial prosthesis is selected that provides proper extension with appropriate collateral ligament balance.

To use either approach safely, flexion contracture should be released before the performance of definitive bone cuts; furthermore, proper collateral ligament balance should be achieved preliminarily. If these have been achieved and either of these techniques has been used properly, then they are nearly identical.

The only major difference is a subtle but complicated point concerning proper relative ligament tension in flexion allowing the natural screw-home internal and external rotation.

Whichever approach is used, the surgeon must be mindful of sources of error. One of the most obvious errors with the standard approach of matching flexion-extension gaps is where the flexion gap has been positioned too far posteriorly. This situation can occur with too "thin" a resection of the posterior femoral condyles or too deep a resection of the proximal tibia. When the knee is brought into extension, the surgeon may find that excessive room already exists in the extension gap before removing any distal femoral bone.

Alternatively, if the flexion gap is made to lie too anteriorly, complex forms of instability may result, with relative instability in gentle or complete flexion.

INTRAOPERATIVE CONSIDERATIONS

Details of careful surgical technique, proper tissue handling, hemostasis, and adequacy of surgical exposure are of great importance. In addition, total knee arthroplasty presents nearly unique challenges in terms of bone-saw technique and in the smooth placement and removal of the instrumentation system. These features of the operative procedure are, however, beyond the planned scope of this chapter.

MANAGEMENT OF DEFORMITY

Cases of major deformity generally involve significant soft tissue imbalance. If this were not the case, then the deformity would be passively correctable to normal alignment.

The soft tissue imbalance can be viewed as a relative tightness of soft tissue on the concave side of the deformity, whereas a relative excess or surplus of soft tissue exists on the convex side. In the case of varus deformity, the medial aspect of the knee represents the tight, concave side, whereas the lateral aspect represents the excess, loose convex side. The opposite is the case for valgus deformity.

It should be appreciated that soft tissue balance in these situations is a problem that is largely independent of bone cutting. The distal femoral and proximal tibial cuts do, however, provide the axial orientation of the femoral and tibial components respectively and thus define the overall axial alignment at the knee once ligament balance has been achieved. If the joint line is to be oriented perpendicular to the mechanical axis, then the tibial cut must be made perpendicular to the shaft of the tibia. The surgeon cannot cut a "little bit more" from the medial compartment in the case of varus to allow fitting the prosthesis, because this will cause the joint line to be tilted on the medial side and the varus deformity will persist. Although the orientation of the cuts is fixed, what the surgeon *can* alter is the relative depth of the cuts.

Second, although any fixed deformity conceivably can be passively corrected by making cuts sufficiently deep (that is, removing enough bone to allow passive correction of the deformity), this type of bone cutting per se does not address the soft tissue imbalance that exists as a separate problem. In many cases of severe deformity soft tissue imbalance will need to be addressed separately and specifically. Balance may be accomplished by (1) releasing the tight side of the deformity, (2) tightening the loose side, (3) accepting some residual soft tissue imbalance, or (4) a combination of any of these.

In dealing with severe deformity the surgeon at the outset has two basic choices. A highly constrained implant may be used, thereby ignoring the consideration of soft tissue balance. Alternatively, whatever reconstruction and soft tissue balance are necessary may be undertaken to implant a relatively unconstrained prosthesis. This second alternative has been my approach in total knee replacement in all but the most unusual of cases. More than 99% of cases are done with a minimally constrained prosthesis, and these cases have included as much as 75 degrees of flexion contracture, postoperative fusions, ankylosis, 30 degrees of varus deformity, 45 degrees of recurvatum, and 65 degrees of valgus deformity. (These limitations do not necessarily represent the maximal extremes amenable to reconstruction, but are rather approximately the extremes encountered to date.)

Flexion contracture

Flexion contracture is a very complicated problem to manage at surgery and, as such, adequate consideration should be given to conservative management preoperatively. Maximal physical therapy, as well as serial casting and bracing, can be considered. In addition, posterior surgical release as a preliminary procedure can be considered in a few select patients.

With persistent flexion deformity, up to 4 mm of distal femoral bone are removed at the beginning of the procedure. Next, it is appropriate, in many cases, to resect what appears to be an anterior tibial osteophyte or an intercondylar tibial prominence.

After the posterior femoral condyles have been resected, and perhaps the proximal tibial plateaus removed, the posterior capsule is divided carefully and, if necessary, the gastrocnemius attach-

ments are elevated from the back of the femur. At this point if full extension with components in place is still not possible, then additional bone resection is contemplated.

Postoperative serial casting can be considered if significant flexion deformity persists and may be expected to be more successful than preoperative casting since the degenerated painful joint surfaces have been removed.

Postoperative splinting of the flexion contracture patient during the first 4 to 7 days after surgery is quite important and is preferred routinely. Continuous passive motion (CPM) is not recommended—at least for the first 3 to 5 days.

Simple bone resection to achieve full extension for fixed flexion contracture invites major collateral instability. This is especially important to realize because the instability may not be appreciated when the knee is forced into maximal extension. Apparent collateral stability may be evident simply because of the posterior soft tissue tether that exists. While forcing maximal extension and attempting varus-valgus stressing, the knee may appear stable. However, even with a few degrees of flexion, major medial and lateral instability will be evident if the knee is observed carefully.

Varus and valgus deformities

Management of fixed varus and valgus embodies generally common principles with only a few exceptions. These principles, rather than step-by-step surgical sequence, are presented here. (See more detailed discussions such as those by Insall[2] and by Krackow and Hungerford[1] for the more specific operative maneuvers.)

The true extent of fixed deformity frequently is not ascertainable by weight bearing x-ray films *or* by the apparent passive correctability of the deformity. Bone collapse, or wear, can overstate the deformity on weight bearing x-ray films, and passive correctability says nothing regarding a stretched medial or lateral side. Rather, this true extent is demonstrated when a tension stress is placed across the joint and the relative varus/valgus position or tibiofemoral angle is recorded at the time that the medial and lateral soft tissues are both under tension.[3]

The vast majority of patients with varus or valgus deformities can be managed by surgical release of the tight, concave side of their deformity. Typically this release is performed on the medial tibial side in varus patients and on the lateral femoral side in patients with valgus deformity.

Ideally, ligament balance, that is, necessary releases, should be performed before bone cuts (distal femur and posterior tibia) so that excessive resection is avoided. That is, a tibial cut made before soft tissue release may, after that release, require an excessively thick prosthesis to fill the resulting bone gap.

Incomplete release on the concave side of the deformity leads, after proper bone resection and prosthetic implantation, to the appearance of ligamentous laxity on the opposite convex side. Attempts to treat this laxity by placement of progressively thicker tibial components either are futile or lead to the development of flexion contracture.

This resulting "convex-side" instability is really well tolerated on the lateral side of varus cases and less well tolerated on the medial side of the valgus cases.

Although a set sequence of soft tissue releases for these deformities is often prescribed, it is more important to examine each situation individually and release in sequence the tightest structures remaining.

The effectiveness of collateral release in some severe cases can be impeded by an intact posterior cruciate ligament. This tendency will be accentuated in patients whose convex side actually is stretched.

Consideration can be given to performing ligament tightening procedures on the convex side of long-standing deformities wherein this convex side has stretched significantly (Figs. 29-2 and 29-6). Similarly, ligamentous tightening can be performed successfully on severe, rigid deformities where achievement of satisfactory balance appears otherwise impossible intraoperatively (Fig. 29-6). Patients with severely overcorrected valgus high tibial osteotomies may have this deformity.

Although seemingly complex, ligamentous tightening procedures may, in fact, be less arduous than extensive release procedures. Their difficulty, however, may be compounded by the asymmetric osteoporosis mentioned earlier. Soft tissue fixation to bone in such cases, as well as others, has been improved by the introduction of a presumably original soft tissue stitch designed to minimize potential for pullout while being easy

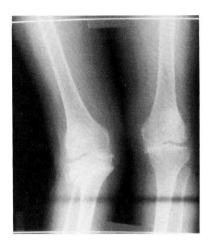

Fig. 29-6. Severe valgus deformity evident on long-standing x-ray films in a patient with malunited high tibial osteotomy of the right knee.

to place into broad flat tissues. This stitch is also relatively free of the bunching or purse-stringing effects of a Bunnell-type suture (Fig. 29-7).

Cases with severe deformity secondary to fracture, malunion, or bowing a short distance from the joint line but within the proximate one third of the affected bone, may more properly require concurrent or subsequent osteotomy to achieve proper alignment.

Postoperative management of patients with deformity undergoing only release of the "tight" side is strictly routine. For those undergoing ligamentous advancement (approximately only 5% of the cases on our service), immobilization in a hinged knee–immobilizer apparatus is employed except during physical therapy and specific exercise periods each day at home. At these times the patient exercises the knee without any external protection.

Patellar alignment

As the surgeon approaches the completion of the knee arthroplasty, it is absolutely imperative to check the tracking of the patella with placement of the trial component and after final fixation of the actual implant. If subluxation or inappropriate tightness is present, then lateral release should be performed.

If, at this stage, the surgeon is cementing a prosthesis, then typically the tourniquet has been reinflated. The surgeon must be mindful that lateral release can leave troublesome bleeders.

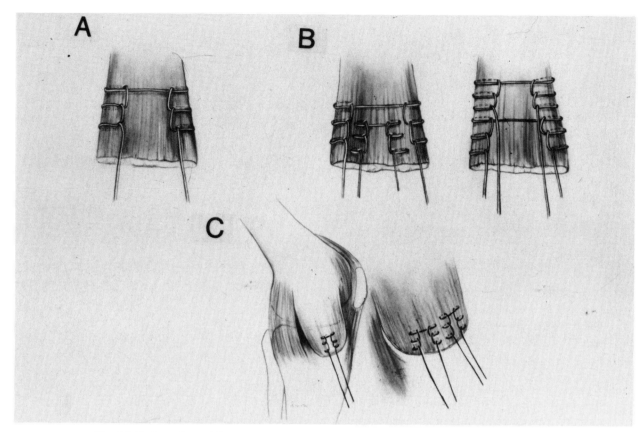

Fig. 29-7. Capsule and ligament suture used to facilitate soft tissue attachment to bone. **A,** Single suture in the ligament or patellar tendon-like material. **B,** Two forms of placement of a double suture. **C,** Placement of the suture in the medial collateral and adjacent medial capsule. The locking-loop character of the suture tightens around the longitudinal bundles of tendinous and ligamentous material resisting pullout. Furthermore, the spatial orientation of the suture is such that the purse stringing or bunching effect seen with the Bunnell type of stitch is not experienced with this technique.

In the most extreme cases, tibial tubercle transposition may need to be considered, although I have not found this necessary in even a large series.

SUMMARY

This chapter has outlined the considerations that must be made preoperatively—assessing the difficulty of the procedure at hand, intelligently selecting the prosthesis to be used, planning the patient's alignment, and understanding the instrumentation to be used.

Intraoperatively the surgeon must work with an adequate, yet careful, surgical exposure, and a safe and effective saw technique. In addition, the surgeon must understand and manage any major, fixed deformity and ensure proper patellar tracking.

REFERENCES
1. Hungerford, D.S., Krackow, K.A., and Kenna, R.V.: Total knee arthroplasty: A comprehensive approach, Baltimore, 1984, Williams & Wilkins.
2. Insall, J.N.: Surgery of the knee, New York, 1985, Churchill Livingstone, Inc.
3. Krackow, K.A.: Approaches to planning lower extremity alignment for total knee arthroplasty and osteotomy about the knee, Advances in Orthop. Surg., **7:**69-88, 1983.

Chapter 30

Resection arthroplasty: an alternative to arthrodesis for salvage of the infected total knee arthroplasty

HERBERT KAUFER

LARRY S. MATTHEWS

Deep infection, one of the most dreaded complications of total knee arthroplasty, occurs in 1% to 20% of cases.[2-7,10] In almost all cases thorough debridement and removal of all foreign bodies are a prerequisite for control of the infection. Cure of the infection with preservation of a functioning prosthesis is extremely rare.[5,9]

Although it is generally agreed that arthrodesis is the best reconstruction for control of the gross instability that follows prosthesis removal, successful bony arthrodesis following removal of an infected total knee prosthesis is difficult to achieve.[1,8] Failure of fusion has been reported in up to 80% of cases.[2,5] Furthermore, a stiff limb in full extension can be a major handicap, especially in severely disabled individuals with multiarticular arthritis who may be obliged to spend nearly all of their time either sitting or recumbent, and some patients refuse to have an arthrodesis performed.

For these reasons, we have, over the past 12 years, treated 30 infected total knee arthroplasties in 28 patients by thorough debridement and removal of the prosthesis. No formal attempt was made to achieve a bony arthrodesis.

MATERIAL AND METHOD

Nineteen marginally ambulatory patients (21 knees) with very limited ambulatory potential had their infected total knee converted to a resection arthroplasty because it was anticipated that their severe disability, caused by multiarticular arthritis, would have been increased by an arthrodesis in extension. Nine patients (nine knees) were treated with a resection arthroplasty because they refused the arthrodesis that had been recommended. Prior incision and drainage procedures combined with systemic antibiotics had failed to control systemic and local signs of sepsis in all 28 patients. Twelve patients (14 knees) had multiarticular rheumatoid arthritis, 15 had degenerative arthritis, and one had multiarticular neuropathic arthropathy. The infected prostheses were nine geometric, eight spherocentric, four geotibial retainer, three Herbert, two Marmor, one Bechtol, one Townley, one Guepar, and one Walldius.

The operation consisted of a thorough debridement of all infected tissue and removal of all foreign bodies including the prosthesis and cement, but no formal attempt was made to achieve an arthrodesis. Nineteen knees were closed over drains and 11 were packed open; three of these had redebridement on at least one occasion.

Transarticular Steinman pins were used in five knees for initial stability and were removed 2 to 4 weeks after surgery. Suture loops passed through drill holes in the distal femur and proximal tibia to approximate the bones and eliminate dead space were used in 18 knees. The sutures provided initial stability and facilitated cast application with the limb in satisfactory alignment. Seven knees had no internal fixation at the time of their resection arthroplasty.

Postoperatively, all limbs were immobilized in a long-leg plaster cast for 4 to 10 months. Precise positioning, with the tibia securely on the end of the femur and the limb aligned in 7 degrees valgus, 15 degrees flexion, and correct rotation are essential to optimize function of the resection arthroplasty. All patients received specific systemic antibiotics as indicated by sensitivity studies for at least 4 weeks or until systemic signs were absent and the wound was benign. The infecting organism was coagulase-positive *Staphylococcus aureus* in 14 knees, coagulase-negative *Staphylococcus aureus* in seven, and multiple organisms in five; no organisms were recovered in four. Systemic antibiotics used were cephalasporin alone in 15 knees, cephalasporin combined with one or more other systemic antibiotics in six knees, and other antibiotics (penicillin, ampicillin, erythromycin, vancomycin, nafcillin, and aminoglycosides) for nine knees. The duration of antibiotic treatment ranged from 2 to 40 months (average 12.75 months).

Weight bearing, as tolerated in the cast, was encouraged as soon as possible. Almost all patients were full weight bearing by the third postoperative week. When the wound had healed and sufficient stability had occurred, the cast was removed. Duration of cast support ranged from 3 to fourteen months (average 7.0 months). If necessary, after the cast was discontinued, external bracing was used.

If, after a trial of function, the resection arthroplasty proved to be unsatisfactory, then a secondary arthrodesis was performed, using a curved trochanter to malleolus intramedullary nail. Secondary arthrodesis was performed in six knees; all were successful. Successful reimplantation of a knee prosthesis was done in one case with cement containing 1½ g of cefamandole per unit of Simplex. Excellent function and stability with 80 degrees of painless motion and no recurrence of sepsis have been achieved in this case with a 20-month follow-up.

RESULTS

Systemic signs of sepsis were controlled in all patients. Twelve knees (40%) healed primarily and have remained free of drainage. Ten knees (33%) drained for 3 to 6 months (average 4.6 months), then healed, and have remained free of drainage. A total of 25 knees (83%) had no drainage at their final follow-up evaluation, and five knees (17%) continue to have small amounts of intermittent drainage at final follow-up, ranging from 2 to 7 years. All are free of signs of systemic sepsis.

Following resection arthroplasty, three patients developed a spontaneous bony ankylosis of the knee in good position. One had rheumatoid arthritis and a medial compartment Marmor arthroplasty. Arthrodesis was apparent 9 months after resection arthroplasty. Another had degenerative arthritis and a geometric prosthesis. Arthrodesis was apparent 11 months after resection arthroplasty. The third had degenerative arthritis and a Townley prosthesis. Arthrodesis was apparent 14 months after the resection arthroplasty. These three patients are all effective, functional independent walkers.

Fourteen patients with a successful resection arthroplasty (two Marmor, one Townley, five geometric, two Herbert, three spherocentric, and one Waldius) are effective functional walkers. Seven have rheumatoid arthritis, six have degenerative arthritis, and one has neuropathic arthropathy. All have a useful arc of knee motion ranging from 20 to 90 degrees (average 40 degrees). Five have sufficient stability to bear full weight with no external limb support (Fig. 30-1). Seven use a long double upright leg brace with a drop lock knee when walking, and two prefer a universal knee splint. All 14 use some hand-held walking aid; four a walker, two crutches, and eight use a single cane. Because of other involved joints or other disease, all 14 patients are severely disabled and walk very little. They spend most of their time sitting. All are convinced that their disability would have been increased by a solid arthrodesis in full extension.

Five patients (six knees), four with rheumatoid arthritis and one with degenerative arthritis (three geometric, two Herbert, one Spherocentric), cannot walk at all. Two of these patients (three knees; two geometric and one Spherocentric) could not walk at all before their prosthetic arthroplasty.

The remaining three (three knees; one geometric, two Herbert) had been severely disabled and were only marginal walkers before prosthetic arthroplasty. Because of multiarticular or associated disease (hemiplegia, cardiopulmonary in-

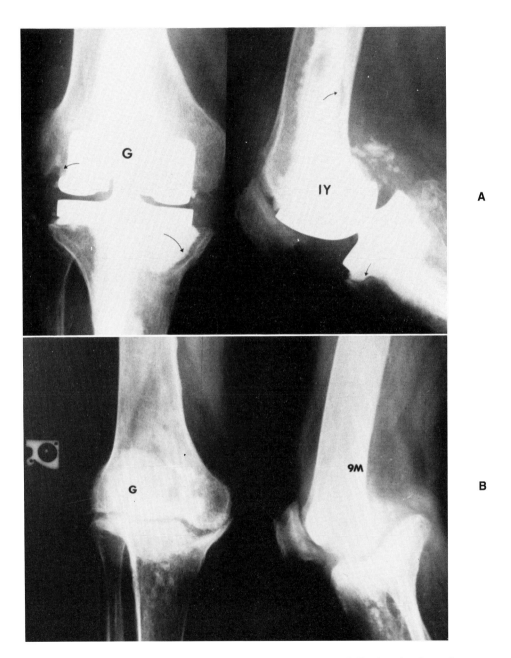

Fig. 30-1. A, Infected spherocentric knee arthroplasty 1 year following implantation. Note septic bone resorption areas *(arrows)* located along the cement-bone surface. **B,** 9 months after resection arthroplasty. The wound was closed primarily. Systemic signs of sepsis cleared rapidly, and there was no wound drainage. At 9 months the limb was free of local signs of inflammation.

Continued.

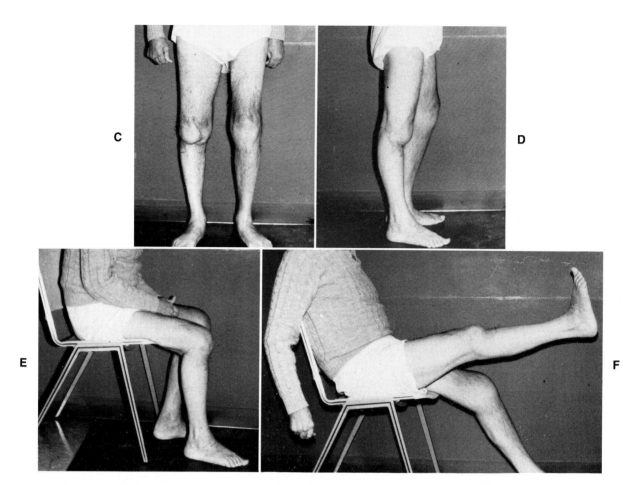

Fig. 30-1, Cont'd. C, AP view of the patient 1 year after resection arthroplasty. Although there is slight varus alignment, overall limb alignment is satisfactory. **D,** Side view of the patient at that time, bearing weight on the resection arthroplasty, shows a small amount of hyperextension. The limb, however, is sufficiently stable to bear full weight without external supports. **E,** The sitting patient demonstrating an 85-degree flexion range of the resection arthroplasty. **F,** Full active extension of the resection arthroplasty against gravity is demonstrated.

sufficiency), these patients would have been non-walkers even with a solid fusion, and their sitting comfort and function would have been impaired by a stiff knee in full extension.

Six patients, all with degenerative arthritis (one Spherocentric, one Guepar, one Waldius, one geotibial retainer, one Herbert, and one Bechtol) had their infection controlled and were free of drainage but, even with bracing, had what they considered to be unacceptable instability (Fig. 30-2). These patients had a secondary elective arthrodesis procedure performed with a trochanter to malleolus intramedullary nail 3 to 14

months after resection arthroplasty (average 10.5 months).

The secondary arthrodeses were done in limbs free of drainage and sepsis at the time of the arthrodesis, and no external immobilization was necessary. Distant bone grafts were not used. All achieved solid bony arthrodesis in good position. Five of the arthrodeses healed primarily. In one, drainage recurred, persisted for 3 months, and then cleared. All six patients that required secondary arthrodesis had relatively minor prearthroplasty disability. All six have been free of drainage for more than 1 year.

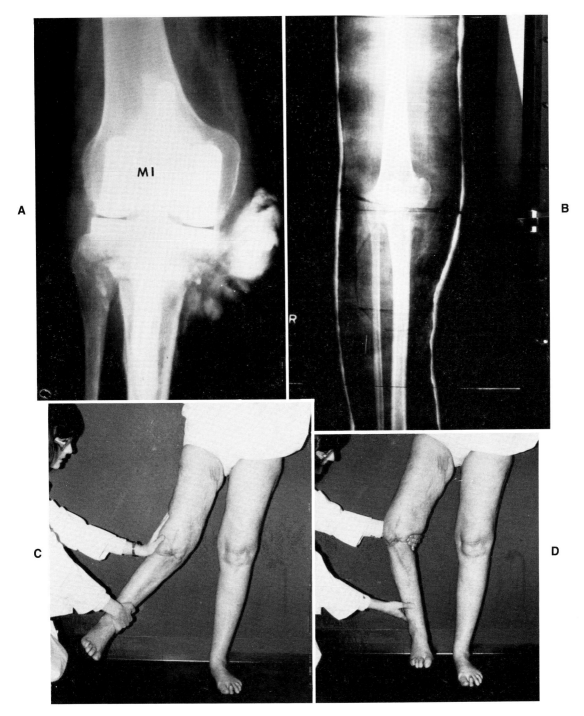

Fig. 30-2. A, Sinogram of an infected spherocentric total knee prosthesis in a patient with posttraumatic arthritis demonstrating a large soft tissue abcess cavity that communicates directly with the prosthesis. **B,** The limb in a cast immediately following resection arthroplasty demonstrates complete removal of the prosthesis and all cement. There is excellent limb alignment. **C,** The patient 1 year after resection arthroplasty. A valgus-producing strain displaces the limb into valgus. **D,** Under a varus-producing strain the limb deforms into varus. The total arc of varus-valgus motion was 45 degrees. This severe instability could not be satisfactorily controlled by a brace.

Continued.

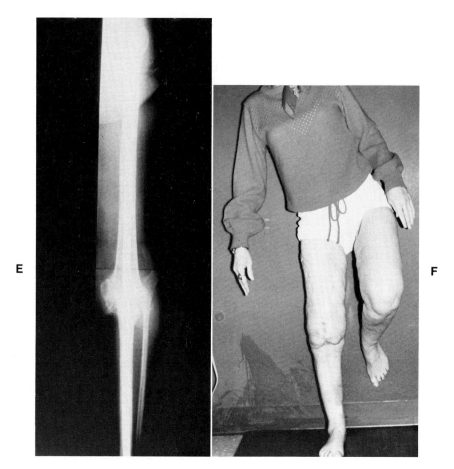

Fig. 30-2, Cont'd. E, After intramedullary arthrodesis, the limb is immediately stable in good alignment. Note the intramedullary Kuntschner nail extending from the tip of the greater trochanter to the malleolar region of the tibia. **F,** The patient 1 year following intramedullary arthrodesis demonstrates her ability to bear full weight on the limb without external support or hand assists.

Nine knees now have a solid bony arthrodesis in good position (three spontaneous, six after a second procedure). They have shortening ranging from 2 cm to 6 cm (average 4 cm). They are symptom-free, have no drainage, walk well, and are satisfied. All had relatively minimal prearthroplasty disability and had refused the arthrodesis that had been recommended initially. The six patients who had an opportunity to try the resection arthroplasty and found it unsatisfactory for their functional needs were better prepared psychologically for the arthrodesis and more satisfied with it than patients who have a successful one-stage arthrodesis procedure for salvage of an infected total knee.

DISCUSSION

Resection arthroplasty has been successful in controlling systemic sepsis in all patients and has yielded a dry limb, free of drainage, in 25 of 30 knees (83%). Neither the type of arthritis (rheumatoid, degenerative, neuropathic), nor the infecting organism, nor the type of infected prosthesis is a reliable predictor of success or failure following resection arthroplasty. All prostheses, ranging from the minimally constrained resurfacing type to the highly constrained intramedullary type (see Fig. 30-1), can be treated successfully by resection arthroplasty. At least one successful resection arthroplasty was seen with each type of prosthesis encountered in this study.

Patients with the most severe preprosthetic arthroplasty disability are most likely to be satisfied with the function of a resection arthroplasty. Of 12 such patients, eight are effective, functional, independent walkers with knee flexion-extension range from 20 to 90 degrees. Four are nonwalkers. Nine (eight walkers and one nonwalker) of the 12 patients have no drainage. Three (two nonwalkers and one walker) have persistent drainage but no systemic sepsis.

Stability of the limb is most likely to be unsatisfactory in relatively minimally disabled patients with monoarticular osteoarthritic disease. All six patients who underwent a secondary arthrodesis had osteoarthritis and relatively minimal preprosthetic arthroplasty disability. In patients such as these resection arthroplasty should be considered the first stage of a two-stage arthrodesis.

The advantages of a two-stage arthrodesis are that it permits the arthrodesis to be performed electively on a dry limb, free of sepsis, at the time of the arthrodesis procedure. The two-stage procedure also gives the patient an opportunity to experience the function of a resection arthroplasty. If it is found inadequate, the patient will be better prepared psychologically for an arthrodesis and more likely to be satisfied with it than a patient who has arthrodesis performed as a single procedure combined with prosthesis removal.

SUMMARY

1. Arthrodesis remains the procedure of choice for salvage of an infected total knee arthroplasty in patients with relatively minor preprosthetic arthroplasty disability.

2. Patients with very severe preprosthetic disability resulting from multiarticular disease or other systemic disease may be treated best by a resection arthroplasty. Systemic sepsis can be eliminated in almost all patients, and drainage can be eliminated in most.

3. Those patients who find the stability of a resection arthroplasty inadequate for their needs can have a secondary arthrodesis performed with an intramedullary rod, which yields a high probability of success. External immobilization is not necessary.

4. The advantages of a two-stage arthrodesis are that it is an elective procedure, performed in a limb free of sepsis. The patient has been psychologically prepared for the arthrodesis, and the two-stage procedure has a high probability of success.

5. Neither the underlying diagnosis, nor the infecting organism, nor the type of infected prosthesis is a reliable predictor of success or failure of either a resection arthroplasty or a second-stage arthrodesis.

REFERENCES

1. Bigliana, L.U., Rosenwasser, M.P., Caulo, N., Schink, M.M., Bassett, C., and Andrew, L.: The use of pulsing electromagnetic fields to achieve arthrodesis of the knee following failed total knee arthroplasty, J. Bone Joint Surg. **65A:**480-485, 1983.
2. Broderson, M.P., Fitzgerald, R.H., Peterson, L.F.A., Coventry, M.B., and Bryan, R.S.: Arthrodesis of the knee following failed total knee arthroplasty, J. Bone Joint Surg. **61A:**181-185, 1979.
3. Deburge, A.: GUEPAR, GUEPAR hinge prosthesis, Clin. Orthop. **120:**47-53, Oct. 1976.
4. Gristina, A.G., and Kolkin, J.: Total joint replacement and sepsis, J. Bone Joint Surg. **65A:**128-134, 1983.
5. Hagemann, W.F., Woods, G.W., and Tullos, H.S.: Arthrodesis in failed total knee replacement, J. Bone Joint Surg. **60A:**790-794, 1978.
6. Insall, J.N., Ranawat, C.S., Aglietti, P., and Shine, J.: A comparison of four models of total knee replacement prosthesis, J. Bone Joint Surg. **58A:**754-765, 1976.
7. Kaufer, H., Irvine, G., and Matthews, L.S.: Intramedullary arthrodesis of the knee, Orthop. Trans. **7**(3):547-548, 1983.
8. Phillips, H.T., and Mears, D.C.: Knee fusion with external skeletal fixation after an infected hinge prosthesis, Clin. Orthop. **151:**147-152, 1980.
9. Salibian, A.H., and Anzel, S.H.: Salvage of an infected total knee prosthesis with medial and lateral gastrocnemius muscle flaps, J. Bone Joint Surg. **65A:**681:684, 1983.
10. Salvati, E.A., Robinson, R.P., Zeno, S.M., Koslin, B.L., Brause, B.D., and Wilson, P.D., Jr.: Infection rates after 3175 total hip and total knee replacements performed with and without a horizontal unidirectional filtered air flow system, J. Bone Joint Surg. **64A:**525-535, 1982.

Chapter 31

Revision of total knee replacement

JOHN N. INSALL

CAUSES

The most common reason for revision of total knee replacement is sepsis. Most septic prostheses can be revised successfully by using a two-stage implantation technique. Although this topic is discussed in Chapter 34, the technical aspects of revising a septic prosthesis are the same as for aseptic revisions. Other causes of failure of primary arthroplasty[3,10] are component loosening, malalignment and malposition of components, subluxation, dislocation, ligament imbalance, fractures adjoining the components,[2] lack of motion, patellar subluxation, and on rare occasions unexplained pain.

Component loosening

At one time component loosening was the most frequent cause of failure,[7] but with modern designs of prostheses and improved technique this has become much less common,[6,8] and loosening rates of less than 5% after 10 years now can be expected.[5] Properly positioned bone cuts, resection of minimal tibial bone, and alignment of the knee in 5 to 10 degrees of valgus are essential.[9]

Subluxation, dislocation, and instability

The tension of the soft tissues should be attended to during the primary arthroplasty. The most frequent fault is failure to balance the collateral soft tissues in extension so that there is unequal tension, resulting in either medial or lateral instability. In cruciate-removing designs, posterior subluxation in flexion can occur if the flexion gap is too loose. Conversely, in cruciate-retaining designs, loss of flexion resulting from excessive tension in the posterior cruciate liga-

ment may occur when the flexion gap is too small or when the joint axis of the prosthesis is proximal to the original. Rotary instability is unusual and is a result of either rotary malposition of the tibial component or, occasionally, excessive tension in the iliotibial tract.

Malposition

The overall alignment of the limb may be satisfactory, but the individual components may be malpositioned. The usual combination is excessive varus of the tibial component accompanied by excessive valgus of the femoral component, which can cause patellar subluxation. Rotary malposition of the tibial component leading to lateral placement of the tibial tubercle also can cause patellar subluxation.

Patellar dislocation

Patellar dislocation can result from the causes just discussed or from imbalance of the components of the quadriceps muscle. Component revision usually is not required unless there is accompanying malposition. A proximal realignment, that is, extensive lateral release including the lower fibers of vastus lateralis with advancement of vastus medialis, usually will control dislocation. In my view a tibial tubercle transposition never should be done; it is better to reposition the tibial component to achieve the same effect. *Avulsion of the tibial tubercle* often follows tibial tubercle transposition, or it may follow retraction during the primary arthroplasty. Once avulsed, the tibial tubercle is difficult to reattach because the bone is osteoporotic and does not hold staples and screws very well.

290

Fractures adjoining the prosthetic components

Fractures adjoining the prosthetic components may, on occasion, be treated best by revision, although often it is possible to treat the fractures by traction or by open reduction and internal fixation. When a component revision is required, custom devices incorporating intramedullary rods are usually the best solution (Fig. 31-1).

Flexion contracture and loss of motion can be treated by revision of the components. Extra bone removal from the femur is required to correct the flexion contracture. Loss of motion may result from peripatellar and intraarticular adhesions or excessive tension in the posterior cruciate ligament, causing the knee to "hinge open."

Unexplained pain may be caused by latent sepsis, and sometimes removal of the components to

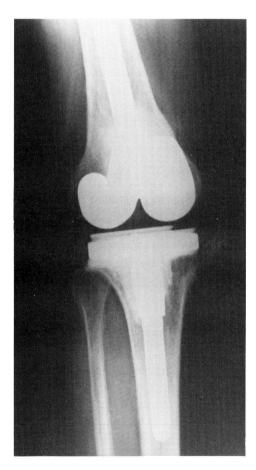

Fig. 31-1. An intramedullary rod incorporated into the femoral component may be used to transfix a supracondylar fracture adjoining a prosthesis. It is not necessary to cement the intramedullary rod into the diaphysis of the femur.

obtain cultures from the interface is the only way of diagnosis. However, when unexplained pain is present, caution is advised because the results of revision are likely to be equally unsatisfactory.

PREOPERATIVE PLANNING

The surgeon must have a clear conception of the operative aims. How is the knee to be exposed? Is it necessary to replace both components? How will the components be removed? What kind of prosthesis is needed for revision? Will a bone graft be required? Are special components required? Can the soft tissues be balanced or will a constrained prosthesis be needed? Finally, is there a possibility of sepsis, and should a two-stage procedure be done to obtain definitive tissue examination and cultures?

EXPOSURE

There will, of course, be previous scars on the knee. If these scars are longitudinal and placed more or less centrally, they can be used for revision. Unfortunately, some of the skin incisions may be placed too far medially or too far laterally to be useful for revision; therefore a new incision must be made. The patient should be made aware of the possibility of skin necrosis in such cases. Transverse skin incisions seldom cause a problem. When possible, it is best to use all or part of the previous skin incision, but the surgeon should beware of excessive undermining. If the knee possesses reasonable motion, a standard capsular incision, which also should be straight or nearly so, can be used.

Exposure in revision operations is more difficult than primary arthroplasty, and the danger of avulsing the tibial tubercle is greater, especially when preoperative flexion is restricted. To minimize the risk, the periosteal incision distally should be placed 1 cm medial to the tibial tubercle, allowing a periosteal cuff to be raised contiguous with the patellar ligament and extending distally down the tibia. This extra tissue provides some additional support and protects against patellar ligament avulsion. Reestablishment of the medial and lateral patellar gutters is helpful, and a synovectomy may aid in loosening the quadriceps expansion and in everting the patella. Medial dissection around the upper tibia beneath the superficial medial ligament allows the tibial component to be delivered anteriorly. If these measures fail to expose the knee properly, a turndown of the quadriceps tendon[1] should be done by making a second incision from the apex of the quadriceps tendon at an angle of 45 degrees into the vastus lateralis. The quadriceps tendon and the patella then are turned laterally and distally, allowing the knee to flex.

Removal of components

Removal of the components sometimes can be a difficult task, particularly if the prosthetic design has firmly fixed intramedullary stems. The principle is to remove the existing prosthesis while causing little damage to the bone stock (often easier said than done). Porous-coated prostheses, especially when used with cement, often cannot be extracted without significant bone loss. Pressurized cement techniques also increase bone loss. The best way of removing a cemented component is to separate the prosthesis from the cement, which is then removed painstakingly with sharp osteotomes in combination with a high-speed low-torque drill. Polyethylene components can be removed by cutting beneath the component with a saw to divide fixation pegs or lugs that are then removed separately. A sliding hammer with specially fabricated attachments to grasp the prosthesis has proved extremely helpful in removing metal or metal-backed components.

When revising for aseptic causes, removal of all cement particles is not as essential as for septic revision. When debris has accumulated within the joint, a synovectomy is advisable. Granulation tissue or fibrous membrane should be removed carefully from the bony surfaces. The posterior capsular recess is often obliterated and should be restored by stripping the capsule with a periosteal elevator or by sharp dissection. It is my opinion that cruciate-substituting designs are best for revision procedures; usually the cruciate ligaments are excised. When the components are being removed, the bone ends should be sufficiently mobilized to give good visualization.

Management of bone defects

Usually when the components have been removed, irregular bony surfaces remain, and it may be tempting to flatten projections to produce a more uniform surface for the insertion of the new prosthesis. I believe that this is not wise and all viable bone should be preserved. Defects may be filled in a variety of ways.

Cement

Contained defects that are surrounded by bone or contained within a new prosthetic component may be filled with cement, but wedge defects are not suitable for this method because the cement may crack, extrude, and lead to prosthetic loosening. Reinforcement of such defects with malleable titanium mesh gives some increased strength and has been used successfully by us for many years. However, I now feel that there are two superior methods of compensating for defects.

Bone grafts. In revision procedures, bone from the knee region itself often is not available and must be obtained either from the iliac crest or the bone bank. The grafts may be held with screws (Fig. 31-2, *A*) or threaded Kirschner wires (Fig. 31-2, *B*). Sometimes the graft may be fashioned so that it self-locks in the defect without need for extra support. When the bone defects are very large, it is usually necessary to use bone bank femoral head grafts; these are useful for filling "trumpet" defects (Fig. 31-3, *A* and *B*).

Custom components. Custom components are available from the manufacturers but take 2 to 3 months to make. The surgeon must specify the components required. Those most commonly needed are discussed here.

1. I prefer to use intramedullary stems such as fluted Sampson rods of a diameter calculated to fit the diaphyseal canal. The length and diameter are calculated from anteroposterior and lateral radiographs. Fluted rods, if a good press fit is obtained, need not be cemented (Fig. 31-4, *A*, and *B*). In fact I prefer not to use cement in the intramedullary canal and use it mostly to level the bone ends.

2. Wedges, either half or full, often are required to compensate for asymmetric defects of the tibia. Wedges of 15 to 20 degrees are most commonly required (Fig. 31-5).

3. In addition to intramedullary stems, the femoral component may need posterior or distal augmentation. Distal augmentation may be required only on one side when the femoral defect is asymmetric.

4. A range of tibial polyethylene components should be ordered and may be attached to the metal tray at the time of surgery.

5. The posterior stabilized type of articulation is most suitable for revision procedures,

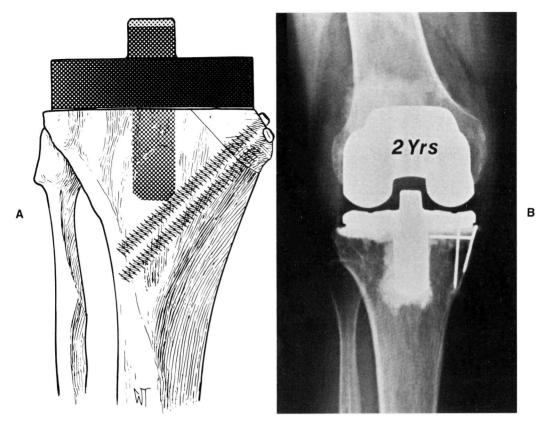

Fig. 31-2. Bone grafts used to fill asymmetric defects of the femur may be held by screws **(A)** or threaded Kirschner wires **(B).**

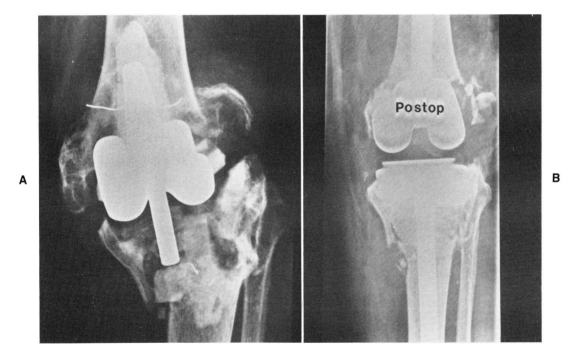

Fig. 31-3. Sometimes loosening of the components is associated with massive bone destruction as in this loose Attenborough knee **(A).** A femoral head bone bank graft was used to fill the tibial defect **(B).** Although the Attenborough knee prosthesis is a stabilizing design, the articulation of the revision prosthesis was a condylar type.

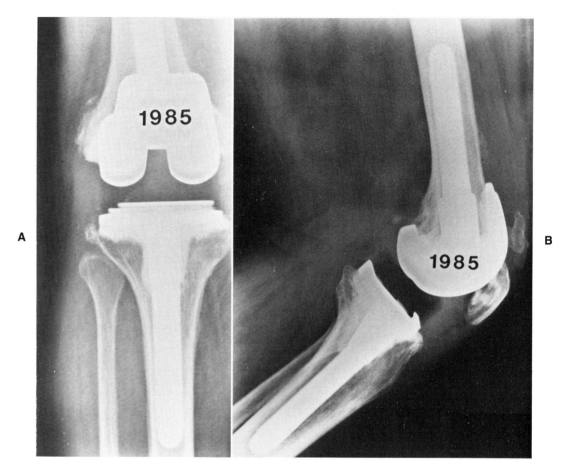

Fig. 31-4. In this revision operation, uncemented fluted rods were used on both components. Cement was used at the distal end of the femur and proximal end of tibia as a filler. By leaving the stems uncemented, extraction in case of infection would not be difficult. Because sepsis is now the primary cause for revision surgery, fixation is regarded as a compromise between security and ease of removal.

although occasionally a Total Condylar Type III or constrained design will be needed. The surgeon should specify which of these two is required, as well as the size of the components. It is not always possible to estimate exactly the required size, although 66 mm components are used most often for male patients and 58 mm components are used most often for females. Overly large components will not fit; when in doubt, the surgeon should order the smaller of the components considered.

Ligament balance

Knee arthroplasties often fail because of malalignment or imperfect ligament balance. The failure usually can be corrected by soft tissue release performed by releasing a sleeve of tissue from the medial tibia when the imbalance is varus or from the lateral femur when the imbalance is valgus. Additional space between the bone ends will be created and must be considered when planning the operation and ordering custom components. Even when the previous prosthesis was of a constrained type, such as a Guepar, Spherocentric, or Attenborough model, a relatively unconstrained posterior stabilized design can be used successfully for the revision, provided that the soft tissues are balanced. Therefore a clear understanding of the techniques and principles of soft tissue release is a prerequisite of successful revision surgery. Occasionally, albeit

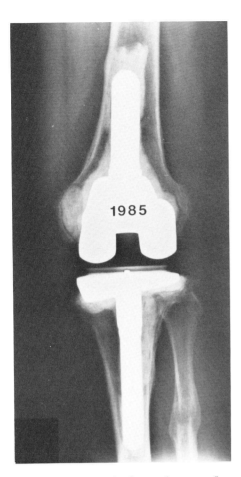

Fig. 31-5. This radiograph shows the use of a medial wedge on the tibial component to fill an asymmetric defect left after removal of the previous prosthesis. In this case because of massive bone loss, particularly on the femoral side, it was believed necessary to cement the stems. Intramedullary bone plugs have been used to plug the canals of the femur and tibia.

rarely, adequate soft tissue support is not present; only then should a more constrained design such as the Total Condylar III be used.

CHOICE OF PROSTHESIS

It is apparent that the posterior stabilized condylar knee is used for the majority of my revision arthroplasties. The more constrained Total Condylar III design is used only rarely. A linked design is considered necessary only for cases with paralytic recurvatum. (Knee reconstruction after excision of tumors is excluded from this discussion.) The surgeon should be clear that the need for a *stem* (to enhance bone fixation) by no means implies the need for *constraint* (to substitute for

inadequate soft tissue support). Stems very often are needed for revision operations; constraint rarely is needed in the articulation. Although it used to be true that constrained designs possessed stems and unconstrained prostheses did not, it is true no longer. Most surface replacements can be obtained with an intramedullary stem.

Fixation

At The Hospital for Special Surgery we have little experience with uncemented prostheses and none with porous ingrowth types. We have on occasion used press-fit designs with intramedullary Sampson rods with bone grafts but without cement. These all have been multiple revision cases with massive bone loss, and our reasoning has been to avoid difficulties of extraction in case postoperative infection occurs. More often we prefer to use cement as a grouting material at the bone ends but avoid its presence in the metaphysis or diaphysis of the femur and tibia. Antibiotic-impregnated cement is desirable for high-risk revision cases.

Postoperative regimen

Unless the quadriceps turndown has been done for the exposure, the postoperative program does not differ from primary arthroplasty. Turndown exposure requires a minimum of 3 weeks of immobilization in extension before beginning flexion, although weight bearing can be started during this period.

When the exposure has been uncomplicated, I begin the continuous passive motion in the recovery room and start weight bearing on the second or third postoperative day. Weight bearing is progressed as tolerated. The patient is discharged walking with a cane and after approximately 90 degrees of knee flexion is obtained. Manipulation with the patient under anesthesia is considered when knee flexion is not satisfactory at the end of 2 weeks. It is my practice to perform routine venography 5 days after surgery and to administer an anticoagulant with warfarin to patients with clots. Heparin is avoided except when large clots are found in the femoral vein or a symptomatic pulmonary embolus occurs. The danger of hemiarthrosis with heparin is considerable.

Intravenous antibiotics are given after revision surgery until cultures are proved negative after 5 days.

Complications

The complications of revision arthroplasty do not differ greatly from those of the primary procedure. Venographic evidence of thrombophlebitis is found in about 50% of the cases, and a change in the lung scan is found in about 10% of the patients. These are treated with warfarin therapy for 2 months.

The most frequent postoperative complications are urinary retention in men and urinary tract infections in women. In male patients with marked urinary frequency before surgery, consideration should be given to a transurethral prostatectomy before proceeding with the revision surgery.

Extensor mechanism weakness is more likely in revision surgery. Tibial tubercle avulsion may occur during the exposure and should be looked for and avoided by performing a quadriceps turndown in difficult cases.

We have not found postoperative instability to be a significant problem. Unlike primary procedures, some stretching can be expected. Therefore we advise that a slight flexion contracture (5 to 10 degrees) should be present at the end of the revision.

RESULTS

The results of revision surgery are seldom quite as good as primary arthroplasty.[4] Most patients experience some degree of pain, although the reason may not be apparent. The range of motion tends to be less, and extensor weakness is more frequent. Postoperative deep infection occurs more often. Radiolucent lines at the cement-bone interface are the rule rather than the exception.

In a study[4] of the results of 72 revision total knee arthroplasties, 38 knees (53%) were rated excellent, 26 knees (36%) good, 4 knees (5.5%) fair, and 4 knees (5.5%) poor. The prostheses used were the Total Condylar I in 7 knees, the Total Condylar III prosthesis in 3 knees, the posterior stabilized prosthesis in 32 knees, and a custom prosthesis with a posterior stabilized articulation in 16 knees. The average range of motion was 96 degrees; 13.8% had an extension lag of 5 to 10 degrees, and 2.7% had an extension lag of 10 to 20 degrees.

Thus, although the 89% rated good or excellent in follow-up is almost the same as in primary arthroplasty, relatively more knees are in the good category and fewer are in the excellent category.

REFERENCES

1. Coonse, K., and Adams, J.D.: A new operative approach to the knee joint, Surg. Gynecol. Obstet. **77**:344, 1943.
2. Hirsh, D.M., Bhalla, S., and Roffman, M.: Supracondylar fracture of the femur following total knee replacement: Report of four cases, J. Bone Joint Surg. **63A**:162, 1981.
3. Hood, R.W., and Insall, J.N.: Total knee revision arthroplasty: Indications, surgical techniques, and results, Orthop. Trans. **5**:412, 1981.
4. Insall, J.N., and Dethmers, D.A.: Revision of total knee arthroplasty, Clin. Orthop. **170**:123, 1982.
5. Insall, J.N., and Kelly, M.: The total condylar prosthesis, Clin. Orthop. (In press.)
6. Insall, J.N., Lachiewicz, P.F., and Burstein, A.H.: The posterior stabilized condylar prosthesis: A modification of the total condylar design; two to four year clinical experience, J. Bone Joint Surg. **64A**:1317, 1982.
7. Insall, J.N., Ranawat, C.S., Aglietti, P., and Shine, J.: A comparison of four models of total knee replacement prostheses, J. Bone Joint Surg. **58A**:754, 1976.
8. Insall, J.N., Scott, W.N., and Ranawat, C.S.: The total condylar knee prosthesis: A report of two hundred and twenty cases, J. Bone Joint Surg. **61A**:173, 1979.
9. Lotke, P.A., and Ecker, M.L.: Influence of positioning of prosthesis in total knee replacement, J. Bone Joint Surg. **59A**:77, 1977.
10. Thornhill, T.S., Hood, R.W., Dalziel, R.E., Ewald, F.C., Insall, J.N., and Sledge, C.B.: Knee revision in failed non-infected total knee arthroplasty—The Robert B. Brigham and Hospital for Special Surgery Experience, Orthop. Trans. **6**:368, 1982.

Chapter 32

Revision total knee arthroplasty: indications and contraindications

HERBERT KAUFER

LARRY S. MATTHEWS

Orthopaedists traditionally have expected failure of total knee arthroplasty to occur earlier and more frequently than failure of total hip arthroplasty.* However, recent experience has shown that the reliability and longevity gap between total hip arthroplasty and total knee arthroplasty has progressively narrowed and may no longer exist. In the experience of some, total knee arthroplasty is as reliable and durable as hip replacement.[3,11,14]

Although infection is the most feared mode of total knee arthroplasty failure, sterile failure is far more common.† Progressive sterile loosening is the single, most commonly reported indication for revision total knee arthroplasty; however, Insall has stated that he no longer considers loosening to be a major knee replacement problem. In his experience, difficulty with the patella has become the most common local problem after total replacement.[12] Excluding infection, postoperative problems for which revision surgery may be considered are:

1. Patellar problems, such as lateral or medial subluxation, tracking aberrations, patellar ligament disruption, and patellar fracture with or without disruption of the extensor mechanism
2. Limited range of motion
3. Deformity, either varus or valgus, flexion

contracture or hyperextension, or combinations
4. Instability of the femoral tibial joint
5. Loosening that leads to pain, deformity, or instability

CONTRAINDICATIONS

Revision total knee arthroplasty is a difficult, time-consuming operative procedure, associated with more frequent and more severe complications and with lesser-quality results than primary total knee arthroplasty.[2,4,25] The symptomatic and functional indications for revision total knee arthroplasty therefore should be more compelling than the indications for a primary procedure. A patient who, after surgery for knee replacement, does not have an optimal result, but whose symptoms or disability are less than would be considered an adequate indication for primary knee replacement surgery should be treated nonoperatively.

Large, healthy young individuals with single-joint disease are poor candidates for an initial total knee arthroplasty. If such a patient has a failed arthroplasty, the error should not be compounded by revising a total knee that should not have been done in the first place. Total knee arthroplasty failure in such patients is best treated nonoperatively or by conversion to an arthrodesis (Fig. 32-1), the procedure that probably should have been done initially.

Many cases of residual pain or mild instability following total knee arthroplasty can be treated

---

*References 4,6,7,9,15,18,21.
†References 4,9,10,21,23,25.

297

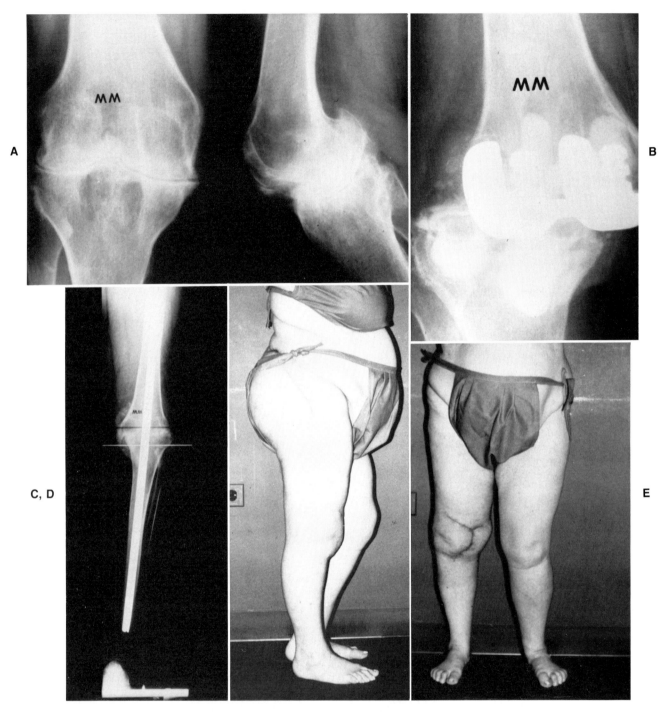

Fig. 32-1. A, Preoperative radiograph of the knee of a 42-year-old woman with severe posttraumatic arthritis. This is the only joint abnormality in this patient who is otherwise in robust good health. She weighs 252 pounds. **B,** AP radiograph of a Bechtol total knee that had been implanted 1 year earlier. It is dislocated in the first postoperative month and has been painful and unstable ever since. **C,** Radiograph 1 year following intramedullary arthrodesis showing secure fusion. **D,** The patient, now 44 years old, bearing full weight on her arthrodesed knee. **E,** AP view of the patient, showing acceptable limb alignment. Vigorous, heavy, young individuals with single-joint disease can be expected to do poorly with total knee replacement. In such patients nonprosthetic approaches to the abnormal knee are preferred.

by oral medications, limitation of activity, brace support, and a walking stick. Revision total knee replacement should be reserved for those patients whose symptoms cannot be controlled adequately by nonoperative means and whose symptoms or disability is sufficiently compelling to warrant the increased hazards and uncertainty associated with a revision total knee replacement.

Malalignment of the limb, malalignment of the prosthetic components, and poor cement technique are total knee arthroplasty deficiencies that increase the probability of future loosening; but alone they do not adequately account for *current* symptoms. Revision arthroplasty in patients with only these findings is highly unlikely to result in symptom relief and is far more likely to increase rather than decrease symptoms. Revision total knee arthroplasty rarely relieves symptoms in patients with unexplained pain; these patients should not be treated operatively, especially if there is no objective evidence of a localized problem such as effusion, edema, crepitus, or instability.

Symptomatic patellofemoral problems that cannot be managed nonoperatively are best treated by patellar mechanism realignment, repair, or both, depending on the nature of the symptom-producing problem. Symptomatic patellofemoral problems, if associated with either significant deviation of the limb from the normal weight-bearing axis or with significant rotational malalignment of the tibia relative to the femur, may be alleviated by a revision total knee arthroplasty. Knees with marked instability or component loosening can benefit from revision total knee arthroplasty.

Additional contraindication for revision total knee arthroplasty include active sepsis and poor quality tissue. Critical tissues in order of decreasing importance are (1) skin, (2) muscle, especially the extensor mechanism, (3) ligaments, and (4) bone.

Very poor quality skin either absolutely contraindicates a revision total knee arthroplasty or requires preliminary pedicle coverage to provide adequate skin through which the procedure can be performed. This is often best done with a gastrocnemius myocutaneous flap or a gastrocnemius muscle flap. Both the medial and lateral heads of gastrocnemius are suitable for this purpose.[22,24] The medial head of gastrocnemius is preferable because it is a bit easier to mobilize and tends to be somewhat longer. However, if the medial head is scarred or in some other way unsuitable, then the lateral head can be mobilized and used in a very similar way. Occasionally, the soft tissue deficiency on the anterior aspect of the knee joint can be so large that both the medial and lateral heads of gastrocnemius are necessary in order to provide adequate soft tissue covering.[22] If possible, the revision total knee operation should not be performed at the same time as the gastrocnemius muscle or myocutaneous flap. The soft tissue coverage procedure should be healed and secure before the revision total knee arthoplasty procedure.

Poor-quality musculature presents a considerable problem for revision total knee arthroplasty and may require prolonged or permanent postrevision bracing but does not constitute an absolute contraindication to revision surgery. Successful total knee replacement has been done in limbs with profound flaccid quadriceps paralysis and even in some with spastic paralysis of thigh muscles.

Mechanical problems that may lead to clinical failure of a total knee arthroplasty include instability, loosening, metaphyseal bone loss, malinsertion of prosthetic components, and residual deformity. If the mechanical failure is not associated with severe pain, revision total knee arthroplasty may not be necessary. Symptoms resulting from instability and loosening often can be successfully managed by bracing (Fig. 32-2). If bracing fails to produce adequate symptom relief or if bracing is not acceptable to the patient, then revision total knee arthroplasty should be considered.

In the process of preoperative planning, the surgeon must consider local factors such as the condition of overlying soft tissue, location, size and direction of previous operative scars, deficiency of local bone stock, and deficiency of supporting soft tissue, specifically extensor mechanism, capsule, and ligaments.

INDICATIONS

Very poor quality ligaments may call for revision to an arthrodesis or for a revision prosthesis with intrinsic stability. There is a limit to ligament release procedures in order to establish ligament balance. Ligament release procedures lengthen the limb. In severe cases, actual intraarticular lengthening of the limb of more than 1 inch can create extensor mechanism problems by displacing the patella distal to the articular surface of the

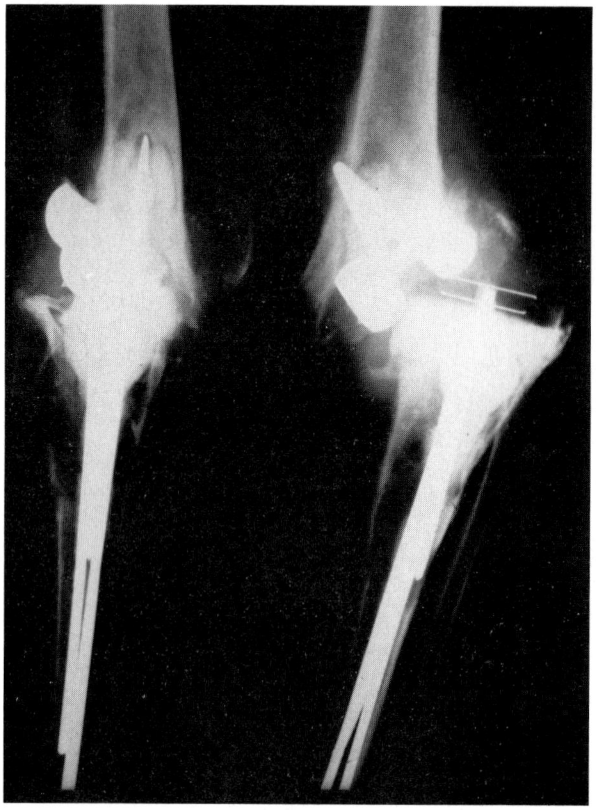

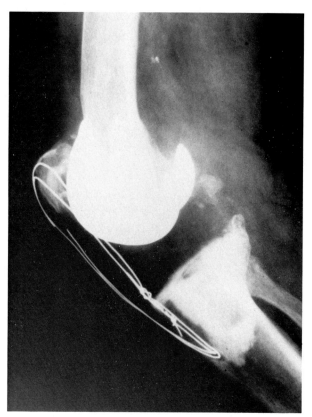

A

Fig. 32-2. This 76-year-old man with severe cardiac disease has an obvious dislocation and gross component loosening. However, pain was not a serious problem. His major knee complaint was giving way and instability, which was solved with a long double upright brace. No operation was done. The braced limb served him satisfactorily for 3 years, at which time he died of cardiac disease.

Fig. 32-3. A, Extensive ligament release procedures required use of a thick tibial component, which resulted in displacement of the patella distal to the patellar articulating surface of the femur. In an attempt to deal with this problem, the operating surgeon performed a patellar ligament lengthening procedure, which has restored the patella to its desired position, articulating with the distal femur.

femur and may lead to peroneal or tibial nerve–stretch palsy or even circulatory compromise (Fig. 32-3). In order to avoid these potential problems, an intrinsically stable prosthesis is preferable to intraarticular lengthening of the limb in excess of 1 inch.

Painful total knee arthroplasty failure associated with loosening, deformity, malinsertion of the initial prosthesis, mild degrees of instability, or mild degrees of metaphyseal bone loss usually can be managed by revision total knee arthroplasty using a nonlinked resurfacing prosthesis of the semiconstrained type.[2,4,25] Failure of total knee arthroplasty associated with severe degrees of ligament insufficiency, severe degrees of metaphyseal bone loss, or combined instability and bone loss, are often best managed by revision to

an intrinsically stable prosthesis[16,27] (Figs. 32-3 and 32-4).

Uni-axial hinge prostheses are now generally agreed to be both unacceptable and unnecessary for total knee arthroplasty. Currently available intrinsically stable knee prostheses capable of multi-axial rotation include the Kinematic rotating hinge,[27] the Attenborough,[1,26] the Noiles,[5,8] the Lacey,[17] and the Spherocentric.[16] Of these, only the Spherocentric has a documented, acceptable clinical performance in large numbers of patients with follow-up of more than 4 years.[16] The Spherocentric prosthesis therefore is considered to be the prosthesis of choice for revision total knee arthroplasty in those knees in which an intrinsically stable prosthesis is desirable (Figs. 32-3 and 32-4).

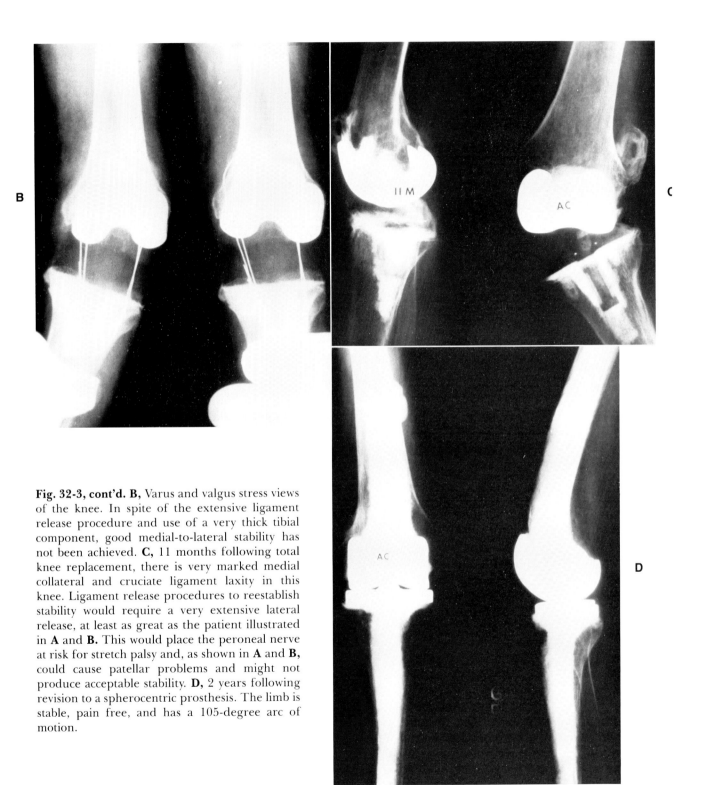

Fig. 32-3, cont'd. B, Varus and valgus stress views of the knee. In spite of the extensive ligament release procedure and use of a very thick tibial component, good medial-to-lateral stability has not been achieved. **C,** 11 months following total knee replacement, there is very marked medial collateral and cruciate ligament laxity in this knee. Ligament release procedures to reestablish stability would require a very extensive lateral release, at least as great as the patient illustrated in **A** and **B.** This would place the peroneal nerve at risk for stretch palsy and, as shown in **A** and **B,** could cause patellar problems and might not produce acceptable stability. **D,** 2 years following revision to a spherocentric prosthesis. The limb is stable, pain free, and has a 105-degree arc of motion.

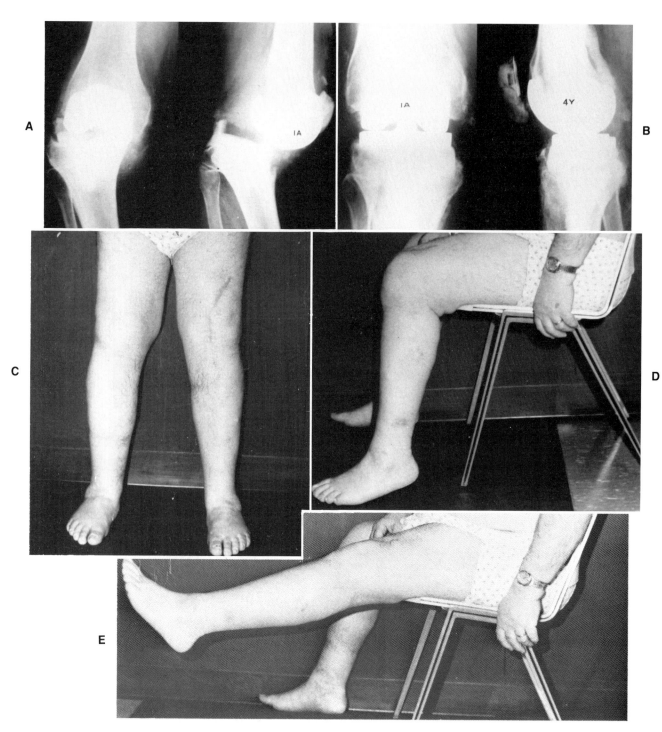

Fig. 32-4. A, AP and lateral radiographs of a revision total condylar type of total knee arthroplasty that had been performed to salvage a previously placed prosthesis that failed because of instability and loosening. Both components are secure with nothing to suggest loosening. The limb is severely deformed in varus and hyperextension. The knee is dislocated with the tibia posterior to the femur. **B,** AP and lateral radiographs of the second revision, this time using the spherocentric prosthesis. 4 years after surgery the knee is well aligned, stable, and pain free. There is a small, limited, lucent line at the tibial cement mass and at the patellar cement mass. Note the large medial proximal tibial cement mass used to overcome the medial tibial metaphyseal defect produced by prior surgery. **C,** AP view of the patient 4 years postoperative showing a well-aligned limb. **D,** Lateral view of the seated patient demonstrating the 85-degree arc of flexion. **E,** Lateral view of the patient demonstrating full active extension against gravity.

SPHEROCENTRIC ARTHROPLASTY

The Spherocentric prosthesis is specifically indicated for revision of failed total knee arthroplasty in which instability is so great that intraarticular lengthening in excess of 1 inch would be required to reestablish ligament balance by ligament release procedures. If the degree of instability is less severe, then revision surgery can be accomplished successfully with a variety of prostheses, using tibial and femoral components of sufficient thickness to fill the space created by the ligament balancing–release procedures.[2,4,25]

Procedure

The operative procedure for a Spherocentric total knee revision is performed through the previous operative scar. Circumferential subperiosteal exposure of the proximal tibia and distal femur is essential. The previously inserted prosthesis should be removed along with all cement and any membrane that may have developed between cement and bone. If a patellar surface had been installed, it need not be removed or exchanged unless it is loose or in some other way mechanically unsatisfactory. If so, the patellar surface should be removed and replaced with a patellar surface that is compatible with the spherocentric patellar flange. The universal patellar dome and the Spherocentric patellar surface are both compatible with the spherocentric patellar flange. Care must be taken to remove no additional bone from either the distal femur or proximal tibia. It is often necessary to use a considerable cement buildup to provide for adequate contact between the prosthetic components and the remaining bone. In order to improve the area of contact between the prosthesis and the bone, a large cement buildup is much preferred over a large bone resection[13] (Fig. 32-4).

Precise limb alignment to reestablish the normal mechanical axis is as important with the Spherocentric prosthesis as it is with any knee replacement procedure.[16,19] Once the tibial and femoral components have been cemented in place and the prosthesis has been assembled by snapping the plastic socket over the tibial sphere and into the femoral cavity, the limb will have perfect stability and a free 120-degree arc of flexion and extension. With an extensive extensor mechanism realignment or reconstruction, postoperative cast immobilization may be desirable. Otherwise, postoperative treatment need not differ from that of a conventional total knee replacement.

Results

Our experience with Spherocentric arthroplasty for revision of failed total knees consists of 68 knees with follow-up of 2 to 8 years. Femoral stem length varied from 4 to 12 inches and tibial stem length varied from 4 to 9-inches. All prostheses had a patellar flange on the femoral component. Of the 68 knees 30 had a polyethylene patellar surface cemented in place. Average postoperative motion was 97 degrees (range 40 to 120 degrees). Excellent initial stability was achieved in all cases. One postoperative infection occurred, which cleared following prosthetic removal and conversion to a resection arthroplasty. Only 21 of the 68 knees show no area of radiolucency. The remaining 47 knees, at some point along the cement bone interface, show a radiolucent zone at least 1 mm wide. The lucent zone is complete around five components in four knees. There has been no case of revision for loosening in this group of patients. One patient sustained a femur fracture at the tip of a 9 inch femoral stem that progressed to a nonunion. It was treated by re-revision with a 12-inch stem. The 3-year follow-up after re-revision was most satisfactory with excellent stability, a 90-degree arc of knee motion, and a securely healed femur fracture.

Patellar problems were the most common source of symptoms following revision Spherocentric arthroplasty. Six knees developed a lateral patellar subluxation. Three of the six had no symptoms associated with the subluxation, which was noted as an incidental radiographic finding. The remaining three had an extensor lag and/or patellofemoral discomfort. An additional four knees developed patellar ligament rupture or avulsion, resulting in proximal migration of the patella and a postoperative extension lag. None of the patients with patellofemoral problems has been reoperated on because of these complaints. They are being treated by oral analgesics, a walking stick, and limitation of activity.

Five knees developed postoperative progressive hyperextension resulting from instability caused by deformation of the plastic components within the Spherocentric prosthesis. Two of these patients were reoperated on, and the deformed plastic components were removed and replaced. The procedure resulted in only temporary control of their instability, which gradually returned. The cemented metal components of these prostheses have remained securely fixed. One of the patients has been lost to follow-up; however, four of these patients are currently being managed by long double upright braces to control hyperextension and medial-lateral instability of their limbs. Although they remain independent walkers, they have persistent instability and a chronic joint effusion but very little pain. Their limbs are quite similar to those observed in patients with neuropathic arthropathy of the knee. Although none has tertiary syphilis, congenital indifference to pain, or any other detectable neurologic abnormality, they may represent a variant of neuropathic arthropathy.

DISCUSSION

The long-stemmed Spherocentric prosthesis with patellar flange has proved to be a highly satisfactory and reliable prosthesis for revision of failed total knee arthroplasty with gross ligamentous instability, severe degrees of metaphyseal bone loss, or combinations of the two.

Many patients with symptoms or disability following total knee arthroplasty are best managed nonoperatively. Only those whose symptoms or disability is very severe, (as severe or more severe than the symptoms that lead to the initial prosthetic arthroplasty) should be considered for revision total knee surgery. In the vast majority successful revision can be accomplished using modern nonlinked resurfacing prostheses.

Revision using an intrinsically stable linked prosthesis should be considered in only the most unstable knees in which ligament balance by ligament release procedures would require intraarticular lengthening of the limb in excess of 1 inch. In failed total knee arthroplasty with this degree of instability, an intrinsically stable prosthesis is preferable. In our opinion the Spherocentric prosthesis is the prosthesis of choice for those cases in which an intrinsically stable prosthesis is indicated.

REFERENCES

1. Attenborough, C.G.: The Attenborough total knee replacement, J. Bone Joint Surg. **60B:**320-326, 1978.
2. Bryan, R.S., and Rand, J.A.: Revision total knee arthroplasty, Clin. Orthop. **170:**116-122, 1982.
3. Buchanan, J.R., Greer, R.B. III, Bowman, L.S., Shearer, A. and Gallagher, K.: Clinical experience with the variable axis total knee replacement, J. Bone Joint Surg. **64A:**337-346, 1982.
4. Cameron, H.U., and Hunter, G.A.: Failure in total knee arthroplasty, mechanisms, revisions and results, Clin. Orthop. **170:**141-146, 1982.
5. Connolly, J.F., Neumann, R., Jardon, O.M., and Shindell, R.: Superior migration of the Noiles total knee prosthesis, paper presented at the Association of Bone and Joint Surgeons meeting, Southamptom, Bermuda, May 14, 1985.
6. Cracchiolo, A. III, Benson, M., Finerman, G.A.M., Horacek, K., and Amstutz, H.C.: A prospective comparative clinical analysis of the first-generation knee replacements, polycentric vs. geometric knee arthroplasty, Clin. Orthop. **145:**37-46, 1979.
7. Deburge, A.: GUEPAR, GUEPAR hinge prosthesis, Clin. Orthop. **120:**47-53, 1976.
8. Flynn, L.M.: The Noiles hinge knee prosthesis with axial rotation, Orthopaedics, **2:**602-609, 1979.
9. Goldberg, V.M., and Henderson, B.T.: The Freeman-Swanson I.C.L.H. total knee arthroplasty: Complications and problems, J. Bone Joint Surg. **62A:**1338-1344, 1980.
10. Gristina, A.G., and Kolkin, J.: Total joint replacement and sepsis, J. Bone Joint Surg. **65A:**128-134, 1983.
11. Hungerford, D.S., and Krachow, K.: Total joint arthroplasty of the knee, Clin. Orthop. **192:**23-33, 1985.
12. Insall, J., Binazzi, R., Soudry, M., and Mestriner, L.A.: Total knee arthroplasty, Clin. Orthop. **192:**13-22, 1985.
13. Insall, J., and Dethmers, D.A.: Revision of total knee arthroplasty, Clin. Orthop. **170:**123-130, 1982.
14. Insall, J. Hood, R.M., Flawn, L.B., and Sullivan, D.J.: The total condylar knee prosthesis in gonarthrosis, J. Bone Joint Surg. **65A:**619-828, 1983.
15. Insall, J.N., Ranawat, C.S., Aglietti, P., and Shine, J.: A comparison of four models of total knee replacement prosthesis, J. Bone Joint Surg. **58A:**754-765, 1976.
16. Kaufer, H., and Matthews, L.S.: Spherocentric arthroplasty of the knee, J. Bone Joint Surg. **63A:**545-559, 1981.
17. Lacey, A.: Lacey total knee, Dow Corning-Wright, Data Sheet L, pp. 095-0009, 1981.
18. Lewallen, D.G., Bryan R.S., and Peterson, L.F.A.: Polycentric total knee arthroplasty, J. Bone Joint Surg. **66A:**1211-1218, 1984.
19. Lotke, P.A., and Ecker: Influence of positioning of prosthesis in total knee replacement, J. Bone Joint Surg. **59A:**77-79, 1977.
20. Marmor, L.: Unicompartmental and total knee arthroplasty, Clin. Orthop. **192:**75-81, 1985.
21. Murray, D.G., Wilde, A.H., Werner, F., and Foster, D.: Herbert total knee prosthesis: Combined laboratory and clinical assessment, J. Bone Joint Surg. **59A:**1026-1032, 1977.
22. Salibian, A.H., and Anzel, S.H.: Salvage of an infected total knee prosthesis with medial and lateral gastrocnemius muscle flaps, J. Bone Joint Surg. **65A:**681-684, 1983.
23. Salvati, E.A., Robinson, R.D., Zeno, S.M., Koslin, B.L., Brause, B.D., and Wilson, P.D., Jr.: Infection rates after 3175 total hip and total knee replacements performed with and without a horizontal unidirectional filtered air flow system, J. Bone Joint Surg. **64A:**525-535, 1982.
24. Sanders, R., and O'Neill, T.: The gastrocnemius myocutaneous flap used as a cover for the exposed knee prosthesis, J. Bone Joint Surg. **63B**(3):383-386, 1981.
25. Thornhill, T.S., Dalziel, R.W., and Sledge, C.B.: Alternatives to arthrodesis for the failed total knee arthroplasty, Clin. Orthop. **170:**131-140, 1982.
26. Vanhegan, J.A.D., Dabrowski, W., and Arden, G.P.: A review of 100 Attenborough stabilized gliding knee prostheses, J. Bone Joint Surg. **61B:**445-450, 1979.
27. Walker, P.S., Emerson, R., Potter, T., Scott, R., Thomas, W.H., and Turner, R.H.: The kinematic rotating hinge, Orthop. Clin. North Am. **13**(1):187-199, 1982.

Chapter 33

Revision total knee arthroplasty

JAMES A. RAND

LOWELL F.A. PETERSON

RICHARD S. BRYAN

DUANE M. ILSTRUP

The initial prosthetic designs used for total knee arthroplasty resulted in numerous failures.[27,32] Failure resulting in reoperation in a large series has been as high as 15%,[33] and salvage of the failed arthroplasty, especially in infection, usually has been by arthrodesis.[37] Revision has been reported by several authors,* but few detailed analyses of a large number of cases have been published. The incidence of revision has ranged from 2%[1] to 13%.[13]

CURRENT EXPERIENCE

The records of patients who underwent revision knee arthroplasty at the Mayo Clinic between 1970 and 1980 were reviewed. Patients with initial revisions in the presence of active infection or malignancy were excluded, as were patients whose reoperation did not require component replacement. Fifteen patients were excluded because of active infection at the initial revision, 11 because of operations performed elsewhere for whom information was inadequate, six because of death shortly after arthroplasty, and nine because of inadequate information in the records. A total of 427 knees (386 patients) remained for evaluation. An additional 28 patients died, and 11 were lost to follow-up within 2 years after revision. These 39 patients were not included in the evaluation of the success of revision at 2 years but

were included in the actuarial analysis of prosthetic survival.

The initial arthroplasty was performed at the Mayo Clinic in 330 knees and at other institutions in 97 knees. During the same time interval, 5643 total knee arthroplasties were performed at the Mayo Clinic for a known incidence of revision of 5.8%. This figure represents a minimal revision rate, since it excludes our patients who have been revised elsewhere without our knowledge. Of the 427 knees with initial arthroplasties, 357 (83.6%) knees had one revision, 60 (14.1%) required two revisions, and 10 (2.3%) had three revisions.

The revision rate of 5.8% that was found in the current study reflects experience with the early-generation prostheses. The geometric prosthesis and polycentric prosthesis constituted 88% of the initial Mayo Clinic total knee arthroplasties that required revision. These prostheses are now rarely used.

Women comprised 56% of the patients, and ages ranged from 20 to 88 years with a mean of 61. Right knees were involved in 53% of the procedures and left knees in 47%. Both knees were replaced in 53% of the patients, but only 41 bilateral revision procedures were performed. Of these knees 40% had been operated before the initial knee arthroplasty with a synovectomy in 15%, upper tibial osteotomy in 13.7%, medial meniscectomy in 11.5%, cheilectomy and debridement in 10.5%, patellectomy in 9.9%, and a tibial plateau prosthesis in 4.7%. Osteoarthritis was

*References 1,5,6,8,11-14,20,26,27,31,37-40.

present in 61%, rheumatoid arthritis in 28%, and posttraumatic arthritis in 0.5%, with the remaining patients having various diagnoses, including ancient septic arthritis, avascular necrosis, and hemophiliac arthropathy. In some patients with initial surgery elsewhere, the underlying diagnosis was not known.

Of the initial arthroplasties 75% were performed between 1972 and 1976, using the first prototype knee-replacement systems. The knees were divided into three groups for analysis: group 1 included the entire 427 knees; group 2 comprised the 330 knees initially operated on at our clinic, and group 3 involved the 97 knees initially operated on at other institutions.

Statistical analysis was performed using the log-rank test,[21,24] and the prosthesis survival was estimated using a nonparametric estimation of survival.[17]

The time intervals between revisions are shown in Table 33-1. Follow-up from the initial arthroplasty was 6.8 ± 2.3 years in group 1, 7.1 ± 2.4 years in group 2, and 5.8 ± 1.7 years in group 3. Follow-up from the last revision was 3.7 ± 1.7 years in group 1, 3.8 ± 1.7 years in group 2, and 3.6 ± 1.6 years in group 3.

The types of the initial and subsequent revision prostheses used are listed in Table 33-2. In group

1, 37% of the initial prostheses were geometric and 41% polycentric. In group 2, 39% were geometric and 50% polycentric. In the same time interval, 1635 geometric and 1761 polycentric prostheses were implanted at the Mayo Clinic. There was a tendency to use a more constrained prosthesis for each subsequent revision procedure (Table 33-2).

MECHANISMS OF FAILURE

Total knee arthroplasty may fail by a variety of mechanisms. Failure may be related to prosthetic design, patient selection, surgical technique, or combinations of these factors.[14] Early prosthetic designs resulted in areas of stress concentration, resulting in implant subsidence, loosening, or occasionally implant breakage.[23,27] Current prosthetic designs employ a femoral component with an anterior flange and a metal reinforced tibial component. Failure from errors in prosthetic design alone currently are infrequent.

Patient selection is important. An intelligent, cooperative individual who will follow advised levels in restriction of activity is essential. Obesity and osteoarthritis have been suggested as important reasons for prosthetic failure.[10,11,37] Prosthesis survival was evaluated from the first to the second revision with respect to patient weight and diagnosis. Body weight was normalized to ideal weight using the Metropolitan Life Insurance Company statistics for ideal body weight. Any patient weighing more than 20% above ideal weight was considered to be overweight. Prosthesis survival was slightly improved ($P<0.07$) in the ideal-weight group over that in the overweight group (Fig. 33-1). In patients with rheumatoid arthritis, the prosthesis survival probability was

Table 33-1. Time intervals to revision (M ± SD yr)

Revision	Mayo Clinic	Elsewhere	Overall
1	2.9 ± 2.1	1.6 ± 1.1	2.6 ± 2.0
2	2.2 ± 1.7	1.5 ± 1.3	1.9 ± 1.6
3	1.8 ± 1.8	2.4 ± 2.0	2.0 ± 1.8

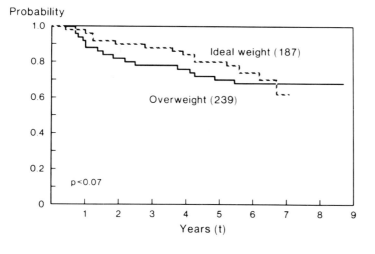

Fig. 33-1. Prosthesis survival rates according to body weight. Overweight is 20% above ideal weight.

Table 33-2. Prosthesis types for revision total knee arthroplasty

Type	Initial			First revision			Second revision			Third revision		
	Mayo	Elsewhere	Overall	Mayo	Elsewhere	Overall	Mayo	Elsewhere	Overall	Mayo	Elsewhere	Overall
Polycentric	164	10	174	44	2	46	2	1	3			
Geometric	128	31	159	94	18	112	8	1	9			
Freeman	1	1	2	1	—	1						
Marmor	2	13	15	—	2	2	—	1	1	—	1	1
Duopatellar	—	1	1	1	—	1						
Gustilo	1	1	2									
RAM				—	1	1						
UCI	1	5	6	1	—	1						
Townley	—	7	7									
Unicompartmental polycentric	20	2	22	2	1	3						
Unicompartmental geometric	2	—	2									
Unicompartmental Marmor	1	8	9	—	1	1						
Total Condylar	1	2	3	23	12	35	2	3	5	2	—	2
Cruciate condylar	2	—	2	33	10	43	3	2	5	1	—	1
Anametric condylar	4	—	4	17	5	22	1	2	3			
Total Condylar II				2	3	5	1	—	1			
Total Condylar III				2	2	4	2	1	3			
Kinematic stabilizer				4	—	4	—	2	2	1	—	1
Kinematic rotating hinge				4	4	8	5	4	9	—	1	1
Spherocentric	1	1	2	6	4	10	2	1	3	—	1	1
Tavernetti	1	—	1	28	5	33	4	1	5	1	—	1
Zimmer offset hinge	—	1	1	1	—	1						
Guepar	1	—	1	50	21	71	10	2	12			
Guepar custom				1	1	2				—	1	1
Herbert				2	—	2						
Walldius	—	2	2	11	1	12	2	2	4	1	—	1
Walldius custom				2	1	3	1	2	3			
Sheehan				1	1	2	—	1	1			
Unknown	—	12	12									
TOTAL	330	97	427	330	97	427	44	26	70	6	4	10

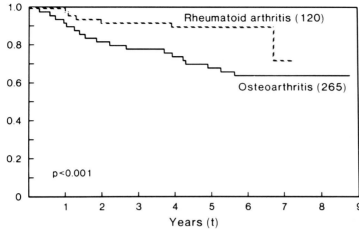

Fig. 33-2. Prosthesis survival rates for rheumatoid knees superior to those for osteoarthritic knees undergoing revision (P <0.001).

Table 33-3. Reasons for revision total knee arthroplasty

Reason	First revision Mayo	First revision Elsewhere	First revision Overall	Second revision Mayo	Second revision Elsewhere	Second revision Overall	Third revision Mayo	Third revision Elsewhere	Third revision Overall
Loosening									
Tibial	174	35	209	13	9	22	2	1	3
Femoral	11	4	15	2	4	6	1	2	3
Both	29	12	41	15	3	18	2	—	2
Instability	114	26	140	9	6	15	0	1	1
Abnormal axial alignment									
Varus	66	14	80	4	5	9			
Valgus	27	8	35	1	2	3			
Component malposition									
Femur	5	2	7	—	4	4			
Tibia	18	3	21	—	1	1	—	1	1
Both	8	3	11	1	—	1			
Patella	2	0	2	2	1	3			
Patellar									
Subluxation	4	—	4	1	—	1			
Dislocation	2	1	3	2	1	3			
Pain of unknown origin	4	7	11	3	0	3			
Suspected sepsis	1	2	3	1	0	1			
Fracture									
Prosthesis	11	3	14	4	2	6	1	—	1
Bone	30	5	35	1	—	1	—	1	1
Both	2	—	2	1	—	1			
Implant settling	6	—	6	1	—	1			
Ankylosis	3	5	8	—	1	2			
Degenerative joint disease in opposite component of									
Unicompartmental	1	1	2						
Residual flexion									
Contracture	14	8	22	2	—	2			

significantly better ($\underline{P}$<0.001) than that in patients with osteoarthritis (Fig. 33-2). This difference may be related to the increased activity level of the patient with osteoarthritis.

Careful surgical technique is essential. The most frequent nonseptic reasons for revision surgery are loosening and instability.* In the current series loosening (especially of the tibial component), instability, and axial malalignment were the most frequent reasons for revision (Table 33-3). Frequently, more than one reason was present for a single knee.

Ligamentous stability of the knee in all planes was evaluated, and any knee with more than mild instability (5mm displacement on clinical examination) in any plane was considered unstable (Table 33-4). Instability was present in approximately one third of all knees before each surgical procedure. At follow-up only 9.1% of the knees were unstable.

Axial alignment was evaluated at each time interval (Table 33-5). Varus malalignment was

*References 1,5,10,15,20,26,27,31,37-40.

Table 33-4. Instability (%) in revision total knee arthroplasty

	Number	Stable	Unstable	Unknown
Preoperative				
Group 1	321	40.3	34.9	24.8
Group 2	317	51.2	44.9	3.9
Group 3	4	3.1	1.0	95.9
First revision				
Group 1	274	39.6	31.6	28.8
Group 2	233	40.0	30.6	29.4
Group 3	41	38.1	35.1	26.8
Second revision				
Group 1	60	47.1	38.6	14.3
Group 2	37	43.2	40.9	15.9
Group 3	23	53.9	34.6	11.5
Third revision				
Group 1	7	30.0	42.9	30.0
Group 2	4	33.3	33.3	33.3
Group 3	3	25.0	50.0	25.0
Latest examination				
Group 1	367	81.3	9.1	9.6
Group 2	281	79.6	10.2	10.2
Group 3	86	87.1	5.4	7.5

Table 33-5. Axial alignment in revision total knee arthroplasty

	Number	Mean ± SD	Malalignment (% of knees)	
			Varus (<5°)	Valgus (>10°)
Preoperative				
Group 1	308	0.4 ± 15.3	63.3	21.1
Group 2	303	0.2 ± 15.6	63.7	20.8
Group 3	5	10.2 ± 12.5	40.0	40.0
First revision				
Group 1	270	1.1 ± 12.4	63.3	17.8
Group 2	209	0.2 ± 11.7	66.0	15.8
Group 3	61	4.1 ± 14.3	54.1	24.6
Second revision				
Group 1	55	0.8 ± 12.7	56.9	20.7
Group 2	36	1.1 ± 13.6	53.9	25.6
Group 3	19	0.3 ± 11.2	63.2	10.5
Third revision				
Group 1	7	−1.1 ± 5.4	72.7	—
Group 2	4	−3.3 ± 5.4	75.0	—
Group 3	3	1.7 ± 4.7	66.7	—
Latest examination				
Group 1	299	3.5 ± 8.6	47.2	6.0
Group 2	229	3.9 ± 9.4	46.7	5.7
Group 3	70	3.5 ± 4.9	48.6	7.1

defined as less than 5 degrees of valgus, and valgus malalignment was defined as greater than 10 degrees of valgus. At follow-up, 48% of the knees were in varus malalignment and 6% were in valgus malalignment.

The importance of axial alignment and its effects on force transfer at the knee have been well documented.[18,19] The quality of the surrounding ligamentous structures and their importance in the transmission of force at the knee also have been emphasized.[10,15,16,34] Therefore failure to correct axial alignment or balance of soft tissue restraints may lead to increased bone-cement interface stress with subsequent prosthetic loosening. These findings emphasize the need for careful patient and prosthesis selection and for correct surgical technique.

FUNCTION

Function after revision surgery was evaluated in regard to the use of ambulatory aids and the distance that the patient could walk without resting. Among the knees with follow-up data, the ability to walk farther than 6 blocks was present after a single revision in 44% of group 1, 43% of group 2, and 48% of group 3; after two revisions in 35% of group 1, 33% of group 2, and 39% of group 3. After three revisions, five of eight patients (Table 33-6) could walk more than 6 blocks. The ability to walk without the use of ambulatory aids was present after a single revision in 55% of group 1, 56% of group 2, and 54% of group 3; after two revisions in 34% of group 1, 30% of group 2, and 40% of group 3. Four of eight patients with three revisions could walk without aids (Table 33-7).

In spite of revision surgery or the number of revisions, the mean range of motion was well maintained (Table 33-8). However, a small number of the patients in the study experienced a loss of knee motion, as indicated by the large standard deviations.

Table 33-6. Ambulatory ability

Revision	Group	>6 Blocks	4-6 Blocks	1-3 Blocks	Indoors	Bed to chair	Unable	No data	Total
One	1	136	39	87	32	4	11	48	357
	2	108	30	72	29	4	8	35	286
	3	28	9	15	3	0	3	13	71
Two	1	17	8	13	8	0	2	12	60
	2	10	6	7	6	0	1	8	38
	3	7	2	6	2	0	1	4	22
Three	1	5	0	1	2	0	0	2	10
	2	3	0	0	1	0	0	2	6
	3	2	0	1	1	0	0	0	4

Table 33-7. Ambulatory aids

Revision	Group	None	Cane—long walks	Cane—full-time	Crutch	Two canes	Two crutches	Walker	Unable	No data	Total
One	1	177	34	51	3	7	26	13	9	37	357
	2	143	24	40	2	7	23	12	6	29	286
	3	34	10	11	1	0	3	1	3	8	71
Two	1	18	8	11	1	2	9	2	2	7	60
	2	10	6	7	0	2	5	2	1	5	38
	3	8	2	4	1	0	4	0	1	2	22
Three	1	4	1	0	0	0	3	0	0	2	10
	2	4	0	0	0	0	0	0	0	2	6
	3	0	1	0	0	0	3	0	0	0	4

Table 33-8. Range of motion (M±SD) in revision total knee arthroplasty

	Number	*Extension*	*Flexion*
Preoperative			
Group 1	323	−9.2 ± 11.1	108.5 ± 19.6
Group 2	318	−9.2 ± 11.1	108.6 ± 19.7
Group 3	5	−9.0 ± 12.4	106.0 ± 15.2
First revision			
Group 1	307	−6.8 ± 10.1	99.3 ± 55.5
Group 2	235	−6.1 ± 9.2	102.8 ± 61.4
Group 3	72	−9.1 ± 12.4	87.9 ± 26.4
Second revision			
Group 1	62	−0.3 ± 9.5	96.9 ± 23.2
Group 2	39	−2.1 ± 9.0	102.0 ± 19.3
Group 3	23	−4.3 ± 9.1	88.4 ± 27.0
Third revision			
Group 1	8	−0.6 ± 8.2	91.9 ± 19.1
Group 2	5	−2.0 ± 7.6	89.0 ± 24.1
Group 3	3	−5.0 ± 8.7	96.7 ± 7.6
Latest examination			
Group 1	386	−1.8 ± 7.3	98.3 ± 45.5
Group 2	296	−1.9 ± 7.2	100.6 ± 50.6
Group 3	90	−1.5 ± 7.7	91.0 ± 20.0

REVISION PROSTHESIS SELECTION

Selection of the appropriate revision prosthesis is important. Hinged-type prostheses, even when used as an initial arthroplasty, have a high failure rate.[1,3] When used for salvage of the failed total knee arthroplasty, hinge prostheses gave less satisfactory results than less constrained prostheses.[3,5] Although the newer rotating hinge prosthesis may provide a satisfactory mode of salvage,[39] our experience with this implant has been unsatisfactory.[29] Good-to-excellent results were obtained in 48% of unconstrained or semiconstrained prostheses, compared to 24% with unlinked hinged prostheses or 21% with linked hinged prostheses.[8]

Statistical analysis using an actuarial estimate of the probability of survival of a functioning revision prosthesis was applied to the different prosthetic types. An actuarial technique for estimating prosthesis survival has been used for the evaluation of total hip and total knee replacement.[9,22,35,36] This technique relies on two assumptions for validity. First, the prosthesis survival rate for the untraced group is equal to that of the traced group.[2,4,17] Second, the rate of

prosthesis failure or patient death is the same for all patients regardless of the time of entry into the study.[2,4,17] Although the second assumption may not be valid for all patients undergoing total knee arthroplasty,[36] an actuarial technique allows the advantages of a larger sample size. The sample is not biased by the exclusion of patients on the basis of an arbitrary duration of follow-up.[2,4] In the present series all 427 knees were included in the actuarial analysis. To avoid problems of different prosthesis survival rates related to the time of surgery, the year of implantation was considered in analyzing the effect of constraint using the older prosthetic types. There were no statistically significant differences in prosthesis survival related to the year of surgery. This finding substantiates the validity of use of actuarial technique.

The highest survival probabilities occurred with the cruciate condylar and anametric prostheses. The lowest survival probabilities were noted when a polycentric prosthesis was utilized for revision (Fig. 33-3). Prosthetic survival among the constrained implants did not vary with implant type (Fig. 33-4).

An estimated 5-year prosthesis survival probability of 75% was seen for the single-revision knees (Fig. 33-5), compared with 62% for knees undergoing two revision procedures (Fig. 33-6). Among the knees with a single revision, there was significantly improved ($P<0.002$) prosthesis survival in group 2 in comparison to group 3 (see Fig. 33-5). There was no significant difference in prosthesis survival probabilities between knees in groups 2 and 3 undergoing two revision procedures.

The effect of prosthetic constraint also was analyzed using actuarial methods. Comparing the older semiconstrained (geometric, polycentric, Freeman, duopatellar, Marmor, UCI, RAM, unicompartmental Marmor) to the older constrained prostheses (Spherocentric, Guepar, Tavernetti, Sheehan, Walldius, Herbert, Zimmer hinge, and Buchholtz hinge) revealed no statistically significant differences in prosthetic survival rates, even when the year of implantation was considered (Fig. 33-7). Survival probabilities among the newer implants were better ($P<0.04$) for the less constrained prostheses (such as the anametric, total condylar, cruciate condylar, and kinematic condylar) than for the more constrained prostheses (Total Condylar II, Total Condylar III,

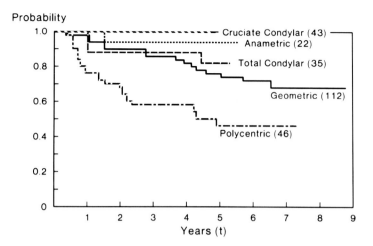

Fig. 33-3. Survival rates for semiconstrained implants in group 1, from first to second revision using actuarial technique. The number of implants is indicated at each survival curve.

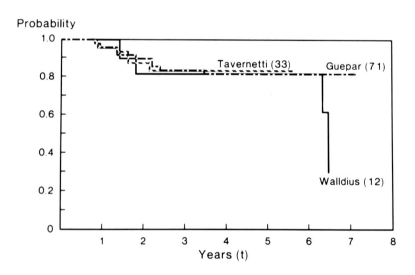

Fig. 33-4. Survival rates for constrained implants in group 1, from first to second revision using actuarial technique. The number of implants is indicated at each survival curve.

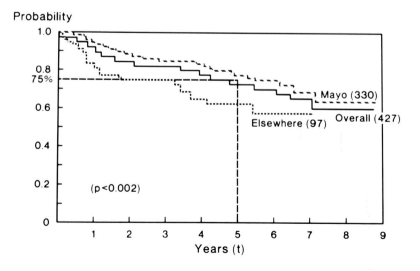

Fig. 33-5. Prosthesis survival rates for knees undergoing one revision. The number of implants is indicated at each survival curve. Prosthesis survival for group 2 superior to that for group 3 ($\underline{P}$ <0.002).

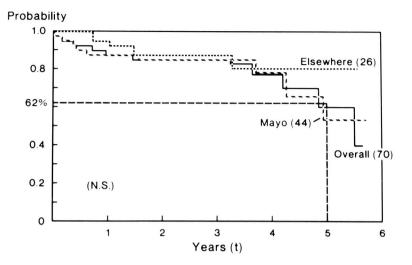

Fig. 33-6. Prosthesis survival rates for knees in group 1 undergoing two revisions. The number of implants is indicated at each survival curve.

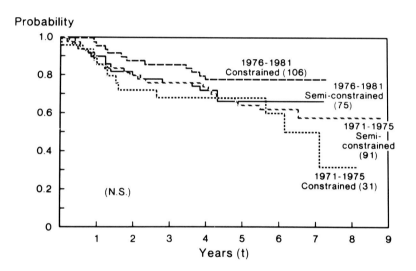

Fig. 33-7. Survival rates for older semiconstrained and constrained implants in group 1 according to year of implantation. The number of implants is indicated at each survival curve.

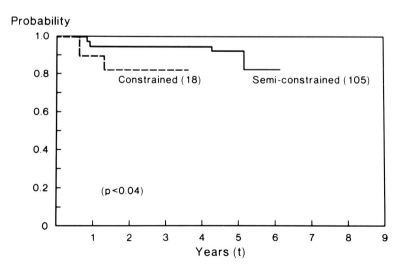

Fig. 33-8. Survival rates in group 1 for the newer semiconstrained implants superior to those for constrained implants ($\underline{P}$ <0.04). The number of implants is indicated at each survival curve.

kinematic stabilizer, and kinematic rotating hinge prosthesis) (Fig. 33-8). The improved estimated prosthesis survival with the newer semiconstrained prostheses may be explained by two mechanisms. First, the less-constrained implant may result in less stress on the bone-cement interface, resulting in a lower incidence of subsequent loosening. Alternatively, the poor survival of the constrained prosthesis simply may represent patient selection. The greater the bone loss and instability, the more likely a surgeon is to use a more constrained prosthesis for salvage. Salvage of the failed constrained implant is also more difficult.[5]

The cruciate condylar prosthesis appears to give the most satisfactory survival curve when used as a revision implant. However, in the current series, only a 67% success rate was achieved in 55 knees using a kinematic condylar, Total Condylar, or cruciate condylar prosthesis. Brady and associates[5] reported satisfactory results using the Total Condylar prosthesis for salvage of the failed total knee arthroplasty. We believe that, in order to minimize bone-cement interface stresses and to preserve bone stock, the least constrained prosthesis that is compatible with satisfactory function should be selected.

Table 33-9. Lucent lines

Location	Width (mm)	Femoral	Tibial
Medial	0-1	0	13 (17.3%)
	1-2	1 (2.3%)	6 (8.0%)
	>2	1 (2.3%)	1 (1.3%)
Anterior	0-1	20 (46.5%)	4 (5.3%)
	1-2	3 (7.0%)	1 (1.3%)
	>2	1 (2.3%)	0
Posterior	0-1	4 (9.3%)	0
	1-2	0	0
	>2	0	0
Medial and lateral	0-1	0	31 (41.3%)
	1-2	1 (2.3%)	12 (16.0%)
	>2	0	0
Anterior and posterior	0-1	4 (9.3%)	0
	1-2	1 (2.3%)	0
	>2	1 (2.3%)	0
General	0-1	1 (2.3%)	0
	1-2	3 (7.0%)	2 (2.7%)
	>2	2 (4.7%)	1 (1.3%)
TOTAL		43	75

LUCENT LINES

The frequency of lucent lines was evaluated only in knees with the newer prosthetic types because the inadequacy of the early generation prostheses has been well documented in the literature. The prostheses studied included the anametric, Total Condylar, Total Condylar II, Total Condylar III, cruciate condylar, kinematic condylar, kinematic stabilizer, and kinematic rotating hinge types. The location and width of the lucent lines were evaluated in detail and analyzed in relation to the clinical results (Table 33-9); 88 knees in 81 patients were reviewed. Follow-up time between the last surgery and the final roentgenogram was a minimum of 1 year, with a mean of 2.8 (1.0 to 6.4) years.

Lucent lines were present in 76 knees (86.4%). Lucent lines were present about 43 femoral and 75 tibial components. Generalized or complete lucent lines were present about six femoral and seven tibial components and about both components in one knee. A lucent line of greater than 2 mm was present about five femoral and two tibial components, and two knees had lucency about both components. In 64 knees with serial roentgenograms, 23 (36%) had progression of lucent lines, as documented by an increase in width or length of the lucent lines. The lines adjoined the femoral component in nine, the tibial component in eight, and both components in six knees. There was no significant correlation between the clinical result and the presence or absence of a lucent line, or its width.

The significance of lucent lines after total knee arthroplasty is unclear. Lucent lines have been noted after initial arthroplasty in 80% of geometric,[33] 22% of Total Condylar,[15] 45% of duopatellar,[34] and 75% of hinge prostheses.[3] Lucent lines greater than 2mm have been reported in 3% of total condylar prostheses.[15] Lucent lines after revision surgery have been reported in 84% of Total Condylar prostheses[12] and 60% of other prostheses.[37,40] In the present series lucent lines were present after revision in 86.4% of the knees with the newer prosthetic types. However, lucent lines greater than 2 mm were noted only in five femoral and two tibial components. Generalized lucent lines were noted in six femoral components and seven tibial components. There was no significant correlation between the presence of lucent lines and the clinical result. Whether the lucent lines will progress to become more symptomatic as the duration of follow-up time increases is unknown, but the findings of progression of the lucent lines in 36% of the knees with serial radiographs in our series are worrisome.

INFECTION

The incidence of positive cultures and the frequency of clinical infection were evaluated. All patients operated on at Mayo Clinic received perioperative antibiotic prophylaxis. The antibiotics used varied during the years of the study in accordance with patient allergies and the preference of the surgeon. Methicillin was most used during the first 5 years of the study and a cephalosporin during the later years. Antibiotics were begun preoperatively and continued for 48 to 72 hours after surgery. If a positive culture was obtained at surgery, the treatment varied with the surgeon and ranged from no treatment to 4 weeks of intravenous antibiotics and subsequent oral antibiotics.

The frequency of infection and positive cultures was evaluated. The incidence of clinical infection in the 427 revision knees was 2.1% (group 2, 2.1%; group 3, 2.0%). For comparison, the overall known incidence of *infection* in 5643 total knee arthroplasties performed at this institution during the same time interval was 1.9%. As part of our standard protocol for total knee replacement, routine cultures were obtained at the time of total knee arthroplasty. The frequency of positive *cultures* was 7.1% at the initial arthroplasty, 11.0% at the first revision, 11.0% at the second, and 8.3% at the third. There was no statistically significant correlation between a positive culture obtained at a previous operation and the subsequent development of a clinical infection.

Infection after total knee arthroplasty has been a difficult problem. Infection rates after non-hinged implants have been between 1.2% and 1.4% with the total condylar prosthesis,[15,16] 1.8% with the geometric prosthesis,[33] and 2.8% with the polycentric prosthesis.[32] Some authors have noted a low correlation,[33] although others have found a significant correlation between a positive operative culture and later prosthetic infection.[32] Infection rates after revision surgery have ranged from 1% to 11%.[13,20] An infection rate of 2.1% in the current series compares favorably with the infection rate of 1.9% in our overall total knee arthroplasty series covering the same time interval. There was no significant correlation between a positive culture obtained at a previous opera-

tion and subsequent clinical infection. The importance of treating incidental cultures obtained at surgery remains controversial.

SUCCESS OF REVISION

A successful result was defined as only mild or no pain, knee flexion to at least 90 degrees, and mild or no instability. When all three criteria were not met, the result was considered unsuccessful. Success was evaluated for all knees. Results are reported for those knees with at least 2 years of follow-up after the last revision (Table 33-10). For knees that were lost to follow-up within 2 years, the assessment of success was based on the last examination. At 2 years a successful result was achieved in 59.6% after a single revision, 51.9% after two revisions, and 50.0% after three revisions.

The results of prosthetic revision for failed total knee arthroplasty reported in the literature are difficult to assess because of variations in criteria for success. Dupont and associates emphasized the importance of pain relief and at least 80 degrees of knee flexion for a successful result.[11] They achieved success in 65% of 103 revision knees.[11] Satisfactory results were obtained in 80% of 116 revisions by Hood and Insall[12] and 89% of 72 knees by Insall and Dethmers.[14] Satisfactory results were obtained in terms of pain relief in 81% of knees, and 81% did not require a subsequent revision surgery in the

Table 33-10. Success after revision total knee arthroplasty

	Lost with less than 2-year follow-up		Greater than 2-year follow-up	
	Number	*Percent*	*Number*	*Percent*
One revision				
Group 1	28	53.6	329	59.6
Group 2	20	54	266	59.7
Group 3	8	75	63	58.7
Two revisions				
Group 1	6	33.3	54	51.9
Group 2	2	100	36	55.6
Group 3	4	0	18	44.4
Three revisions				
Group 1			10	50
Group 2			6	50
Group 3			4	50

series of Kim and Finerman.[20] Satisfactory results were obtained in five of seven knees reported by Ducheyne and associates,[10] seven of ten knees by Ahlberg and Lunden,[1] and nine of 17 knees by Bargar and associates.[3] Good or excellent results of only 30% in 73 revisions was reported by Hunter and coworkers[13] and 37% by Cameron and Hunter.[8] In the present series the relatively poor success rate reflects the deficiencies of the prostheses used for arthroplasty and revision during the early experience with knee arthroplasty. Many failed arthroplasties were salvaged with constrained hinges and other implants that are no longer used. This series should be considered as worst-experience data. The prosthesis survival rate of the newer semiconstrained implants appears to be improving and should continue to do so.

TECHNIQUE OF REVISION

The technique of revision involves nine basic steps: (1) definition of the reason or reasons for failure, (2) assessment of the remaining bone stock and ligaments, (3) determination of the presence or absence of sepsis, (4) removal of the implant, cement, and fibrous membrane, (5) preparation of the bone surfaces, (6) correction of alignment and soft tissue balancing, (7) insertion of the revision prosthesis, (8) postoperative rehabilitation, and (9) patient education.

The reason or reasons for failure must be determined so that the errors that led to failure of the initial arthroplasty are not repeated. The quality and quantity of the remaining bone stock and the integrity of the soft tissues must be assessed because these factors will affect the choice of the revision prosthesis, as well as the ability for salvage. A functioning extensor mechanism and, preferably, intact collateral ligaments are essential for a satisfactory result. Adequate quality and quantity of bone stock must be present or be substituted by a custom prosthesis or bone grafting. Ligament stability, which can be restored, must be evaluated to achieve the proper tensioning of the revision arthroplasty.

The presence of sepsis must be carefully assessed by bone scanning, knee aspiration, hematologic studies, and, finally, by exploration of the knee. This discussion focuses only on the management of the nonseptic revision, but other clinicians have reported on the techniques of assessment.[25,28,29]

Removal of an implant that is not loose may be difficult; a high-speed cutting instrument such as the Midas Rex is invaluable. Dissection should be performed between the implant and cement to preserve bone stock. Occasionally metal-backed components may need to be sectioned with a diamond saw to facilitate their removal. All loose cement should be removed, but some secure cement may be left in situ if its removal would jeopardize bone stock. An interposed fibrous membrane will be present between the bone and cement and should be completely removed. Removal of the prosthesis can be extremely difficult. The surgeon needs to assess thoroughly the order of disassembly, since certain types of prostheses must be taken apart in a reverse manner to their assembly. This procedure is particularly appropriate when considering hinged prostheses or fully constrained prostheses.

Preparation of the bone surface consists of thorough lavage with a high-speed pulsating lavage such as the Water Pik. Lavage removes any remaining loose debris, allows visualization of any remaining cement or fibrous membrane, and leaves a satisfactory surface for the new cement. Areas of sclerotic bone may be penetrated more effectively with new cement by placing several small drill holes in the bone.

Correction of alignment and soft tissue balancing in both flexion and extension must be obtained. Revision instrumentation that relies on the mechanical axis of the limb is available and facilitates this procedure. Excessive scar tissue should be excised to allow soft tissue gliding, but the extensor mechanism and collateral ligaments must be preserved. The stability of the knee and tracking of the patella must be assessed with the provisional components seated and the extensor mechanism reduced.

Standard or revision total knee arthroplasty components may be used. Occasionally a custom prosthetic replacement is necessary. A wide selection of prosthetic components that are compatible must be available. However, custom prosthetic replacement of the proximal tibia below the attachment of the patellar tendon in not advised. Their use here results in severe, uncontrolled flexion deformity. A custom prosthetic replacement of the distal femur is possible because the limb below the knee has its functioning extensor and flexor mechanisms present. We try to use the least-constrained prosthesis possible. Various forms of posterior stabilizing prostheses are most helpful, and it is only rarely necessary to use a fully constrained prosthesis. Occasionally only one portion of the prosthesis need be replaced. Therefore a careful assessment of prosthetic component compatibility should be performed preoperatively and be available at the time of surgery.

In the presence of satisfactory bone stock, insertion of the revision prosthesis does not differ from primary arthroplasty. If a prosthesis with an intramedullary stem is used, more effective cement fixation can be obtained by using techniques adapted from total hip arthroplasty. Plugging of the intramedullary canal, lavage of the intramedullary canal, and pressure injection of the cement will result in a more homogenous column of cement to support the prosthesis. The tibial and femoral implants should be cemented separately, usually beginning with the tibial side. Insertion of the femoral trial component followed by extension of the knee will further pressurize the tibial cement.

Resumption of motion is more difficult following revision surgery. Therefore continuous passive motion is extremely helpful during the early postoperative period, and a carefully supervised program of physical therapy is invaluable. The rehabilitation program may be modified depending on the type of surgical approach and the need for ligamentous reconstruction. A Coonse-Adams turndown of the extensor mechanism should be protected from active extension for 6 weeks. Collateral ligament repair or reconstruction should be protected by a brace for 6 weeks to prevent excessive varus or valgus stresses.

Patient education is essential. The level of activity of the patient must be supervised to obtain longevity of the implant. Avoidance of heavy lifting (greater than 30 pounds), kneeling, impact loading, and sudden changes in direction, acceleration, or deceleration are important. Some difficult revisions with poor bone stock may require protection with a cane indefinitely.

The current interest in noncemented implant fixation offers some hope for the future with patients who are unlikely to be salvaged by cemented implants. In patients who have massive loss of bone, the use of biologic fixation combined with intramedullary stems and bone grafting, although still experimental, appears to offer the best hope of salvage. The design of replacements to reconstitute the normal relationships in regard to ligament and muscular tension is possible, and gradually the components are becoming available in practice.

SUMMARY

Careful attention to axial alignment, soft tissue balance, and stability will minimize prosthetic failure. In revision arthroplasty a prosthesis designed to replace bone loss with the least constraint possible should be used. In the current series revision of the noninfected failed total knee arthroplasty has provided satisfactory results in 50% to 60% of the patients. We believe that use of the newer implants and instrumentation will improve results markedly.

REFERENCES

1. Ahlberg, A., and Lunden, A.: Secondary operations after knee joint replacement, Clin. Orthop. **156:**170-174, 1981.
2. Armitage, P.: Statistical methods in medical research, Oxford, England, 1971, Blackwell Scientific Publications, Ltd.
3. Bargar, W.L., Cracchiolo, A. III, and Amstutz, H.C.: Results with the constrained total knee prosthesis in treating severely disabled patients and patients with failed total knee replacements, J. Bone Joint Surg. **62A:**504-512, 1980.
4. Berkson, J., and Gage, R.P.: Specific methods of calculating survival rates of patients with cancer. In Pack, G.T., and Ariel, I.M., editors: Treatment of cancer and allied diseases, ed. 2, New York, 1958, Paul B. Hoeber.
5. Brady, T.A., Ranawat, C., Kettelkamp, D.B., and Rapp, G.F.: Salvage of the failed total knee arthroplasty (abstract), Orthop. Trans. **1:**101-102, 1977.
6. Bryan, R.S., and Rand, J.A.: Revision total knee arthroplasty, Clin. Orthop. **170:**116-122, 1982.
7. Bryan, R.S., and Rand, J.A.: Revision of total knee arthroplasty. In Ranawat, C.S., editor: Total condylar knee arthoplasty, New York, Springer-Verlag, 1985.
8. Cameron, H.U., and Hunter, G.A.: Failure in total knee arthroplasty: Mechanisms, revisions, and results, Clin. Orthop. **170:**141-146, 1982.
9. Dobbs, H.S.: Survivorship of total hip replacements, J. Bone Joint Surg. **62B:**168-173, 1980.
10. Ducheyne, P., Kagan, A. II, and Lacy, J.A.: Failure of total knee arthroplasty due to loosening and deformation of the tibial component, J. Bone Joint Surg. **60A:**384-391, 1978.
11. Dupont, J.A., Campbell, E.D., Jr., and Lumsden, R.M. III.: Total knee arthroplasty revisions (abstract), Orthop. Trans. **4:**321-322, 1980.
12. Hood, R.W., and Insall, J.N.: Total knee revision arthroplasty: Indications, surgical techniques, and results (abstract), Orthop. Trans. **5:**412-413, 1981.
13. Hunter, G.A., Cameron, H.U., Welsh, R.P., and Bailey, W.H.: The natural history of the failed knee replacement (abstract), Orthop. Trans. **4:**389, 1980.
14. Insall, J.N., and Dethmers, D.A.: Revision of total knee arthroplasty, Clin. Orthop. **170:**123-130, 1982.

15. Insall, J., Scott, W.N., and Ranawat, C.S.: The total condylar knee prosthesis: A report of two hundred and twenty cases, J. Bone Joint Surg. **61A:**173-180, 1979.

16. Insall, J., Tria, A.J., and Scott, W.N.: The total condylar knee prosthesis: The first five years, Clin. Orthop. **145:** 69-77, 1979.

17. Kaplan, E.L., and Meier, P.: Nonparametric estimation from incomplete observations, J. Am. Stat. Assoc. **53:**457-481, 1958.

18. Kettelkamp, D.B., and Chao, E.Y.: A method for quantitative analysis of medial and lateral compression forces at the knee during standing, Clin. Orthop. **83:**202-213, 1972.

19. Kettelkamp, D.B., and Nasca, R.: Biomechanics and knee replacement arthroplasty, Clin. Orthop. **94:**8-14, 1973.

20. Kim, L., and Finerman, G.A.M.: Results of revisions for aseptic failed knee arthroplasties, Orthop. Trans. **7:**535, 1983.

21. Kurnow, R.N., Brass, W., Pike, M.C., Cox, D.R., Durbin, J., Hill, I.D., Stuart, A., and Gehan, E.: Discussion. J. R. Stat. Soc. (A), **135:**199-207, 1972.

22. Lettin, A.W.F., Kavanagh, T.G., Craig, D., and Scales, J.T.: Assessment of the survival and the clinical results of stanmore total knee replacements, J. Bone Joint Surg. **66B:**355-361, 1984.

23. Nogi, J., Caldwell, J.W., Kavzlanich, J.J., and Thompson, R.C., Jr.: Load testing of geometric and polycentric total knee replacement, Clin. Orthop. **114:**235-242, 1976.

24. Peto, R., and Peto, J.: Asymptomatically efficient rank invariant test procedures, J. R. Stat. Soc. **135(A):**185-198, 1972.

25. Rand, J.A., and Bryan, R.S.: Reimplantation for the salvage of an infected total knee arthroplasty, J. Bone Joint Surg. **65A:**1081-1086, 1983.

26. Rand, J.A., and Bryan, R.S.: Revision after total knee arthroplasty, Orthop. Clin. North Am. **13:**201-212, 1982.

27. Rand, J.A., and Coventry, M.B.: Stress fractures after total knee arthroplasty, J. Bone Joint Surg. **62A:**226-233, 1980.

28. Rand, J.A., Morrey, B.F., and Bryan, R.S.: Management of the infected total joint arthroplasty, Orthop. Clin. North Am. **15:**491-504, 1984.

29. Rand, J.A., Stauffer, R.N., and Chao, E.Y.S.: Kinematic rotating hinge total knee arthroplasty, Paper presented to the American Academy of Orthopaedic Surgeons, Las Vegas, 1985.

30. Rand, J.A., Morrey, B.F., Bryan, R.S., and Westholm, F.: Management of the infected total knee arthroplasty, Clin. Orthop., April 1986.

31. Samuelson, K.M., Freeman, M.A.R., and Day, W.H.: Salvage of failed total knee replacements: Is a hinge necessary? (abstract), Orthop. Trans. **4:**98-99, 1980.

32. Skolnick, M.D., Bryan, R.S., Peterson, L.F.A., Combs, J.J., Jr., and Ilstrup, D.M.: Polycentric total knee arthroplasty: A two-year follow-up study, J. Bone Joint Surg. **58A:**743-780, 1976.

33. Skolnick, M.D., Coventry, M.B., and Ilstrup, D.M.: Geometric total knee arthroplasty: A two year follow-up study, J. Bone Joint Surg. **58A:**749-753, 1976.

34. Sledge, C.B., and Ewald, F.C.: Total knee arthroplasty experience at the Robert Breck Brigham Hospital, Clin. Orthop. **145:**78-84, 1979.

35. Surin, V.V., and Sundholm, K.: Survival of patients and prostheses after total hip arthroplasty, Clin. Orthop. **177:**148-153, 1983.

36. Tew, M., and Waugh, W.: Estimating the survival time of knee replacements, J. Bone Joint Surg. **64B:**579-582, 1982.

37. Thornhill, T.S., Hood, R.W., Batte, N.J., Msika, C., and Sledge, C.B.: Knee revision in failed non-infected total knee arthroplasties—The Robert Breck Brigham Hospital and Hospital for Special Surgery experience (abstract), Orthop. Trans. **6:**368, 1982.

38. Turner, R.H.: Revision of total knee replacement implants: Surgical techniques and available implants (abstract), Orthop. Trans. **4:**89, 1980.

39. Turner, R.H., Murray, W.R., Emerson, R.H., Scheller, A.D., Scott, R.D., and Walker, P.: The kinematic rotating hinge for revision knee arthroplasty (abstract), Orthop. Trans. **6:**370, 1982.

40. Wertzberger, K.L., and Bryan, R.S.: Analysis of failed total knee arthroplasty, excluding infection, undergoing re-operation (abstract), Orthop. Trans. **3:**265-266, 1979.

Chapter 34

Infection of total knee arthroplasty

JOHN N. INSALL

Wound infections are customarily described as superficial or deep. Since the term "superficial infection" lacks clarity, we prefer to describe wound drainage that can be either culture negative or culture positive in nature. This description allows inclusion of hematoma and disorders of primary skin healing such as necrosis. Wound drainage in my experience has only an occasional association with deep infection, although of course sometimes one can lead to the other.

Wound drainage is seldom of lasting consequence but may delay rehabilitation and prolong hospitalization. Deep periprosthetic infection, on the other hand, is a catastrophe. In my unit, deep infection is now the major cause of failure of total knee replacement, outnumbering all other causes.

Infections usually are described as early or late. A somewhat arbitrary definition of a late infection is one occurring more than 3 months after initial surgery. In truth many late infections are often early ones, and only the diagnosis is "late."

Causes of deep infection

Early infections usually result from contamination during surgery but in rare instances may follow wound drainage or skin necrosis. Therefore when there is failure of primary wound healing, motion should be stopped to prevent deep contamination.

The cause of a late infection is often obscure. Metastatic infections[1,3,4] may be associated with infection at sites remote from the knee, such as teeth, ulcers, lungs, gastrointestinal tract, and genitourinary tract. In these cases seeding on to the prosthetic knee occurs most likely through transient bacteremia. However, often such a cause is not discernible, and in these cases the surgeon must suspect that the infection was introduced at the time of surgery but remained dormant.

Healing incidence and presentation

The incidence of deep infection (early and late) is about 1%. In spite of routine antibiotic prophylaxis, modern operating theaters, and improved surgical technique, surgical infection has not been eliminated. Because patients are often elderly and obese, and have other medical conditions, a predisposition to failure of wound healing exists, particularly in rheumatoid arthritis. Metastatic infections can be reduced by patient education, and prophylactic antibiotics should be taken to cover dental procedures and to treat obvious infections elsewhere in the body that may put the prosthesis at risk.

DIAGNOSIS

Early infections should be suspected when the patient's preoperative course is abnormal. Obviously, experience helps in this recognition, given the wide variation of patient recovery. Persistent fever and excessive swelling and pain beyond the first week usually are cause for concern. The sedimentation rate and white count may be helpful, but when there is doubt aspiration of the joint is indicated.

The diagnosis of a late infection can be elusive.[8] A painful total knee arthroplasty without detectable mechanical cause should indicate infection until proved otherwise. The recommended procedure to establish the presence of infection is a knee aspiration performed under strict aseptic precautions. The fluid aspirated is sent immediately to the bacteriology laboratory for sensitivity tests, direct smear, Gram stain, and anaerobic, microbacterial, and fungal cultures. Occasionally the infecting organism can be an indolent kind of bacteria. To increase the chances of bacterial growth, the aspirate should be inoculated as soon as possible in the appropriate broth and culture medium. A transport system with a culture medium to support the bacteria during the time of transport is recommended.

If enough fluid is aspirated from the knee, a complete cell count and differential also may give valuable information. If the complete count shows more than 25,000 polymorphonuclear leukocytes per milliliter and if the differential count is more than 75% of these white cells, infection should be suspected. Obviously the higher the number of polymorphonuclear leukocytes, the greater the possibility of infection. Fluid also should be sent for glucose and protein levels. In the normal synovial fluid the protein levels are about one third of serum levels, whereas in infection they approach serum levels. Glucose values in synovial fluid are similar to those of plasma. In the presence of infection synovial glucose values are lowered because of the presence of organisms that use sugar in their metabolism. Thus measures of low glucose and high protein are compatible with infection.

If the diagnosis is still unclear once all this information is gathered and if the clinical suspicion of infection is strong, an open biopsy is indicated. At surgery a thorough debridement is done; frozen tissue sections, complete Gram stains, cultures of the tissue, and the macroscopic appearance of the wound also should provide diagnostic information. In suspected early infections the prosthetic components should be left in situ. However, when the infection is late, the components should be removed because positive cultures may be obtained only from the interface of the prosthesis, cement, and bone (Fig. 34-1).

I condemn procrastination and the prolonged use of oral antibiotics, particularly when infection is only suspected and not confirmed by bacteriologic evidence. The result is likely to be an indolent subclinical infection and a painful prosthesis. In addition, subsequent cultures of the organism may become very difficult to obtain even after the components have been removed, so that proper and appropriate antibiotic therapy is impossible and ultimate salvage of the arthroplasty by reimplantation of another prosthesis is much less likely.

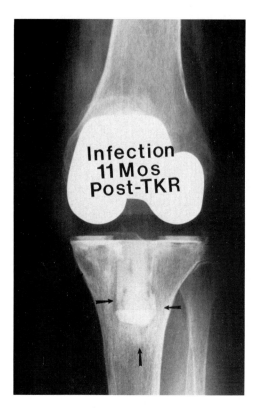

Fig. 34-1. Although radiographs often are not helpful in the diagnosis of late infection, the presence of a complete or patchy radiolucency around the components is highly suspicious of infection. In this case aspiration fluid from the knee cultured *Pseudomonas* organisms. However, even when cultures of the joint fluid prove negative, we recommend exploration and removal of the components whenever radiographic appearance such as this is present.

I have no experience in the use of radioisotopes to differentiate mechanical loosening from septic loosening in total knee replacement, although this procedure has been used in the diagnosis of infected total hip arthroplasties.

TREATMENT

I do not believe that infections complicating total knee replacements should be treated with antibiotic therapy alone, which may transiently suppress the symptoms of infection. This treatment may be indicated only as a temporary measure if surgery is contraindicated because of medical reasons or if the patient does not accept surgery. Antibiotic therapy alone is unlikely to cure the infectious process. Furthermore, its use can complicate the problem by selecting resistant strains.

Early infection

When the diagnosis of infection is made early in the postoperative phase, particularly when the patient is still hospitalized, incision, drainage, and debridement are indicated, leaving the components in situ. The wound is closed over wide-bore suction drains that are removed at 36 hours. I do not favor closed-suction irrigation because of the risk of exogenous suprainfection. Intravenous antibiotic therapy is begun in the manner described later. After 2 weeks the wound is inspected and reaspirated under strict aseptic conditions. If the wound is benign and the cultures are negative, antibiotic therapy is continued for a further 4 weeks; if not, reoperation with removal of the prosthetic components and all cement is performed.

Late infection

I believe that the treatment for proved or suspected late deep infection is thorough debridement of the involved tissues and removal of the prosthetic components with acrylic cement. Adequate preoperative planning is necessary, and the availability of special instruments is recommended. Removal of the prosthetic components and acrylic cement can be a difficult task because, if the septic process is recent, the prosthetic components most likely will not be loose. Therefore removal of the tight interdigitation between the bone and cement will demand a laborious, patient, and meticulous technique to prevent unnecessary loss of bone stock. After the debridement the bone ends are allowed to come into contact to reduce dead space. To maintain close apposition in case reimplantation is not possible, a single absorbable suture is passed through the medial-tibial and femoral cortices and loosely tied. Wide-bore suction drains are introduced, the wound is closed, and a heavily padded dressing with plaster splint reinforcement is applied.

According to the patient's response to antibiotic therapy the future options are (1) prolonged immobilization to produce a painless pseudarthrosis, (2) arthrodesis,[5] and (3) reimplantation of another prosthesis.[6,7]

When the response to antibiotic therapy is favorable and the patient is willing and robust enough to undergo a second surgical procedure, my recommendation is to reimplant another prosthesis. The procedure may not be suitable for surgeons without extensive experience or for every patient with a deep infection. The proper

timing of reimplantation after antibiotic therapy must be based on the appearance of the wound. When doubt about the appearance exists, an aspiration should be done, antibiotics should be discontinued, and the wound should be observed for a few weeks before making a decision. Experience is required to make the correct judgment concerning the timing of the reimplantation. However, if the tissue about the wound appear benign with no edema or inflammation and if there is no pain, then reimplantation can proceed. When the knee is exposed, Gram stains of the wound exudate are done, and the tissue specimen is sent for examination of a frozen section. If any organisms are found or if the presence of polymorphonuclear leukocytes suggests acute inflammation, the wound is closed without proceeding further. If the surgeon has any doubt about the condition of the tissues, it is better to discontinue the procedure and await further cultures.

Technically, reimplantation is feasible for at least 3 months after removal of the components. Beyond this time soft tissue contracture makes exposure very difficult, and restoration of worthwhile motion is unlikely. I recommend the posterior stabilized condylar prosthesis (Fig. 34-2) for reimplantation because the posterior cruciate ligament is usually absent and correct spacing between the femur and the tibia during flexion and extension is difficult to obtain. Posterior subluxation in flexion may occur if a total condylar type prosthesis is used, and the fit in flexion is loose. The posterior stabilized prosthesis can be used even when the previous device was hinged, because an adequate soft tissue sleeve around the joint is usually present. It is desirable to avoid the use of an intramedullary stem for reimplantation because such devices[2] are difficult to remove should the infection recur. However, a total condylar III prosthesis sometimes may be needed to obtain medial-lateral stability.

The final selection of the prosthesis to be used for reimplantation can be made during the operation. When obvious and pronounced loss of bone stock exists, custom components with or without intramedullary stems may be needed. When the reimplantation is especially difficult, a turndown of the quadriceps mechanism (modified Coonse-Adams) is needed. Some periosteal dissection of the collateral ligament attachments to the femur sometimes may be needed to skeletonize the lower femur and aid exposure. It is important to

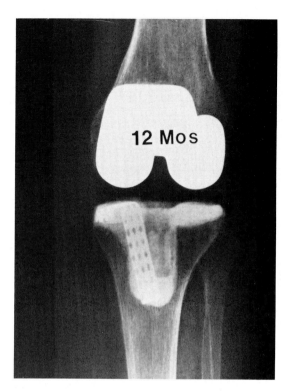

Fig. 34-2. The 12-month radiograph after reimplantation of the infected knee shown in Fig. 34-1. The reimplantation was the posterior stabilized condylar prosthesis, and reinforcement with titanium wire mesh was used for a small medial tibial bony defect.

reestablish the normal posterior recess by stripping the posterior capsule from the back of the femur as the knee is flexed. After a prolonged reimplatation time, capsular and skin closure may be difficult; on occasion we have found it necessary to excise the patella to aid in soft tissue closure.

Medical management of infection

Antibiotic management is critical. An infectious disease consultant should orchestrate the selection, dosages, and synergistic combinations of drugs on the basis of serum bactericidal levels determined periodically during treatment. The antibiotics should be selected to maintain adequate bactericidal levels with the least toxicity.

My medical colleagues and I believe that intravenous therapy is necessary; therefore continued hospitalization is required. All patients are given parenteral antibiotics for at least 6 weeks after removal of the prosthesis. Our antimicrobial regimens were designed on the basis of quantitative in vivo sensitivity studies in which the minimum bactericidal concentrations of a variety of antibiotics were determined for each infecting organism. Once therapy has been instituted, its adequacy is confirmed by testing the serum bactericidal titers using a serial twofold tube-dilution method to determine the ability of increasingly dilute concentrations of the patient's serum to kill the infecting organism. The test was terminated at the highest dilution of serum that caused 99% destruction of a standard inoculum of the infecting organism. A serum bactericidal level of 1 to 8 or greater was set arbitrarily as the adequate antibiotic level to resolve the infection, on the basis of the accepted effectiveness of similar titers in the treatment of bacterial endocarditis.

The initial antibiotic treatment may require changing to obtain adequate serum levels. For example, a *Staphylococcus aureus* infection in one patient was treated serially with nafcillin, vancomycin, nafcillin, and finally ampicillin. Another *Staphylococcus aureus* infection was treated initially with cephalothin for 5 days and then with nafcillin and gentamicin for 6 weeks. Drug synergy was exploited to treat relatively resistant organisms. A mixed infection was treated with three drugs given simultaneously, vancomycin, cefazolin, and clindamycin.

In some cases antibiotic therapy may be discontinued for 1 to 2 weeks before reimplantation to observe the patient for signs of recurrence and to ensure that the culture of the tissue specimen obtained at operation would not be influenced by antibiotic suppression. At the time of reimplantation, prophylactic antibiotics are withheld until operative specimens have been obtained for culture. The usual prophylactic antibiotic regimen (cephalothin or oxacillin) is given after reimplantation because it is assumed that the original infection has resolved and only routine prophylaxis is required. All antibiotics are discontinued 3 to 8 days after reimplantation if the cultures of the specimens obtained at reoperation show no growth.

We have not had complications attributable to antibiotic therapy. The patients were monitored for signs of leukopenia and renal dysfunction and for auditory dysfunction when ototoxic drugs are used.

RESULTS

In the years 1977 to 1983, we treated 43 infected knee arthroplasties on the Knee Service.

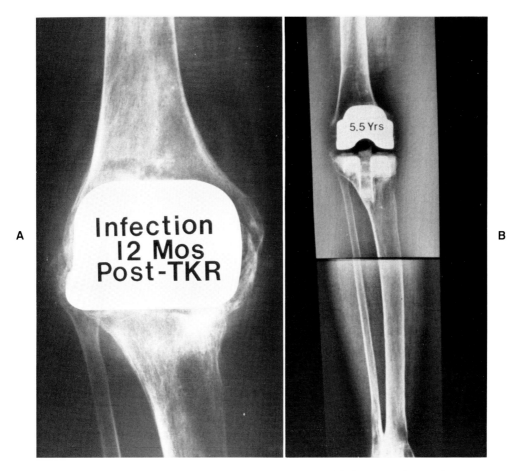

Fig. 34-3. Chronic infection since the time of surgery had led to subsidence of the tibial component. **A,** At the time of reimplantation it was found impossible to close the capsular layer even though extra-small prosthetic components were used. To obtain closure a patellectomy was necessary. **B,** Radiograph showing the appearance 5½ years after reimplantation. The range of motion in the knee is from 0 to 90 degrees. Extension is full without a lag in spite of the patellectomy, but muscle strength is reduced so the patient uses a cane when walking.

After removal of the prosthesis and performance of antibiotic therapy according to the outlined protocol, 30 knees were judged suitable for reimplantation, which was performed after an interval ranging from 6 to 10 weeks following removal. These patients now have a follow-up period of 1 to 7 years. According to the knee rating form used at The Hospital for Special Surgery, the results are excellent in 15 knees (47%), good in 10 knees (31%), fair in 6 knees (19%), and poor in 1 knee (3%). The one poor result was a result of a recurrent infection, the only one in our series to date. The six knees with the fair results showed no evidence of infection at the time of follow-up; this rating resulted from extensor mechanism weakness and extension lag.

I have on occasion mentioned patellectomy to obtain soft tissue closure (Fig. 34-3, *A* and *B*); also contributing to an extension lag is the need to turn down the quadriceps for exposure during reimplantation. Were it not for this deficiency, these six knees would have had a good rating, because in other respects the reconstruction was satisfactory. These results following reimplantation are comparable to our results of revision surgery for aseptic causes.

Eleven knees were excluded from the reimplantation protocol either because the patient refused the treatment, the infecting organism was refractory to antibiotic therapy, or gross sepsis could not be controlled. In two of these the prosthesis was removed, resulting in a pseudarthrosis (one painless and one painful). In two cases with late infections of Guepar prosthesis the tissues were so devitalized that high thigh amputation was required to control the sepsis. In one knee the prosthesis was eventually removed and successfully reimplanted. Of the remaining six knees, three had active sepsis with draining sinuses at the time of review and three patients died of other causes while on antibiotic suppression.

It is our experience that the best treatment for an infected prosthesis is removal and reimplantation whenever possible. When the protocol cannot be followed, retention of a functioning arthroplasty has been unusual.

REFERENCES

1. Artz, T.D., Macys, J., Salvati, E.A., Jacobs, B., and Wilson, P.D., Jr.: Hematogenous infection of total hip replacements: A report of four cases, J. Bone Joint Surg. **57A:** 1024, 1975.
2. Bargar, W.L., Cracchiolo, A. III, and Amstutz, H.C.: Results with the constrained total knee prosthesis in treating severly disabled patients and patients with failed total knee replacements, J. Bone Joint Surg. **62A:**504, 1980.
3. Cruess, R.L., Bickel, W.S., and von Kessler, K.L.C.: Infections in total hips secondary to a primary source elsewhere, Clin. Orthop. **106:**99, 1975.
4. D'Ambrosia, R.D., Shoji, H., and Heater, R.: Secondarily infected total joint replacements by hematogenous spread, J. Bone Joint Surg. **58A:**450, 1976.
5. Hagemann, W.F., Woods, G.W., and Tullos, H.S.: Arthrodesis in failed total knee replacement, J. Bone Joint Surg. **60A:**790, 1978.
6. Insall, J.N., Thompson, F.M., and Brause, B.D.: Two-stage reimplantation for the salvage of infected total knee arthroplasty, J. Bone Joint Surg. **65A:**1088, 1983.
7. Salvati, E.A., Brause, B.D., Chekofsky, K.M., Wilson, P.D., Jr., Thompson, F.M., Insall, J.N., and Ranawat, C.S.: Reimplantation in infected total joint arthroplasty, Orthop. Trans. **5:**449, 1981.
8. Salvati, E.A., and Insall, J.N.: The management of sepsis in total knee replacement. In Savastano, A.A., editor: Total knee replacement, New York, 1980, Appleton-Century-Crofts.

Chapter 35

Knee arthrodesis

JAMES A. RAND

Until recently treatment of the severely damaged knee from arthritis, infection, or severe ligamentous instability was by arthrodesis. With the advent of total knee arthroplasty, prosthetic replacement has become the more common mode of initial management. However, with the increasing number of arthroplasties and extended time in use, prosthetic failure has become a problem. Prosthetic failure may occur by a wide variety of mechanisms including loosening, instability, implant settling, bone fracture, prosthesis fracture, malalignment, malposition, and infection.*

Infection has remained a major unsolved problem. The infection rate in large series of total knee arthroplasties has ranged from a low of 1% with a resurfacing prosthesis to as high as 16.0% with a kinematic rotating hinge.[49,77] Between 1970 and 1983 7308 total knee arthroplasties were performed at the Mayo Clinic with an overall infection rate of 1.51%.[75]

FACTORS PREDISPOSING TO INFECTION

A variety of factors has been suggested as predisposing to prosthetic infection. On an experimental basis, Blomgren and Lundgren have found surrounding the implant and cement a decreased tissue vitality that impairs local defense mechanisms.[4,5] Particulate metal debris, especially chromium and cobalt, appears to impair local defense mechanisms and results in a foreign body response.[61,73] Petty and Green found that low concentrations of polymethylmethacrylate in vitro inhibit leukocyte chemotaxis, phagocytosis, and killing ability.[35,68,69,70] On a clinical basis several factors have been associated with postoperative infection. A history of ancient septic arthritis, rheumatoid arthritis, previous surgery on the affected knee, or concurrent sepsis elsewhere in the body have all been implicated in postoperative infection.* High-dose corticosteroids either systemically or intraarticularly have been implicated in postoperative infection.[37,86,90] Any factor that impairs the well-being of the host, such as diabetes mellitus, poor nutrition, old age, or obesity, may increase the potential for infection.[37] Prolonged preoperative hospitalization may allow colonization of the skin with antibiotic-resistant organisms, making antibiotic prophylaxis less effective.[66]

Careful surgical technique is of utmost importance. Any time there is failure of primary wound healing, whether resulting from skin necrosis, wound dehiscence, or need to evacuate a postoperative hematoma, there is a potentially increased risk for infection.[70] In addition, the size of the foreign body may be important, because there is an increased incidence of infection surrounding large, articulating metal implants.[2]

The surgical environment cannot be ignored. Any factor that leads to increased operative contamination of the wound potentially increases the risk of infection. Therefore the duration of surgery, frequency of air exchange, dress of the personnel, and the use of laminar air flow become important variables.[30,66,83]

*References 1, 6, 20, 26, 33, 39, 51, 80, 84, 85, 87.

*References 13, 30, 37, 46, 47, 70, 90.

SALVAGE OPTIONS

Regardless of the technique of salvage chosen, the objectives for management of the infected total knee arthroplasty remain the same. There must be eradication of the infection, limb salvage, preservation of all bone stock to allow whatever reconstructive procedure is chosen, and maintenance of a functional extremity. Eradication of the infection is the first priority. An infected arthroplasty can lead to generalized sepsis and a fatal outcome. Surgical debridement remains the mainstay of therapy. Systemic antibiotics alone are rarely of value.[49,82]

A variety of options is available for management of the infected total knee arthroplasty. Early surgical debridement within the first 24 to 48 hours following the onset of infection may occasionally salvage a prosthesis. Reimplantation appears to be most valuable when used in the presence of a low-virulence microorganism and when performed as a delayed technique.[48,74] Resection arthroplasty in our experience has proved to be unpredictable and frequently requires the use of a brace for support.[26,51,52] Amputation should be reserved for those individuals with life-threatening sepsis or sepsis combined with massive bone loss. Arthrodesis provides a painless stable base of support but at the expense of knee motion.

INDICATIONS FOR ARTHRODESIS

The classical indications for knee arthrodesis have included infection, tumor, severe ligamentous instability, paralysis, severe bone loss, and neuropathic arthropathy.* Recently, failure of total knee arthroplasty has been added to this list.† Relative contraindications to arthrodesis include ipsilateral ankle or hip disease, severe segmental bone loss, contralateral leg amputation, and bilateral knee disease.[17] It is interesting that Charnley noted 11 patients who were satisfied with a bilateral knee arthrodesis.[17]

Perhaps, in the presence of one of these relative contraindications to arthrodesis, reimplantation or resection arthroplasty should be pursued more vigorously.

---

*References 9, 14, 19, 22, 23, 27, 31, 32, 42-44, 62, 64, 88, 94.
†References 3, 12, 24, 25, 28, 36, 38, 40, 50, 55, 56, 71, 75, 78, 92, 93, 95-98.

PROBLEMS WITH ARTHRODESIS

The problems inherent with arthrodesis as a salvage for the failed total knee arthroplasty are those of bone loss, shortening, and gait disturbance.[40,60] If infection is also present, the surgeon has the additional problems of soft tissue management and eradication of the infection. Hankin and associates have studied experimentally the quantity of bone remaining for arthrodesis following a variety of failed total knee arthroplasties.[40] The least bone was sacrificed by a polycentric and the most with a Walldius hinge. The largest interface remained following a Townley prosthesis. However, once additional bone was removed to allow knee arthrodesis, the total quantity of bone removed varied only 55 mm among the various prosthetic types.[38] Shortening ranged from 3.0 to 3.5 cm.[40] In clinical studies shortening has ranged from a low of 3 cm to as much as 7.5 cm.[95] Knee arthrodesis also results in an increased energy expenditure for normal ambulation.[60]

TECHNICAL FACTORS

A careful technique of arthrodesis is essential. Adequate bone apposition is the key. Ideally, there should be healthy, vascular cancellous bone opposed to healthy, vascular cancellous bone. Projections of bone may exist that can be made to interdigitate, such as following a geometric or polycentric arthroplasty, and the patella is an excellent source for local bone graft. Some of the easiest circumstances in which to obtain arthrodesis follow a resurfacing prosthesis with minimal loss of bone stock. However, in the case of a hinged arthroplasty or any prosthesis with a large intramedullary stem, only a small shell of cortical bone may remain, resulting in poor bone contact (Fig. 35-1). In these cases, the surgeon should consider additional cancellous bone grafting to improve the surfaces for bone apposition combined with prolonged immobilization. Bone grafting may be performed either at the time of delayed wound closure or as a Papineau technique.[56] The bone graft should be placed peripherally about the arthrodesis site to allow revascularization from the surrounding soft tissues, because the intramedullary circulation has been compromised by the previous prosthesis and cement (Fig. 35-2).

The optimal position of knee arthrodesis has been suggested as slight flexion.[17] In view of the

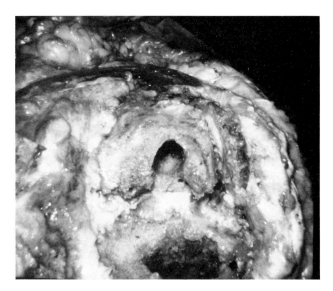

Fig. 35-1. The small rim of cortical bone remaining after removal of a total knee arthroplasty with an intramedullary stem.

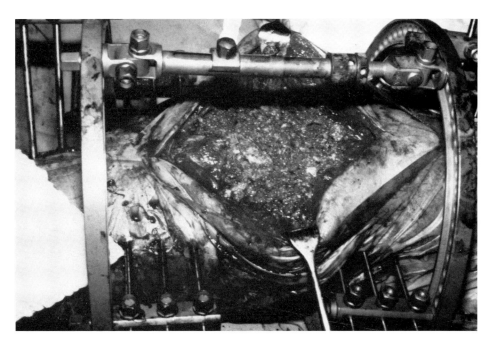

Fig. 35-2. Peripheral placement of combined autogenous iliac and homogenous bone graft about the arthrodesis site.

degree of shortening that occurs, the optimal position is closer to full extension and should be no more than 20 degrees. A position of 5 to 10 degrees of flexion is generally satisfactory.

Adequate wound management is essential. Thorough debridement of all infected granulation tissue and removal of the prosthesis and all cement are required. Delayed wound closure is most predictable, but occasionally primary wound closure may be acceptable following an extensive debridement procedure. If closed suction irrigation is used to help control hematoma formation, it should not be continued for more than 24 to 48 hours to prevent the risk of superinfection.

A variety of techniques has been used in primary knee arthrodesis, including intramedullary nails, plates, pins, and external fixation.* In the Mayo experience a successful arthrodesis was achieved following a failed total knee arthroplasty in 39 of 45 cases using external fixation, compared to two of three with crossed pins, one of two with a plate, and one of three with a cast alone.[12] The importance of adequate fixation has been recognized. Hankin and associates have found an improved success rate of arthrodesis using a two-pin rather than a single-pin Charnley clamp.[40] Similar results were reported by Knutson and associates, with 25 of 43 arthrodeses that were successful with multiple pin fixation, compared to 11 of 36 with a single-pin Charnley clamp.[55] External fixation remains our technique of choice because it allows wound management, does minimal damage to the bone vascularity that has already been compromised by the previous prosthesis and cement, and allows the application of compression across the bone surfaces.† The disadvantages of external fixation are possible pin-tract infection, neurovascular injury during pin insertion, and difficulty in providing anteroposterior stability.‡

Chao and coworkers from our biomechanics laboratory have studied the bending stiffness of a variety of external fixation devices.[11] Regardless of the device chosen with uniplanar pin fixation, there is poor rigidity in the anteroposterior bending mode. We have modified our technique based on this information to include an anterior frame and half pins to help control these forces. A successful result using biplanar external fixation in six of seven knees has been reported by Brooker and Hanson,[13] and an improved success rate with biplanar external fixation has been reported by Rothacker and Cabanela, with union occurring in six of six cases with biplanar external fixation compared to 31 of 37 cases with uniplanar pin fixation.[78]

SURGICAL TECHNIQUE

The technique for knee arthrodesis using external fixation consists of four basic steps: (1) removal of the prosthesis, (2) preparation of the bony bed, (3) application of the external fixator, and (4) bone grafting if necessary. The surgical approach should use preexisting surgical incisions whenever feasible to prevent areas of skin necrosis between the old and new incisions. A longitudinal anteromedial approach is ideal.

Removal of the implant may be relatively easy if it is loose. However, in the case of a secure component, a high-speed cutting instrument such as a Midas Rex has proved invaluable. Dissection should be made in the plane between the prosthesis and cement to prevent loss of bone stock. In a case of metal-backed components, it may be necessary occasionally to transect the metal component to remove it without damage to the bone. All cement, from the surface of the bone and from an intramedullary location, should be removed. Retained cement can act as a stress riser, as well as a source for residual sepsis in the future. An interposed fibrous membrane that will be present at the bone-cement interface and any infected granulation tissue must be thoroughly removed. A high-speed pulsating lavage should be used to prepare the bone surfaces because this will allow identification of any retained fragments of cement or fibrous membrane.

Correct alignment consists of a correct mechanical axis with the knee in slight flexion of no more than 20 degrees. Alignment can be determined best by placing a radiographic marker over the hip before surgery. This will allow intraoperative definition of the mechanical axis of the limb by palpating the previously placed radiographic marker, as well as the center of the ankle. The mechanical axis should extend from the center of the femoral head to the center of the ankle and pass through the center of the knee.

---

*References 7-9, 15-18, 36, 41, 53, 54, 57, 59, 63, 67, 72, 79, 89.
†References 16-18, 53, 63, 78, 89.
‡References 16-18, 53, 63, 78, 89.

Standard total knee arthroplasty instrumentation also is very helpful in preparing the bony bed. To obtain healthy vascular cancellous bone, 2 to 3 mm of the proximal tibia, as well as the distal femur, should be resected. A tibial cutting guide is used to make a transverse cut on the tibia in both the coronal and sagittal planes, removing 2 mm of bone. Some residual defects that can be bone grafted may be left, but a stable peripheral cortical rim should be preserved.

The knee is placed in the proper degree of flexion and alignment, and, by using a distal femoral cutting guide, an osteotomy of the distal femur is performed. Approximately 2 to 3 mm of bone are removed from the distal femur to expose a healthy, vascular cancellous bed. The bone ends are then approximated and should be stable with correct alignment.

The external fixator may be applied. Three transfixing pins are used in the distal femur and three in the proximal tibia, all with a threaded central portion. A 5 mm titanium pin is best because it provides the greatest rigidity of fixation. The femoral pins are placed from the medial side and the tibial pins from the lateral side to prevent impingement on neurovascular structures. The Ace-Fischer apparatus uses a cannula for pin placement through the soft tissues to bone. The central obturator is removed and the hole for the pin predrilled. This procedure minimizes thermal necrosis of the bone and subsequent pin-tract problems.[29,91] All the pins should be parallel. To prevent tethering of the soft tissues by the pins, traction should be applied to the soft tissues at the time of pin insertion.

After the pins have been placed, the semicircular rings are attached to the pins, and three connecting bars are used to join the two rings. One connecting bar is placed anteriorly in the midline and the other two bars are placed posteriorly. The rings should be placed so that they extend posterior to the pin sites to allow the connecting bars to be placed posterior to the axis of the limb. The three connecting bars are then compressed. Only hand tightening is required to obtain a considerable amount of force, and some plastic deformation of the pins will occur. Once the apparatus has been assembled, alignment again should be checked. Some anteroposterior instability will remain before application of the anterior pins. Two anterior half pins are placed in the distal femur, and two half pins are placed in the proximal tibia and connected to the semicircular rings. In the case of a hinge prosthesis, poor bone stock will exist and the anterior half pins should be placed on the outside of the ring. In the case of a resurfacing prosthesis, the anterior half pins may be placed on the inside of the ring.

Bone grafting now may be performed. If extensive loss of intramedullary bone has occurred, as in the case of a hinged prosthesis, cancellous bone grafting about the periphery of the arthrodesis should be performed. A combination of autogenous iliac cancellous bone and homogenous bone from the bone bank is finely ground in a bone mill. In the case of a resurfacing prosthesis with remaining small bony defects, there may be little or no need for bone grafting. The patella can be used as a source of bone graft to fill small defects in the proximal tibia or distal femur before application of the external fixator.

Suction drains are placed in the wound, and the wound is closed in the routine manner. A bulky Robert-Jones dressing is used for the first 4 to 5 days and then may be removed, routine pin-site care then may begin.

ANTIBIOTICS

Systemic antibiotics based on culture reports are administered intravenously for 4 weeks. Additional oral antibiotics are administered for a variable period of time. The antibiotic regimen chosen should be bactericidal and achieve adequate bone and soft tissue concentrations; therapy should be monitored based on serum antibiotic levels.[10]

TIME TO UNION

The time to arthrodesis following the failed total knee arthroplasty which has ranged from a low of 2.5 months following a resurfacing prosthesis to 22 months with a hinged arthroplasty,[23,93] depends on the prosthesis type and the extent of previous surgery. Our technique is to maintain external fixation for 2 to 3 months until bone union is believed to be occurring, followed by a cylinder cast for 2 to 4 months. Additional bracing may be required until the arthrodesis is solid. Since it is often difficult to determine when bone union has occurred, tomography is of value in this decision.

ILLUSTRATIVE CASE

A 74-year-old woman with osteoarthritis had a right kinematic condylar total knee arthroplasty

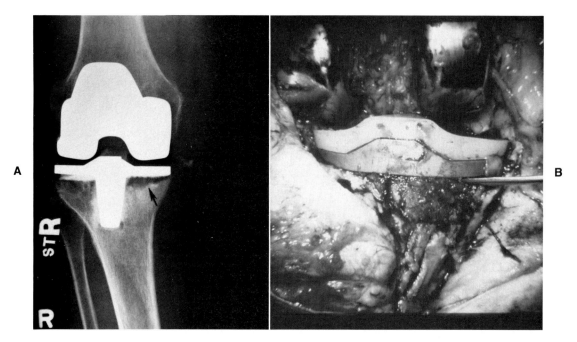

Fig. 35-3. A, AP radiograph. **B,** Surgical appearance of a kinematic condylar total knee arthroplasty with a *Pseudomonas aeruginosa* infection. There is infected granulation tissue beneath the medial aspect of the tibial component.

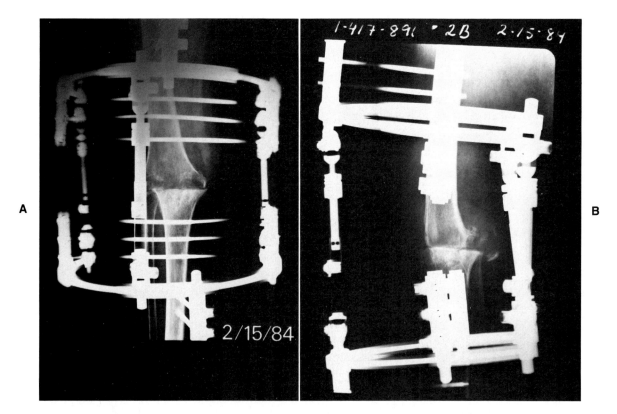

Fig. 35-4. A, AP radiograph. **B,** Lateral radiograph. **C,** Clinical appearance after arthrodesis with a biplanar Ace-Fisher apparatus.

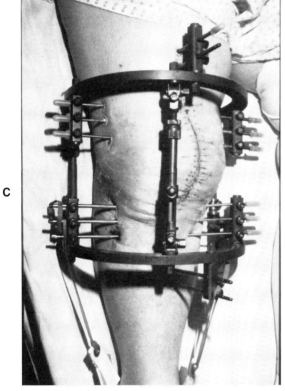

Fig. 35-4, Cont'd. For legend see p. 330.

performed 2 months previously. She developed an infection with *Pseudomonas aerginosa*. When she was referred to the Mayo Clinic, she had obvious infection with an area of advancing osteolysis beneath the tibial component, which is indicative of infected granulation tissue (Fig. 35-3). The implant, cement, and granulation tissue were removed, and arthrodesis was performed with a biplanar Ace-Fischer external fixator (Fig. 35-4). She received 4 weeks of intravenous antibiotics. At 2 months the external fixator was removed and a cylinder cast was applied for an additional 6 weeks. There was union of the arthrodesis 6 months after surgery (Fig. 35-5).

RESULTS OF ARTHRODESIS

The results of compression arthrodesis of the knee for the failed total knee arthroplasty vary considerably,* and are generally better following a resurfacing prosthesis than following a hinged arthroplasty (Table 35-1). In the Mayo series an 81% success rate was achieved following a resurfacing prosthesis compared to a 56% success rate following a hinged arthroplasty.[12] Combined re-

*References 3, 12, 21, 38, 45, 55, 70, 81, 95.

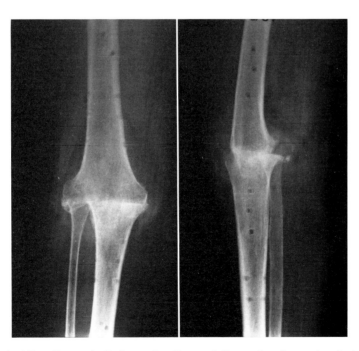

Fig. 35-5. A, AP radiograph. **B,** Lateral radiograph 6 months after arthrodesis. There is union in a satisfactory position.

Table 35-1. Comparison of results

Author	Prosthesis	Success
Petty	Resurfacing	4/6
Hageman	Resurfacing	7/10
Brodersen	Resurfacing	29/36
Vahvanen	Resurfacing	4/8
Knutson	Resurfacing	30/44
Debruge	Hinged	3/14
Hui	Hinged	2/3
Hageman	Hinged	4/7
Brodersen	Hinged	5/9
Salvati	Various	4/14
Knutson	Constrained	22/43

sults of the multiple series in the literature using compression arthrodesis of the knee following a failed total knee arthroplasty reveal a success rate of 73% for a resurfacing prosthesis, 43% for a hinged arthroplasty, or 58% overall. This must be compared to a 95% to 98% success rate for primary compression arthrodesis of the knee.[16-18]

COMPLICATIONS

The complications associated with compression arthrodesis of the knee for the failed total knee arthroplasty are those related to the technique, such as pin-tract infection, neurovascular injury, and malalignment—which should be preventable —and the complications of ipsilateral limb fracture and failure of arthrodesis. Minor pin-tract inflammation and drainage are not infrequent; however, serious pin-tract infection occurred in only one patient in the Mayo series.[12] Pin-tract problems can be minimized by predrilling the pins, and adequate soft tissue releases adjacent to the pin sites.[29,34,58] Ipsilateral limb fracture complicates treatment of 10% to 15% of patients following arthrodesis and probably reflects a long lever arm acting at the fracture site.[91] Stress risers, such as pin tracts either with or without the pin in place, and retained fragments of cement may be contributing factors. Retained cement is also detrimental because it can act as a residual source of sepsis.

The most frequent complication is failure of arthrodesis. The etiology of failure has generally been that of bone loss, persistent sepsis, or re-

peated manipulation leading to loss of bone apposition.[12] If repeat attempts at arthrodesis are performed, shortening may be severe (up to 7.5 cm in Vahvanen's series); the overall success rate for repeat knee arthrodesis is approximately 50%.[55,75,95]

A recent review of the Mayo Clinic experience with arthrodesis for the failed total knee arthroplasty revealed failure in 25 of 120 attempts or 21%.[75] The criterion for failure was no union 1 year after the initial surgical procedure or reoperation to obtain union.[76] A successful arthrodesis occurred in 5 of 14 initial attempts, 4 of 8 second attempts, and 1 of 2 third attempts; a single fourth attempt at arthrodesis was unsuccessful.[75] The most frequent reasons for failure were bone loss and poor bone apposition. However, seven initial attempts at arthrodeses failed for no obvious reason. The reason for the initial attempts at arthrodesis was sepsis in 20 of the 25 knees, but subsequent attempts at arthrodesis were related primarily to pain and instability resulting from pseudarthrosis.[75]

Functional results in terms of pain relief and walking ability were better for those knees that obtained union than for those that had a persistent nonunion.[75] No patient with union had moderate or severe pain in comparison to five patients with nonunion.[75] Five patients with nonunion were either unable to walk or limited to indoors only compared to none in the union group.[75] Knutson, and associates found that 38 of 39 patients with successful union were satisfied compared to only 14 satisfied patients of 20 who had a persistent nonunion following attempted arthrodesis.[55] Therefore the failed arthrodesis is functionally disabling.

Salvage techniques for the failed arthrodesis include bone grafting alone, bone grafting combined with a repeat course of external fixation, internal fixation with a plate or intramedullary nail, and/or electrical stimulation. Internal fixation is performed best once there is no longer evidence of active sepsis. Dual compression plates are an excellent internal fixation technique.[57] Intramedullary arthrodesis has been reported successful in 14 patients following a failed total knee arthroplasty by Kaufer and associates.[36,50,95] A combination of an intramedullary nail and external fixation with a Charnley clamp has been reported successful in five knees.[25] External coil electrical stimulation has been reported successful in salvaging the failed knee arthrodesis in 85% of patients with union occurring within 5.9 months.[3] Little attention has been paid to the use of percutaneous electrodes for electrical stimulation. Sometimes combinations of these techniques are useful as the plan of initial management in the case of a difficult arthrodesis with loss of bone stock.

SUMMARY

Thorough excision of all scarred and infected tissues with careful contouring of the bone ends to ensure adequate bone apposition should be performed. Cancellous bone grafts placed about the periphery of the arthrodesis should be considered in the case of loss of bone stock to improve the surfaces for bone apposition. Rigid biplanar external fixation should be used to obtain a compression arthrodesis combined with prolonged immobilization. Unfortunately, some patients will require permanent bracing.

REFERENCES

1. Ahlberg, A., and Lunden, A.: Secondary operations after knee joint replacement, Clin. Orthop. **156:**170-174, 1981.
2. Arden, C.P.: Total replacement of the knee, Proc. Aust. Orthop. Assoc. J. Bone Joint Surg. **57B:**119-120, 1975.
3. Bigliani, L.U., Rosenwasser, M.P., Caulo, N., Schink, N.M., and Bassett, C.A.L.: The use of pulsing electromagnetic fields to achieve arthrodesis of the knee following failed total knee arthroplasty, J. Bone Joint Surg. **65A:**480-485, 1983.
4. Blomgren, G., and Lindgren, U.: The susceptibility of total joint replacement to hematogenous infection in the early postoperative period, Clin. Orthop. **151:**308-312, 1980.
5. Blomgren, G., Lundquist, H., Nord, C.E., and Lindgren, U.: Late anaerobic hematogenous infection of experimental total joint replacement, J. Bone Joint Surg. **63B:**614-618, 1981.
6. Borden, L.: Infection in total knee replacement, Paper presented at the thirty-second annual meeting of the American Academy of Orthopaedic Surgeons, Phoenix, Oct. 29, 1983.
7. Bosworth, D.M.: Knee fusion by the use of a three-flanged nail, J. Bone Joint Surg. **28**(3):550-554, 1946.
8. Brashear, H.R.: The value of the intramedullary nail for knee fusion particularly for the charcot joint, Am. J. Surg. **87:**64-65, 1954.
9. Brattstrom, H., and Brattstrom, J.: Long-term results in knee arthrodesis in rheumatoid arthritis, Acta Rheum. Scand. **17:**86-93, 1971.
10. Brause, B.D.: Infected total knee replacement, Orthop. Clin. North Am. **13:**245-249, 1982.
11. Briggs, B.T., and Chao, E.Y.S.: The mechanical performance of the standard Hoffmann-Vidal external fixation apparatus, J. Bone Joint Surg. **64A:**566-573, 1982.
12. Brodersen, M.P., Fitzgerald, R.H., Peterson, L.F.A., Coventry, M.B., and Bryan, R.S.: Arthrodesis of the knee following failed total knee arthroplasty, J. Bone Joint Surg. **61A:**181-186, 1979.
13. Brooker, A.F., Jr., and Hansen, N.M., Jr.: The biplane frame, Clin. Orthop. **160:**163-167, 1981.
14. Bryan, R.S., and Brodersen, M.P.: Arthrodesis of the knee joint. In Evarts, C.M., editor: Surgery of the musculoskeletal system, vol. 3, New York, 1983, Churchill Livingstone, Inc.
15. Chapchal, G.: Intramedullary pinning for arthrodesis of the knee joint, J. Bone Joint Surg. **30:**734, 1948.
16. Charnley, J.: Positive pressure in arthrodesis of the knee joint, J. Bone Joint Surg. **30B:**478-486, 1948.
17. Charnley, J.: Arthrodesis of the knee, Clin. Orthop. **18:**37-42, 1960.
18. Charnley, J., and Baker, S.L.: Compression arthrodesis of the knee: A clinical and histological study, J. Bone Joint Surg. **34B:**187-199, 1952.
19. Cleveland, M.: Operative fusion of the unstable or flail knee due to anterior poliomyelitis: A study of the late results, J. Bone Joint Surg. **14:**525-534, 1932.
20. D'Ambrosia, R.D., Shoji, H., and Heater, R.: Secondarily infected total joint replacement by hematogenous spread, J. Bone Joint Surg. **58A:**450-453, 1976.
21. Deburge, A., and GUEPAR: Guepar hinge prosthesis, Clin. Orthop. **120:**47-53, 1976.
22. Dee, R.: The case for arthrodesis of the knee, Orthop. Clin. North Am. **10**(1):249-261, 1979.
23. Drennan, D.B., and Maylahn, D.J.: Important factors in achieving arthrodesis of the Charcot knee, J. Bone Joint Surg. **53A:**1180-1193, 1971.
24. Drinker, H., Potter, T.A., Turner, R.H., and Thomas, W.H.: Arthrodesis for failed knee arthroplasty, Orthop. Trans. **13**(3):302, 1979.
25. Fahmy, N.R.M.: A technique for difficult arthrodesis of the knee, J. Bone Joint Surg. **66B:**367-370, 1984.
26. Falahee, M.H., Kaufer, H., and Matthews, L.S.: Resection arthroplasty of the infected total knee arthroplasty, Paper presented at the thirty-fourth annual meeting of the American Academy of Orthopaedic Surgeons, Las Vegas, Jan. 25, 1985.
27. Fett, H.C., and Zorn, E.L.: Compression arthrodesis of the knee, J. Bone Joint Surg. **35:**172-177, 1953.
28. Fidler, M.W.: Knee arthrodesis following prosthesis removal: Use of the Wagner apparatus, J. Bone Joint Surg. **65B:**29-31, 1983.
29. Fisher, D.A.: The Hoffman external fixator: Technique of application. In Brooker, A.F., and Edwards, C.C., editors: External fixation: the current state of the art, Baltimore, 1979, Williams & Wilkins.
30. Fitzgerald, R.H., and Kelly, P.J.: Total joint arthroplasty, Biologic causes of failure, Mayo Clin. Proc. **54:**590-596, 1979.
31. Freeman, M.A.R., and Charnley, J.: Arthrodesis. In Freeman, M.A.R., editor, Arthritis of the knee: Clinical features and surgical management, Berlin, 1980, Springer-Verlag.
32. Frymeyer, J.W., and Hoagland, F.T.: The role of arthrodesis in reconstruction of the knee, Clin. Orthop. **101:**82-92, 1974.

33. Glynn, M.K., and Sheehan, J.M.: An analysis of the causes of deep infection after hip and knee arthroplasties, Clin. Orthop. **178:**202-206, 1983.

34. Green, D.P., Parkes, J.C. II, and Stinchfield, F.E.: Arthrodesis of the knee: A follow-up study, J. Bone Joint Surg. **49A:**1065-1078, 1967.

35. Green, S.A.: The effect of methacrylate on phagocytosis, J. Bone Joint Surg. **57A:**583, 1975.

36. Griend, R.V.: Arthrodesis of the knee with intramedullary fixation, Clin. Orthop. **181:**146-150, 1983.

37. Gristina, A.G., and Kolkin, J.: Current concepts review: Total joint replacement and sepsis, J. Bone Joint Surg. **65A:**128-134, 1983.

38. Hageman, W.F., Woods, G.W., and Tullos, H.G.: Arthrodesis in failed total knee replacement, J. Bone Joint Surg. **60A:**790-794, 1978.

39. Hall, A.J.: Late infection about a total knee prosthesis, J. Bone Joint Surg. **56B:**144-147, 1974.

40. Hankin, F., Louie, K.W., and Matthews, L.S.: The effect of total knee arthroplasty prostheses design on the potential for salvage arthrodesis: Measurements of volumes, lengths and trabecular bone contact areas, Clin. Orthop. **155:**52-58, 1981.

41. Hatt, R.N.: The central bone graft in joint arthrodesis, Arch. Surg. **46:**664-665, 1943.

42. Henderson, M.S., and Fortin, H.J.: Tuberculosis of the knee joint in the Adult, J. Bone Joint Surg. **9:**700-710, 1927.

43. Hibbs, R.A.: An operation for stiffening the knee joint with report of cases from the service of the New York Orthopedic Hospital, Ann. Surg. **53:**404-407, 1911.

44. Hibbs, R.A.: The treatment of tuberculosis of the joints of the lower extremities by operative fusion, J. Bone Joint Surg. **12:**749-754, 1930.

45. Hui, F.C., and Fitzgerald, R.H.: Hinged total knee arthroplasty, J. Bone Joint Surg. **62A:**513-519, 1980.

46. Inman, R.D., Gallegos, B.D., Redecha, P.B., and Christian, C.L.: Clinical and microbial features of prosthetic joint infection, Am. J. Med. **77:**47-53, 1984.

47. Insall, J.N.: Infection in total knee arthroplasty. In Frankel, V.H., editor: Instructional course lectures: The American Academy of Orthopaedic Surgeons, St. Louis, 1982, The C. V. Mosby Co.

48. Insall, J.N., Hood, R.W., Flawn, L.B., and Sullivan, D.J.: The total condylar knee prosthesis in gonarthrosis, J. Bone Joint Surg. **65A:**619-628, 1983.

49. Insall, J.N., Thompson, F.M., and Brause, B.D.: Two-stage reimplantation for the salvage of infected total knee arthroplasty, J. Bone Joint Surg. **65A:**1087-1098, 1983.

50. Kaufer, H., Irvine, G., and Matthews, L.S.: Intramedullary arthrodesis of the knee, Orthop. Trans. **7:**416, 1983.

51. Kaufer, H., and Matthews, L.S.: Spherocentric arthroplasty of the knee, J. Bone Joint Surg. **63A:**545-559, 1981.

52. Kaufer, H., and Matthews, L.S.: Resection arthroplasty for salvage of the infected total knee arthroplasty, American Academy of Orthopaedic Surgeons, instructional course, Anaheim, Calif., Feb. 13, 1984.

53. Key, J.A.: Positive pressure in arthrodesis for tuberculosis of the knee joint, South. Med. J. **25:**909, 1932.

54. Key, J.A.: Arthrodesis of the knee with a large central autogenous bone peg, South. Med. J. **30:**574-579, 1937.

55. Knutson, K., Hovelius, L., Lindstrand, A., and Lidgren, L.: Arthrodesis after failed knee arthroplasty, Clin. Orthop. **191:**202-211, 1984.

56. Lortat-Jacob, A., Lelong, P., Benoit, J., and Ramadier, J.O.: Arthrodesis of the knee after removal of infected knee prostheses, Orthop. Trans. **3:**29, 1979.

57. Lucas, D.B., and Murray, W.R.: Arthrodesis of the knee by double plating, J. Bone Joint Surg. **43A:**795-808, 1961.

58. Matthews, L.S., Green, C.A., and Goldstein, S.A.: The thermal effects of skeletal fixation-pin insertion in bone, J. Bone Joint Surg. **66A:**1077-1083, 1984.

59. Mazet, R., Jr., and Urist, M.R.: Arthrodesis of the knee with intramedullary nail fixation, Clin. Orthop. **18:**43-53, 1960.

60. Mazzetti, R.F.: Effect of immobilization of the knee on energy expenditure during walking, J. Bone Joint Surg. **42:**533, 1960.

61. Merrit, K.: Implant site infection rates with porous and dense material, J. Biomed. Mat. Res. **13:**101-108, 1978.

62. Moore, F.H., and Smillie, I.S.: Arthrodesis of the knee joint, Clin. Orthop. **13:**215-221, 1959.

63. Morris, H.D., and Mosiman, R.S.: Arthrodesis of the knee: A comparison of the compression method with the non-compression method, J. Bone Joint Surg. **33A:**982-987, 1951.

64. Nelson, C.L., and Evarts, C.M.: Arthroplasty and arthrodesis of the knee joint, Orthop. Clin. North Am. **2**(1):245-264, 1971.

65. Nelson, J.P.: Total knee arthroplasty infection—A review of seventeen cases, Orthop. Trans. **6:**477, 1982.

66. Nelson, J.P.: Asepsis and perioperative infection and prevention: Orthopedic perspectives, Infections in surgery, 39-41, vol. 2, no. 1, 1983.

67. Nesse, L.: Arthrodesis of the knee using two plates, Acta Orthop. Scand. **49:**636, 1978.

68. Petty, W.: The effect of methylmethacrylate on chemotaxis of polymorphonuclear leukocytes, J. Bone Joint Surg. **60A:**492-498, 1978.

69. Petty, W.: The effect of methylmethacrylate on bacterial phagocytosis and killing by human polymorphonuclear leukocytes, J. Bone Joint Surg. **60A:**752-757, 1978.

70. Petty, W., Bryan, R.S., Coventry, M.B., and Peterson, L.F.A.: Infection after total knee arthroplasty, Orthop. Clin. North Am. **6:**1005-1014, 1975.

71. Phillips, H.T., and Mears, D.C.: Knee fusion with external skeletal fixation after an infected hinge prosthesis: A case report, Clin. Orthop. **151:**147, 1980.

72. Potter, T.A.: Fusion of the destroyed arthritic knee compression arthrodesis vs. intramedullary rod technique, Surg. Clin. North Am. **49**(4):939-945, 1969.

73. Rae, T.: A study on the effects of particulate metals of orthopedic interest on murine macrophages in vitro, J. Bone Joint Surg. **57B:**444-450, 1975.

74. Rand, J.A., and Bryan, R.S.: Reimplantation for the salvage of an infected total knee arthroplasty, J. Bone Joint Surg. **65A:**1081-1086, 1983.

75. Rand, J.A., and Bryan, R.S.: The outcome of failed knee arthrodesis following total knee arthroplasty, Clin. Orthop. (In press.)

76. Rand, J.A., Morrey, B.F., and Bryan, R.S.: Management of infected total joint arthroplasty, Orthop. Clin. North Am. **15:**491-504, 1984.

77. Rand, J.A., Stauffer, R.N., and Chao, E.Y.S.: Kinematic rotating hinge total knee arthroplasty, Paper presented at the thirty-fourth annual meeting of the American Academy of Orthopaedic Surgeons, Las Vegas, Jan. 25, 1986.
78. Rothacker, G.W., and Cabenela, M.E.: External fixation for arthrodesis of the knee and ankle, Clin. Orthop. **180:**101-108, 1983.
79. Salenius, P., and Kivilaakso, R.: Follow-up examination of a series of arthrodesis of the knee joint, Acta Orthop. Scand. **39:**91-100, 1968.
80. Salibian, A.M., and Anzel, S.H.: Salvage of an infected total knee prosthesis with medial and lateral gastrocnemius muscle flaps, J. Bone Joint Surg. **65A:**681-684, 1983.
81. Salvati, E.A., Braun, B.D., Chekofsky, K.M., and Wilson, P.D.: Reimplantation in infection: An eleven year experience, Orthop. Trans. **5:**370, 1981.
82. Salvati, E.A., and Insall, J.N.: The management of sepsis in total knee replacement. In Savastono, A.A., editor: Total knee replacement, East Norwalk, Conn., 1980, Appleton-Century-Crofts.
83. Salvati, E.A., Robinson, R.P., Zeno, S.M., Koslin, B.L., Braun, D.B., and Wilson, P.D.: Infection rates after 3,175 total hip and total knee replacements performed with and without a horizontal undirectional filtered air-flow system, J. Bone Joint Surg. **64A:**525-535, 1982.
84. Sanders, R., and O'Neill, T.: The gastrocnemius myocutaneous flap used as a cover for the exposed knee prosthesis, J. Bone Joint Surg. **63B:**383-386, 1981.
85. Schurman, D.J.: The management of the infected total knee replacement, Orthop. Trans. **6:**477, 1982.
86. Schurman, D.J., Johnson, L., and Amstutz, H.C.: Knee joint infections with *Staphylococcus aureus* and *Micrococcus* species, J. Bone Joint Surg. **57A:**40-49, 1975.
87. Shea, G., Wynn, J., and Arden, G.P.: A study of the results of the removal of total knee prostheses, J. Bone Joint Surg. **63B:**287, 1981.
88. Siller, T.N.: Arthrodesis in the treatment of degenerative arthritis of the knee. In Cruess, R.L. and Mitchell, N.S., editors: Surgical management of degenerative arthritis of the lower limb, Philadelphia, 1975, Lea & Febiger.
89. Stewart, M.B., and Bland, W.C.: Compression in arthrodesis: a comparative study of methods of fusion of the knee in ninety-three cases, J. Bone Joint Surg. **40A:**585-606, 1958.
90. Stinchfield, F.E., Bigliani, L.U., Neu, H.C., Goss, T.P., and Foster, C.R.: Late hematogenous infections of total joint replacements, J. Bone Joint Surg. **62A:**1345-1350, 1980.
91. Stoltz, M.R., and Ganz, R.: Fracture after arthrodesis of the hip and knee, Clin. Orthop. **115:**177-181, 1976.
92. Stulberg, S.D.: Arthrodesis in failed total knee replacements, Orthop. Clin. North Am. **13:**213-224, 1982.
93. Thornhill, T.S., Dalziel, R.W., and Sledge, C.B.: Alternatives to arthrodesis for the failed total knee arthroplasty, Clin. Orthop. **170:**131-140, 1982.
94. Toumey, J.W.: Knee joint tuberculosis: Two hundred twenty-two patients treated by operative fusion, Surg. Gynecol. Obstet. **68:**1029-1037, 1939.
95. Vahvanen, V.: Arthrodesis in failed knee replacement in eight rheumatoid patients, Ann. Chir. Gyn. **68:**57-62, 1979.
96. Wade, P.J.F., and Denham, R.A.: Arthrodesis of the knee after failed knee replacement, J. Bone Joint Surg. **66B:**362-366, 1984.
97. Walker, R.H., and Schruman, D.J.: Management of infected total knee replacements, Clin. Orthop. **186:**81-89, 1984.
98. Woods, C.W., Lioberger, D.R., and Tulls, H.S.: Failed total knee arthroplasty, Clin. Orthop. **173:**184-190, 1983.

Section VI

THE FOOT

Chapter 36

Hallux valgus

ROGER A. MANN

In the Instructional Course Lecture series in 1982, I presented an in-depth discussion of the etiology and treatment of hallux valgus.[3] The treatment that was carried out for the typical bunion deformity was the DuVries modification of the McBride procedure, which resulted in approximately 90% good and excellent results. However, in the review of 100 cases there was an 11% incidence of hallux varus associated with this procedure. Of these 11 cases, seven had a varus deformity of 4 degrees or less and represented only a radiographic finding, not a clinical problem (Fig. 36-1). The other four cases had a significant degree of varus, averaging 16 degrees. The etiology of the hallux varus resulted mainly from the muscle imbalance created by the excision of the lateral sesamoid and the subsequent failure of the lateral capsular tissue to reform a competent capsule. If the proximal phalanx was slightly overcorrected and the lateral capsule failed to adequately reconstitute itself, the potential to form a hallux varus was present. Because of this potential, a careful reevaluation of the procedure was undertaken in an attempt to reduce the incidence of this possible complication. This chapter presents the pathologic, anatomic, and biomechanical factors considered in modifying the operative procedure.

PATHOLOGIC ANATOMY

The typical hallux valgus deformity results from lateral deviation of the proximal phalanx on the first metatarsal head. This deviation results in certain changes about the metatarsophalangeal joint and metatarsal shaft (Fig. 36-2). A soft tissue contracture consisting of the lateral joint capsule, the adductor hallucis, and the transverse metatar-

sal ligament develops on the lateral aspect of the first metatarsophalangeal joint (Fig. 36-3). Fixation of the proximal phalanx in the laterally deviated position results in progressive attenuation of the medial capsular tissues, formation of a medial eminence of varying degrees, and increased medial deviation of the first metatarsal shaft.

No muscle inserts into the metatarsal head per se, but rather the muscles pass by the head to insert into the proximal or distal phalanx. The first metatarsal head thus is suspended by a sling

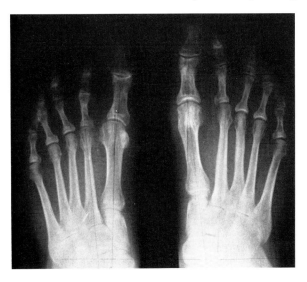

Fig. 36-1. Radiograph demonstrating the results after the correction of a hallux valgus using the DuVries modification of the McBride procedure. The lateral sesamoid has been removed, and there is slight overcorrection of the metatarsophalangeal joint. Although technically this is considered a varus deformity, from a clinical standpoint the function of the great toe is normal.

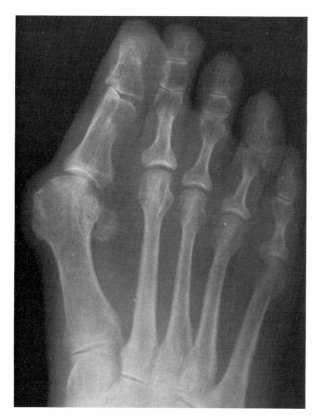

Fig. 36-2. A typical hallux valgus deformity, which consists of lateral deviation of the proximal phalanx on the metatarsal head. This results in a contracture of the capsular tissues on the lateral aspect of the joint, attenuation of the capsular tissues on the medial side of the joint, medial migration of the metatarsal head off the sesamoids, and pronation of the great toe.

of muscles passing about it (Fig. 36-4). In the normal state the sesamoids are centered beneath the first metatarsal head and held in place by the capsular ligaments and the crista beneath the metatarsal head, along the medial side by the abductor hallucis, and along the lateral side by the adductor hallucis. In the pathologic state in which the metatarsal head deviates medially by the pressure exerted by the laterally drifting proximal phalanx, the muscles that normally act to stabilize the metatarsophalangeal joint actually become deforming forces. Once this muscle group becomes unstabilized, it tends to increase the valgus deformity rather than prevent it. The long flexor and extensor tendons likewise act to

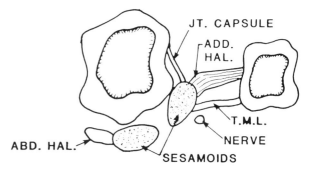

Fig. 36-3. A cross section of the first and second metatarsal heads demonstrating the contracture that is present on the lateral side of the metatarsophalangeal joint, which consists of the joint capsule, the adductor hallucis, and the transverse metatarsal ligament.

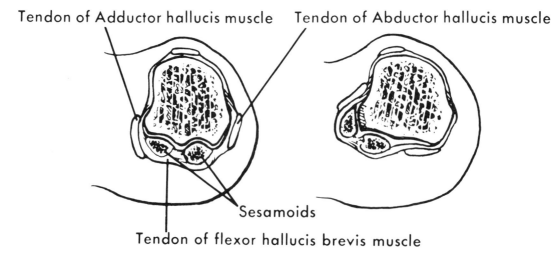

Fig. 36-4. The metatarsal head is held in place by tendons that pass by it. *Left,* In the normal state these structures stabilize the metatarsophalangeal joint. *Right,* In the pathologic state they tend to accentuate the deformity.

stabilize the first metatarsophalangeal joint when properly aligned, but in the pathologic state these become bow-strung laterally at the metatarsophalangeal joint and also contribute to the instability of the metatarsophalangeal joint.

The pronation of the proximal phalanx that occurs in the more advanced stages of the deformity is brought about by the metatarsal head moving medially off the sesamoids. As this occurs, the sesamoid sling, which inserts into the base of the proximal phalanx, remains in place. As the metatarsal head moves off the sling and the abductor hallucis slides under the metatarsal head, the proximal phalanx rotates on its axis into a pronated position as the medial aspect of the metatarsal head attenuates the medial joint capsule. The pivot point for this rotation is the insertion of the adductor hallucis into the proximal phalanx. Unless the sesamoids are brought back under the first metatarsal when carrying out the hallux valgus correction, the pronation remains.

SURGICAL CONSIDERATIONS

Based on these pathologic changes, the repair of the hallux valgus deformity is dependent on four essential steps.

1. Adequate release of the soft tissue contracture on the lateral side of the metatarsophalangeal joint, which includes the release of the lateral joint capsule, the adductor hallucis muscle, and the transverse metatarsal ligament
2. Removal of the medial eminence in line with the medial aspect of the first metatarsal shaft
3. Plication of the medial capsular structures to maintain the proximal phalanx in satisfactory alignment
4. Realignment of the first and second metatarsal shafts, either by the use of the soft tissue procedure alone or by the addition of an osteotomy at the base of the first metatarsal

If any of these four steps is not adequately carried out, a recurrent hallux valgus deformity is possible.

The repair, which has evolved over a period of time, is a modification of the soft tissue procedures advocated by McBride,[2] Silver,[4] and DuVries,[1] to which an osteotomy in the proximal portion of the metatarsal is used in approximately 80% of cases to correct residual metatarsus primus varus. The procedure is based on correcting the anatomic deformity while maintaining the stability of the joint and preserving the length of the first metatarsal. The main advantage of this surgical approach is that it anatomically corrects the hallux valgus deformity while not exposing the patient to a significant risk by creating a muscle imbalance about the first metatarsophalangeal joint, postoperative displacement, or shortening of a metatarsal osteotomy.

The changes made in the previously published procedure include leaving the fibular sesamoid in place, which provides greater stability to the sesamoid sling and helps prevent a hallux varus deformity from occurring. Since the fibular sesamoid is left in place, the transverse metatarsal ligament, which passes from the base of the second metatarsal into the lateral aspect of the sesamoid, must be sectioned to free the sesamoid sling and to relieve the contracture that is present on the lateral side of the metatarsophalangeal joint. If this release is not carried out, the sesamoids cannot be realigned beneath the metatarsal head and a recurrence of the deformity is possible. The last change in the procedure is to perform a proximal metatarsal osteotomy in approximately 80% of cases. The addition of the metatarsal osteotomy corrects the metatarsus varus and therefore the intermetatarsal angle to such an extent that it permits the realignment of the first metatarsophalangeal joint to occur and to remain corrected. The correction of the metatarsus varus into the normal anatomic range results in little or no stress against the hallux, which might bring about a recurrence of the deformity.

The crescentic-shaped osteotomy was selected because it creates a long, thin osteotomy through the cancellous portion of the metatarsal. The osteotomy site is through almost 2.0 to 2.5 cm of cancellous bone and is quite stable once a pin or screw is placed across it. Little or no chance exists for any displacement of the osteotomy site despite the fact that the patients are walked in a firm dressing and in a wooden shoe from the first day after surgery.

The procedure can be carried out in all age-groups, from juveniles through the seventh or eighth decade of life. It is contraindicated in patients who have advanced degenerative arthritis, significant hallux rigidus, or an irregularly shaped metatarsophalangeal joint that would preclude rotation of the proximal phalanx on the metatarsal head; in patients who have a significant lateral deviation of the articular surface of the metatarsal head; and in patients with spasticity secondary to cerebral palsy or stroke.

PATIENT SELECTION FOR HALLUS VALGUS REPAIR

The most important factor in the treatment of a patient with a hallux valgus deformity is proper conservative management. The patient should be instructed concerning the nature of the problem and counseled regarding the proper shoe, which should be broad toed and low heeled with a sufficient toe box area. If a patient is comfortable and accepts wearing this type of shoe, I believe that this is preferable to surgical correction. However, if the patient continues to have discomfort, then surgical correction should be made available.

I believe that only on rare occasions should a hallux valgus be corrected solely for cosmetic reasons. In my experience it is unusual to see a patient with a hallux valgus deformity develop degenerative arthritis at the metatarsophalangeal joint as a result of the hallux valgus. Therefore hallux valgus surgery should not be performed on feet with minimal deformities, because of fear of developing degenerative changes in the future. It is also important to carefully explain the nature of the surgery, so that the patient has an adequate understanding of the hazards of surgery and the expected outcome. Many female patients believe that, through surgery, the foot will become significantly narrower and they can resume wearing pointed, high-heeled shoes. In my experience about 60% to 70% of patients can return to unrestricted shoe wear after bunion surgery, but conversely 30% to 40% cannot, and patients should be made aware of this.

SURGICAL TECHNIQUE
Release of the lateral contracture

1. A midline incision is made through the dorsal aspect of the first interspace and carried down through the subcutaneous tissue and fat into the adventitious bursa between the first and second metatarsal heads. It is important to keep the incision in the midline to avoid the superficial branches of the deep peroneal nerve in the web space. A Weitlaner now is inserted into the wound to spread the metatarsal heads apart and to identify the underlying adductor hallucis tendon (Fig. 36-5, *A*).

2. The adductor hallucis tendon is detached along its superior border from its insertion along

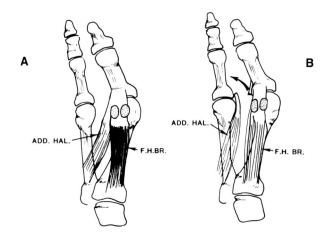

Fig. 36-5. Diagram of the muscles inserting into the plantar lateral aspect of the proximal phalanx of the first toe. The method by which the adductor hallucis tendon is released from its insertion into the base of the proximal phalanx and along the lateral aspect of the sesamoid until the fleshy portion of the flexor hallucis brevis is encountered.

the lateral aspect of the joint capsule. The line of this incision then is carried distally to the base of the proximal phalanx, and the adductor tendon is detached from its insertion into the base of the proximal phalanx. The adductor tendon next is detached from its insertion along the lateral aspect of the fibular sesamoid until the fleshy muscle fibers of the flexor hallucis brevis muscle are encountered (Fig. 36-5, *B*). Once this has been accomplished, the fibular sesamoid is freed of its soft tissue attachment and is held in place only by the transverse metatarsal ligament. The Weitlaner now is inserted into a deeper level to pry the metatarsal heads apart as far as possible, placing the transverse metatarsal ligament under tension.

3. The transverse metatarsal ligament, which passes from the second metatarsal into the plantar lateral aspect of the fibular sesamoid, now is carefully identified with a freer and then cut (Fig. 36-6). While cutting this structure, care must be taken to avoid injury to the common digital nerve and vessel to the first web space, which lie just below the ligament. The Weitlaner now is removed and the lateral joint capsule is identified.

4. The lateral joint capsule is torn at this time by bringing the great toe into about 40 degrees of varus. If the lateral capsule is too strong to be torn with firm, gentle pressure, the capsule is perforated with the tip of a knife until it gives way.

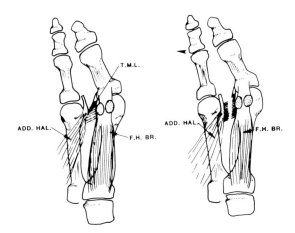

Fig. 36-6. Diagram of the insertion of the transverse metatarsal ligament into the lateral sesamoid. *Right,* The transverse metatarsal ligament has been released. When performing this release, caution must be exercised to avoid disrupting the underlying common digital nerve to the first web space.

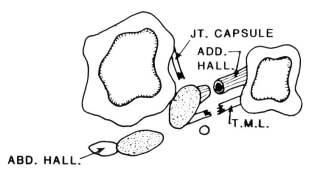

Fig. 36-7. A cross-sectional diagram through the first and second metatarsals demonstrating the tissues that have been released to relieve the lateral joint contracture.

At this point the release of the contracted tissues on the lateral side of the metatarsophalangeal joint is complete (Fig. 36-7). The importance of this part of the procedure cannot be overemphasized. Unless the lateral contracture is adequately released, the sesamoids will not be mobilized, and therefore they cannot be realigned beneath the first metatarsal head. If realignment does not occur, a satisfactory long-term result cannot be achieved.

Repair of the medial side of the metatarsophalangeal joint

1. The joint capsule is exposed through a 5 cm longitudinal incision centered over the midpor-tion of the metatarsophalangeal joint.

2. A dorsal and plantar flap is developed carefully along the capsular plane. By taking a full-thickness flap, the dorsal and plantar digital nerves are swept out of the way as the flap is developed.

3. A vertical capsulotomy is performed in the medial joint capsule. The initial incision in the capsule is made 2 to 3 mm proximal to the base of the proximal phalanx and carried down into the joint. The second incision, approximately 5 to 8 mm more proximal than the first, is made parallel to the initial incision (Fig. 36-8). These two capsular incisions then are brought together on the plantar aspect by a V, ending at the medial margin of the tibial sesamoid. Dorsally a V is created, ending approximately 0.5 cm medial to the extensor hallucis longus tendon. The size of the wedge of the capsule that is removed is dependent on the deformity that is present. If the surgeon has any doubt about the width of the capsule to be removed, it is important to remove too little capsule rather than too much.

4. The medial capsular tissue now is carefully stripped off the medial eminence. This dissection is begun on the plantar medial aspect of the joint and brought up dorsally. If the capsular tissue is believed to be too tight over the medial eminence, a horizontal cut along the superior medial aspect of the metatarsal head helps to mobilize the medial capsule into a flap based proximally and plantarly. When this dissection is carried out, the proximal periosteal attachment of the capsule must not be detached or the flap will be mobilized and cannot be used for the repair unless reattached to bone.

5. The medial eminence now is excised with the use of an osteotome or power saw. The excision of the medial eminence begins 1 mm medial to the sagittal sulcus and is carried out in line with the medial aspect of the metatarsal shaft. Before the medial eminence is removed, the x-ray film must be observed carefully so that the line of the excision of the medial eminence is in line with the medial aspect of the metatarsal shaft. In this manner an excessive amount of metatarsal head will not be removed inadvertently (Fig. 36-9).

The preparation of the medial aspect of the metatarsophalangeal joint now has been completed, and an evaluation of the mobility of the first metatarsal shaft needs to be made.

The surgeon now must decide whether an

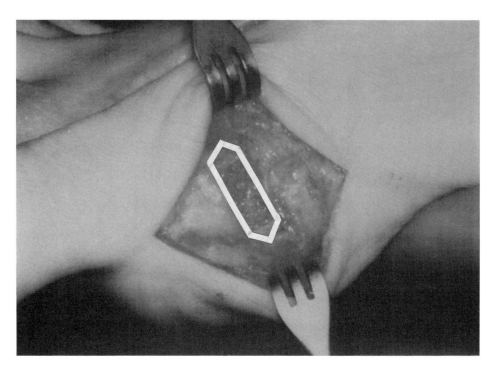

Fig. 36-8. Photograph of the medial aspect of the first metatarsophalangeal joint. The shape of the medial capsule to be excised is outlined. The width of the excised area varies from 3 to 8 mm, depending on the degree of deformity.

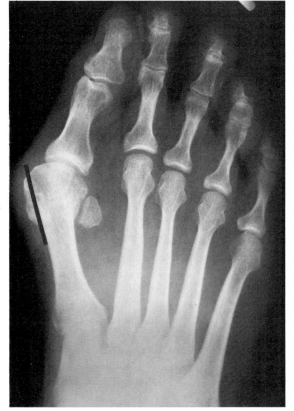

Fig. 36-9. The medial eminence should be excised in line with the medial aspect of the metatarsal shaft. **A,** Line of excision of the medial eminence in a patient with a large prominence. **B,** Line of excision of the medial eminence in a patient with a small prominence. **C,** Excessive excision of the medial eminence, resulting in a hallux varus deformity.

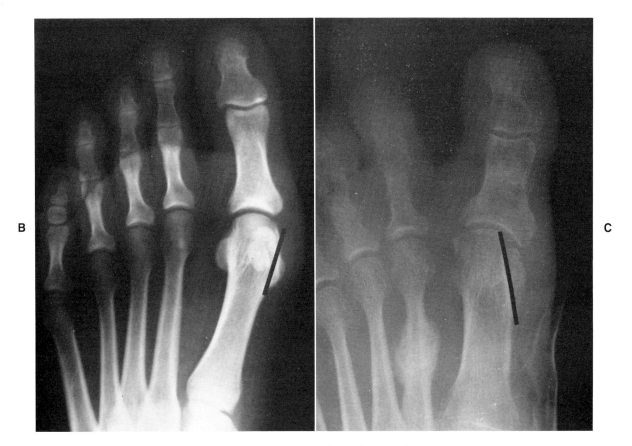

Fig. 36-9, Cont'd. For legend see p. 344.

osteotomy of the base of the first metatarsal is necessary to realign the first and second metatarsals (to correct a fixed metatarsus varus). In approximately 20% of patients the first metatarsal corrects to the second metatarsal once the soft tissue portion of the procedure has been carried out. In approximately 80% of patients an osteotomy of the base of the first metatarsal is necessary to realign the first and second metatarsals. If the first metatarsal is not brought back into satisfactory alignment in relation to the second metatarsal and remains in a fixed varus position, a satisfactory long-term result will not occur (Fig. 36-10) because the first metatarsal is still in a varus position. Although the soft tissue correction initially maintains the hallux in satisfactory alignment, in time the deformity will recur because the metatarsus varus is still present.

The decision concerning whether an osteotomy is necessary depends on the case of realigning the first metatarsal to the second metatarsal. This determination is made by gently pushing on the medial side of the first metatarsal head and seeing whether it corrects to the second metatarsal head with little or no pressure, and then has a tendency to remain there (Fig. 36-11). If there is any tendency for the first and second metatarsals to spread apart, then it is necessary to perform an osteotomy. If the first metatarsal literally "sits" next to the second, demonstrating little or no propensity to spring medially once again, then an osteotomy is not necessary. If any doubt exists in the surgeon's mind, I believe it is better to do an osteotomy than not to do one.

Metatarsal osteotomy

1. The base of the first metatarsal is exposed through a 2.5 cm dorsal incision made just medial to the extensor hallucis longus tendon. The metatarsocuneiform joint is identified for orientation purposes.

2. The osteotomy should be approximately 5

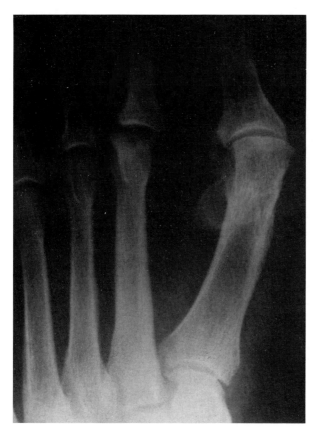

Fig. 36-10. A recurrent hallux valgus as a result of the failure to correct the intermetatarsal angle at the time of the distal soft tissue procedure.

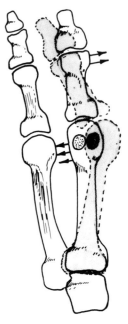

Fig. 36-11. After the release of the contracture of the lateral aspect of the metatarsophalangeal joint and preparation of the medial aspect of the joint, a decision has to be made concerning whether the first metatarsal will correct to the second. If the first metatarsal head can be pushed over to the second and will remain there without pressure, no osteotomy is necessary. If, however, there is any tendency for the first metatarsal to again spring medially, a proximal metatarsal osteotomy is indicated.

to 7 mm distal to the metatarsocuneiform joint. A crescentic-shaped osteotomy then is produced, with the apex based proximally. The osteotomy blade that is used is shown in Fig. 36-12.

3. When the osteotomy is cut with the micro-oscillating saw and curved blade, the plane of the osteotomy passes from dorsal to volar in such a manner that the blade is perpendicular neither to the metatarsal shaft nor the plantar aspect of the foot but rather is in a plane between these two guidelines.

4. When the osteotomy is produced in this manner, the metatarsal shaft can be literally rolled around within the crescent-shaped osteotomy to realign the first and second metatarsals. The osteotomy itself is placed within cancellous bone that is approximately 2.0 to 2.5 cm in thickness, and as a result a great deal of stability is present at the osteotomy site to resist displacement in all planes. After the osteotomy is pro-

duced, and after the osteotomy site is mobilized, the first metatarsal head can be brought next to the second. Once this occurs the first metatarsophalangeal joint usually is well aligned.

The four steps in the hallux valgus repair now have been completed. These four steps consist of:

1. Release of the contracture of the lateral aspect of the first metatarsophalangeal joint
2. Preparation of the capsule on the medial side of the metatarsophalangeal joint
3. Excision of the medial eminence
4. A basal osteotomy of the first metatarsal

After these steps are complete, these structures must be reconstructed to correct the hallux valgus deformity.

Reconstruction of the hallux valgus deformity

1. At the initial incision in the first web space, three sutures are placed between the first and second metatarsal heads, incorporating the ad-

base of the osteotomy approximately 1.5 mm medial to the lateral cortex of the osteotomy site, while the metatarsal head is displaced laterally so that it lies next to the second metatarsal. The base of the osteotomy site is stabilized using a neurologic freer to hold it in position so that, as the pressure from the pin is applied to the metatarsal, it does not displace (Fig. 36-13).

The osteotomy site is fixed using a 5/64-inch smooth Steinmann pin, which is driven across the osteotomy site and into the tarsal bones approximately 4 to 5 cm. Once this procedure is achieved, the first and second metatarsals are properly aligned. Although the osteotomy site is not rigidly fixed by the single pin, the pin provides enough stability so that when postoperative dressings are applied, unwanted displacement of the osteotomy site rarely occurs. The pin is cut off, leaving it to protrude about 0.5 cm from the skin. If the surgeon desires, this osteotomy site can be stabilized with a screw that should be long enough to pass into the tarsal bones.

4. The first metatarsophalangeal joint is placed into proper alignment by having the assistant hold the great toe in neutral position relative to dorsiflexion and plantar flexion; the toe is derotated so that any pronation is corrected, and in approximately 0 to 5 degrees of varus. The derotation of the toe is important because it places the sesamoids, which are attached to the base of the proximal phalanx, beneath the metatarsal head, so that as the surgeon repairs the medial capsule, the medial aspect of the tibial sesamoid can be observed. If this does not occur, there is some residual pronation of the great toe secondary to some uncorrected contracture that needs to be identified and corrected. Four sutures of number 00 chromic are placed into the medial capsular structures. This step of the procedure is extremely important, and since the plantar half of the joint capsule is thicker and stronger than the dorsal half, it is imperative that at least three sutures be placed into the plantar half of the capsule. Once this has been accomplished, the sutures are tied and the toe should be in satisfactory alignment. If an inadequate amount of medial joint capsule has been removed, then it is necessary to remove the sutures, excise more capsular tissue, and replicate the medial joint capsule. If the medial joint capsule has not been shortened sufficiently to align the toe at surgery, it certainly will not contract after surgery to

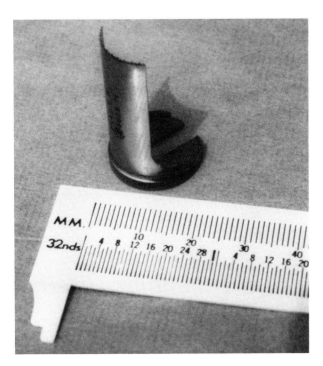

Fig. 36-12. The curved osteotomy blade that is recommended to carry out the proximal metatarsal osteotomy. (The blade is produced by Hall Zimmer, catalog number 5053-71.)

ductor tendon. These sutures help to bring the first and second metatarsal heads together, but, more important, they also bring the detached portion of the adductor hallucis tendon off the bottom of the foot into a position between the metatarsal heads. In this manner, I believe, the adductor hallucis tendon will help form and reinforce the capsule on the lateral aspect of the first metatarsophalangeal joint. Number 00 chromic sutures are used to carry out this repair.

2. If a metatarsal osteotomy has been performed, it is fixed at this point; but if a metatarsal osteotomy has not been necessary, this step is omitted and the surgeon proceeds with the plication of the medial capsular tissues (no. 4).

3. To fix the osteotomy site, a 3 mm incision is made over the medial aspect of the first metatarsal, approximately 1 cm distal to the osteotomy site. A 1/16 inch drill bit is used to make a hole in the medial cortex of the first metatarsal. The drill hole is created because it is easier to place a pin across the osteotomy site with the tip of it starting in a predrilled hole. The first metatarsal is held in its corrected position by displacing the

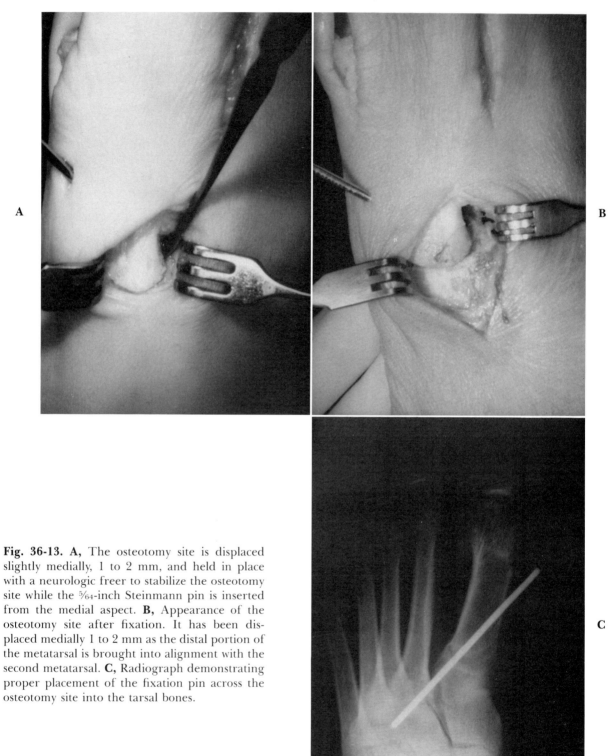

Fig. 36-13. A, The osteotomy site is displaced slightly medially, 1 to 2 mm, and held in place with a neurologic freer to stabilize the osteotomy site while the 5/64-inch Steinmann pin is inserted from the medial aspect. **B,** Appearance of the osteotomy site after fixation. It has been displaced medially 1 to 2 mm as the distal portion of the metatarsal is brought into alignment with the second metatarsal. **C,** Radiograph demonstrating proper placement of the fixation pin across the osteotomy site into the tarsal bones.

achieve satisfactory alignment.

5. The sutures in the first web space now are tied and the skin is closed. I prefer to close the skin with a single layer of interrupted sutures.

6. A firm compression dressing is applied for approximately 12 to 18 hours. On the following day the dressing is changed from a large, bulky, compression dressing to a firm dressing that consists of 2-inch Kling applied as a spica around the forefoot and great toe. This dressing is reinforced with 0.5-inch regular adhesive tape. The dressing, which is changed weekly for 8 weeks, is applied so as to bind the metatarsal heads together and then hold the great toe in satisfactory alignment (Fig. 36-14). During this period the patient is walked in a wooden shoe as tolerated. Even if patients have had an osteotomy, they are ambulated in a wooden shoe the day following the surgery. The main advantage of changing the dressings on a weekly basis is that the alignment of the toe can be constantly monitored so that it will not drift into an abnormal position. I do not like to use a cast because, as the postoperative swelling subsides, it may not support the hallux and the alignment of the great toe may be altered.

The dressings are removed after 8 weeks, and the patient is started on active range-of-motion exercises. It usually will take an average of 4 to 6 weeks before the patient can comfortably wear regular shoes, although at times persistent swelling, which may last for many months, can be a problem.

The pin fixing the osteotomy site usually is left in place for 4 weeks and then removed. Occasionally the pin will loosen and back out after only 2 to 3 weeks, but the premature loss of the fixation usually does not result in loss of position, probably because the firm dressing about the metatarsal head prevents displacement. There has been neither any problem with dorsal displacement of the osteotomy site nor any significant shortening of the first metatarsal, since no bone is removed at the time of the osteotomy. No patient developed a transfer lesion beneath the second or third metatarsal head after surgery.

RESULTS

In a recent review of 50 patients the soft tissue procedure and the proximal metatarsal osteotomy produced the corrections described in Table 36-1.

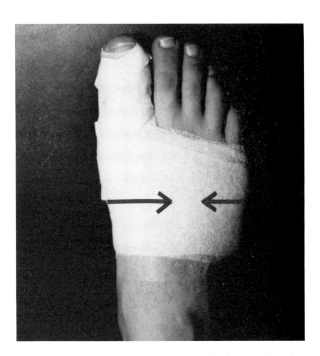

Fig. 36-14. The postoperative ambulatory dressing consists of 2-inch Kling and 0.5-inch adhesive tape. It is applied to tightly bind the metatarsal heads together (*arrows*) and then wrapped around the great toe to hold it in neutral position to allow proper capsular healing. When this dressing is applied, it is important that there is no residual pronation left in the great toe.

Table 36-1. Results of soft tissue procedure and proximal metatarsal osteotomy

	Preoperative deformity		Postoperative deformity	
	Halux valgus	Intermetatarsal angle	Hallux valgus	Intermetatarsal angle
Less than 20 degrees (3 cases)	20	8	6	3
21 to 39 degrees (35 cases)	31	12.3	9	3.4
Greater than 40 degrees (12 cases)	44	16.3	14	7.7

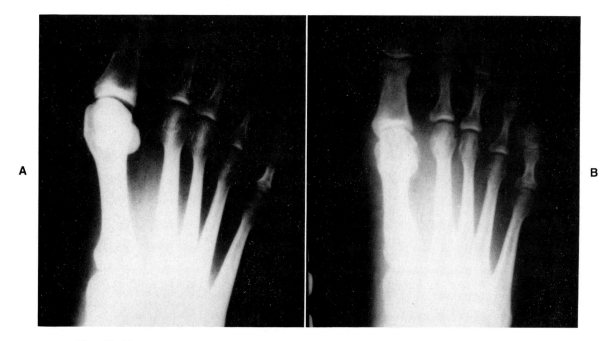

Fig. 36-15. A, Preoperative radiograph of a 20-degree hallux valgus deformity. **B,** Postoperative radiograph demonstrating satisfactory alignment.

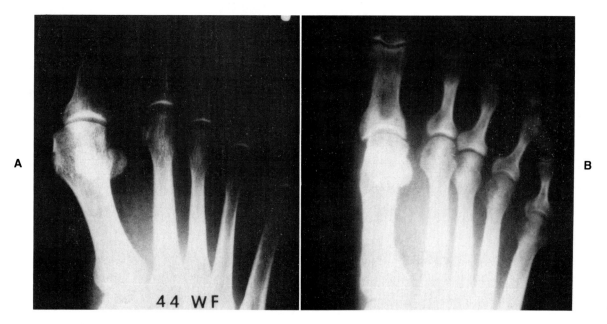

Fig. 36-16. A, Preoperative radiograph of a hallux valgus deformity of 33 degrees. **B,** Postoperative radiograph demonstrating satisfactory correction of the deformity.

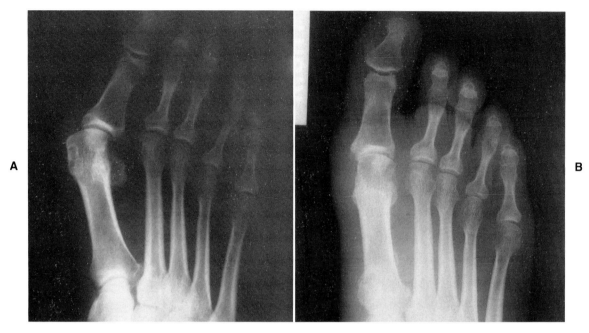

Fig. 36-17. A, Preoperative radiograph of a hallux valgus deformity of 45 degrees. **B,** Postoperative radiograph demonstrating satisfactory alignment.

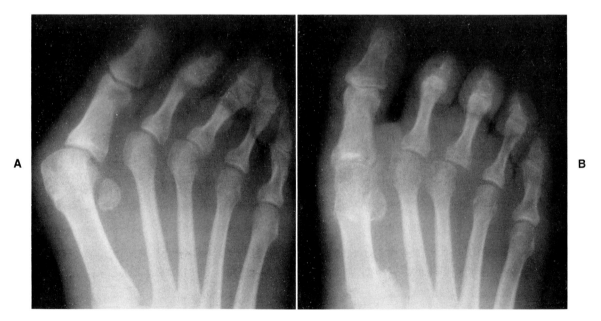

Fig. 36-18. A, Preoperative radiograph demonstrating a hallux valgus deformity of 52 degrees. **B,** Postoperative radiograph demonstrating satisfactory correction. A negative intermetatarsal angle has been created, since the lesser metatarsals (in particular two and three) are in an adducted position.

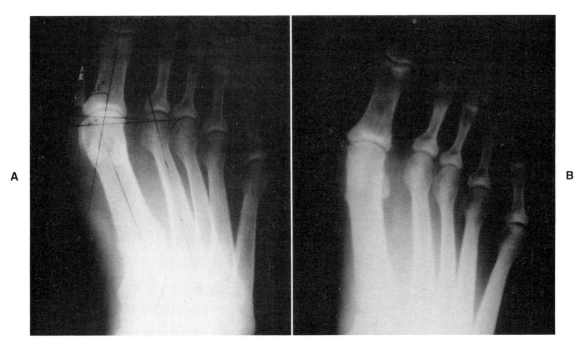

Fig. 36-19. A, Preoperative radiograph of a 32-degree hallux valgus deformity. **B,** Postoperative radiograph demonstrating a residual 24-degree deformity but correction of the intermetatarsal angle. This has occurred because the articular surface of the metatarsal head is facing laterally, and as a result an Akin procedure must be added to the surgery to bring about a straight hallux.

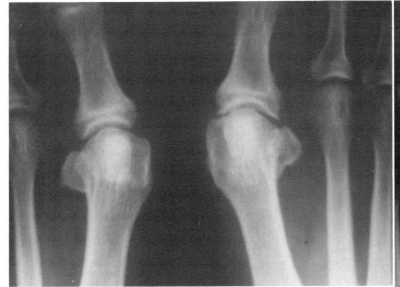

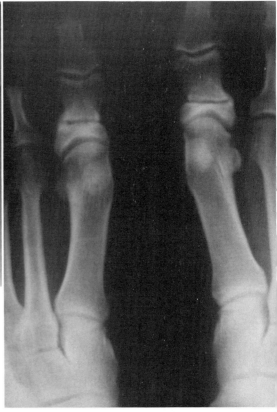

Fig. 36-20. A, Preoperative radiograph demonstrating an irregular metatarsal head. In the presence of an irregularly shaped metatarsal head, a soft tissue procedure is contraindicated. **B,** Satisfactory correction of the hallux valgus deformity after an excision of the medial eminence, plication of the medial capsule, and an Akin procedure.

Preceding are examples of corrections that can be obtained using the soft tissue procedure and an osteotomy in a patient with a 20-degree deformity (Fig. 36-15), a 33-degree deformity (Fig. 36-16), a 45-degree deformity (Fig. 36-17), and a 52-degree deformity (Fig. 36-18).

If the first metatarsal head is laterally deviated, a soft tissue procedure and osteotomy will not produce an adequate correction (Fig. 36-19). This is because the two articular surfaces will line up in a congruent manner, but since the articular surface of the metatarsal head faces laterally, so will the hallux. In this case an Akin procedure is required to bring about a complete correction.

The soft tissue procedure is contraindicated in a patient with an irregularly shaped metatarsal head (Fig. 36-20). Since the joint surfaces are already congruent in their irregular way, any attempt to rotate the proximal phalanx about the metatarsal head will result in an incongruent situation and a failure of the procedure. In such cases the medial eminence should be removed and the medial capsule plicated. An Akin procedure then is used to correct the residual deformity.

REFERENCES

1. DuVries, H.L.: Surgery of the foot, St. Louis, 1959, The C.V. Mosby Co.
2. McBride, E.D.: A conservative operation for bunions, J. Bone Joint Surg. **10:**735, 1928.
3. Mann, R.A.: Hallux Valgus: In Frankel, V.F., editor: Instructional course lectures: The American Academy of Orthopaedic Surgeons, vol. 31, St. Louis, 1982, The C.V. Mosby Co.
4. Silver, D.: The operative treatment of hallux valgus, J. Bone Joint Surg. **5:**225, 1923.

FRACTURES

Chapter 37

Impending pathologic fractures from metastatic malignancy: evaluation and management

KEVIN D. HARRINGTON

It has been estimated that 90% of patients dying from disseminated malignancy will have bony metastases demonstrable by careful post-mortem examination. Probably fewer than half of these patients have experienced bone symptoms, and fewer than 10% had suffered a pathologic fracture through a tumor focus before their deaths. Nevertheless, because the development of a fracture is so devastating to a cancer patient, increasing emphasis is being placed on attempts to determine which metastases are likely to produce fractures and how individual lesions may best be managed to avoid this complication.

HISTOMECHANICS

A common misconception is that only lytic metastases are likely to supply sufficient bone to result in a fracture and that the new bone that is laid down by blastic foci actually may increase cortical strength in many instances or at least make the bone locally harder. There is in fact no statistical or histologic basis for this belief. A long bone with blastic metastases may seem harder from the viewpoint of the surgeon attempting to attach hardware to it, but it lacks most of the strength and plasticity of normal bone. Approximately 60% of pathologic long bone fractures occur through breast carcinoma metastases despite the fact that more than half of these metastases are primarily blastic. Prostatic carcinoma, which almost invariably produces blastic bony metastases, nevertheless ranks high as a cause of long bone pathologic fractures.

Experimental evidence suggests that epithelial cells from breast, prostate, bladder, and certain lung carcinomas have the capacity to form bone within metastatic foci.[8] These metastatic tumor cells apparently produce an osteoblast-stimulating factor while forming a fibrous stroma developing around the tumor.[10,14] It seems likely that the two phenomena are synchronous and that the stroma so formed affords a suitable matrix for ossification in the presence of the osteoprogenitor cells produced by the tumor.

Certainly most tumor metastases have the secondary capacity to stimulate endosteal trabecular and even periosteal new bone formation by causing adjacent normal bone to respond to stress while being weakened by tumor lysis (see Fig. 37-2, *A*). This phenomenon is similar only qualitatively to callus repair of a traumatic fracture but differs markedly in a quantitative sense because of the poor strength of the callus. The reactive bone has a haphazard configuration histologically, lacking the parallelism of the bone fibers seen in normal stress-responsive lamellar bone. Although often appearing almost normal radiographically, these blastic foci are markedly weaker than normal bone and have an only slightly lower predisposition to pathologic fracture than do more obvious lytic foci (see Figs. 37-9, *D*, and 37-10, *B*).

Lytic bony metastases appear to weaken bone principally by two mechanisms. The first and quantitatively the most important is mediated by way of osteoclasts. Galasko demonstrated clearly that osteoclast proliferation occurred within 24

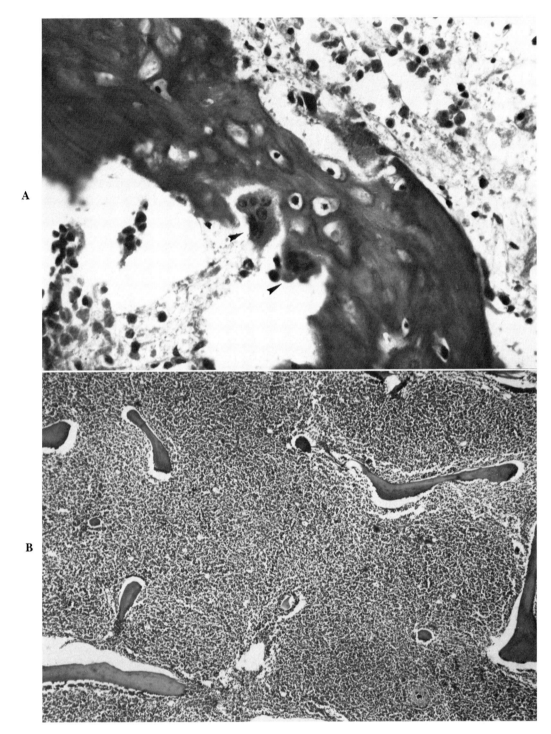

Fig. 37-1. A, High-power photomicrograph of a biopsy taken at the site of a pathologic fracture in a patient with metastatic breast carcinoma. Malignant cells are apparent in the soft tissue stoma adjacent to mature trabecular bone. Active resorption of bone is being caused by large multinucleated osteoclasts (*arrows*), which are not malignant. **B,** Low-power photomicrograph of tissue taken from the site of a pathologic fracture in a patient with a malignant lypmphoma. No osteoclasts are apparent, but extensive destruction of cortical bone has occurred. The densely packed malignant round cells appear to be causing bone lysis by direct resorption.

hours of inoculation of experimental animals with cancer cell strains.[10] Similar histologic changes are seen in the majority of human skeletal metastases and are as pronounced in highly cellular tumors as in relatively acellular sclerotic metastases. The phenomenon is seen in host bone immediately adjacent to tumor foci, separated from the tumor cells by the type of reactive fiber stroma already described. The osteoclasts are not malignant cells but rather concentrate in response to some tumor stimulus. Bone resorption occurs in lacunae around each osteoclast. Osteoclastic destruction of the cortex extends to the periosteal surface, the osteoclasts always preceding the tumor itself (Fig. 37-1, *A*).

It appears that such osteoclastic proliferation is mediated by way of an osteoclast activating factor (OAF) secreted by the tumor.[7,11,13]

Leukocytes concentrating at the tumor host margin also are capable of producing an OAF.[22] This phenomenon appears to play a particular role in osteoclasis around myelomatous and lymphomatous tumors. A similar phenomenon, however, occurs with many metastatic carcinomas, particularly breast carcinomas, where the OAF is secreted not directly by leukocytes but rather via prostaglandins, particularly PGE_2.

The production of these osteoclastic prostaglandins can be inhibited experimentally by certain nonsteroidal antiinflammatory drugs, particularly indomethacin,[12] although the drug's efficacy has not been demonstrated consistently in clinical situations in humans. If these agents are to play a role in the control of lytic bony metastases, it is likely that it will need to be before extensive cortical erosion has occurred and while osteoclastic activity is still prominent.

Once cortical bone destruction has extended through from the endosteal to the periosteal surface, the remaining spicules are densely encased by tumor cells and osteoclasts have in fact disappeared. At this point, the tumor cells alone apparently can destroy bone directly via immediate bone resorption[22] or by the secretion of bone-degrading enzymes[14] (Fig. 37-1, *B*).

BIOMECHANICS

From a biomechanical viewpoint, it is obvious that cortical defects weaken bone, especially with regard to torsional stresses. There are two general categories of cortical defects: those with a dimension less than the diameter of the bone and those with a dimension in excess of that diameter.

The smaller defect, termed a stress riser, weakens the bone by creating an uneven distribution of stresses in a loaded bone. Such a stress riser can decrease bone strength by 60% to 70%.[24]

The larger defect, termed an open-section defect, has a more profound effect on decreasing shear and torque-loading resistance. In normal bone under torsion loading, the shear stresses are more evenly distributed through the cross section (Fig. 37-2, *H*). The stress distribution in the closed section is radically altered by a large defect. Because the open section does not have a continuous outer surface, only the shear stress developed at the periphery of the section can resist the applied torque (Fig. 37-2, *I*). Consequently, the mass of bone resisting any given load is greatly decreased. Torsional testing of human adult tibiae with open-section defects shows a 90% reduction in load to failure and in energy storage to failure.[24]

INDICATIONS FOR INTERNAL FIXATION

The means of assessment of these biomechanical factors for any given patient is the conventional anteroposterior and lateral radiograph (Fig. 37-3, *A* and *B*). Fidler has demonstrated a technique estimating the percentage of cortical bone destruction at any level of a long bone using these two views alone (Fig. 37-3, *C-E*), and it is my experience that the technique usually is as accurate a prognosticator of impending pathologic fracture as is a cross-sectional CT scan. However, when cortical destruction progresses in a patchy or spiral distribution, it may be difficult to assess the circumferential bone loss accurately by this technique and a cross-sectional CT scan of the extremity may be more accurate (Fig. 37-4).

Once tumor lysis has progressed to the point that 50% or more of the cortex has been destroyed at any given level, the incidence of spontaneous pathologic fracture increases dramatically (Fig. 37-5). In the proximal femur, a lytic lesion in excess of 2.5 cm on either the anteroposterior or lateral view almost always can be seen to have an associated cortical disruption in excess of 50%, although it may be difficult to demonstrate such cortical destruction by a lateral radiograph because of the difficulty of obtaining such an x-ray view in a patient with a painful hip (Fig. 37-6, *A* and *B*).

The finding of a pathologic avulsion fracture of the lesser trochanter also suggests that at least 50% of the femoral cortex has been destroyed

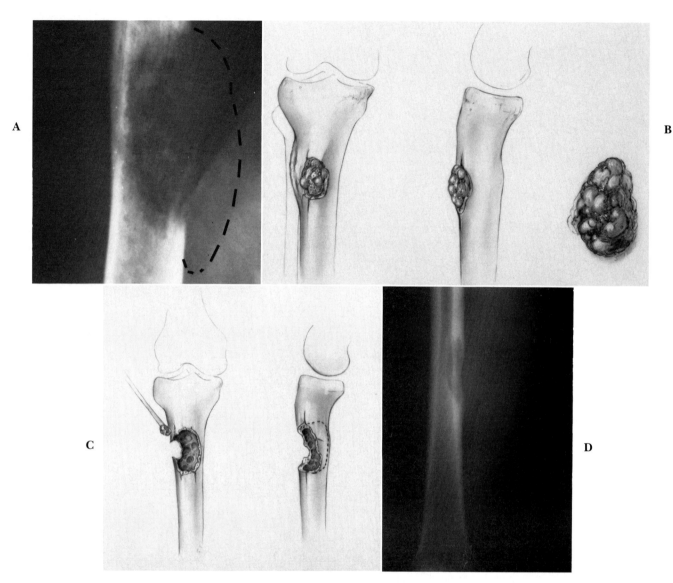

Fig. 37-2. A, Most radiographic pictures of metastases show focal destruction and surrounding patchy lysis. This appearance of a lesion radiographically suggests that there is little reactive host bone formation walling the tumor process (unlike Fig. 37-3, **A** and **B**), although there is evidence of periosteal new bone formed in response to the stress of an impending fracture. Often such lesions will have broken through the cortex by the time they become symptomatic, although the conventional radiographs usually do not demonstrate the soft tissue mass. This x-ray film of the distal femur of a patient with multiple myeloma shows an ill-defined extension of tumor lysis well beyond the confines of the cortical defect. Some minimal reactive bone has formed along the opposite cortex but is of little structural significance. At surgery, a large extracortical soft tissue mass was found (*dotted lines*), although the mass was not apparent radiographically. **B,** Schematic rendering of such a lesion (here in the proximal tibia) as it would be seen at surgery. The tumor tissue typically is soft, multiply lobulated, and moderately vascular. **C,** After curettage of the defect and removal of structurally inadequate bone, the cavity typically is twice the size of the lesion first appreciated radiographically. The extent of cortical destruction is also well in excess of that anticipated preoperatively. **D,** Lesion of the femoral diaphysis in a patient with metastatic breast carcinoma. The lesion appeared well circumscribed radiographically and involved approximately 60% of the circumferential cortex when measured by the technique shown in Fig. 37-3, **C-E.**

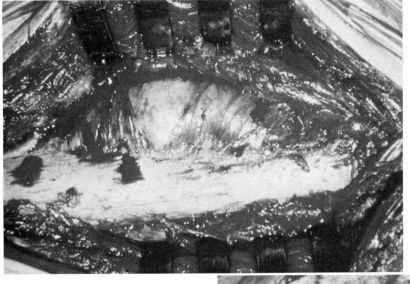

E

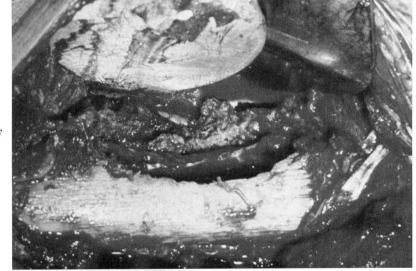

F

G

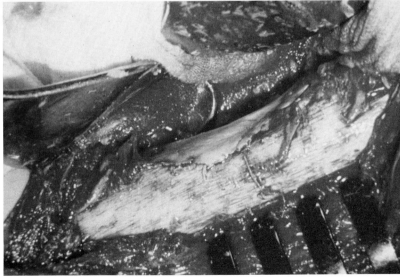

Fig. 37-2, cont'd. E, At surgery an unsuspected large exophytic mass was encountered emerging from the cortical defect. **F,** At curettage of the lesion, the extent of the cortical destruction was apparent. **G,** After closed Kuntscher nail fixation of the femur, the cortical defect and adjacent intramedullary canal were packed with methylmethacrylate in an effort to reduce the localized stress riser created by a large open-section defect in the cortex.

Continued.

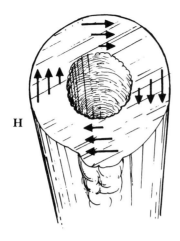 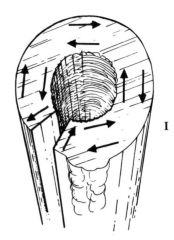

Fig. 37-2, cont'd. H, Under torsional loading the distribution of shear stress in a cross section of intact bone is symmetric and linearly a function of the radius. **I,** An open-section defect causes a redistribution of stresses. Only the stress vectors at the periphery of the cross section are able to resist the tortionally applied load. Thus an open-section defect severely reduces the ability of the bone to carry torsional load. (**H** and **I,** From Pugh, J., et al., J.B. Lippincott, Inc.)

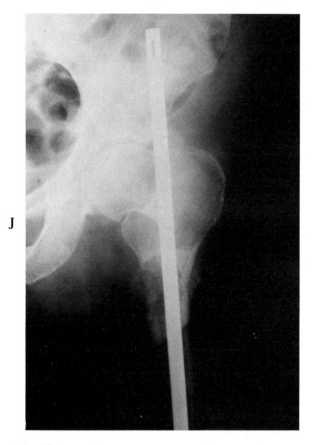

Fig. 37-2, cont'd. J, Another reason for packing large lytic lesions with methylmethacrylate at the time of internal fixation is to avoid the sort of shortening apparent here, which cannot be obviated by fixation with an intramedullary device alone.

locally and that the patient has a significant chance of developing a pathologic fracture across the femur at the intertrochanteric or subtrochanteric level (Fig. 37-7).[2]

Based on these observations, it is possible to establish relative criteria for prophylactic internal stabilization of impending pathologic fractures.[1,9,14,16,18] These criteria include:

1. A destructive lesion involving more than 50% of the cortical bone circumferentially
2. A lytic lesion of the proximal femur larger than 2.5 cm
3. A lesion of the proximal femur associated with avulsion of the lesser trochanter

It is important to realize that many of these lytic lesions will not be painful before the development of the fracture. Fidler found that less than half of such patients experienced local pain before the fracture occurred.[9]

Unfortunately, all of these criteria are based on the assessment of lytic lesions where the size of the tumor focus or the extent of its destruction can be determined radiographically. In fact, the majority of bony metastases ultimately resulting in pathologic fractures combine both blastic and lytic changes or show radiographic evidence of diffuse or difficult to quantify lytic changes; thus it is easy to underestimate the actual extent of tumor lysis (Figs. 37-2, *A-G,* and 37-8, *A* and *B*). Radionuclide scans using technetium-99 accu-

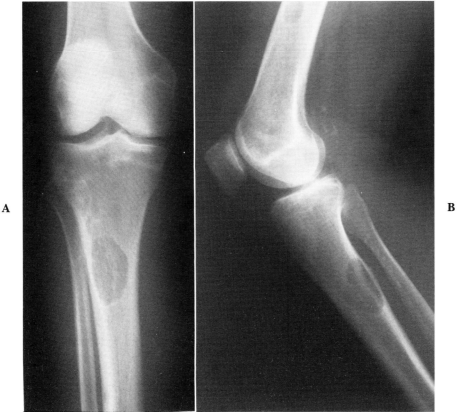

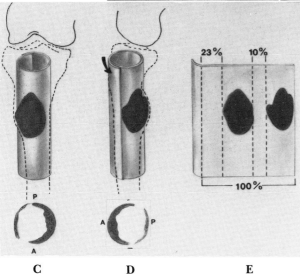

Fig. 37-3. A and **B,** Well-circumscribed lytic myelomatous lesion of the proximal tibia with a similar but smaller focus apparent in the distal femur. Although the lesion's distinct margin and the surrounding reactive bone suggest that it is only slowly progressive, the extent of cortical destruction and persistent pain with weight bearing indicated a need for prophylactic internal fixation. With such well-circumscribed lesions, the extent of cortical destruction can be estimated with surprising accuracy from conventional anteroposterior and lateral radiographs by using the method of Fidler.[9] A sheet of paper is rolled into a tube approximating the shaft of the affected long bone. The lesion outlined is copied from the anteroposterior radiograph onto the front of the tube (**C**). The tube is then turned 90 degrees, and the outline from the lateral radiograph is copied (**D**). When the sheet is unfurled (**E**), an accurate assessment can be made of the extent of circumferential cortical destruction. In this instance, only 33% of the circumferential cortex remains intact. As noted in Table 37-1, this patient is at high risk for a spontaneous pathologic fracture and should have prophylactic fixation.

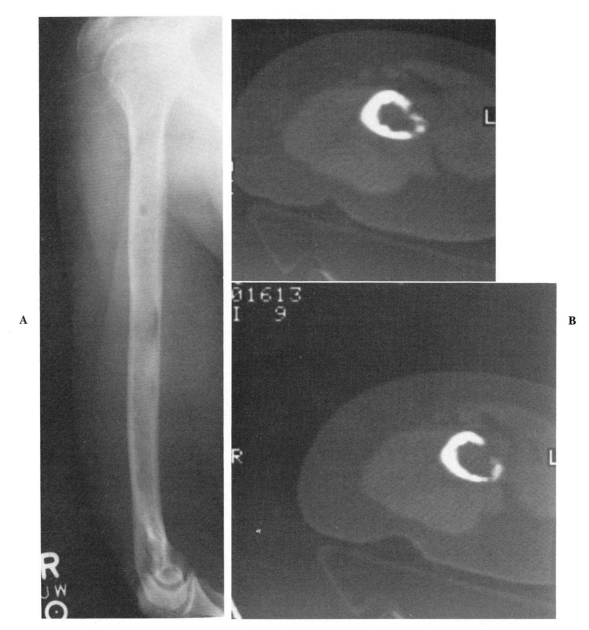

Fig. 37-4. A, A partially circumscribed myelomatous lesion of the midhumeral diaphysis. Although some cortical destruction is apparent, neither an anteroposterior nor this lateral view suggested that the cortical loss was in excess of 20%. **B,** Because of persistent pain in the area with even the slightest stress on the arm, and because of progressive radial neuralgia, a computerized tomographic scan was obtained. This reveals at least 50% loss of circumferential cortex and suggests the presence of an exophytic soft tissue mass arising from the cortical defect. At operation destruction of approximately 50% of the circumferential cortex was apparent and a large soft tissue tumor was noted that had partially encompassed the radial nerve. The tumor was debulked, and prophylactic fixation using an ASIF plate reinforced by methylmethacrylate was accomplished. The patient, who experienced prompt relief of pain and recovery of neurologic function, remains symptom-free 19 months after surgery.

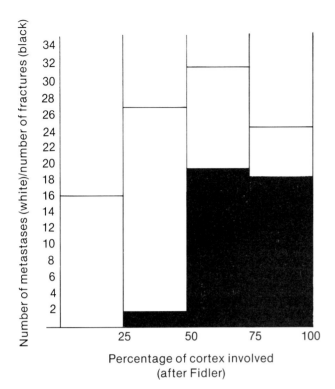

Fig. 37-5. Incidence of spontaneous pathologic fracture in metastatic malignancy.

rately demonstrate the presence of skeletal metastases in over 90% of cases, but such scans are not particularly useful in attempting to quantitate the extent of bone destruction or, more important, the likelihood of a pathologic fracture developing. Because technetium-99 uptake initially is dependent on local blood flow to bone and later dependent on local osteoblastic activity, slowly or rapidly progressive lytic lesions provoking minimal response from adjacent host osteocytes often appear deceptively quiet on bone scan (Fig. 37-9, *A* and *B*). Myeloma, lymphoma, and colon metastases often behave in this way. Galium scanning has offered no improvement in diagnostic accuracy over conventional technetium-99 bone scans.

For patients who experience focal limb pain that is aggravated by weight bearing, where conventional radiographs, CT scans, or tomograms do not demonstrate a clear-cut risk of impending fracture, a combination of these studies with radioisotope scanning affords a better concept of the balance between tumor aggressiveness and host response. Such patients are treated typically by local irradiation therapy, and in most instances

---

INDICATIONS FOR PROPHYLACTIC FIXATION OF IMPENDING LONG BONE FRACTURES

1. Cortical bone destruction of 50% or more
2. Lesion of 2.5 cm or more of proximal femur
3. Pathologic avulsion fracture of the lesser trochanter
4. Persisting stress pain despite irradiation

---

effective pain control can be achieved. However, the physician must realize that the initial response of bone to irradiation is focal hyperemia leading to a localized osteoporosis, which actually weakens the host bone temporarily. For the first 10 to 18 days after beginning a course of radiotherapy, the patient actually is at a higher risk of fracturing through the tumor focus than before radiation was commenced. Patients may frequently incur long bone fractures while transferring to or from the radiotherapy table after 2 weeks of a projected 4-week course of treatment.

The vagaries of assessing fracture risk in patients with mixed blastic and lytic lesions and the increase in risk of fracture created by the initial response to irradiation prompt the establishment of another relative indication for prophylactic fixation. This is the presence of persistent or increasing local pain, particularly when aggravated by weight bearing, despite completion of at least 2 weeks of radiotherapy (see box). Most such patients probably have microfractures that will progress to displacement even in the face of restricted weight bearing if the bone is not internally splinted (Fig. 37-9, *C-E*).

HEALING

Tong and associates[25] report that up to 58% of patients with long bone lesions treated by irradiation but without prophylactic fixation suffered late recurrences of pain despite initial complete relief. In addition, 26% of these patients suffered pathologic fractures after the completion of a full course (average 4050 rads) of radiotherapy. These figures reinforce concern about the existence of unrecognized microfractures that may progress to frank displacement, perhaps after adequate radiation therapy. They also raise concern that, even if the destructive tumor process is ablated by irradiation, the open section defects or

Text continued on p. 372.

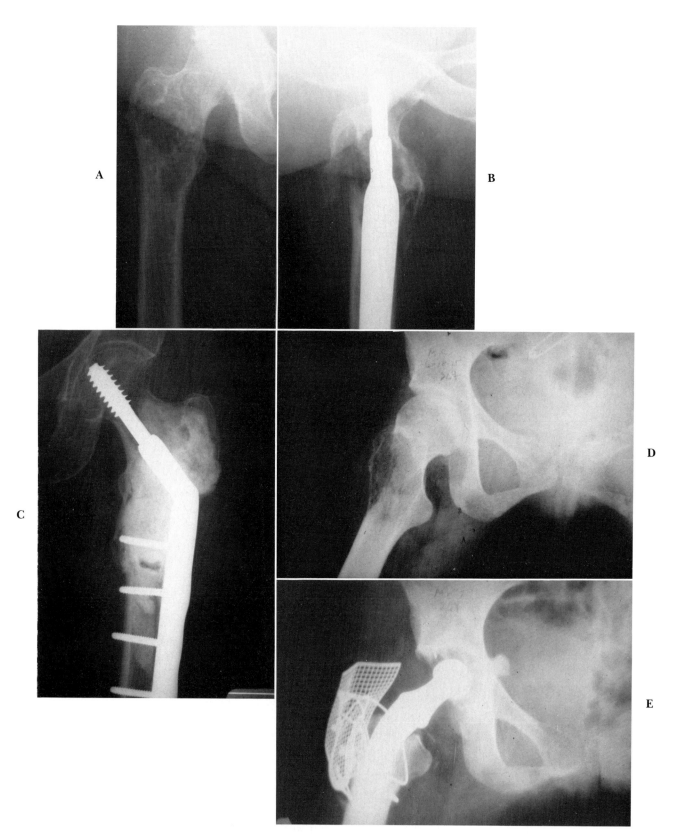

Fig. 37-6. For legend see opposite page.

Fig. 37-6. A, An extensive lytic metastasis at least 3 cm in diameter involving the proximal femur (carcinoma of the breast). Neither this view nor a "frogleg" lateral view revealed definite cortical destruction. **B,** Because of the lesion's size, prophylactic fixation was accomplished before the area was irradiated. An intraoperative true lateral view after fixation clearly demonstrates extensive destruction of the anterior cortex. The lesion healed after irradiation, and the patient remains alive and pain free 5 years after surgery. **C,** Expansile lytic lesion of the proximal femur associated with expansion of the medullary canal and marked thinning of the cortex. Methylmethacrylate filling the lesion (and the medullary canal proximal and distal to the lesion) greatly enhances prophylactic fixation with a compression hip screw. Ideally, the acrylic cement should extend proximally up to the level of the threads of the hip screw and distally to incorporate at least the second screw of the sideplate. An artificial buttress thus is created, effectively resisting compression loads and the tendency for the proximal femur to angulate into varus. Such fixation also complements the resistance to shear and torque forces that are primarily afforded by the hip screw. **D,** A similar expansile lytic lesion of the proximal femur in a 26-year-old female with metastatic breast cancer. **E,** Other than attempting prophylactic internal fixation of this femur, the surgeon chose to resect the proximal head and neck and to perform a total hip arthroplasty. Wire mesh was used to secure the abductor muscles to the shaft, because the greater trochanter had been destroyed by tumor. Total hip replacement in preference to internal fixation is favored by many surgeons who believe that the technique obviates further concerns about the permanency of internal fixation in the face of questionable bony union after radiation. (**D** and **E** from Habermann, E.T., et al.: Clin. Orthop. **169:**70, 1982.)

Fig. 37-7. A, A pathologic avulsion fracture of the lesser trochanter in a patient with metastatic carcinoma of the breast. Although the femoral neck and subtrochanteric region appeared unaffected by metastases, the lesser trochanter fracture was considered an ominous warning of impending fracture of the proximal femur. **B,** The technitium scan revealed markedly increased uptake in the intertrochanteric femur. The patient refused prophylactic stabilization of the femur and 2 weeks later suffered a spontaneous intertrochanteric fracture when she rolled over in bed.

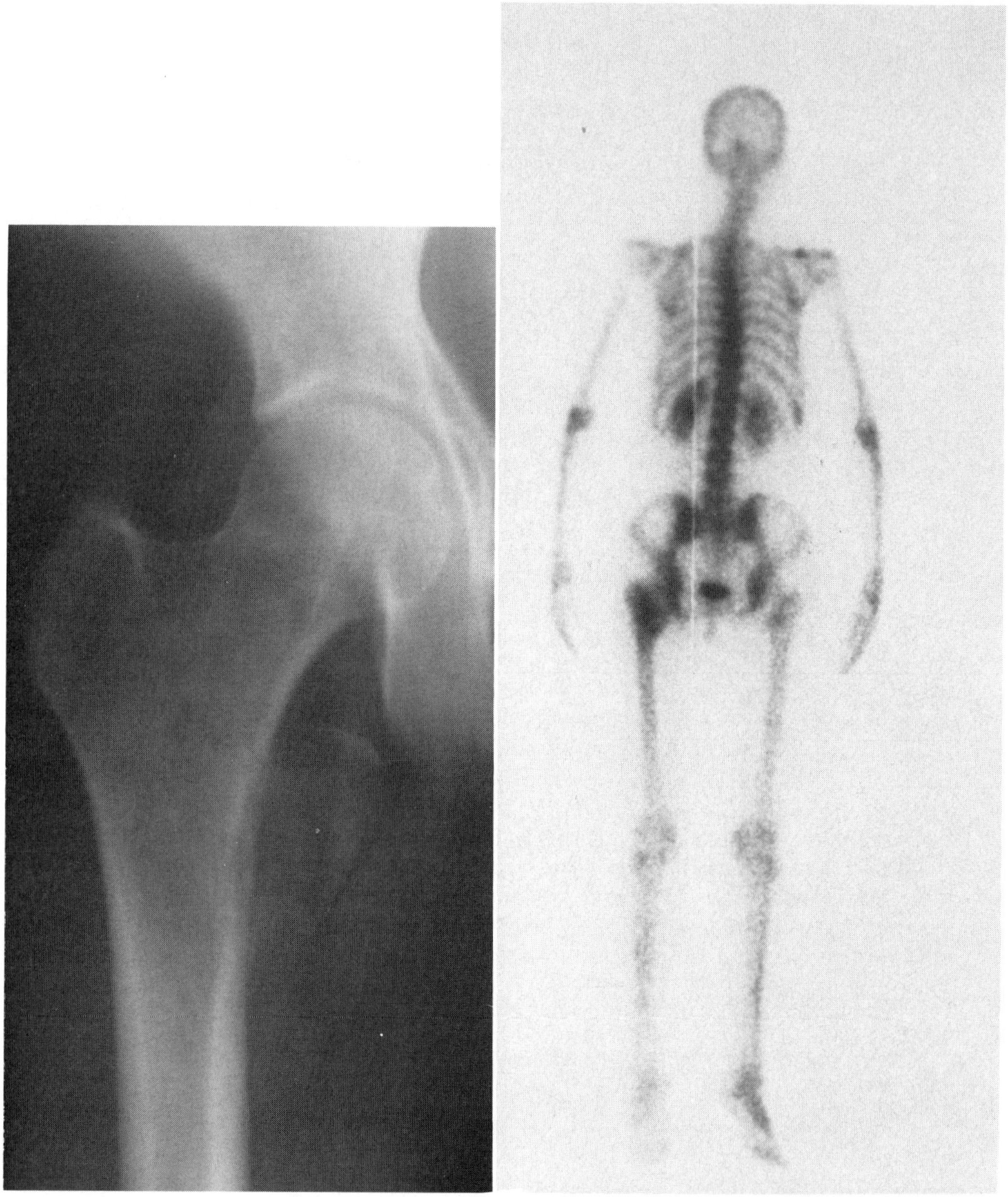

B

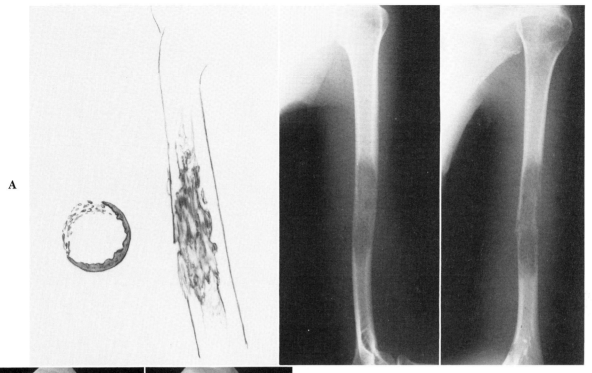

A

C

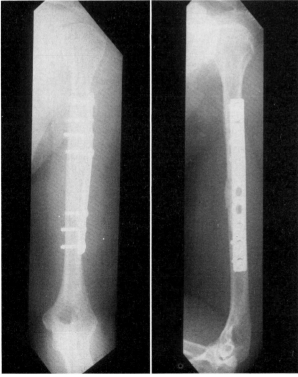

D   **E**

Fig. 37-8. A, Some metastases appear as diffusely reticulated lytic lesions with poorly defined margins. Typically the extent of bony destruction is underestimated unless a cross-sectional CT scan is obtained to demonstrate the loss of cortical continuity. The tipoff to an impending fracture is persistence of pain, particularly with stress to the bone, which persists despite adequate irradiation. **B,** A 33-year old female with metastatic carcinoma of the breast and extensive reticulated lysis of the humeral diaphysis. The lesion remained painful despite adequate irradiation, suggesting the presence of cortical microfractures not apparent radiographically. The patient's oncologist recommended against prophylactic fixation, hoping her bone pain would resolve with chemotherapy alone. **C,** 2 months later a frank pathologic fracture is apparent, unfortunately having occurred during transcontinental air travel. The fracture was complicated by a radial nerve palsy persisting 3 months. **D** and **E,** After open fixation and radial neurolysis, the patient was pain free within 10 days. She enjoyed excellent fracture stability, despite the absence of true bony union, until her death 26 months after surgery.

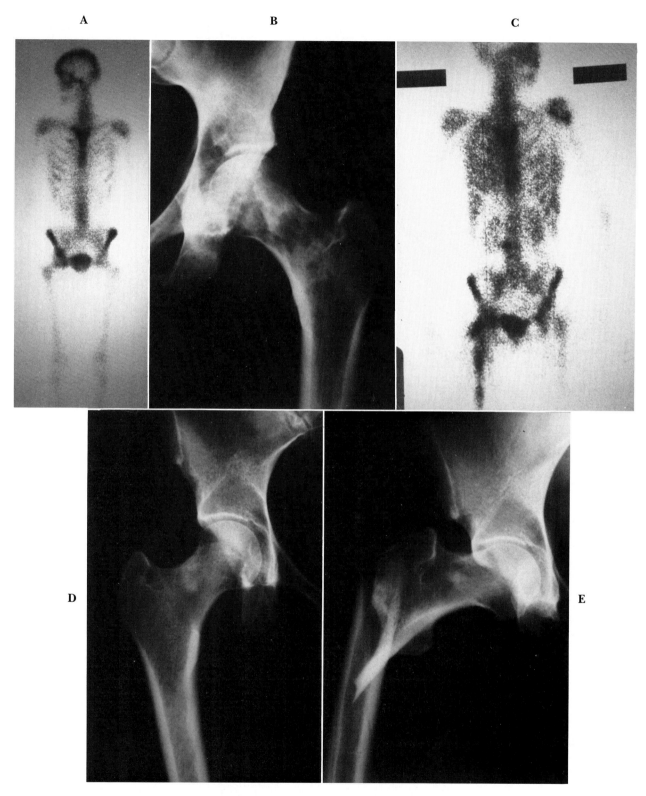

Fig. 37-9. For legend see opposite page.

Fig. 37-9. A technitium bone scan reflects both blood flow through bone (during the initial vascular phase of the scan) and osteoblastic activity (during the late or secondary phase). Metastatic lesions stimulating minimal increase in blood flow or osteoblastic reaction will appear misleadingly quiet by scan despite aggressive bone destruction apparent radiographically. **A,** A technitium bone scan of a patient with left hip pain. Increased uptake was described in the opposite right supraacetabular region, but the scan did not suggest the extent of metastatic disease, which was subsequently revealed by the radiograph (**B**), in the left proximal femur. **B,** An anteroposterior view of the left hip shows extensive lytic destruction of the femoral neck. A spontaneous pathologic fracture occurred through this area 3 days after the x-ray film was obtained. **C,** Conversely, intensive hypervascularity and/or osteoblastic activity in bone, suggestive of an aggressive neoplastic process, may not be reflected by discernible changes on conventional radiographs until there is at least 75% destruction of bone locally. This is a technitium scan of a patient with pain in the right hip. Markedly increased uptake is apparent in the proximal half of the right femur. **D,** An x-ray film of the right hip taken at the same time reveals only a small blastic focus in the femoral neck. The extent of lysis in the subtrochanteric area is not apparent. **E,** A subtrochanteric pathologic fracture occurred as the patient was being lifted off the x-ray table. At surgery there was extensive cortical lysis as suggested by the bone scan.

Fig. 37-10. A case demonstrating postirradiation heterotopic ossification or calcification within a metastatic focus mimicking true bone healing. **A,** A lytic lesion in the subtrochanteric region of the left femur is apparent in a patient with metastatic carcinoma of the breast. **B,** After the lesion was irradiated with 4000 rads, the radiograph was interpreted as showing bone healing, but in fact merely demonstrated calcification within the tumor focus.

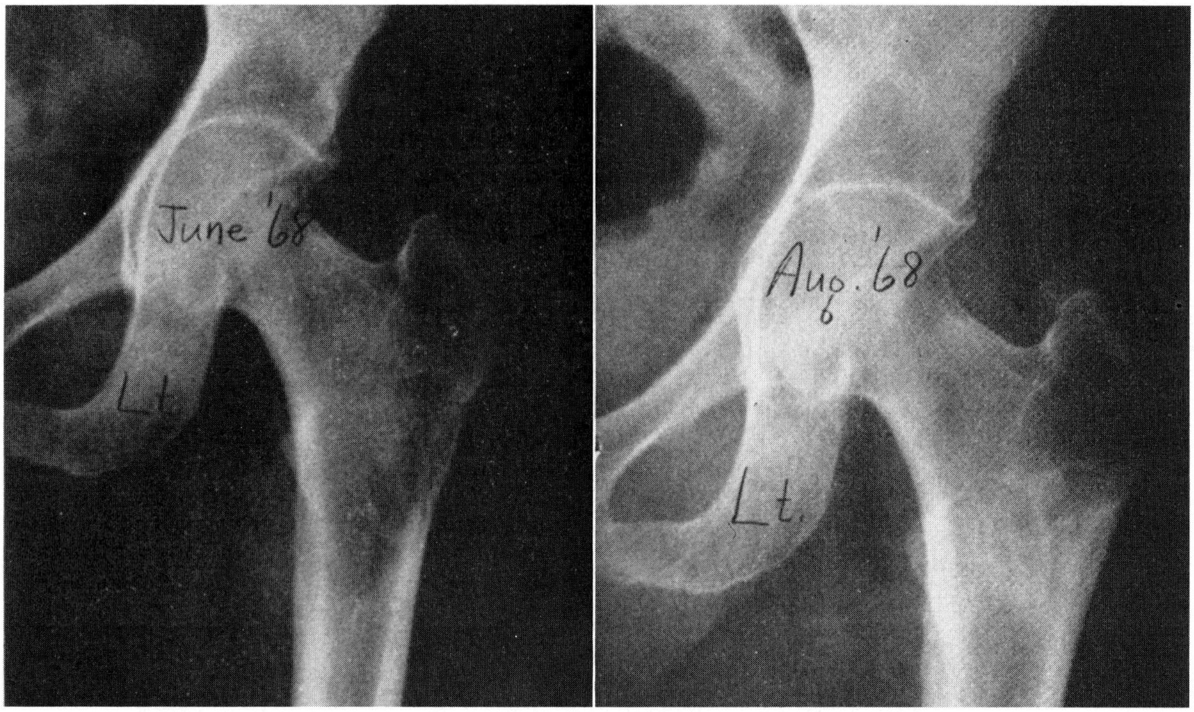

stress risers originally created in cortical bone by the tumor remain and that these predispose to eventual fracture even in the absence of active tumor lysis.

Various radiotherapists[3,4,25] also have raised the question of how frequently lytic lesions actually reossify following completion of radiation and why there appears to be a large disparity clinically between the high rate of healing and reossification of lytic lesions, and the low incidence of bony union if a pathologic fracture occurs through that lesion. Although Beals[1] estimated that only 4% of lytic breast metastases reossify, most other workers have reported an incidence of 65% to 85% reossification under similar circumstances so long as a fracture has not ensued.[6,17,23] Although some changes radiographically interpreted as reossification may actually represent the formation of heterotopic ossification within the lesion (Fig. 37-10), in the great majority of instances replacement of the lesion by mature organized bone does occur.

This reparative process following irradiation has been summarized by Matsubayashi.[21] Initially there is evidence of degeneration and necrosis of cancer cells followed by replacement with proliferative fibrous tissue. Collagen fibers then aggregate within a loose but richly vascularized fibrous stroma. These fluffy strands of aggregated collagen gradually become calcified, and finally woven bone trabeculae appear that eventually mature into lamellar bone.

If a pathologic fracture supervenes during this reparative process, a totally different pathway for healing exists. Normally, fractures heal by the formation of a bridging callus, which develops through the network of organizing hematoma and gradually is differentiated into fibrocartilage, then into hyaline cartilage, and eventually is replaced by bone. As noted, this process is in marked contrast to a lytic metastasis, which appears to occur primarily as a result of direct osteogenesis. The chondrogenetic phase of healing (the formation of fibrocartilage and its evolution into hyaline cartilage) required for the healing of a pathologic fracture—but not for the

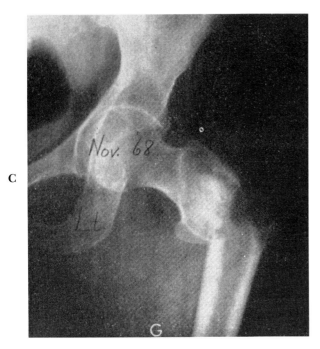

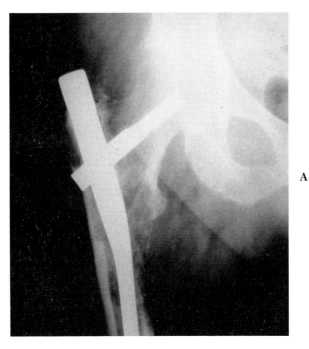

Fig. 37-10, cont'd. C, The patient remained ambulatory despite hip pain and 3 months later suffered a displaced pathologic fracture through the original lytic focus. Considering the size and location of the lesion and the fact that it remained painful with weight bearing after irradiation, prophylactic internal fixation should have been performed. (From Blake, D.D., J.B. Lippincott, Inc.)

Fig. 37-11. A, A 63-year-old female with metastatic carcinoma of the breast and large lytic metastases in the subtrochanteric femur. The impending pathologic fracture was prophylactically fixed closed with a Zickel nail and need not be exposed. Adjunctive fixation by methylmethacrylate is not necessary.

Continued.

filling in of a lytic defect—is extremely sensitive to radiation. Bonarigo and Rubin[4] demonstrated experimentally that radiation in excess of 2500 rads seriously interfered with the chondrogenetic phase of fracture healing yet caused minimal interference with osteoblastic proliferation. For this reason, nonunion of a fracture often occurs after radiation, whereas osteogenesis continues healing through a nonfractured lytic area. Here again is a strong argument for prophylactic internal fixation of lytic lesions at high risk for fracture before such a fracture occurs (Fig. 37-11, *A* and *B*).

TECHNIQUES OF PROPHYLACTIC INTERNAL FIXATION

Once the decision has been made to fix an impending fracture internally, the surgeon must review several general technical considerations critical to the success of the procedure.

1. Every effort should be made to prevent the occurrence of a fracture during the operative procedure to avoid the concomitant higher risk of nonunion.

2. Soft tissue surrounding the bone should be disturbed as little as possible to preserve the periosteal blood supply. This is particularly important because the endosteal circulation usually has been disrupted locally by the tumor process.

3. Where large thin-walled lesions exist or where the intramedullary canal varies greatly in size (Fig. 37-11, *D*), closed intramedullary nailing techniques should be augmented by direct reinforcement of the lesion using methylmethacrylate. This will enhance fixation of the distal long bone, particularly with regard to the torsional stability, and will also prevent shortening of the bone. The use of an intralocking intramedullary device that is specifically designed to prevent shortening, such as the Grosse-Kempf nail, also may be considered. However, the use of this device is technically much more demanding than conventional intramedullary fixation and is not as secure a method of preventing late shortening of the long bone if bony union does not occur ultimately.

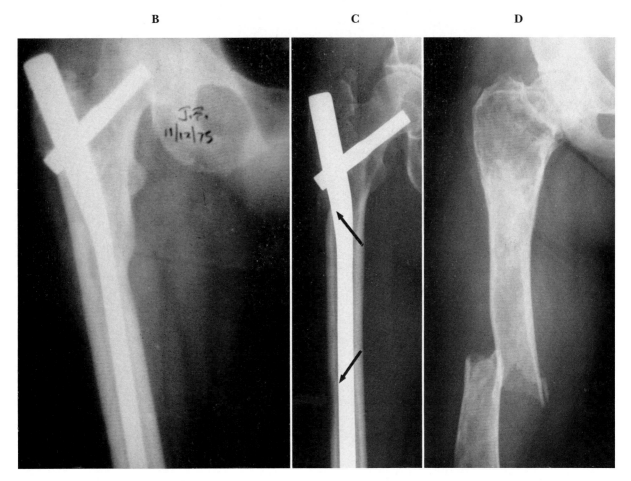

B **C** **D**

Fig. 37-11, cont'd. B, Fracture through the lesion was prevented by prophylactic fixation, and 5 months after surgery, despite local irradiation, the lesion was healed completely. (From Habermann, E.T.) **C,** Another example of an ideal use for the Zickel nail. An extensive lytic foxus in the subtrochanteric region (*arrow*) of the femur has been reinforced prophylactically and, by the same technique, a lesion of the femoral diaphysis with moderate destruction has been stabilized (*arrow*). In this circumstance closed insertion of the Zickel nail components could be accomplished without the necessity of using intramedullary methylmethacrylate. **D,** This unusual situation of a patient with widespread metastases from renal carcinoma with cortical destruction and deformity involved almost the entire femur. This patient had been encouraged to have prophylactic fixation using a Zickel nail but had refused surgical intervention even after the fracture occurred. Prophylactic fixation using an intramedullary rod before the fracture had occurred would not have been appropriate because a major stress riser would have been created at the base of the femoral neck and in the intertrochanteric region of the femur and a fracture through that area would have ensued. Once the fracture occurred, a Zickel nail still would have been ideal for fixation but rotational stability of the distal femur could only have been achieved by extensive curettage of the medullary canal and packing the canal with methylmethacrylate around the distal end of the nail. The distal canal would have been filled with cement in a liquid state and the fracture then reduced with the nail inserted the length of the canal before polymerization occurred.

A

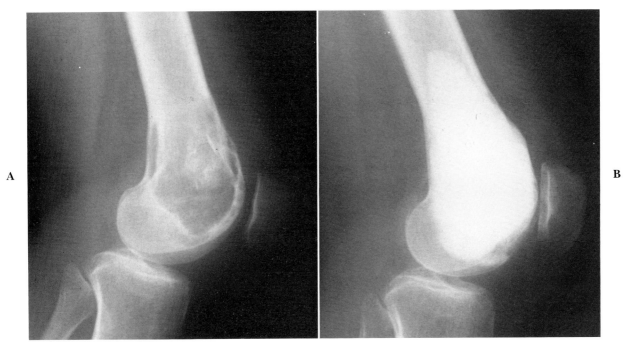

B

Fig. 37-12. A, Occasionally, extensive metaphyseal or epiphyseal destructive defects have insufficient bone proximal or distal to the lesional margins to allow conventional prophylactic fixation. **B,** The technique of intralesional curettage and filling of the defect with methylmethacrylate can be used to prevent subchondral fractures, bony collapse, and disruption of the joint surface. The lesion then can be irradiated with impunity. The presence of methylmethacrylate within the tumor cavity, even if radio-opaque, does not interfere with the efficacy of irradiation. Moreover, irradiation does not change the mechanical properties of the cement.

4. Where defects extend through the full thickness of cortical bone, these defects should be plugged by acrylic cement at the time of fixation to minimize the significance of stress risers or open section defects (Fig. 37-2, *H* and *I*).

5. Lesions that have not been irradiated before fixation should have as much tumor tissue as possible debulked before fixation to enhance the efficacy of subsequent irradiation (Fig. 37-2, *D-G*).

6. Lesions appearing likely to be highly vascular should be considered for arteriographic evaluation and possible emobilization before open curettage.

Lesions of the femoral neck or of the intertrochanteric area of the proximal femur are treated best by fixation with the use of a compression hip screw and side plate. Intramedullary devices such as the Zickel nail, although affording better prophylaxis against subsequent fracture of the subtrochanteric area, do not reinforce the femoral neck adequately if there is tumor lysis extending significantly into that area. I have reviewed the x-ray films of three patients with such lesions reinforced by a Zickel nail, each of whom suffered a subsequent fracture through the subcapital portion of the femoral neck just proximal to the tip of the cross-fixation pin.

Patients with impending intertrochanteric or femoral neck fracture are positioned on a fracture table, and a guide pin is inserted into the midportion of the femoral head and neck under image intensification. A 2 cm by 2 cm lateral cortical window is created, and the corkscrew portion of a compression hip screw is inserted over the guide pin under direct vision as proximally as possible so that its tip lies in the immediately subchondral bone of the femoral head. As much tumor tissue as possible is removed from the intertrochanteric lesion both proximal and distal to the cortical window. A four- or five-hole side plate is articulated with the corkscrew, while care is taken to avoid undue sheer or torque stress across the weakened bone thereby creating a fracture. Once the surgeon is comfortable that the sideplate can be positioned easily over the screw, the sideplate is removed and the cavity filled with methylmethacrylate injected under pressure and filling its entire confines. Ideally, the cement extends proximally to the level of the hip screw threads and distally to the level of the first or second sideplate screw (Fig. 37-6, *C*). A sideplate should be chosen of sufficient length to allow bicortical fixation by at least three screws below the distal extent of the tumor cavity.

Haberman,[14] Lane,[20] and Sim[18] all have advocated resection of the proximal femur where intertrochanteric lesions create a high risk of fracture. The upper femur is thereby replaced by a proximal femoral prosthesis, often necessitating acetabular prosthetic replacement as well (Fig. 37-6, *D* and *E*). Biopsy of the acetabular bone at the time of surgery often reveals evidence of metastases, and Haberman has used this indication to replace both sides of the joint.[14]

Such replacement (rather than fixation) of proximal lesions obviates fears of late local tumor recurrence or fixation-device failure. However, the technique requires the surgeon to maintain a large stock of proximal femoral prostheses. It also subjects the patient to much more operative time and blood loss than does prophylactic fixation, and it introduces risk of acetabular loosening, hip dislocation, trochanteric avulsion, or nonunion, which are not encountered after internal fixation. For these reasons I still advocate fixation techniques for all but the most severely destroyed proximal femora.

Subtrochanteric lesions are stabilized best by using a Zickel nail inserted while the patient is in the lateral decubitus position. This position allows the affected leg to be positioned freely for insertion of the nail through the tip of the greater trochanter. I have found that attempts to insert the Zickel nail while the patient is supine on the fracture table necessitates forceful adduction and often rotation of the affected limb, thus predisposing to a fracture through weakened subtrochanteric bone where much of that stress is concentrated.

Many subtrochanteric lesions can be effectively fixed prophylactically with the Zickel nail alone, inserted by a closed technique and without augmentation by intramedullary methylmethacrylate (Fig. 37-11, *C*). However, when large cortical defects exist in the subtrochanteric area, I believe that these should be filled with acrylic cement, polymerizing in situ in an effort to restore cortical continuity and thereby reduce local stress potentially productive of a subsequent fracture (Fig.

37-2, *H* and *I*). This requires local exposure of the tumor focus, but it offers the additional advantage that extensive debulking of the tumor mass can be established as well, thereby enhancing the efficacy of subsequent radiation therapy. Others have performed such fixation without filling the defect with cement and have reported good results with a low incidence of late refracture (Fig. 37-11, *A* and *B*).[14]

Lesions of the femoral shaft usually can be fixed internally by closed intramedullary nailing with the patient in the lateral decubitus position. Again, however, when large defects exist, particularly associated with marked cortical thinning or open defects, it may be necessary to expose these areas, remove tissue within the cavity, and fill the resulting defect with acrylic cement. This procedure prevents the all-too-common complication during later weight bearing that bone about the tumor focus collapses, the proximal shaft fragment slides over the nail to impact over the distal fragment, and femoral shortening with proximal nail protrusion results (Fig. 37-2, *J*). Under these circumstances an alternative method of preventing shortening and maintaining the principles of closed intramedullary fixation is to use an interlocking nail with cross fixation well proximal and distal to the area of tumor lysis. However, a potential disadvantage of this fixation technique is that, if the lytic lesion does not ossify ultimately, the relatively fragile cross-fixation screws eventually will loosen or break.

If a risk does not seem to exist that shortening will occur by telescoping of the major fragments about the intramedullary rod, a conventional closed rodding technique should be accomplished and no attempt should be made to fill the lytic defect with methylmethacrylate. There is no effective way to augment the fixation by methylmethacrylate unless the lytic focus is approached directly surgically, tumor tissue is removed under direct vision, and the cavity is filled with cement. Low-viscosity acrylic cement can be injected down the full length of the femoral shaft within the intramedullary rod, but in my opinion the cement adds little if any ancillary stability under these circumstances.

Large thin-walled lytic metastases in the distal femur are uncommon, but when present they are especially challenging because of the difficulty of accomplishing fixation of the narrow distal fragment. If sufficient bone of the femoral condyle remains, an angulated condylar plate can be used, augmenting the fixation by packing methyl-methacrylate into the debrided cavity of the lytic metastasis. Again, care should be taken to use a blade plate of sufficient length to allow at least two and preferably three screws to transfix intact cortices about the confines of the lesion.

Occasionally a metastatic focus may aggressively destroy bone right up to the subchondral bone of the femoral condylar articular cartilage (Fig. 37-12). Because all cartilage is resistant to tumor invasion,[19] it is extremely unlikely that the malignant process will invade the knee joint unless a pathologic fracture has occurred. These lesions are best managed by curettage through a cortical window followed by packing of the tumor cavity with cement without attempted reinforcement by any metal-fixation device. Care must be taken to prevent extrusion of liquid cement into the knee joint through even a small fracture defect. Intraoperative radiographs should be obtained, and if cement is noted in the joint it should be removed through a small arthrotomy.

Large aneurysmal lesions of the distal femur, particularly those from myeloma or from retro-perotoneal malignancies, often should be studied arteriographically before surgery because of the high likelihood of their being hypervascular and the consequent risk of intractable intraoperative blood loss. Embolization of such lesions by free fat or by Gelfoam strips soaked in thrombin is indicated for particularly vascular lesions, especially if those lesions have been irradiated. There is some evidence that the effectiveness of radiation administered after such embolization may be lessened by the temporarily diminished oxygen tension in the tumor caused by its embolization.

As already noted, Haberman has taken biopsies of radiographically normal–appearing periacetabular bone in many breast carcinoma patients who have recognizable proximal femoral lesions and has found a high incidence of metastases. Under these circumstances he often has advocated prophylactic acetabular replacement. My own experience suggests that the great majority of such metastases can be controlled by focal irradiation and that they will not progress to fracture or even—in most instances—become symptomatic. However, occasional patients will develop intractable acetabular pain unresponsive to radiotherapy and aggravated by the stress of weight bearing. These individuals should be considered to have microfractures of the acetabular bone and to have a high risk of a central acetab-

ular fracture if a joint replacement and stabilization is not performed (Fig. 37-13). In most instances, the extent of bone destruction encountered at surgery and the technical requirements for joint stabilization far exceed what might be anticipated from preoperative roentgenograms.[16] It is the presence of pain on weight bearing even after the completion of an adequate course of radiation that is the clearest indicator of the need for prophylactic acetabular reconstruction.

Lytic lesions of the humerus generally are considered to have a minimal risk of fracture simply because the humerus is not ordinarily subjected to weight bearing. However, because patients with widespread metastases often are required to use assistive devices such as canes, crutches, or a walker, necessitated by concomitant metastases of the spine or lower extremities, the humerus may in effect become a weight-bearing bone and require similarly aggressive prophylaxis.

By far the most common focus for impending humeral fractures is the mid-diaphysis. Typically, lesions that are focal and have minimal risk of shortening are best managed by closed intramedullary fixation using a humeral Kuntscher nail.

Where a large lesion with extension-bone destruction exists, fixation by a long compression bone plate is advisable (Figs. 37-4 and 37-8). Although the application of such a plate requires a more difficult anatomic dissection that encompasses some risk to the radial nerve, the advantages of the technique far outweigh its disadvantages: (1) the tumor focus can be entered, debulked, and filled with methylmethacrylate and (2) fixation by heavy plate augmented by acrylic protects not only against shortening of the humerus but also against the development of a subsequent fracture secondary to a distraction force. It must be remembered that the usual stresses on the upper extremity long bones involve distraction and not compression. I have seen three instances where such forces caused a distraction through a lytic focus despite internal splintage by an intramedullary rod.

Distal humeral lesions are the most difficult to fix prophylactically for several reasons: (1) the thin bone at the olecranon fossa prevents direct axial intramedullary fixation or fixation by a blade plate, (2) one or both epicondyles are frequently involved, thereby obviating adequate fixation by a Y or T plate of the type used for

Fig. 37-13. A, Destructive lesion of the supraacetabular bone in a 51-year-old female 11 years after a mastectomy for breast carcinoma. The patient was asymptomatic, and this film was obtained as part of an intravenous pylogram study for the evaluation of chronic pylonephritis. No further evaluation of the patient's hip disease was undertaken, but she was given prophylactic irradiation (4500 rads) because of the changes on x-ray film. **B,** 3 months later the patient was running to catch a bus and suddenly suffered a minimally painful superior-central fracture dislocation of the hip. Previously noted changes in the supraacetabular region are minimally apparent after irradiation. This fracture was managed by total hip reconstruction, stabilizing the acetabular component by the use of a protrusio cup and Steinmann pins inserted across the sacroiliac joint.

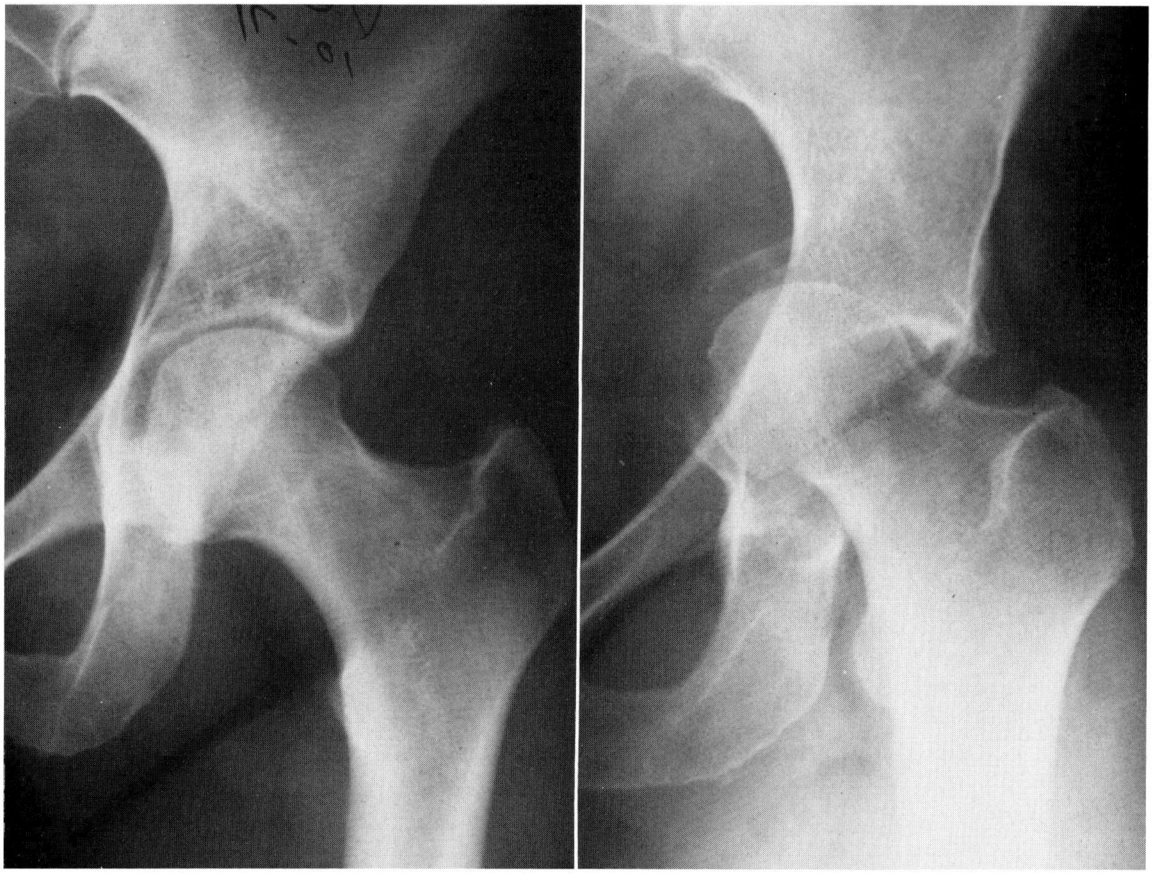

Fig. 37-14. A and **B,** Another extensive area of reticulated lysis, here involving the distal humerus. A spontaneous fracture occurred as the patient was transferred from the x-ray table. **C** and **D,** Because of the distal extent of bone destruction, including a portion of the medial epicondyle (*arrow*), fixation was accomplished by using Rush rods inserted retrograde and reinforced by methylmethacrylate packed into the curetted lesion. The fixation, although appearing somewhat tenuous, has remained secure in the absence of bony union for 24 months after surgery.

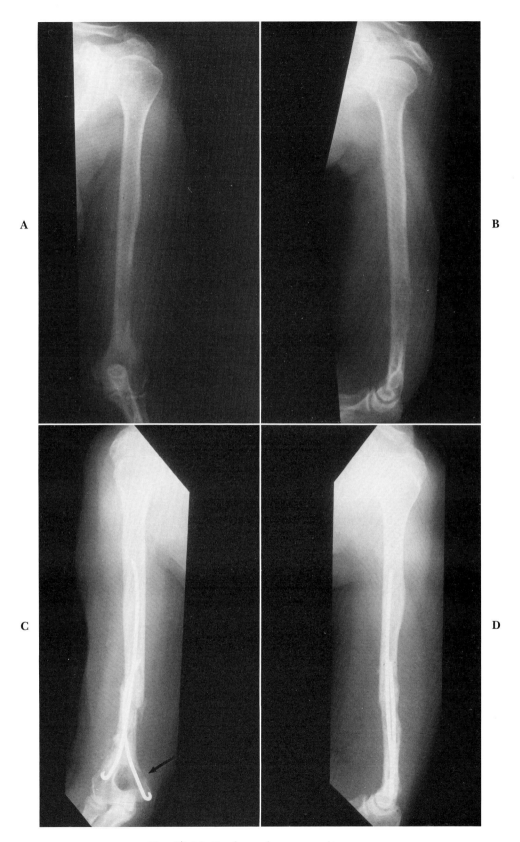

Fig. 37-14. For legend see opposite page.

traumatic supracondylar or intracondylar fractures (Fig. 37-14, *A* and *B*), and (3) early elbow motion is essential to minimize upper extremity disability for these patients who often depend so greatly on walking aids. Because of these difficulties the most effective method for fixation includes local debridement of the tumor focus and packing the resulting defect with acrylic cement after first stabilizing the distal humerus by using Rush rods inserted percutaneously and retrogradely through remaining intact bone of the epicondyles (Fig. 37-14, *C* and *D*).

Whether prophylactic fixation of spinal metastases ever is indicated is difficult to determine. Spinal metastases are extremely common, particularly from lesions such as breast carcinoma, hypernephroma, colon carcinoma, prostatic carcinoma, and myeloma. Pathologic compression fractures also are common under such circumstances, but the great majority become inherently stable just as do vertebral compression fractures occurring in women who have osteoporosis without malignant disease. It is not difficult to predict which vertebrae are likely to fracture, particularly if one obtains a cross-sectional CT scan, but the magnitude and risks of the operation required for "prophylactic" stabilization of these lesions generally preclude such a procedure for the spine. However, an exception is the destructive tumor that has not only created a risk of fracture but also has resulted in a progressive neurologic compromise necessitating anterior decompression. In such an instance, spinal cord or root decompression can be accomplished by resecting much of the remaining bone of the vertebral body, and vertebral replacement and stabilization can be achieved by using methylmethacrylate and distraction rod fixation.[15,17]

SUMMARY

Both lytic and blastic long bone metastases are at risk to develop pathologic fractures in instances where more than 50% of the circumferential cortical bone has been destroyed or where the pain with weight-bearing stresses persists, increases, or recurs despite adequate local irradiation. Moreover, those most commonly encountered lesions of the proximal femur are at high risk to fracture if they are in excess of 2.5 cm in any dimension or if they are associated with avulsion of the lesser trochanter.

Such lesions should be treated aggressively by prophylactic internal fixation. This will avoid the development of a secondary fracture with its concomitantly high risk that true bony healing will not occur even with adequate fixation.

When internal fixation is chosen for a large metastasis with extensive cortical destruction, that fixation should be augmented by debulking of the lesion and by packing it with methylmethacrylate polymerizing in situ. Such an expedient not only improves the efficacy of subsequent radiotherapy but also prevents shortening of the bone with weight bearing while enhancing the torque capacity and sheer resistance inherent in the metal fixation device.

REFERENCES

1. Beals, R.K., Lawton, G.D., and Snell, W.E.: Prophylactic internal fixation of the femur in metastatic breast cancer, Cancer **28:**1350, 1971.
2. Bertin, K.C., Horstman, J., and Coleman, S.S.: Metastatic malignant disease: Isolated fracture of the greater trochanter in adults, J. Bone Joint Surg. **66A:**770, June 1984.
3. Blake, D.D.: Radiation tretment of metastatic bone disease, Clin. Orthop. **73:**89, 1970.
4. Bonarigo, B.C., and Rubin, P.: Nonunion of pathologic fracture after radiation therapy, Radiology **88:**889, 1967.
5. Burstein, A.H., Currey, J., Frankel, V.H., Heiple, K.G., Linseth, P., and Vessely, J.C.: Bone strength: The effect of screw holes, J. Bone Joint Surg. **54A:**1143, 1972.
6. Cheng, D.S., Seitz, C.B., and Eyre, H.J.: Nonoperative management of femoral, humeral, and acetabular metastases in patients with breast carcinoma, Cancer **45:**1533, 1980.
7. Cramer, S.F., Fried, L., and Carter, K.J.: The cellular basis of metastatic bone disease in patients with lung cancer, Cancer **48:**2649, 1981.
8. Enneking, W.F.: Metastatic carcinoma. In Musculoskeletal tumor surgery, New York, 1982 Churchill Livingstone, Inc.
9. Fidler, M.: Prophylactic internal fixation of secondary neoplastic deposits in long bones, Br. Med. J. **1:**341, 1973.
10. Galasko, C.S.B.: The pathological basis for skeletal scintigraphy, J. Bone Joint Surg. **57B:**353, 1975.
11. Galasko, C.S.B.: Mechanisms of bone destruction in the development of skeletal metastases, Nature **263:**507, 1976.
12. Galasko, C.S.B., Rawlings, R., and Bennett, A.: Prostaglandins, osteoclasts, and bone destruction produced by VX2 carcinoma in rabbits: Effects of administering indomethacin at different doses and times, Br. J. Cancer **40:**360, 1979.
13. Galasko, C.S.B.: Mechanisms of lytic and blastic metastatic disease of bone, Clin. Orthop. **169:**20, 1982.
14. Haberman, E.T., Sachs, R., Stern, R.E., Hirsh, D.M., and Anderson, W.J.: The pathology and treatment of metastatic disease of the femur, Clin. Orthop. **169:**70, 1982.

15. Harrington, K.D.: The use of methylmethacrylate for vertebral-body replacement and anterior stabilization of pathological fracture-dislocations of the spine due to metastatic malignant disease, J. Bone Joint Surg. **63A:**36-44, 1981.
16. Harrington, K.D.: New trends in the management of lower extremity metastases, Clin. Orthop. **169:**53, 1982.
17. Harrington, K.D.: Anterior cord decompression and spine stabilization for patients with metastatic lesions of the spine, J. Neurosurg. **61:**107, 1984.
18. Harrington, K.D., Sim, F.H., Enis, J.E., Johnston, J.O., Dick, H.M., and Gristin, A.G.: Methylmethacrylate as an adjunct in the internal fixation of pathological fractures, J. Bone Joint Surg. **58A:**1047, 1976.
19. Kuettner, K.E., and Pauli, B.U.: Resistance of cartilage to normal and neoplastic invasion. In Horton, J.E., editor: Mechanisms of localized bone loss (Special Supplement to Calcif. Tissue Res.) 251, 1978.
20. Lane, J.M., Sculco, T.P., and Zolan, S.: Treatment of pathological fractures of the hip by endoprosthetic replacement, J. Bone Joint Surg. **62A:**954, 1980.
21. Matsubayashi, T.: The reparative process of metastatic bone lesions after radiotherapy, Japanese J. Clin. Oncol. **11**(Suppl.):253, 1981.
22. Mundy, G.R., and Raisz, L.G.: Big and little forms of osteoclast activating factor, J. Clin. Invest. **60:**122, 1977.
23. Parrish, F.F., and Murray, J.A.: Surgical treatment for secondary neoplastic fractures: A retrospective study of ninety-six patients, J. Bone Joint Surg. **52A:**665, 1970.
24. Pugh, J., Sherry, H.S., Futterman, B., and Frankel, V.H.: Biomechanics of pathologic fractures, Clin. Orthop. **169:**109, 1982.
25. Tong, D., Gillick, L., and Hendrickson, F.R.: The palliation of symptomtic osseus metastases, Cancer **50:**893, 1982.

Chapter 38

Surgical management of acetabular fractures

JOEL M. MATTA

EMILE LETOURNEL

BRUCE D. BROWNER

Surgical management of acetabular fractures is a relatively recent development in the orthopaedic literature. Levine[10] reported open reduction of an acetabular fracture through an anterior approach, Epstein and Thompson[15] reported open reduction for posterior dislocations associated with acetabular fracture, and Knight[5] and Smith recommended open reduction of acetabulum fractures and described an effective reduction technique.

Judet became unhappy with the results of closed treatment of acetabulum fractures and first attempted open reduction in 1954. His early attempts were through the Kocher-Langenbeck approach and for the most part produced unsatisfactory results. When Letournel became Judet's resident in May 1956, he was asked to work on the project of open reduction of acetabulum fractures and to develop surgical approaches. A number of the standard hip approaches were tried, including the Kocher-Langenbeck, the Smith-Peterson, and the modified Ollier approach. By 1958 it was Letournel's conclusion that the primary problem was at that time not the surgical access to the hip, but the inability of Judet and Letournel to understand the x-ray films. Letournel therefore undertook anatomic studies—combined with radiologic studies of the innominate bone—to understand the various fracture types. His radiologic work was completed in 1960 with a thesis involving the radiologic study of 75 fracture cases.[6,7] From this thesis has come the standard radiographic interpretation techniques that are most useful today. Subse-

quently Letournel developed the ilioinguinal and extended iliofemoral approaches as specialized approaches to acetabulum fractures.

RADIOLOGY AND CLASSIFICATION

Initial radiographic evaluation should be done on a standard x-ray table. Attempts to take x-ray films with portable machines with the patient in

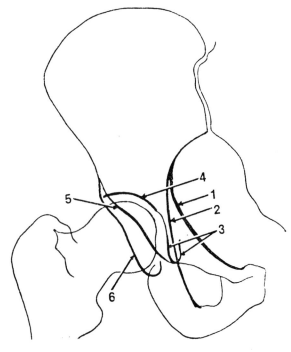

Fig. 38-1. AP view. *1*, Iliopectineal line; *2*, ilioischial line; *3*, roentgenographic—U; *4*, roof; *5*, anterior rim; *6*, posterior rim.

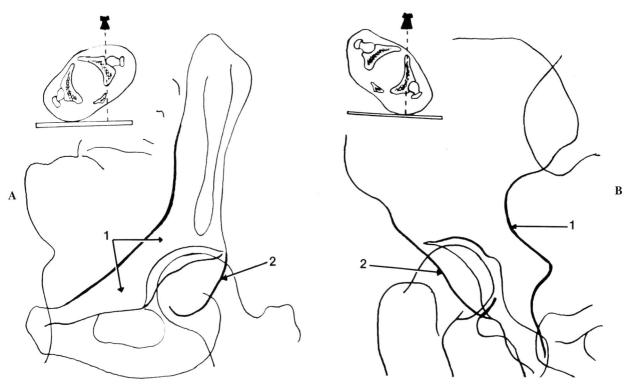

Fig. 38-2. A, Obturator oblique view. *1,* Anterior column; *2,* posterior rim. **B,** Iliac oblique view. *1,* Posterior column; *2,* anterior rim.

traction usually are accompanied by poor radiographic images. An AP pelvis x-ray film and 45-degree oblique views of the pelvis form the standard radiographic examination.[4] The AP view should be examined for disruption of the standard radiographic lines of the pelvis and acetabulum (Fig. 38-1). A useful technique is to draw the lines of the pelvis using tracing paper placed over the x-ray films.

As the clinician becomes proficient in radiographic interpretation, examination of the AP view should lead to the proper fracture classification in the majority of cases. Independent disruption of the posterior rim indicates a posterior wall fracture. Independent disruption of the ilioischial line and posterior rim indicates a posterior column or associated posterior column and posterior wall fracture. Independent disruption of the iliopectoneal line and anterior rim indicates an anterior column or anterior wall fracture. However, if the iliopectoneal line, ilioischial line, and anterior and posterior rims are disrupted together, if a portion of the roof remains attached to the ileum, and if the obturator foramin is

intact, the diagnosis is a transverse fracture or an associated transverse, posterior wall fracture. With the addition of an obturator foramin fracture (usually through the inferior public ramus), the diagnosis is a T-shaped fracture. Involvement of all of the radiographic landmarks of the acetabulum, as well as a fracture through the iliac wing and a fracture of the obturator foramin, indicates a both-column fracture.

The 45-degree oblique views are examined after interpretation of the AP view. The obturator oblique view further delineates involvement of the anterior column and the posterior rim of the acetabulum (Fig. 38-2, *A*). The iliac oblique view further delineates involvement of the posterior column and the anterior rim of the acetabulum (Fig. 38-2, *B*).

The three standard views should be supplemented by a CT scan of the pelvis if possible. The CT scan can help answer specific questions that remain following interpretation of the plain films.[3] The CT scan is particularly useful for detecting occult fractures through the sacrum, minimally displaced or incomplete fractures

---

CLASSIFICATION OF JUDET AND LETOURNEL

SIMPLE FRACTURE TYPES

Posterior wall
Posterior column
Anterior wall
Anterior column
Transverse

ASSOCIATED FRACTURE TYPES

Posterior column and
   posterior wall
Transverse and
   posterior wall
Associated anterior and
   posterior hemitransverse
T-shaped
Both column

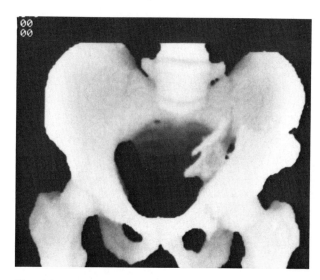

Fig. 38-3. Three-dimensional CT scan of a displaced both-column fracture.

through the iliac wing, and displaying fractures through the quadrilateral surface, as well as in the diagnosis of loose bodies within the joint and rotational displacement of the anterior and posterior column. The CT scan, however, should not be interpreted alone without the AP and oblique views. The CT scan can also be deceptive in several respects. It may be interpreted erroneously as showing loose bodies within the acetabulum when the physician is simply seeing a cross section through the small end point of a larger fracture fragment. Another possible misinterpretation is that of extreme comminution, which often appears to be present near the lower portion of the anterior column despite a simple fracture configuration. Recently the technique of three-dimensional imaging from CT scanning has become available. This technique gives the clinician a three-dimensional picture of the fracture and helps in the overall understanding of the fracture pattern and displacement (Fig. 38-3).

Following the radiographic examination the surgeon should be able to classify the fracture properly and draw the fracture lines on an innominate bone (see box).[9]

INDICATION FOR SURGERY

It is our belief that open reduction and internal fixation is indicated for the majority of displaced acetabulum fractures. The goal at surgery is to obtain reduction of the innominate bone, as well as the articular surface of the acetabulum. A minority of displaced fractures, which fall into two categories, will predictably have a satisfactory prognosis. The first category is fractures involving only a small or prognostically insignificant portion of the acetabulum.[12] An example would be a very low anterior column fracture involving only the pubic portion of the acetabulum. The second category is the moderately displaced complete both-column fracture in which a secondary or apparent congruence is present despite displacement of the articular surface.[9]

Surgery usually is performed 48 hours after the injury, when the initial bleeding from the injury has been controlled. Surgery before 10 days have elapsed is advisable to avoid undue difficulty in reduction. It is important to examine the patient carefully for associated soft tissue injuries such as abrasions, wounds, and subcutaneous hematomas that can increase the risk of infection.

SURGICAL APPROACHES

No one surgical approach has been found satisfactory for all acetabulum fractures. Therefore the surgeon must be knowledgeable about several surgical approaches for ideal access to the various fracture types. With accurate preoperative x-ray film interpretation and thorough knowledge of the capabilities of each surgical approach, a single approach that will allow reduction and fixation of the entire fracture almost always can be selected. Combined surgical approaches that are performed successively are needed at times although they should be the exception.

Surgical approaches found to be consistently useful for acetabulum fractures are the Kocher-Langenbeck approach, the ilioinguinal approach, and the extended iliofemoral approach, all of which are normally performed on a fracture table with the patient in either the prone, supine, or lateral position respectively. Mears[13] advocates the use of a triradiate surgical approach using a modified type of Ollier incision. The final aspect of this approach is similar to the extended ilio-femoral approach.

The Kocher-Langenbeck approach gives access to the retroacetabular surface of the innominate bone from the ischium to the greater sciatic notch. By removal of the trochanter or abductor tendons from the trochanter, access to the inferior iliac wing as far anterior as the anterior inferior iliac spine is possible. Proximal access along the iliac wing is limited by the superior gluteal neurovascular bundle. Access to the quadrilateral surface is possible by palpation through the greater sciatic notch. This incision splits the gluteus maximus muscle and the fascia lata over the lateral aspect of the femur (Fig. 38-4, *A*). The tendons of the piriformis and obturator internis are identified and transected at their trochanteric insertion. These muscles expose respectively the

greater and lesser sciatic notches. The quadratus femoris should be left intact at its femoral attachment to protect the ascending branch of the medial femoral circumflex artery. Visualization of the interior of the joint may be obtained through a capsulotomy performed along the acetabular rim (Fig. 38-4, *B*).

The ilioinguinal approach provides access primarily to the internal aspect of the innominate bone. This includes the anterior sacroiliac joint, the internal iliac fossa, the entire pelvic brim, the superior pubic ramus, and the quadrilateral surface. Access is also possible to the anterior portion of the external iliac wing. The incision starts posterior to the lateralmost convexity of the iliac crest and proceeds along the crest to the anterior superior iliac spine and then medially across the lower abdomen to a point 2 cm proximal to the symphysis pubis (Fig. 38-5, *A*). The iliacus and abdominal muscles are released from the iliac crest and internal iliac fossa. The inguinal canal is opened on its internal and external aspect, and the abdominal muscles, as well as transversalis fascia, are mobilized proximally from the inguinal ligament. The various structures crossing the inguinal ligament—including the spermatic cord, external iliac vessels, iliopsoas, and femoral nerve—are identified and mobilized to allow retraction for reduction and fixation of the differ-

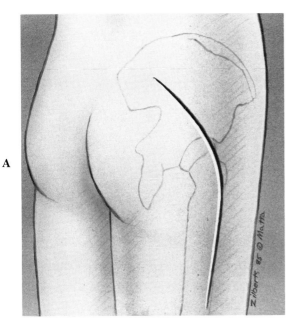

A

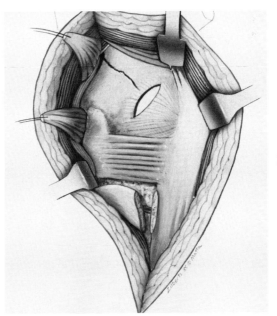

B

Fig. 38-4. A, Kocher-Langenbeck approach surgical incision. **B,** Final exposure of retroacetabular surface.

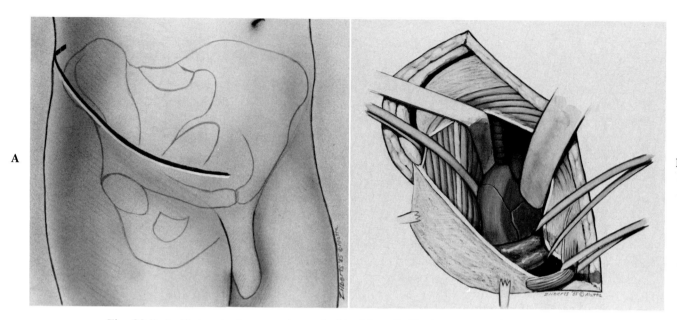

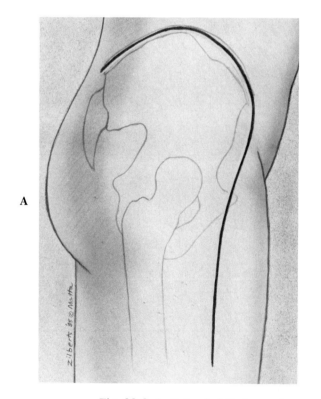

Fig. 38-5. A, Ilioinguinal approach surgical incision. **B,** Final exposure with retraction of iliopsoas and femoral nerve lateral and external iliac vessels medial.

A

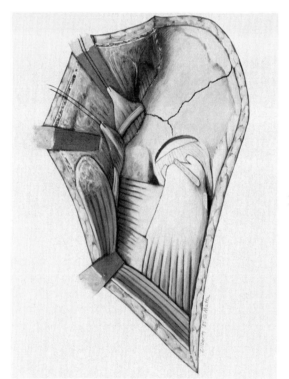

B

Fig. 38-6. A, Extended iliofemoral approach incision. **B,** Final exposure of innominate bone external aspect.

ent portions of the innominate bone.

In this approach it is necessary to work in several intervals or windows bounded by the structures crossing the inguinal ligament (Fig. 38-5, *B*). Although reduction and fixation can at times be difficult and deceptive through this approach, the advantages include a cosmetic scar and minimal muscle stripping from the innominate bone, which leads to low surgical morbidity and almost no ectopic bone formation.

The extended iliofemoral approach primarily gives access to the external aspect of the innominate bone, exposing the entire external aspect of the iliac wing and retroacetabular surface. A limited access to the internal aspect is also possible through exposure of the internal iliac fossa as far distally as the pectoneal eminence. The incision follows the iliac crest from the posterior superior spine to the anterior superior spine and then is directed distally along the anterolateral thigh (Fig. 38-6, *A*). The approach proceeds through a logical neurovascular interval, reflecting the superior and inferior gluteal innervated muscles posteriorly and the femoral nerve innervated muscles medially. The tensor fascia lata and gluteus medius and minimus muscles are reflected posteriorly from their iliac origin, and their tendons of insertion are transected at the greater trochanter. The piriformis and obturator internis tendons are transected at the trochanter as in the Kocher-Langenbeck approach (Fig. 38-6, *B*).

Exposure of the internal aspect of the innominate bone is obtained by detaching and iliacus and abdominal muscles from the iliac crest and the sartorius muscle and inguinal ligament from the anterior superior iliac spine. The rectus femoris origin also may be detached at its reflected and direct heads. A very good visualization of the internal aspect of the joint is possible when a capsulotomy is performed in combination with this approach. Depending on the fracture pattern encountered, the surgeon must be careful in stripping both sides of the iliac wing to prevent devascularization of portions of the iliac wing or anterior column. This approach provides the best simultaneous access to the anterior and posterior column, and it is useful for old fractures in which fracture callus must be removed or osteotomy performed. The use of this approach is limited to the most difficult cases because the period of postoperative rehabilitation is the longest and the incidence of ectopic bone formation the highest.

TECHNIQUES OF REDUCTION AND FIXATION

For the operation the patient is placed on a fracture table in either the prone, supine, or lateral position depending on the surgical approach and is placed in traction through a distal femoral pin. The knee is kept in a flexed position to relax the sciatic nerve. During surgery lateral traction should be available through a mechanical device attached to the table. If the patient is in the prone or supine position, a screw that is inserted into the greater trochanter is pulled in a lateral direction with the mechanical device attached to the table. With the patient is in the lateral position, the peroneal post can be raised or lowered to achieve a lateral traction effect. Intraoperative traction removes the femoral head from its displaced intrapelvic position to allow reduction of the fracture fragments. Distraction of the femoral head from the acetabulum also provides visualization of the interior of the joint. Fractures of the contralateral superior and inferior pubic rami may prevent use of the fracture table because distal traction can cause the peroneal post to deform the inferior pelvic ring.

An alternative to the use of the fracture table is to place an A0 femoral distractor between the iliac wing and the proximal femur. The fracture table is most useful when the Kocher-Langenbeck or ilioinguinal approaches are used.

A variety of reduction forceps should be available to accommodate different portions of the innominate bone (Fig. 38-7). Pointed reduction forceps that gain good purchase on the flat surface of the bone are quite useful and also may be applied to shallow drill holes placed on the surface of the bone. Forceps that can gain purchase on screw heads protruding above the bony surface can be very useful for reduction. By the surgeon's manipulation of two screws placed to either side of a fracture line, a fracture may be distracted, translated in shear, or closed with considerable compressive force.

As the surgeon undertakes reduction of the fracture, the diastasis or translational displacement of a fracture usually is immediately apparent. The rotational displacement of the fracture often is perceived less easily, however, and must always be corrected in addition to the displacement. Rotation of the posterior column often can be controlled by a femoral head corkscrew type extractor inserted into the ischial tuberosity. Rotation of the anterior column often

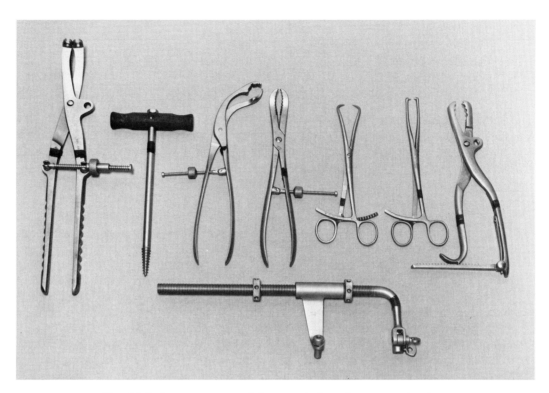

Fig. 38-7. Instruments used for acetabulum fracture reduction.

can be controlled by a Farabeuf reduction forceps placed astride the anterior border of the innominate bone at the level of the anterior-inferior iliac spine. We have independently and collectively endeavored to design reduction clamps especially proportioned to the reduction problems of the innominate bone; however, this design problem remains far from solved.

Appreciation of the fracture configuration and reduction of the fracture remain the primary problems facing the surgeon. Fracture reduction usually cannot be achieved at a single step. It is necessary to proceed by reduction of single fracture fragments to intact portions of the pelvis and then build on the previously assembled parts. It is very important that the initial reductions of even extraarticular fragments be performed as precisely as possible. Initial small errors in reduction will magnify progressively as the reduction proceeds to further fragments.

Performing the reductions of small separate fragments should not be ignored. Extraarticular free fragments often will be present along the iliac crest, the pelvic brim, and the greater sciatic notch. Reduction of these fragments often provides a key to reduction of the larger segments

and aids in the final stability. The final articular reduction is not always directly visualized. Special problems such as incarcerated fragments and articular impaction should be identified preoperatively and often can be corrected by manipulation between fracture fragments.

Fracture fixation normally is performed with a combination of interfragmentary screws and plates and rarely with screws alone (Fig. 38-8), although when beginning the fixation it is often useful to assemble the fracture provisionally with screws alone. Screws between main fracture fragments usually are placed as lag screws, which provide interfragmentary compression and thereby enhance stability.[14]

Screws should be available in several diameters from 3.5 mm to 6.5 mm and up to 110 mm in length. Plates should be available in a variety of lengths and contourable in all directions. Precurved plates also can be quite useful for placement along the pelvic brim or paralleling the rim of the acetabulum. The plates usually are fixed with 3.5 mm diameter screws. Screws for the plates may include lag screws traversing between major fragments. Care should be taken to avoid penetration of the joint with screws. This often

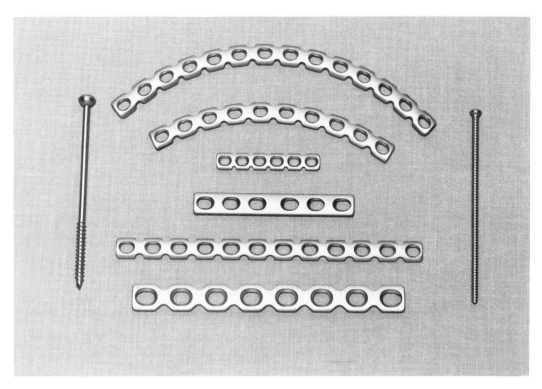

Fig. 38-8. Screws and plates used for acetabulum fracture fixation.

can occur more easily than suspected and is most prone to happen with screws placed into the retroacetabular surface or along the pelvic brim.

REDUCTION AND FIXATION OF INDIVIDUAL FRACTURE TYPES

The posterior wall fracture is approached through the Kocher-Langenbeck approach (Fig. 38-9, *A*). Reduction and fixation of this fracture is most commonly performed with the patient in the lateral position on a standard table. The leg is draped free and the hip redislocated during the procedure to inspect the joint for incarcerated fragments that often are present after a posterior dislocation.[1,2] Following concentric reduction of the femoral head with the acetabulum, the femoral head is used as a stint to position the posterior wall fragments. The surgeon should be aware of marginal impaction of the articular surface that should be corrected by elevation of the fragment and buttressing of the fragment with bone graft or the other surrounding posterior wall fragments. In a great majority of cases the posterior fracture fragments initially are stabilized with screw fixation followed by buttressing of the fragments with a plate parallel to the rim of the

acetabulum. If screw fixation alone is used there is a distinct possibility for loss of fixation after surgery.

Posterior column fractures are approached through the Kocher-Langenbeck incision with the patient in the prone position (Fig. 38-9, *B*). A fracture table aids in reduction through distal and lateral distraction of the femoral head. Fracture displacement usually is controlled best by a clamp gripping a screw on either side of the fracture site. Rotation of the fracture can be controlled with a lever placed into the ischial tuberosity. The displacement is easily appreciated visually. The rotation is best judged by placing a finger in the greater sciatic notch and palpating the quadrilateral surface. A smooth quadrilateral surface indicates correction of the rotational displacement of the posterior column.

Transverse fractures normally are approached from the posterior with the patient in the prone position on the fracture table (Fig. 38-10, *A*). The appearance of the fracture on the retroacetabular surface will be the same as a posterior column fracture. Again, displacement is controlled best with the two-screw technique, and rotation is controlled with the corkscrew lever placed into

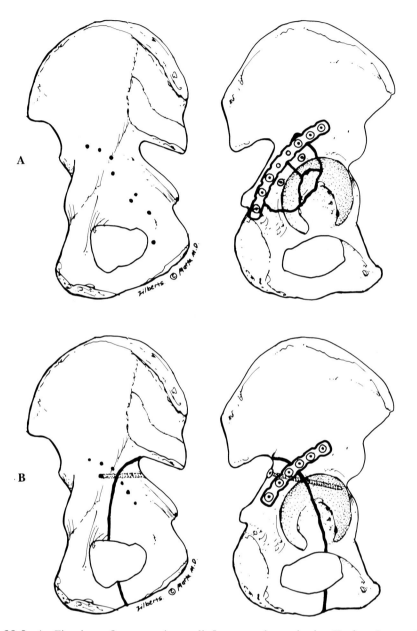

Fig. 38-9. A, Fixation of a posterior wall fracture through the Kocher-Langenbeck approach. **B,** Fixation of a posterior column fracture through the Kocher-Langenbeck approach.

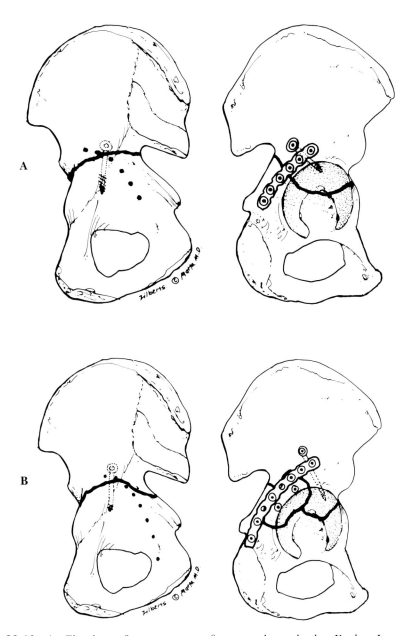

Fig. 38-10. A, Fixation of a transverse fracture through the Kocher-Langenbeck approach. **B,** Fixation of an associated transverse and posterior wall fracture through the Kocher-Langenbeck approach.

Continued.

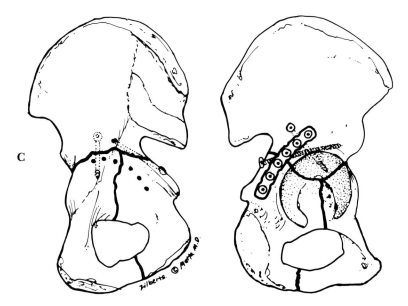

Fig. 38-10, cont'd. C, Fixation of a T-shaped fracture through the Kocher-Langenbeck approach.

the ischial tuberosity. Reduction must be satisfactory as visualized on the retroacetabular surface and palpated along the quadrilateral surface. A minority of transverse fractures have more displacement anteriorly than posteriorly and proceed from a position of high anterior to low posterior. These fractures are best reduced through the ilioinguinal approach.

A majority of transverse plus posterior wall fractures can be approached through the Kocher-Langenbeck approach with prone positioning on the fracture table (Fig. 38-10, *B*). Since these fractures often are associated with posterior dislocation and incarcerated fragments, it is necessary to distract the femoral head and thoroughly inspect the interior of the joint for free fragments. Reduction of the transverse portion of the fracture is performed as for a simple transverse fracture. Provisional fixation is obtained by a screw across the transverse fracture. At this point distraction of the femoral head will show the articular reduction along the anterior portion of the acetabulum and will also show that the lag screw is clear of the joint. Following this, traction is relaxed, seating the femoral head into the acetabulum, and the posterior wall fracture is reduced and fixed with a plate that spans the

transverse fracture, as well as the posterior wall fracture.

If provisional lag-screw fixation is not possible for the transverse fracture, a small plate can be placed along the sciatic notch before reduction of the posterior fragment. Reduction of the transverse fracture can be complicated by a very large posterior wall fracture that includes the anterior border of the sciatic notch. In these cases the reduction can be assessed by visualization of the interior of the acetabulum and palpation of the pelvic brim through the sciatic notch. If great difficulty in reduction is anticipated through the Kocher-Langenbeck approach, the extended iliofemoral approach may be chosen initially.

T-shaped fractures present additional problems over the transverse fracture configurations (Fig. 38-10, *C*). Whereas the transverse fracture has a single ischiopubic segment for the inferior fracture fragment, in the T-shaped fracture a vertical stem divides the ischiopubic segment into separate anterior and posterior column fragments that must be reduced and fixed separately. For most T-shaped fractures we prefer to place the patient in a prone position on the fracture table and use the Kocher-Langenbeck approach. The displacement of the anterior column may be

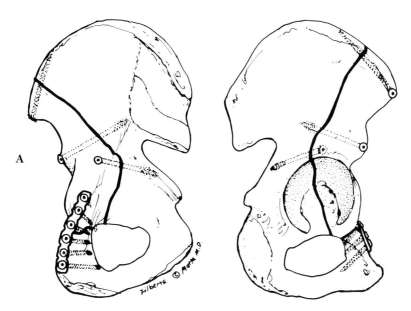

Fig. 38-11. A, Fixation of an anterior column fracture through the ilioinguinal approach.

Continued.

appreciated by distraction of the femoral head and posterior displacement of the posterior column to visualize the anterior column fracture on the acetabular articular surface. Displacement also may be palpated along the pelvic brim with a finger placed in the sciatic notch. While the posterior column is in a displaced position, a bone hook can be placed through the vertical stem of the T and around the pelvic brim. The bone hook can be used to pull the anterior column into position. Then fixation can be performed with a lag screw started posterior and superior to the acetabulum and directed anteriorly and distally into the anterior column. Following this the posterior column can be reduced in the normal fashion.

Another alternative is to first reduce and fix the posterior column, taking care not to place screws into the vertical portion of the T and then reduce the anterior column with a bone reduction clamp or other instrument placed through the sciatic notch to the pelvic brim. If anterior column reduction is found to be impossible through the Kocher-Langenbeck approach, the posterior column alone will be fixed and the patient then turned supine for reduction and fixation of the anterior column through the ilioinguinal ap-

proach. If great difficulties are expected, it is probably best to proceed through the extended iliofemoral approach initially so that the entire reduction may be performed through the single approach. T-shaped fractures that present unusual difficulties include transtectal fractures, fractures in which the anterior column is fractured at two levels, and cases in which contralateral pubic ramus fractures prevent use of the fracture table.

Fractures of the anterior wall and column are approached through the ilioinguinal approach (Fig. 38-11, *A*). The ilioinguinal approach allows exposure of the entire length of the anterior column fracture line so that subtle rotational or angular displacements can be appreciated and corrected. Forceps applied to screw heads are usually less useful along the anterior column, and pointed clamps, as well as simple pressure applied to displaced fracture fragments, become more useful.

In high anterior column fractures, which include the anterior border of the iliac wing, rotational control of the fracture can be obtained through gripping the anterior border of the bone with a clamp. Plate fixation is always necessary for fractures that include only the anterior wall.

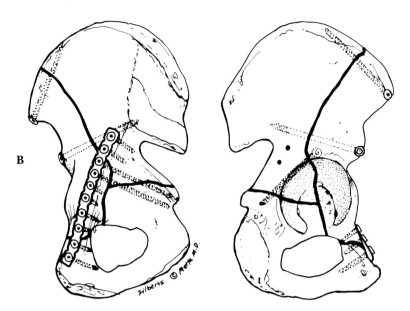

Fig. 38-11, cont'd. B, Fixation of an associated anterior column and posterior hemitransverse fracture through the ilioinguinal approach.

Interfragmentary screw fixation has greater reliability in high anterior column fractures, including the anterior border of the iliac wing. In this case long lag screws may be placed between the two tables of the ileum. Plate fixation still may be necessary, however, at the lower end of the fracture fragment. Screws placed along the pelvic brim should parallel the quadrilateral surface to avoid entering the acetabulum. Long screws whose tips exit near the ischial spine are useful. The pectoneal eminence marks the center of the femoral head, and at this point it is probably advisable to use only very short screws to avoid entering the joint.

For anterior plus posterior hemitransverse fractures the ilioinguinal is the preferred approach (Fig. 38-11, *B*). Anterior column reduction is performed first as described earlier. The posterior column fracture is low and usually not significantly displaced. Reduction of the posterior column will be achieved by simple pressure on the fragment or with pointed clamps along the quadrilateral surface. Fixation will be obtained by long screws that enter at the pelvic brim and parallel the quadrilateral surface distally toward the ischium.

Both-column fractures are, unfortunately, a common fracture pattern and constitute the most difficult fracture on which to achieve a satisfactory reduction and fixation. Both-column fractures detach all segments of the articular surface from the intact portion of the ileum and therefore leave no point of reference of intact cartilage that the surgeon can build on.

The ilioinguinal approach with the patient in supine position on the fracture table is preferred if the entire reduction and fixation is judged to be possible through this approach (Fig. 38-12, *A*). Reduction of the anterior column usually is undertaken first. This is ordinarily accomplished by pressure placed in a posterior and lateral direction along the fractured anterior column. Rotation and displacement also are controlled by a clamp astride the anterior border of the iliac wing. Free fragments along the iliac crest and the pelvic brim are reduced and internally fixed first to aid in judging the reduction. After reduction provisional lag-screw fixation usually can be obtained by screws placed between the tables of the iliac wing.

It may be necessary at this time additionally to place a long curved plate along the pelvic brim to hold the various segments of the anterior column together. As the plate is placed, several screw

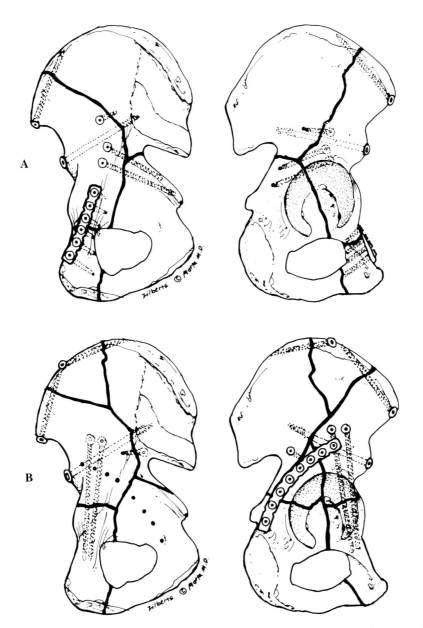

Fig. 38-12. A, Fixation of a both-column fracture through the ilioinguinal approach. **B,** Fixation of a both-column fracture through the extended iliofemoral approach.

holes will be left open and only short screws used in some holes so that the screws in the anterior column do not block the posterior column reduction and fixation.

The posterior column reduction and fixation is achieved through the second window of the ilioinguinal approach, that is, by retracting the iliopsoas and femoral nerve laterally and the external iliac vessels medially to expose the pelvic brim and quadrilateral surface. Simple pressure to the posterior column fragment and application of a pointed clamp from the pelvic brim to the quadrilateral surface can reduce the posterior column.

The posterior column reduction is checked by palpation along the greater sciatic notch from the inner aspect of the pelvis and visualization of the fracture line on the quadrilateral surface. It is normal for almost the entire quadrilateral surface to stay with the posterior column segment. Whether this is the case can be seen readily on the CT scan before surgery. Fixation of the posterior column is carried out by placing lag screws of 50 to 100 mm in length from the pelvic brim into the posterior column. Lag screws often pass through a plate along the pelvic brim. Again, the screws should parallel the quadrilateral surface, and only short screws should be used directly over the pectoneal eminence. After reduction and fixation through the ilioinguinal approach, it is often advisable to check the reduction and screw position with intraoperative image intensification.

Many both-column fractures that are not reducible through the ilioinguinal approach include fractures that have a large displaced segment of the posterior wall, fractures that include part of the sacroiliac joint either through a large posterior column segment or an iliac wing fracture that is very posterior, and fractures more than 2 weeks old that require removal of callus from the fracture lines (Fig. 38-12, *B*). These fractures should be approached through the extended iliofemoral approach. The anterior column usually is reduced and fixed first. However, if the posterior column segment is very large and uncomminuted, it may be best to reduce and fix this first. Pointed clamps or the two-screw technique controls displacement while rotation is controlled in the normal manner.

POSTOPERATIVE CARE

After surgery Hemovac drainage is continued for 24 to 48 hours. Depending on the surgical approach used, it is important to drain the external iliac fossa, the internal iliac fossa, the space adjacent to the quadrilateral surface, and retropubic space of Retzius. The patient is not placed in traction or immobilized after surgery. Gait training is begun at 5 to 7 days following surgery or when symptoms permit. Passive mobilization of the hip is used before ambulation. Weight bearing is limited for the first 8 weeks after surgery and then progressed as tolerated. It is important to emphasize rehabilitation of the hip musculature, particularly the abductors. If the fracture has been reduced satisfactorily and ectopic bone does not develop, the range of motion can be expected to return to 90% of normal.

RESULTS OF OPERATIVE TREATMENT

In 1979 Letournel[8] reported the results of 21 years of experience with acetabular fractures treated surgically. Within 3 weeks of injury 406 fractures were operated on. After surgery the fracture reductions were graded as perfect in 73%, imperfect in 22%, bad in 3.2% and technical failures in 1.7%. Infections occurred in 5.6%, including seven intraarticular infections and sixteen extraarticular infections. Two peaks in the infection incidence occurred. The first occurred in the early cases that were prolonged and laborious, and the second occurred with the early use of the ilioinguinal approach. The sciatic palsy rate was 8.6%, although the rate dropped from 18.4% to 6.5% after the practice of flexing the knee during surgery was initiated. The majority of patients with sciatic palsy recovered enough to have good function without a brace.

Cases available for follow-up at 2 to 21 years totaled 350. Average follow-up was 8.5 years. The clinical results at follow-up were graded very good in 75.5%, good in 8.3%, mediocre in 6.9%, and bad in 9.1%. A very good result followed in 84% of perfect reductions, 55% of imperfect reductions, and 11% of bad reductions. There were very good results after technical failures.

Acetabulum fractures occur primarily in young adult patients as a result of high energy trauma. Significant disability can result from posttraumatic arthritis. Accurate articular reduction correlates best with a satisfactory clinical outcome.[8,11] Use of the foregoing techniques has allowed reductions of displaced fractures and thereby led to improved clinical results.

SUMMARY

We have each experienced a significant learning phase for surgical treatment of these fractures. However, problems of articular reduction remain significant, particularly for complex fractures. It is our opinion that a certain degree of centralization of acetabulum fracture treatment—especially for the associated types—can lead to an improved standard of care overall.

BIBLIOGRAPHY

1. Epstein, H.C.: Open management of fractures of the acetabulum. In The hip: Proceedings of the seventh open scientific meeting of The Hip Society, St. Louis, 1979, The C.V. Mosby Co.
2. Epstein, H.C.: Traumatic dislocations of the hip, Baltimore, 1980, Williams & Wilkins.
3. Harley, J., Mack, L., and Winquist, R.: CT of acetabular Fractures, AJR, **138:**413-417, 1982.
4. Judet, R., Judet, J., and Letournel, E.: Fractures of the acetabulum: Classification and surgical approaches for open reduction, J. Bone Joint Surg. **46A:**1615-1638, 1964.
5. Knight, R.A., and Smith, H.: Central fractures of the acetabulum, J. Bone Joint Surg. **40A:**1-16, 1958.
6. Letournel, E.: Les Fractures du Cotyle. Etude d'une Serie de 75 Cas, medical thesis, Arnette, Paris, 1961.
7. Letournel, E.: Les Fractures du cotyle. Etude d'une Serie de 75 Cas, J. Chir. **82:**47-87, 1961.
8. Letournel, E.: The results of acetabular fractures treated surgically: Twenty-one years experience. In The hip: Proceedings of the seventh open scientific meeting of The Hip Society, St. Louis, 1979, The C.V. Mosby Co.
9. Letournel, E.: Fractures of the acetabulum, New York, 1981, Springer-Verlag.
10. Levine, M.A.: A treatment of central fractures of the acetabulum, J. Bone Joint Surg. **25A:**902-906, 1943.
11. Matta, J., Anderson, L., Epstein, H., and Hendricks, P.: Fractures of the acetabulum: A retrospective analysis, Clin. Orthop. **205:**230-240, 1986.
12. Matta, J., Mehne, D., and Roffi, R.: Fractures of the acetabulum: Early results of a prospective study, Clin. Orthop. **205:**241-250, 1986.
13. Mears, D., and Rubash, H.: Extensile exposure of the pelvis, Contemp. Orthop. **6**(2):21-31, 1983.
14. Muller, M.E., and Allgoer, M.: Manual of internal fixation, New York, 1979, Springer-Verlag.
15. Thompson, V.P., and Epstein, H.L.: Traumatic dislocation of the hip, J. Bone Joint Surg. **33A:**746-778, 1951.

THE SPINE

Chapter 39

Posterior stabilization of thoracic, lumbar, and sacral injuries

PAUL R. MEYER, JR.

This chapter discusses the management of injuries to the thoracic, lumbar, and sacral spine that required stabilization by the posterior surgical approach or were managed conservatively. Other surgical approaches used for spine instrumentation are discussed in Chapter 40.

All injuries discussed were managed acutely, with the median time between injury and admission 8 hours. The mean time between admission and surgery was 10 days (range 0 to 47 days), and the mean time between admission and discharge was 29 days (range 2 to 180 days).

PATIENT POPULATION

Statistics are derived from admission records of patients who sustained injury to the thoracic, lumbar and sacral spine and who were admitted to the Acute Spinal Cord Injury Center at Northwestern University between 1972 and 1985. The locus of injury to the spine was as follows: 224 thoracic spine injuries (T1 to T10), 360 thoracic-lumbar junction injuries (T11 to L2), 57 injuries to the lumbar spine (L3 to L5), and 5 injuries to the sacrum (S1 to S5) (Table 39-1). Of the 646 thoracic, lumbar, and sacral fractures, 374 underwent surgical stabilization (58.04%), of which 306 (81.81%) were stabilized by the posterior approach. Two thirds of the patients were male with a mean age of 29 years (range 8 to 77 years). The principal etiologic mechanisms of injury in this group of patients were (1) falls, (2) motor vehicle accidents, (3) gunshot wounds, (4) motorcycle accidents, and (5) falling objects and other causes (Table 39-2).

STATISTICAL DATA

Orthopaedic literature does describe the occurrence of neurologic deterioration following posterior instrumentation systems concurrent to the management of scoliosis. These complications

Table 39-1. Thoracic-lumbar spine injuries*

	Number	Percent
Thoracic-lumbar fractures	646	32
Thoracic (T_1-T_{10})	224	35
Thoracolumbar junction		
(T_{11}-L_2)	360	56
Lumbar (L_3-L_5)	57	9
Sacral (S_1-S_5)	5	0.7
Nonsurgically managed	272	42
Surgically managed	374	58

*Acute spine injuries (all levels) totaled 2045 at less than 72 hours of trauma from 1972 to 1985.

Table 39-2. Mechanism of spine injury: thoracolumbar (T1-sacral) region

Etiology of injury	Number	Percent
Falls	182	28.17
Auto	163	25.25
Gunshot wound	133	20.59
Other trauma	86	13.31
Motorcycle	51	7.89
Sports	17	2.63
Medical	14	2.17
TOTAL	646	

Table 39-3. Surgical approach: thoracic-lumbar-sacral spine (T1-S5)

Surgical procedure	Number	Percent
Anterior	9	2.41
Posterior	306	81.82
Combined anteroposterior	52	13.90
Anterior, then posterior	5	1.34
Posterior, then anterior	2	0.53
TOTAL	374	

(dysesthesias to complete paraplegia) may be the result of either the introduction of hardware or correction of a spinal deformity.* Although descriptions of neurologic recovery following instrumentation in acute traumatic spine injuries do appear in the literature,[7,8,10,18,25] few papers record loss of neurologic function following instrumentation. The most frequent causes for complications include:

1. Progression of the original injury
2. Neurologic change secondary to surgery but not surgically induced (that is, anesthesia, positioning on the operating table, cardiovascular hypotension during surgery, hypothermia, change in vertebral column alignment, among others)
3. Neurologic change secondary to either direct or indirect alteration in spinal cord vascularity by means of spinal cord distraction (lengthening of the vertebral column with correction of the deformity or manipulation of the spinal cord during the performance of the procedure)
4. No known cause

Of the 646 acute fracture-dislocations of the thoracic, lumbar, and sacral spine admitted to the Acute Spine Injury Center 224 were thoracic spine (T1 to T10) injuries, 360 were injuries to the thoracic-lumbar junction (T11 to L2), 57 were injuries to the lumbar spine (L3 to L5) and 5 injuries to the sacrum (S1 to S5). (see Table 39-1)

Of the 374 (58.04%) thoracic, lumbar, and sacral spine injuries requiring operative intervention, 306 (78%) were stabilized posteriorly, 1.25% anteriorly, 18% by the combined (simultaneous) anteroposterior approach, and the remainder staged (anterior then posterior) (Table 39-3).

For purposes of evaluation, all patients within this study group (thoracic, lumbar, and sacral

*References 2, 3, 9, 12, 13, 17, 23, 24, 26.

spine) were divided into two management groups: conservative and surgical. In the conservative group comparison neurologic examinations between admission and discharge from the acute unit revealed the following (Table 39-4).

1. Of those managed conservatively: at discharge 0.3% revealed degradation in their neurologic status and 6.57% revealed improvement
2. Of those managed surgically: 2.39% revealed some degree of degradation in their postoperative neurologic status and 15.22% demonstrated evidence of one Frankel[5,6,14] grade in neurologic improvement (Table 39-5). Statistically, the surgical data was found to be significant: $p = 0.0080$, chi square = 23.838.

ASSOCIATED MULTISYSTEM INJURIES

As anticipated, blunt, severe trauma to the chest and abdomen frequently produces multiple-system injury. In this series of thoracic, lumbar, and sacral spine injuries, 28% of the patients had injury to one major system other than the vertebral column; 11% had injury to two other systems, 4.8% had injury to three, and 0.6% had four systems injured other than the spine. Within this group, 25% involved injury to the head, 17% with injury to the extremities, 15% with injury to the chest, and 10% with injury to the abdomen.

PATIENT CARE PROTOCOL AND EVALUATION TECHNIQUES

The "catchment area" for the retrieval and receipt of patients with acute spinal cord injuries is from an area of 200 to 300 miles surrounding Chicago. Identified as having sustained a spinal injury, patients are transferred to the Spine Center at Northwestern. As noted, the mean admission time for all patients between June 1972 and July 1985 is 8 hours.[20] Although it has not been demonstrated that steroids are of any benefit to neurologic recovery (except brain injury), in the early years following the development of the Spine Injury Center, dexamethasone (50 mg) was administered within the early minutes to hours following the patient's trauma.[1] This practice has since been discontinued, awaiting the institution of a triple-blind drug study investigating naloxone, thyrotropic-releasing hormone, and dexamethasone (or in combination) in a carefully controlled study.

All acute spine injured patients are evalu-

Table 39-4. Neurologic improvement: conservative vs. surgical management

	Total cases	Total conservative	Conservative Improvement Number	Percent	Degradation Number	Percent	Total surgical	Surgical Improvement Number	Percent	Degradation Number	Percent
No fracture	269	263	28	10.65	1	0.38	6	0	0.00	0	0.00
Cervical	968	611	56	9.17	7	1.15	357	41	11.48	1	0.28
Thoracic	216	137	9	6.57	0	0.00	79	3	3.80	2	2.53
Thoracic-lumbar	348	126	5	3.97	1	0.79	222	43	19.37	6	2.70
Lumbar	54	21	4	19.05	0	0.00	33	5	15.15	0	0.00
Sacral	6	5	1	20.00	0	0.00	1	0	0.00	0	0.00
TOTAL	1861	1163	103	8.86	9	0.77	698	92	13.18	9	1.29

Table 39-5. Frankel neurologic classification*

Discharge neurologic

Admission neurologic	A	B	C	D	E
A					
B			X		
C					
D					Z
E					

*Key: **A,** Absent motor and sensory function, **B,** Absent motor, sensory present, **C,** Motor: active (gravity eliminated), **D,** Motor: active (against gravity)—weak, **E,** Intact: normal motor-sensory function.

Example X: Patient admitted without motor but sensation below level of injury. On discharge patient demonstrated motor function (only with gravity eliminated) (improvement by one grade: B to C). *Example Z:* Patient admitted with active (weak, antigravity) motor function. On discharge patient demonstrated normal motor function (improvement by one grade: D to E).

ated by the orthopaedic, neurosurgery, and respiratory-critical care services in the emergency room on arrival and before transfer to the Spinal Cord Intensive Care Unit. Consultations are obtained from supporting medical and surgical services as indicated. Patients in the emergency room are transferred from the spine board, on which they arrive, to a Stryker frame. The exception to this rule is the multiply traumatized patient with an unstable cervical, thoracic, or lumbar spine injury combined with other medical-surgical conditions (multiple trauma) requiring the use of a kinetic treatment (Roto-Rest) bed.

1. Plain "scout" roentgenograms (anteroposterior and lateral) are performed on the entire spine in the emergency room (Fig. 39-1).
2. Linear tomograms in the anteroposterior

and lateral planes are obtained of the injured segment, on all patients, on the day following admission unless there is need for emergent visualization. Examples of such are a deterioration in neurologic function; an acute (complete) dislocation in the presence of residual neurologic function; or inadequate visualization of the fracture on standard radiographs.

3. Computerized axial tomography is performed in all cases where neural canal compromise is suspected.
4. Although magnetic resonance imaging (MRI) is available, the techniques required for the transfer and management of the acute spine–injured patient, within this new radiologic device, have not been established. One easily identified problem is the use of metal splints and devices on or about such patients, precluding the use of the instrument. It is believed, from the controlled studies performed to date, this new evaluative technique will provide a significant step forward in vertebral column and spinal cord injury assessment.
5. Myelography is performed based on established criteria in the emergency room (see box).

INDICATIONS FOR MYELOGRAPHY
1. Incomplete preoperative data
2. Patients with increasing neurologic deficits
3. Patients who neurologically plateau early
4. Neurologic findings inconsistent with negative radiologic findings
5. Neurologic findings inconsistent with somatosensory evoked potential (SSEP) findings

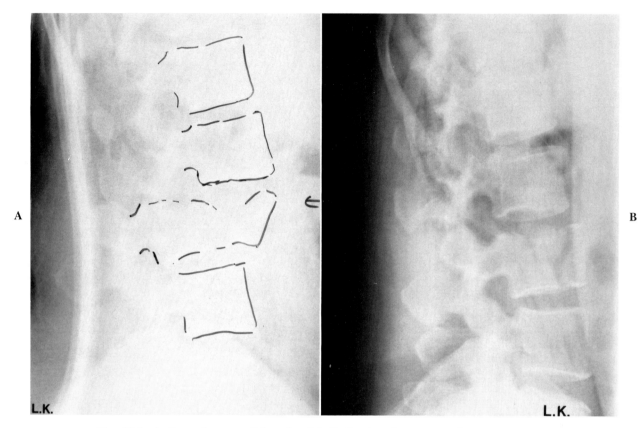

Fig. 39-1. A, Burst fracture dislocation L3. **B,** Stryker frame recumbent reduction L3. Ease of reduction indicative of instability.

6. Preoperative and postoperative cortical somatosensory and dermatomal evoked potentials are obtained routinely on each patient and intraoperatively on all patients having repeatable preoperative waveforms.

7. The "wake up" test is reserved for those situations when a significant variation in the preoperative and the intraoperative evoked potential has occurred and confirmation of continued neurologic function is required.

The mean number of days for which the patient is maintained at bed rest before surgery is 9 to 11 days. The reasons for this lapse in time before the performance of surgery are:

1. The allowance for the subsidence of spinal cord or root edema
2. Organization of fracture hematoma
3. Medical stabilization of the often multiply traumatized patient
4. The careful repeat performance of complete neurologic evaluations, observing for signs of neurologic improvement or deterioration. Emergency surgery under the standing orthopaedic surgery–neurosurgery protocol is indicated *only* in the presence of documented neurologic deterioration

SELECTION CRITERIA: INTERNAL FIXATION DEVICES

An interesting observation over the years concerns the change in philosophy concerning internal fixation, based on new information and new devices. Meyer[19] in 1978, Pinzer and Meyer[21] in 1979, Stauffer in 1975,[22] Jacobs[10] in 1980, and Dunn[4] in 1980 reported on biomechanical characteristics of various internal fixation devices used in the management of fractures of the vertebral column below C7 and the selection criteria for the more appropriate device under certain conditions. As noted, Harrington distraction rods were significantly more rigid than other internal fixation devices then in use (the Luque rods, Jacob's AO rods and Edwards or Wisconsin techniques were not yet developed). While I had worked in a cooperative investigative evaluation study with the developer of the Weiss compres-

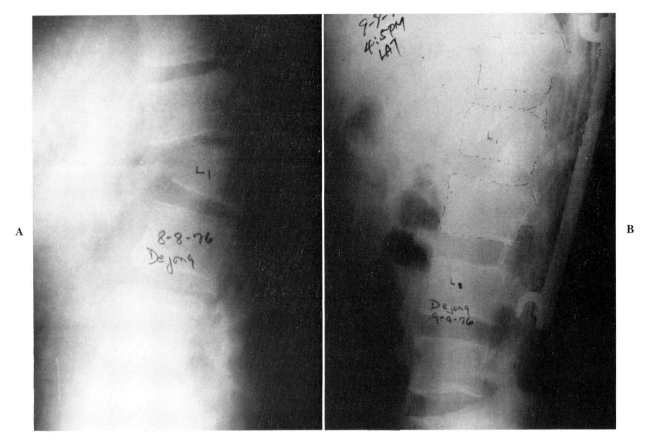

Fig. 39-2. Harrington distraction rods. Fracture-dislocation T12-L1. **A,** Lateral view, preoperative. **B,** Lateral view, postoperative Harrington rods. Note that rod only extends above fracture 2 levels proximally and distally. Recommended technique is three levels.

sion springs, they were found to have very restrictive uses because of their inherent instability under bending and rotational loads. The Weiss compression device was found to be easy to insert and provided stable dynamic compression in those situations where thoracic or lumbar facet dislocation, without fracture, had occurred. Even at that, its instability in rotation and bending was a matter of concern.

Today, Harrington distraction rods are the most frequently used method of internal stabilization (Fig. 39-2). The second most frequently used device is the Luque "segmental instrumentation system."[9,15,24]

Which internal fixation device to use under what circumstances is the single most important question to answer preoperatively. The answer is based on knowledge of the presence of an unstable fracture vs. a stable fracture. Other questions requiring answers are:

1. What internal fixation techniques are available, and what are their indications?
2. Are any of the management options affected by the presence of varying degrees of neurologic dysfunction?
3. What influence might the insertion of an internal fixation device have on an already present neurologic injury?

The insertion of any internal fixation device carries with it a potential hazard of either extending or producing neurologic injury under varying circumstances. Most often this concern accompanies correction of a major spinal deformity, where force or distraction[13] is required in the correction or reduction sufficient to produce vascular embarrassment.

With the introduction of the Luque "segmental spinal instrumentation" technique[15] (Fig. 39-3) as a positive method of gaining vertebral element stability following trauma, new hazards and concerns of iatrogenic neurologic injury during instrumentation (passage of sublaminar wires)

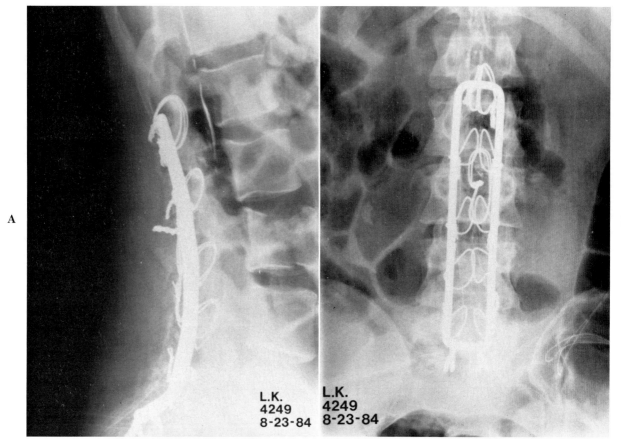

Fig. 39-3. Luque instrumentation with rectangular rods. **A,** Lateral. **B,** Anteroposterior of Fig. 39-1, **A** and **B**. Demonstrates excellent anteroposterior and lateral reduction.

arose. This is of particular concern in the upper thoracic neural canal, where the width of the canal at the T6 level is the size of the tip of the index finger or smaller.

Harrington compression rods

The indications for the use of Harrington compression rods or compression springs are similar insofar as both produce compression, but Harrington compression rods are rigid, producing greater compressive forces across two unstable joints. Compression devices are indicated in those situations where distraction is the primary disruptive force, and compression without gross vertebral column instability (fractures in two of the three columns) is present. With the use of this multilevel rod-hook device, compressive loads can be distributed equally across several levels, reducing the hazard of hyperextension at the fracture site, although it may still occur in the presence of instability within the anterior longitudinal liga-

ment.

A contraindication to the application of Harrington compression rods is the presence of a "unilateral body-pedicle-facet fracture" of a vertebra (Fig. 39-4). The application of a compressive load across the fracture frequently produces an iatrogenic scoliosis (Fig. 39-5). Another relative contraindication is the application of a Harrington compression rod device across a fracture of a vertebral body that demonstrates significant comminution and compression. The application of a compression device across such a fracture will neither correct the deformity nor prevent its collapse (Fig. 39-6).

Harrington distraction rods

Harrington distraction rods are the instrument of choice in:

1. A compression fracture where greater than 30% to 50% of the anterior vertebral body height exists

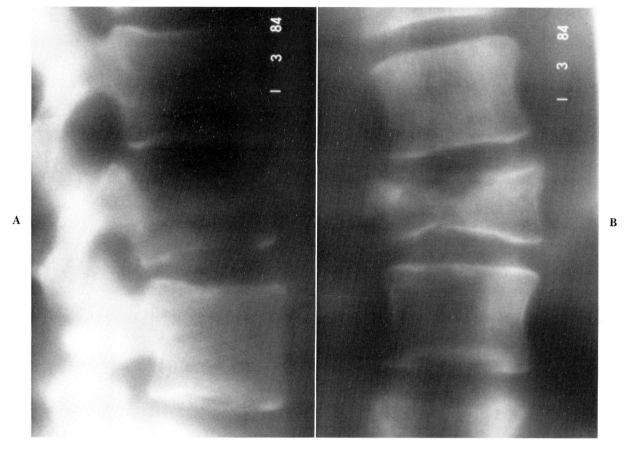

A   B

Fig. 39-4. Compression fracture L3 with unilateral fracture of vertebral body pedicle is an indication for Harrington distraction rods. **A,** Lateral tomogram. **B,** Anteroposterior tomogram.

2. The presence of a burst fracture of a vertebral body
3. Where there is gross spinal malalignment serving as evidence of significant vertebral-ligamentous instability
4. Evidence of tumorous destruction of a vertebral element

A major concern with the use of the Harrington distraction rods is the possibility of overdistraction of the vertebral elements (Fig. 39-7). This can occur as a result of greater than anticipated spinal instability or the application of too great a distraction force. Another concern is the possibility of producing vascular and neural injury to the spinal cord with overdistraction.

Although they are not complications, disadvantages to the Harrington distraction rod device are:

1. The occasional need to bend the rods to have them conform to the shape of the spine, particularly in the area of the kyphotic thoracic spine
2. The need to extend three levels above and below the fracture site (to have two intact lamina above and below the level of the fracture)
3. That with increased spine flexion (presumably after the fractures have healed), the rods frequently dislodge from the lower hooks, requiring their removal. Occasionally they dislodge before fracture healing
4. That with increased activity (again presumably after fracture healing or as evidence of failure of healing) the rods will fatigue fracture at the junction of the shank-ratchett portion of the distraction rod (Fig. 39-8)

Luque rods

There are many advantages to the use of Luque rods. Either the separate or rectangular rods can

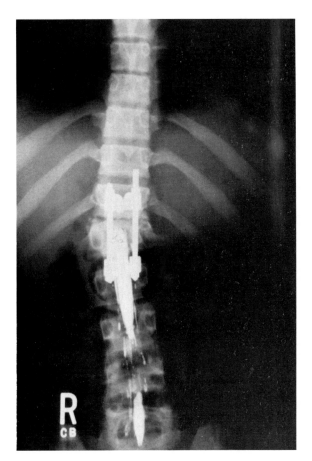

Fig. 39-5. Iatrogenic scoliosis produced by compression with Harrington compression rods across unilateral vertebral body-pedicle-facet fracture L1.

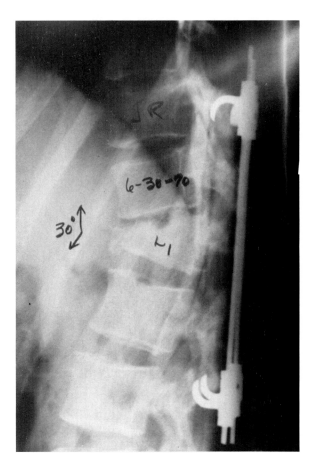

Fig. 39-6. Failure of Harrington compression rods across severe comminuted compression fractures L1 (> 50% loss of anterior vertebral body height). Note that too few hooks were applied to lamina posteriorly and rods cross too few segments.

be bent into the conforming shape of the area of the spine where the surgeon is working or the rods can be bent to have the unstable spine take on a corrected and more proper alignment.

This device is the most rigid of the internal stabilization instruments. Its stability is gained through the rigid fixation obtained by wiring the rods (with sublaminar wires) to each of the posterior elements they cross.

Luque rods can be used with relative safety at every level of the thoracic and lumbar spine when the neurologic injury is complete. They also may be used in those situations where absolute spine stability is required (as with tumor involvement) particularly when there is an attempt to preserve neurologic function (Fig. 39-9). The device (and sublaminar wires) must be used in the thoracic area (between T1 and T10) with extreme care and preferably with spinal cord monitoring. This is because the measured sagittal diameter be-

tween the posterior surface of the vertebra and the inner surface of the neural arch averages 6.0 mm at T3, 6.1 mm at T6 (it can vary as much as 3.7 mm to 7.8 mm), 6.5 mm at T10; 6.9 mm at T11, and 7.4 mm at T12 (with a variance between 3.8 mm to 9.3 mm).[11,16] In the most narrow area of the neural canal lies the thoracic spinal cord and, at T12 to L1, the conus medullaris (known for its intolerence to trauma).

On the other hand, the neural canal in the thoracic-lumbar region of the vertebral column is wider both in the interpedicular and the sagittal distances and contains the lower conus medullaris and the cauda equina (Fig. 39-10), which is quite resistant to permanent trauma. Other than the rigid stability gained by the application of the Luque rods, a major advantage is the ability to "shape" the rods to the curve of the vertebral

Text continued p. 414.

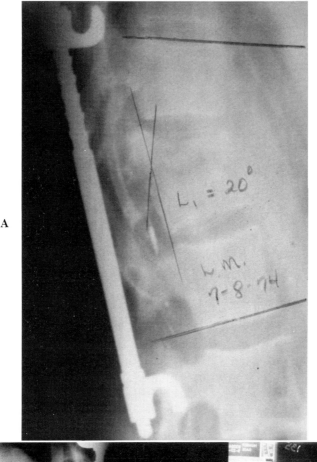

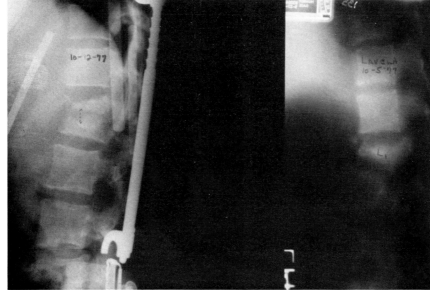

Fig. 39-7. A, Lateral view: burst fracture L1. Note overdistraction of fracture with Harrington distraction rods. **B,** Lateral view: comminuted fracture with compression L1. Note overdistraction of vertebral body with distraction applied to Harrington distraction rods.

Fig. 39-8. Compression fracture L3. **A,** Harrington distraction rods used to stabilize a burst fracture L3 (lateral view). Note shank and ratchett junction at same level as fracture. **B,** Fixation device. Same patient's rods fractured at 11 months after stabilization procedure.

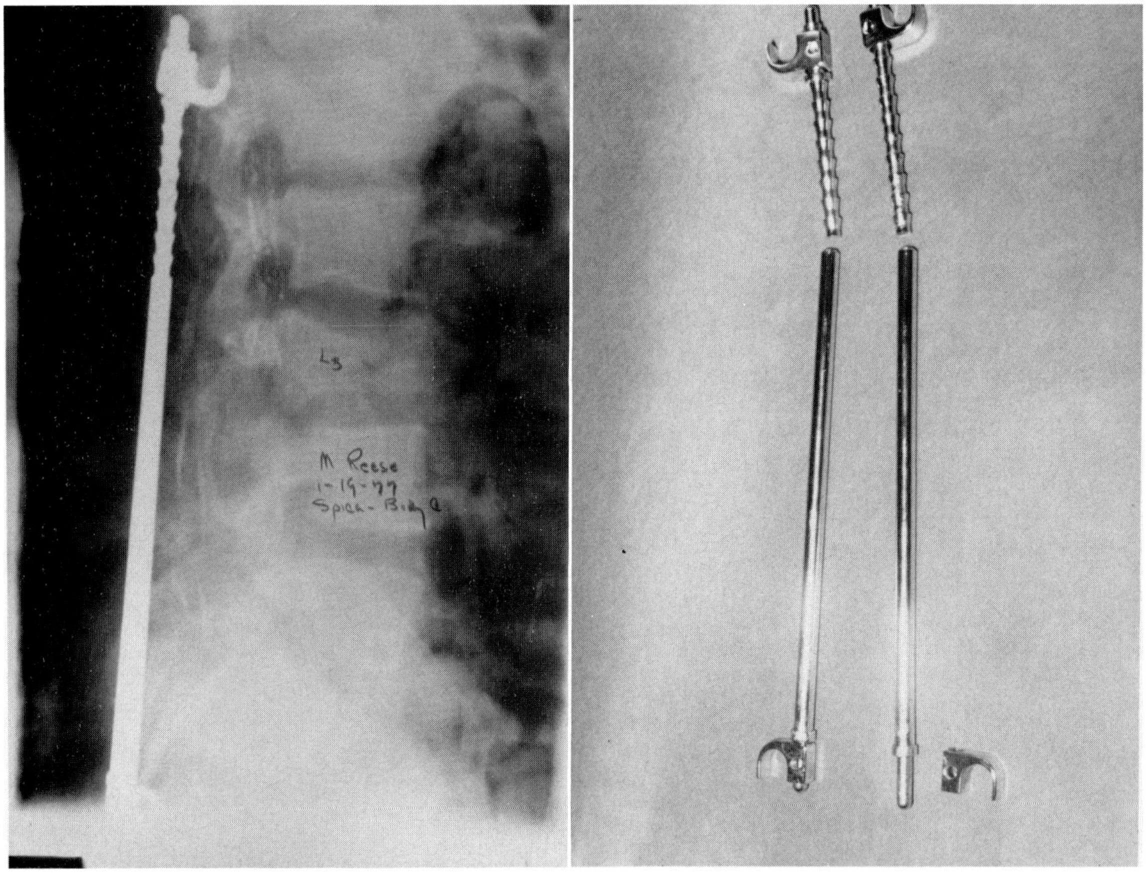

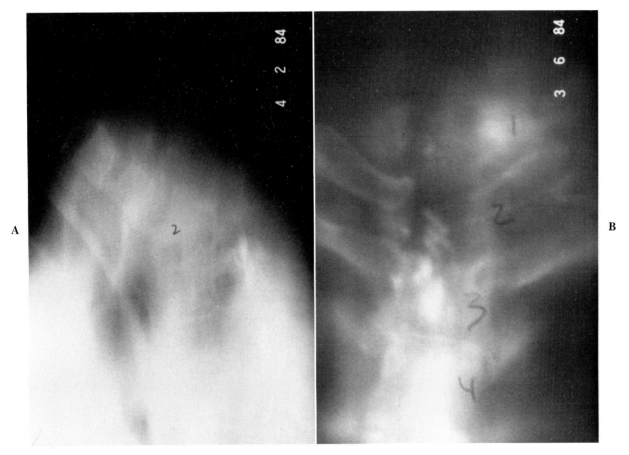

Fig. 39-9. Malignant metastatic tumor to T1 to T3 with impending neurologic loss of function and acute development of cervicothoracic kyphosis. **A,** Lateral view. **B,** AP view revealing laminectomy T1 to T3.

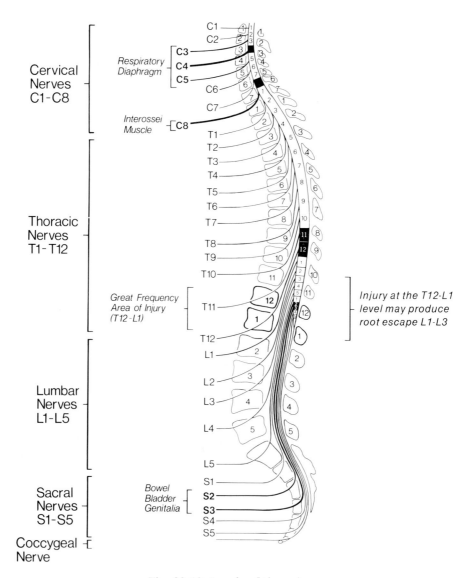

Cervical
Nerves
C1-C8

Thoracic
Nerves
T1-T12

Lumbar
Nerves
L1-L5

Sacral
Nerves
S1-S5

Coccygeal
Nerve

C1
C2
*Respiratory
Diaphragm* [**C3**
C4
C5
C6
C7
*Interossei
Muscle* [C8
T1
T2
T3
T4
T5
T6
T7
T8
T9
T10
*Great Frequency
Area of Injury
(T12-L1)*
T11
1
T12
L1
L2
L3
L4
L5
S1
*Bowel
Bladder
Genitalia* [**S2**
S3
S4
S5

*Injury at the T12-L1
level may produce
root escape L1-L3*

Fig. 39-10. Levels of the spine.

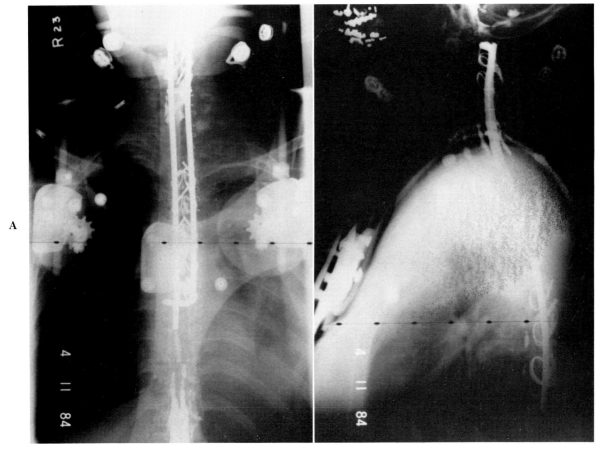

Fig. 39-11. A and **B,** Postoperative Luque rod procedure for metastatic tumor to cervicothoracic spine (T1 to T3). Stabilized with Luque rods C2-T8. Note contour of Luque rods.

column. In many instances bending the rods into an appropriate shape helps in restoring the normal anatomic alignment in that area of the vertebral column (Fig. 39-11).

NUMBER OF FUSED SEGMENTS

The mean number of fused segments per posterior procedure was 5.9 segments. The number of levels instrumented per posterior procedure was 6.2 levels.

INJURY PATTERNS

As shown in Table 39-6, the types of injuries found to occur in the area of the thoracic, lumbar, and sacral spine were the following:

1. 243 (37.6%) fracture dislocations of the thoracic-lumbar spine
2. 231 (35.8%) compression (burst) fractures
3. 26 (4.0%) dislocations
4. 24 (3.7%) fractures of the posterior elements (spinous process and lamina)
5. 119 (18%) other injury patterns

A review of each of these major groups, based on the previous discussion, provides the surgeon with some idea concerning the type of internal fixation device most applicable. Some examples follow.

1. For fracture-dislocations, where neurologic injury is frequently complete, posterior stabilization becomes the primary concern. Depending on

Table 39-6. Thoracic, lumbar, and sacral spine fractures: 1972 to 1985

Type of fracture	Number	Percent
Fracture/dislocation	243	37.79
Compression (burst) fracture	231	35.93
Other	119	18.51
Pure dislocation	26	4.04
Fracture of posterior elements	24	3.73
TOTAL	643	

the length of time the vertebral column or element may have been dislocated, or the extent of spinal instability (one-, two-, or three-column involvement), the surgeon usually can determine which of the fixation devices to use (Harrington distraction rods where distraction force is required or Luque rods where maximal stability is required).

2. In the case of the compression (burst) fracture, the presence or absence of neurologic injury often influences the procedure of choice. For example, where neurologic function is intact, the passage of sublaminar wires (the Luque procedure) is not contraindicated but certainly should be carefully considered, particularly if there has been any indication of neurologic injury. Under those conditions and where the pos-

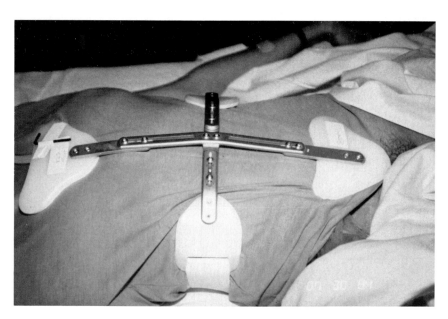

Fig. 39-12. Jewett (Florida) hyperextension orthosis for management of chance fracture L4.

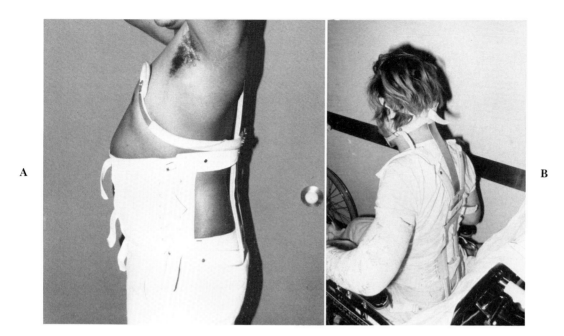

Fig. 39-13. A, Lateral view, Knight-Taylor orthosis with pectoral horns, for thoracic-lumbar fractures below T6. **B,** Knight-Taylor with cervical extension for fractures of T6 and above.

terior wall of the vertebral body demonstrates (tomograms) the presence of bone retropulsion, Harrington distraction rods are indicated. If significantly (incomplete) neurologic compromise exists, the patient is a candidate for anterior decompression and posterior stabilization (staged or simultaneously). Before its removal from the surgical armamentarium, the Dunn[4] apparatus was used under such circumstances, where anterior decompression was required, followed by stabilization.

3. In those situations where injury to the spine results in a pure dislocation, there is evidence of gross vertebral column instability (with forward subluxation of one vertebra on the other, fracture dislocation with a "tear" through the anterior longitudinal ligament). The presence of neurologic injury frequently depends on the extent of the original dislocation. The two or three procedures available for the stabilization of this type of injury are (1) Luque Rods, (2) Harrington distraction rods, (3) Jacobs spinal (AO) rods, and (4) Harrington compression rods.

4. In the case of fractures of the posterior elements where only the spinous process and posterior lamina are involved, internal stabilization generally is not required. What might alter this management schema may be the presence of

other vertebral element injuries, such as ligamentous disruption with vertebral element subluxation. Where internal fixation is not required, one of several types of orthotic devices may be used: the Jewett or Florida orthosis (Fig. 39-12 and 39-14), plastic laminate, or the Knight-Taylor orthosis (Fig. 39-13).

5. On those occasions when several vertebral fractures over several different areas may have occurred, conservative care with extended recumbency (3 to 4 weeks) and an external orthosis are usually all that is indicated if the spine is stable. To determine whether stability exists, flexion-extension radiographs may be required. If the spine is stable, the type of orthosis most frequently used is the Knight-Taylor orthosis with pectoral horns (Fig. 39-13, *A*). If the injury occurs above the level of the sixth thoracic vertebra, a cervical extension is added to the Knight-Taylor orthosis to prevent the development of a kyphotic deformity in the upper segment.

USE OF EVOKED RESPONSE MONITORING DURING SURGERY

Use of the intraoperative somatosensory cortical evoked potential is a reliable method of providing early warning in the prevention of neurologic injury during surgical instrumentation of

Fig. 39-14. Chance fracture L4 managed conservatively by recumbency and Jewett (Florida) hyperextension orthosis. **A,** Lateral view. **B,** AP view.

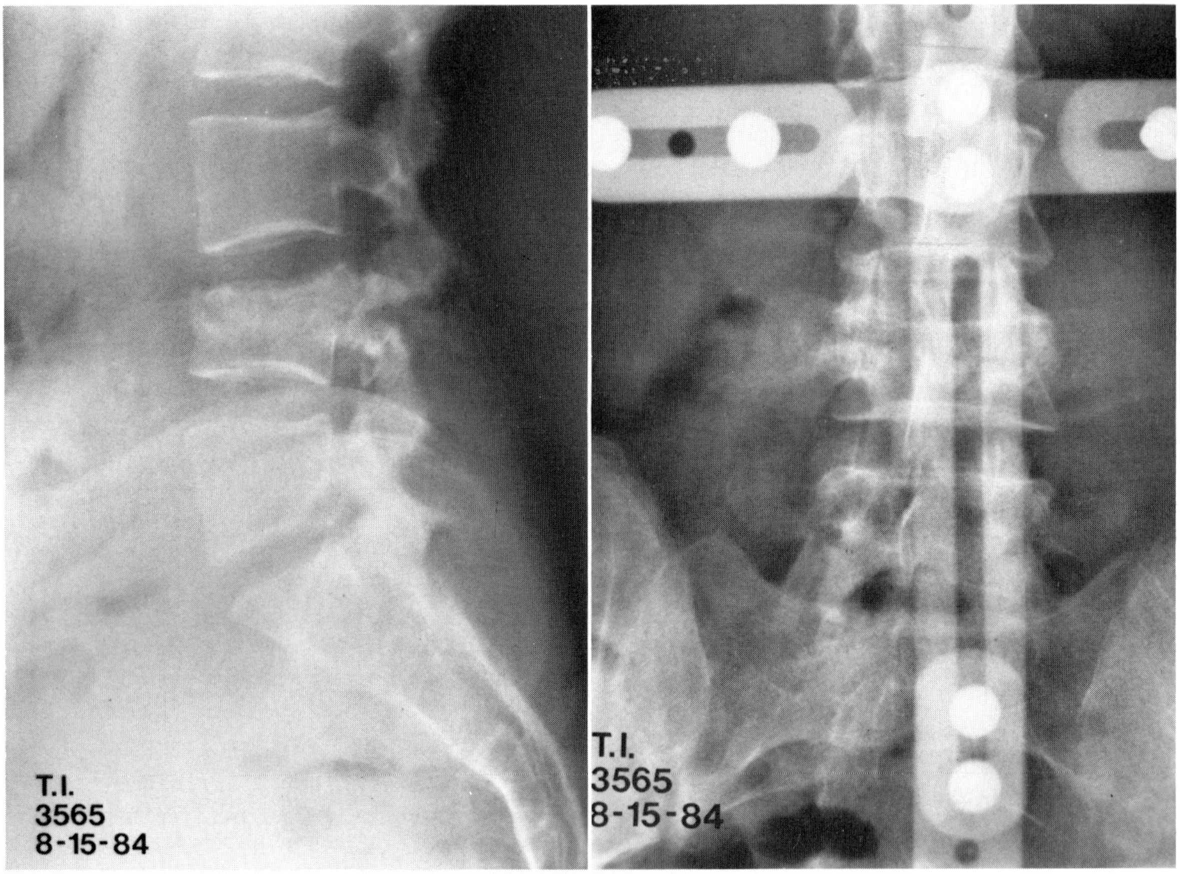

fractures of the spine. When there is evidence of deterioration in repeatable evoked responses, every possible cause for alteration in the wave form must be eliminated. Alterations in evoked responses may result from:

1. Technical failure (electrodes becoming disconnected)
2. Pharmacologic reasons (the administration of various anesthetic agents or drugs)
3. Physiologic reasons (the administration of cold blood, changes in room temperature, changes in body core temperature)

4. Surgical reasons (direct injury to the spinal cord or embarrassment of its vascular supply)

If the cause of concern for the loss of evoked response cannot be accurately identified, three recommendations are:

1. Administer dexamethosone 50 mg stat, IV
2. Perform the "wake-up" test if function is less than preoperative
3. Remove all internal fixation that may have been implanted and wait at least 30 to 60 minutes before proceeding

RESULTS

The primary etiologic causes for fracture-dislocation of the thoracic, lumbar, and sacral area of the vertebral column were falls, motor vehicle accidents, and gunshot wounds. The majority of injuries occurred in the junctional area of T11 through L2 (56%) and the area between T1 and T10 (35%) (Table 39-7).

Of 646 patients with fracture-dislocations of the thoracic, lumbar, and sacral spine, who were admitted within 8 hours of injury to the Acute Spine Injury Center at Northwestern University between June 1972 and July 1985, 374 (58%) underwent surgical stabilization (Table 39-8). The region of the spine most often requiring surgical stabilization was the lumbar spine (82%), followed by the thoracic-lumbar junction (66%).

The surgical approach most frequently used for spine instrumentation was the posterior approach (82%), followed by the combined (simultaneous) anteroposterior approach (14%).

Harrington distraction rods were most frequently used for spine stabilization (41%). Because of the length of the longitudinal study on instrumentation of fractures of the thoracic, lumbar, and sacral spine (13 years), additional devices used include compression springs, Harrington

Table 39-7. Highest fractured vertebra

Level fractured	Number	Percent
T1	13	2.01%
T2	15	2.32%
T3	28	4.33%
T4	34	5.26%
T5	38	5.88%
T6	19	2.94%
T7	29	4.48%
T8	30	4.46%
T9	20	3.09%
T10	33	5.10%
T11	53	8.20%
T12	122	18.88%
L1	116	17.95%
L2	40	6.19%
L3	25	3.86%
L4	17	2.63%
L5	9	1.39%
S1	5	0.77%
TOTAL	646	

Table 39-8. Level of skeletal injury

Level of injury	Number	Percent	Number of operations	Percent of operations
Thoracic (T1-T10)	224	34.67	87	38.83%
Thoracic-lumbar (T11-L2)	360	55.73	239	66.38%
Lumbar (L3-L5)	57	8.83	47	82.45%
Sacrum (S1-S5)	5	0.77	1	20.00%
TOTAL	646		374	58.04%

Table 39-9. Types of instrumentation for thoracic, lumbar, or sacral spine*

Type of surgical instrumentation	Number	Percent
Harrington distraction rod	144	40.79%
Harrington compression rod	2	0.57%
Compression springs	147	41.64%
Luque rods	47	13.32%
Anterior decompression	9	2.55%
Wires	4	1.13%
TOTAL	353	

*Injuries, T1 to S5.

compression rods, Luque rods, and wire, among others (Table 39-9).

SUMMARY

While new spine-stabilizing devices are beginning to appear as alternative methods of providing operative spine stability, a careful review of those methods used by the Spine Injury Service at Northwestern University was undertaken. The method of stabilization most frequently used was the Harrington distraction rod device. With the coming of the Luque rod "segmental instrumentation" technique, improved spine stability was attained, although the attributes of the Harrington distraction system could not be substituted by the Luque system.

A natural spin-off was the combination of the Harrington and the Luque methods of internal fixation (Fig. 39-15). This has been a significant addition to the spine surgeon's surgical armamentarium. Still there are problems of implant stability, for which the Jacobs AO rods were developed, and the need for better correction of the spine's malposition following fracture (Edwards system). Because of the concern for the placement of sublaminar wires beneath the lamina, particularly in the area of the very narrow thoracic neural

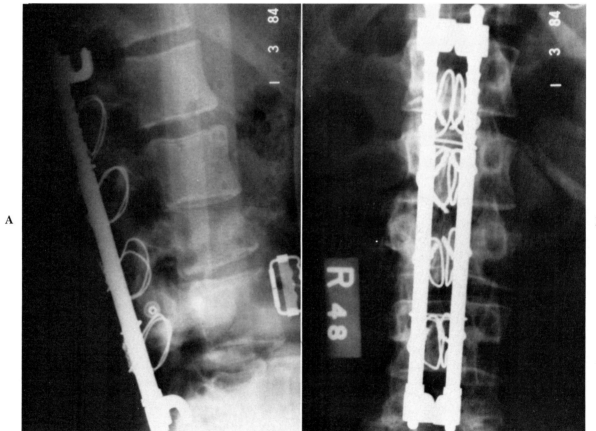

Fig. 39-15. Harrington-Luque rods combination at compression fracture L3. **A,** Lateral view. **B,** Anteroposterior view. Note flattening and loss of lumbar lordotic curve using Harrington distraction rods.

canal, the "Wisconsin" system of spinous process wires was developed. The discussion in this chapter is limited to the statistical data gathered from the management of 646 fracture-dislocations of the spine, of which 374 were surgically managed.

As noted in Table 39-3, there are hazards to the instrumentation of the thoracic, lumbar, and sacral spine. In this surgical group, neurologic deterioration occurred in 2.39%; however, there was evidence of significant "risk-benefit" in surgery, with 15.22% of surgical patients demonstrating neurologic improvement after surgery of at least one Frankel grade. When compared with those patients managed conservatively, 6.57% demonstrated neurologic improvement, whereas only 0.34% demonstrated neurologic deterioration.

REFERENCES

1. Bracken, M.B., Collins, W.F., Freeman, D.F., et al.: Efficacy of methylprednisone in acute spinal cord injury, JAMA **251**(1):45-52, 1984.
2. DeWald, R.L., Faut, M.M., Taddonio, R.F., and Neuwirth, M.G.: Severe lumbosacral spondylolisthesis in adolescents and children: Reduction and staged circumferential fusion, J. Bone Joint Surg. **63A**:619-626, 1981.
3. Duhaime, M., Labelle, P., Lebel, M., Simoneau, R., Poitras, B., Rivard, C.H., and Morton, D.: Treatment of idiopathic scoliosis by the Harrington techniques, Chir-Pediatr. **23**(1):17-22, 1982.
4. Dunn, H.K., Daniels, A.U., and McBride, G.G.: Comparative assessment of spine stability achieved with a new anterior spine fixation device, Orthop. Trans. J. Bone Joint Surg. **4**(2):268-269, 1980.
5. Frankel, H., Hancock, D., Hyslop, G., et al.: The value of postural reduction in the initial management of closed injuries to the spine with paraplegia, paraplegia **7**:179-192, 1969.
6. Frankel, H.L.: Ascending cord lesions in the early stages following spinal injury, Paraplegia **7**:111, 1969.
7. Gertzbein, S.D., MacMichael, D., and Tile, M.: Harrington instrumentation as a method of fixation in fractures of the spine, J. Bone Joint Surg. **64B**(5):526-529, 1982.
8. Hannon, K.M.: Harrington instrumentation in fractures and dislocations of the thoracic and lumbar spine, South. Med. J. **69**(10):1269-1279, 1976.
9. Herring, J.A., and Wenger, D.R.: Segmental spinal instrumentation, Spine **7**(3):285-298, 1982.
10. Jacobs, R.R., Asher, M.A., and Snider, R.K.: Dorso-lumbar spine fractures: Recumbent vs. operative treatment, Paraplegia **18**(6):358-376, 1980.
11. Jirout, J.: Fortschr. Geb. Reontgenstr. Nuklearmed. Erganzungsband, **104**:89, 1966.
12. Leatherman, K.D., and Deckman, R.A.: Two-stage corrective surgery for congenital deformities of the spine, J. Bone Joint Surg. **61B**:324-328, 1979.
13. Letts, R.M., and Hollenberg, C.: Delayed paresis following spinal fusion with Harrington instrumentation, Clin. Orthop. **125**:45-48, 1977.
14. Lucus, J.G., and Ducker, T.B.: Motor classification of spinal cord injuries with mobility, morbidity, and recovery indices, Am. Surg. **45**:151-158, 1979.
15. Luque, E.R., Cassis, N., and Ramirez-Wiella, G.: Segmental spine instrumentation in the treatment of fractures of the thoracolumbar spine, Spine **7**(3):312-317, 1982.
16. Lusted, L.B., and Keats, T.E.: Atlas of roentgenographic measurement, ed. 4, Chicago, 1978, Year Book Medical Publishers, Inc.
17. MacEwen, G.D., Bunnell, W.P., and Sriran, K.: Acute neurological complications in the treatment of scoliosis: A report of the Scoliosis Research Society, J. Bone Joint Surg. **57A**:404-408, 1975.
18. McAfee, D.C., Yuan, H.A., and Lasada, M.A.: The unstable burst fracture, Spine **7**(4):365-373, 1982.
19. Meyer, P.R.: Complications of treatment of fractures of the dorsolumbar spine. In Epps, C., editor: Complications in orthopaedic surgery, vol. 2, Philadelphia, 1978, J.B. Lippincott Co.
20. Meyer, P.R.: The spinal cord injury patient. In Beal, J.M., editor: Critical care for surgical patients, New York, 1982, Macmillan Publishing Co.
21. Pinzer, M.S., Meyer, P.R., et al.: Measurement of internal fixation device support in experimentally produced fractures of the dorsolumbar spine, Orthopaedics **2**(1):28-34, 1979.
22. Stauffer, E.S., and Neil, J.L.: Biomechanical analysis of structural stability of internal fixation in fractures in the thoracolumbar spine, Clin. Orthop. **112**:159-164, 1975.
23. Swank, S., Lonstein, J.E., Moe, J.H., Winter, R.B., and Bradford, D.S.: Surgical treatment of adult scoliosis, J. Bone Joint Surg. **63A**(2):268-287, 1981.
24. Wilbur, R.G., Thompson, G.H., Shaffer, J.W., and Mash, C.L.: Post-operative neurological deficits in segmental spinal instrumentation, J. Bone Joint Surg. **66A**:1178-1187, 1984.
25. Yosipovitch, Z., Robin, G.C., and Maskin, M.: Open reduction of unstable thoracolumbar spinal injuries and fixation with Harrington rods, J. Bone Joint Surg. **59**(8):1003-1015, 1977.
26. Zillke, K., and Pellin, B.: Results of surgical management of scoliosis and kyphoscoliosis in adults, Z. Orthop. **113**(2):157-174, 1975.

Chapter 40

Spinal stenosis

ROBERT E. BOOTH, JR.

For a surgeon trained in the era of the simple laminectomy and disk excision or even in the age of the lumbar fusion, the surgery of spinal stenosis presents some unique conceptual and technical challenges. When properly performed, however, the more extensive procedures necessitated by the pathophysiology of spinal stenosis should yield the same excellent results as simple disk surgery, even though the symptoms may be of greater longevity and the patients of significantly greater age.

The opportunity to pass on the concepts of spinal stenosis surgery to young fellows and residents of varying talents and interests has nurtured the development of certain principles that allow stenosis surgery to be performed simply and effectively with minimal risk to the patient and to the patient's neural elements. As we have learned in the past from such operations as total hip replacement, part of the power of any surgical procedure resides in its capacity to be simplified and organized to yield a good result in the face of a wide spectrum of surgical pathology and a great diversity of surgical skills. In the surgery of the spine, the obverse is also all too true. A decompressive laminectomy that is unsuccessful —often the result of poor control of hemostasis, loss of intraoperative orientation, incomplete understanding of the surgical pathology, or inadequate decompression and stabilization—creates a "failed back" and a pain problem for which there may be no resolution.

An examination of the surgical records of patients whose spinal surgery has been unsuccessful reveals a striking similarity to four problems that often beset the surgical novice. These four areas, which are the topic of this discussion, include the techniques of hemostasis, the princi-

ples of surgical orientation, the concept of what constitutes an adequate decompression of a spinal nerve, and an approach to the appropriate use of spinal stabilization in conjunction with decompressive procedures for spinal stenosis. Perhaps the most direct way to approach these topics is to review the technique of spinal stenosis decompression in light of the principles that have evolved at Pennsylvania Hospital.

TECHNIQUE OF SPINAL STENOSIS

Currently general agreement exists about the positioning of a patient for a lumbar decompressive surgery, since most surgeons use some variation of the position depicted in Fig. 40-1, with the chest and knees supporting the body while the abdomen hangs free.[4,5] This position significantly reduces the intraabdominal pressure and thereby decompresses the epidural veins. The reduction in pressure allows the surgical procedures to be performed with a minimum of hemorrhage to obscure the pathology and the neural elements, and it also reduces the chance of postoperative hemorrhage, which may produce a dreaded epidural hematoma. Elastic stockings provide venous support to the lower extremities. Spinal anesthesia supplements this vascular decompression by adding the effect of a pharmacologic phlebotomy to the surgical position. In 15 years of using this position at Pennsylvania Hospital, we have encountered no specific complications relative to the neurologic surgical posture itself.

It should be noted that in the kneeling position the spine is placed in hyperextension. Although this position admittedly increases the difficulty of performing a laminectomy and decompressing the neural elements and the facet joints, the position of spinal hyperextension most nearly

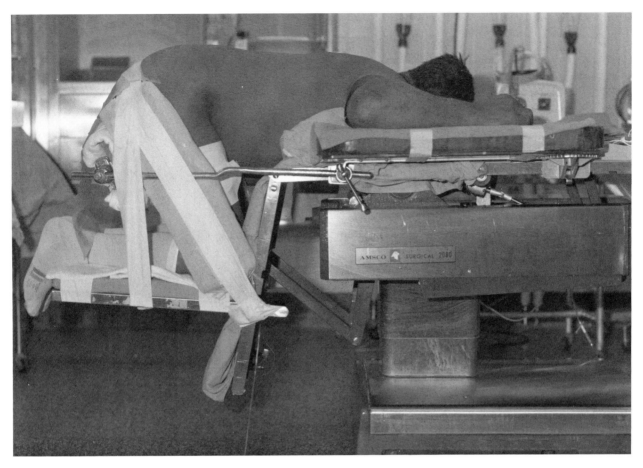

Fig. 40-1. Kneeling position for lumbar spine surgery. Even in the most obese patient the abdomen can be completely free of pressure. ECG pads facilitate cardiac monitoring; ausculation is difficult in this position. Lateral padding. A padded seat cushion served to stabilize and position the patient. Elastic stockings are used to prevent blood pooling in the lower extremities.

reproduces the axial and appendicular symptoms of nerve root compression. Thus if the spine is decompressed in this hyperextended posture, complete relief of pain when the patient is erect and active should be expected.

Localization of the appropriate level for the spinal incision begins with the examination of the anteroposterior x-ray film, which is best viewed as if the patient were facing away from the examiner. A careful search should be made for such spinal anomalies as transitional vertebrae, bifid spinous processes, asymmetric transverse processes, and other structural irregularities that may help identify a specific level. This information can be transferred to the palpation of the posterior spine, which in the kneeling position is relatively subcutaneous even in the most obese patient. Not only does the surgeon palpate for the presence of the spinous processes at the level of the lumbosacral junction, but also for the level of the iliac crest relative to the bony spine because it is the most common landmark. It is important to remember to discount the supplemental thickness of skin, fat, and muscle, which will falsely elevate the apparent level of the iliac crest.

Once a dissection has begun, there is a fairly constant decussation of the fascial fibers of the lumbodorsal fascia at the L5 to S1 interspace, providing an anatomic clue to the site of the lumbosacral junction.

The appropriate level of spinal surgery

The best technique for identifying the appropriate level of spinal surgery, however, remains the exposure of the sacrum through the bottom of the skin incision. Only when the true level of the sacrum is known can the surgeon be confident of a proper orientation within the spine. The ability to palpate the termination of the interlaminar spaces, the hollow sound that the sacrum affords when it is scraped by dissecting instruments, and the palpable alar prominences laterally give great reassurance that the correct level is identified, even when the stenosis is at a higher spinal level such as L3 to L4.

A supplemental technique involves the grasping of the spinous processes with towel clips to demonstrate the presence or absence of motion at the lowest levels of the spine. Finally, the surgeon should have a very low threshold for ordering an intraoperative x-ray film, and use a metallic instrument to mark the levels in question. With the patient in the kneeling position, lateral x-ray films are easy to obtain and relatively clear. It is far better to expend some additional time to confirm the level of surgery than to decompress levels that do not have surgical pathology.

When an incorrect spinal level has been decompressed, the general error is to be too high in the spine, rarely too low. Thus the exploration for the correct level should proceed distally rather than proximally, after the surgeon has reidentified the sacrum and confirmed the orientation.

The initial spinal incision

The initial spinal incision is made in the midline, directly over the spinous processes, which are palpable just beneath the skin. The dissection should be carried down through the subcutaneous fat to the lumbodorsal fascia, which is a very thick structure seen clearly in the anatomic specimen in Fig. 40-2. The lumbodorsal fascia forms a very thick envelope encompassing the erector spinae muscles, coalescing with the psoas fascia anteriorly and the periosteum of the lamina and spinous process medially. It is critical to preserve this envelope of fascia and periosteum by performing a subperiosteal dissection of the bony elements of the spine. This procedure avoids violating the intramuscular veins, it allows for tamponade of the paraspinous veins by post-surgical muscle swelling, and it prevents the surgical field from becoming obscured with blood.

An additional hazard of the kneeling position is that the focus of the final dissection of the spine is at the bottom of the wound, which will collect blood from any unattended vessels higher in the incision. Thus it is a general principle of spinal surgery that blood vessels must be coagulated as they are encountered, at each step of the dissection. Skin and fascial vessels therefore will be addressed before the fascial and subperiosteal dissection begins, and these vessels will be controlled before the spinal canal is opened.

When the subperiosteal dissection of the spinous processes and laminae is begun, instruments such as an electrocautery or periosteal elevator should be angled away from the midline to account for the bulbous enlargement of the tip of the spinous process, which is part of the pathophysiology of spinal degeneration. If this is not done, the instruments would plunge directly anteriorly, entering the paraspinal envelope of fascia and muscle. It is also helpful to dissect the paraspinous musculature from caudad to cephalad, since the oblique insertions of these muscles will serve to keep the dissecting instrument close to the bone, just as the surgeon would dissect the femoral musculature from distal to proximal as well.

At this time instruments should be placed to retract the paraspinous muscles, opening the surgical field and compressing the underlying blood vessels. Many types of self-retaining and hand-held retractors have been devised. The Taylor reverse retractor is favored at our institution because of its safety and simplicity, the ease of transferring the retractor to different spinal levels, and the variability of applied tension when it is controlled by a strip of muslin or gauze connected to the surgeon's foot. These retractors use the facet joint as their point of leverage, and they are inserted easily by sliding the tip of the retractor down the spinous process, out obliquely along the lamina, and out over the edge of the facet joint (Fig. 40-3). This provides sufficient visualization for almost any decompressive procedure.

Some additional bleeding now may be encountered from the small facetal arteries, which course around the medial aspect of each facet joint and provide the primary source of intraoperative bleeding outside the spinal canal itself (Fig. 40-4). These arteries can be safely controlled with electrocautery, because the neural elements are still protected by the bone above them. At this juncture, many surgeons prefer to remove the spinous processes with a large bone biter, occasionally exposing venous lakes within the soft bone of

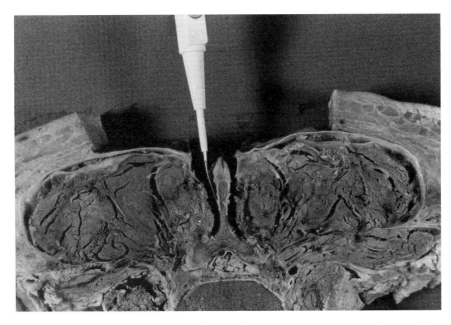

Fig. 40-2. Subperiosteal dissection of the spinous process preserves the envelope of paraspinous muscles and avoids their blood vessels as seen clearly in this transverse section.

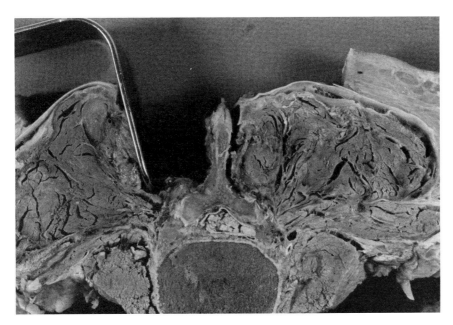

Fig. 40-3. Retractors placed over the lateral facet joint provide excellent visualization and also compress the paraspinous muscle mass, minimizing hemorrhage.

the elderly patient. Even though the laminae may be removed subsequently, the use of bone wax on these areas of hemorrhage will keep the wound dry during laminar excision.

The surgical anatomy

Now, before opening the spinal canal itself, the operating physician should review the surgical anatomy and the planned dissection. In particular, the surgeon should identify and articulate the location of the pedicles, which are the key to the subsequent anatomic dissection (Fig. 40-5). It is around the pedicles that the neural elements will course, by which the nerve roots are numbered, and which will remain even after the rest of the dorsal spinal elements are removed. It is surprisingly easy to become disoriented when the usual posterior bony landmarks have been removed and the spinal canal is completely open.

Specific nerve roots to be decompressed will have been identified in the course of the physical examination and preoperative planning. Although the spinal stenosis syndrome encompasses a wide variety of anatomic variants, each individual nerve root is generally at risk at two areas: in the lateral recess and in the foramen. It is very helpful to articulate the location of these areas before proceeding with further dissection.

Even the most effective periosteal dissection will still leave some short muscle fibers attached to the laminae and ligamentum flavum, and these can be excised with a large curette. This is done with a gentle scraping motion, preferably moving from the lateral area of the facet joint toward the midline of the spinous process so that the final excursion of the instrument does not violate the parafacetal arteries or paraspinous muscle envelope.

When the ligamentum flavum has been cleanly exposed, a small curette then may be used to gently dissect the insertion of the ligament from the under surface of the superior vertebra (Fig. 40-6). Curettes are quite effective at this task, and they enjoy the additional safety of presenting a round bowl to the delicate neural elements beneath. This step, and all subsequent steps to remove the laminae, should be initiated in the midline and then proceed laterally. Even in the most narrow spinal canal, the midline is the last area to become occluded and the safest area to begin a dissection.

When the inferior edge of the lamina has been exposed, a Schlesinger punch is used to begin dissecting the bone of the lamina itself (Fig. 40-7). Again, this step is initiated in the midline and then carried smoothly to the lateral sides of the

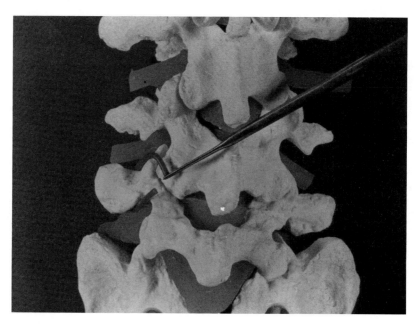

Fig. 40-4. Most debleeding in the extraspinal area results from violation of the small arteries that course from anterior to posterior around the facet joints.

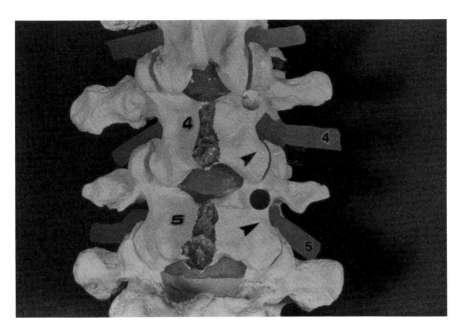

Fig. 40-5. Clear comprehension of the course of the nerves within the spinal canal should be maintained, particularly before the identifying landmarks are dissected. Here the dark circles represent the position of the pedicles deep to the posterior elements of the spine, which are preserved in almost all dissections. The arrows show the areas of greatest jeopardy for the L5 nerve root, proximally in the lateral recess and distally at the foramen.

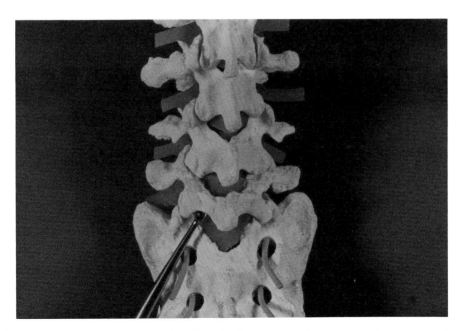

Fig. 40-6. A small curette is used to free the ligamentum flavum from the undersurface of the superior lamina.

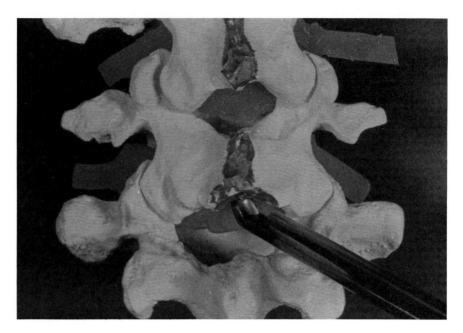

Fig. 40-7. A Schlesinger punch is used to remove the bone of the lamina, beginning the dissection in the midline where the canal is most capacious.

spinal canal. The round bowl of the Schlesinger punch protects the neural elements, particularly if all pressure is directed dorsally. The dura in a patient with true spinal stenosis may be quite thin, and the typical dorsal fat may be absent. In inflammatory spondylopathies such as ankylosing spondylitis, the dura may even be adherent to the anterior surface of the lamina and extreme care must be taken in the dissection. As the laminar dissection proceeds cephalad, curettes or Frazier palpators can be used to ensure that the path ahead is free of such adhesions. The Schlesinger punch should not be rocked from side to side in removing pieces of bone, so that the dura is not abraded or lacerated by the edges of the bony fragments. The ligamentum flavum of the succeeding interspace then can be dissected with the same technique.

The result of this dissection will be a central trough extending proximally and distally over the appropriate levels to be decompressed and extending laterally to the medial edge of the facet joint (Fig. 40-8). The dura will be readily visible, and any bleeding encountered at this point in the epidural vessels should be controlled with bipolar electrocautery, topical coagulants, or sponges. The surgical field again should be completely dried before any further examination of the neural elements.

In patients with a central spinal stenosis, who constitute a very small proportion of those with spinal stenosis seen in the average practice, this dissection will be adequate to alleviate neurologic symptoms. These patients are typically young people with a congenitally narrow spinal canal, usually by virtue of short pedicles.

In the vast majority of patients, however, the area of stenosis is in the lateral recess or foramen, and further dissection is necessary. The first objective is to remove the encroachment on the lateral nerve roots created by the overgrown superior facet joints. An appreciation for this problem is first gained by placing a probe along the path of the nerve root in question. This maneuver, as well as the insertion of all subsequent dissecting instruments, should be done from proximal to distal with the instrument parallel to the nerve root. Although it is tempting to attack the lateral bony elements directly and perpendicular to the axis of the spine, it is possible to grasp or transect the nerve roots themselves. Thus the use of the instruments parallel to the nerves will avoid unfortunate accidents. Initially, residual pieces of ligamentum flavum will be removed, followed by the bony fragments of the hypertrophied superior facet. If the handle of the Schlesinger punch is angled toward the opposite side of the spine, the su-

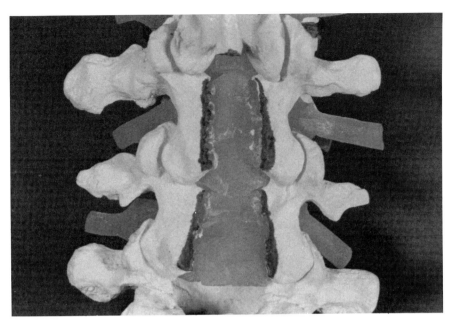

Fig. 40-8. A midline decompression with laminar excision is occasionally sufficient in patients with central spinal stenosis.

perior facet may be undercut quite effectively, removing the encroachment of the lateral recess without destabilizing the facet joint at that level (Fig. 40-9). This can be done throughout the length of the exposed spinal levels, providing a complete release of the lateral recess without jeopardizing spinal stability. This dissection will eliminate the symptoms of spinal stenosis in the vast majority of surgical patients.

Adequacy of spinal decompression

At this juncture it is appropriate to consider the adequacy of spinal decompression. Unfortunately, this is an area where the surgeon must rely heavily on judgment, experience, and the "feel" of the decompressed nerve root. Although much has been written about the appropriate degree of lumbar decompression, the best general guideline is that enunciated by Marvin Tile of Toronto, who has exhorted us to "think nerve". We must not cling to our preconceived and presurgical notions of where the pathology may lie, particularly as it is shown by CT scans and MRI images. Rather we must rely on our tactile and visual senses at the time of surgery to be sure that each nerve root is free from compression in the central spinal canal, the lateral recess, the foramen, and—if necessary—beyond. There is no test or objective criterion by which to judge this situation, and the

surgeon must constantly bear in mind the occasionally delicate balance between complete neural freedom and spinal stability. Nonetheless, no surgical dissection for spinal stenosis should be terminated until the nerve roots at jeopardy are no longer under tension.

Neural decompression

With the central spinal canal and the lateral recess already decompressed, it is the handling of the foraminal and extraforaminal sources of nerve compression that is crucial in the successful treatment of spinal stenosis.[2,3,6] Although any of an enormous variety of anatomic variance may cause foraminal or extra foraminal stenosis, there are four common problems that should always be considered when a nerve root, decompressed to the extent of its lateral recess, fails to move appropriately under direct palpation. The first of these involves the entrapment of the spinal nerve between the superior facet of one vertebra and the posterolateral aspect of the vertebral body of the superadjacent vertebra (Fig. 40-10). To resolve this problem, the surgeon need only undermine further the superior facet or perhaps excise the facet joint itself.

A related problem is seen when the nerve root is caught between the superior facet of one vertebra and the descending pedicle of the verte-

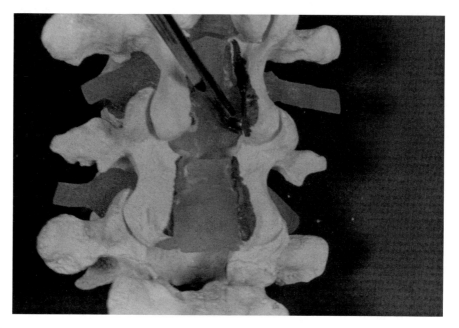

Fig. 40-9. A Schlesinger punch is used to remove portions of the superior facet, thus freeing the lateral recess. Dissecting instruments should be placed in line with the nerves at jeopardy. Angling the Schlesinger punch allows the facet to be undercut with minimal compromise to its stability.

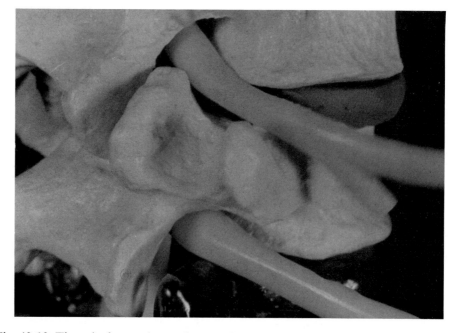

Fig. 40-10. The spinal nerve is seen here under compression between the superior facet of one vertebra and the posterior body of the superior vertebra.

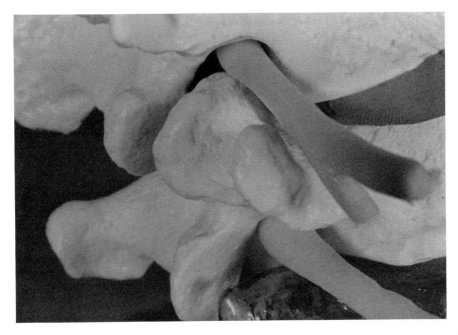

Fig. 40-11. Here the spinal nerve is entrapped between the tip of the superior facet and the pedicle.

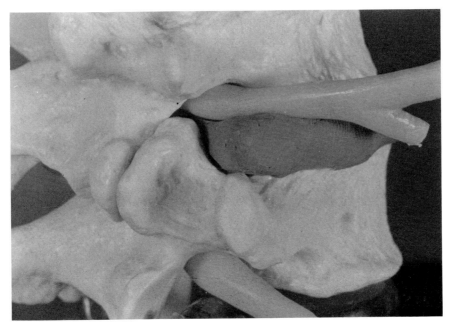

Fig. 40-12. Occasionally the spinal nerve will be compressed between the bulging anulus and the pedicle or osteophytes of the vertebra above.

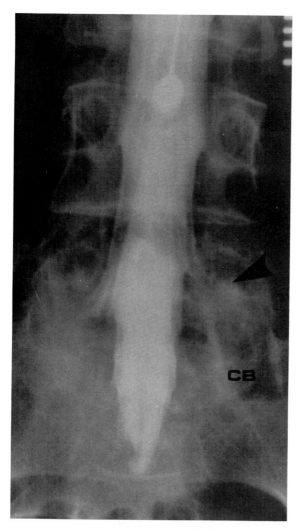

Fig. 40-13. The myelographic findings of an isolated nerve-root compression are sometimes quite subtle. Here the right L5 nerve root is not seen to course as far beneath its pedicle as the root on the opposite side.

bra above (Fig. 40-11). Again, the nerve can be freed by excising the tip of the superior facet or the entire facet joint if necessary.

The third, and perhaps most common, of these lateral syndromes is seen when the nerve root is entrapped between the bulging anulus of the degenerated disc and the pedicle and the vertebral body of the superadjacent vertebra (Fig. 40-12). This is more of a soft tissue problem than the two preceding stenosis patterns and is sometimes difficult to appreciate (Fig. 40-13). It is usually the result of a subanular herniation or severe degeneration and collapse of the intervertebral disk. This problem can be resolved in two

ways. The easiest approach is to excise the lateral anulus, either with a pituitary rongeur or a small knife. The small knife is preferable because it minimizes the fibrosis that may cause the problem to recur (Fig. 40-14). A second approach is to take down the inferomedial aspect of the vertebral pedicle, either with a curette or an osteotome (Fig. 40-15). Certainly both of these techniques are quite delicate, and adequate protection of the neural elements must be provided.

The fourth pattern of neural decompression at the foraminal level occurs in degenerative spondylolisthesis (Fig. 40-16). It is most common at the L4 to L5 level, producing symptoms when the L5 root is caught between the vertebral body of L5 and the advancing inferior facet of L4, which has eroded through the superior facet of the subjacent vertebra. Although these degenerative spondylolistheses will produce a dramatic myelographic defect, often a complete block at L4 to L5, the vertebral body of L4 almost never advances more than one third of the width of the L5 vertebral body. At this point, the L4 inferior facets impinge on the body of L5 and halt the progressive spondylolisthesis. Many articles have discussed the propensity for this problem in patients with a low intercrestal line, but it is seen very commonly throughout maturity. Again, the appropriate response is to free the entrapped nerve root at the sacrifice of part of the facet joint.

Residual spinal stability

It is apparent that the resolution of the more lateral and complex patterns of spinal stenosis usually involves some sacrifice of the facet joints. This brings us to our final consideration, the residual spinal stability when some elements of the posterior spine have been ablated. Again, many attempts to organize this information can be found in the literature, but the best approach remains a simple one. The rule of thumb now accepted among spinal surgeons is to retain the total of one facet joint at each spinal level. That is, a unilateral hemifacetectomy or even complete facetectomy can be performed without significantly compromising the stability of the lumbar spine. A bilateral hemifacetectomy will likewise leave enough facet joint to prevent spondylolisthesis (Figs. 40-17 and 40-18). Bilateral complete facetectomies, however, render the spine unstable and must be treated with a lumbar fusion (Fig. 40-19).

Text continued on p. 435.

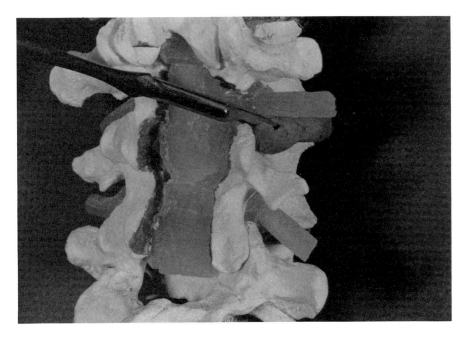

Fig. 40-14. A knife can be used to perform a partial annulectomy, thus freeing the nerve root entrapped between the bulging disk and the superior pedicle body.

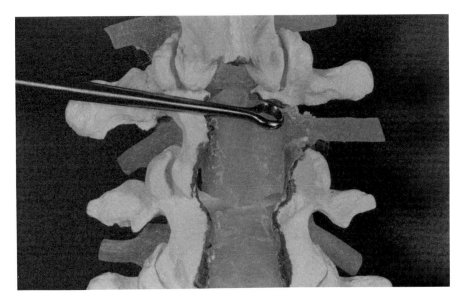

Fig. 40-15. An alternative method of decompression is to remove the inferior medial portion of the pedicle with either a curette or an osteotome.

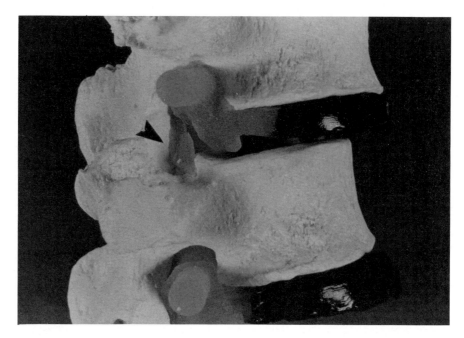

Fig. 40-16. In degenerative spondylolistheses the neural elements are entrapped between the advancing inferior facets of the slipped vertebra and the body of the vertebra below.

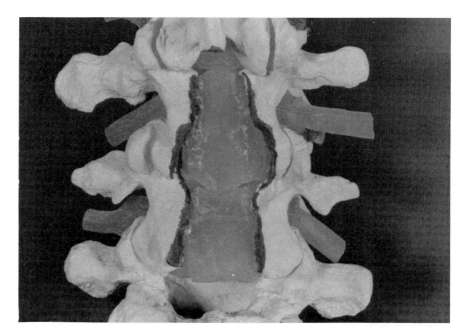

Fig. 40-17. Here both lateral recesses have been decompressed by a hemifacetectomy. Nonetheless, a total of one facet joint remains at this level, and the spine is relatively stable.

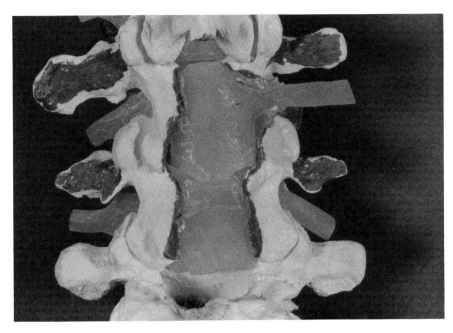

Fig. 40-18. A complete facetectomy on the right and a hemifacetectomy on the left leaves less than the total of one facet joint, and lumbar fusion should be considered.

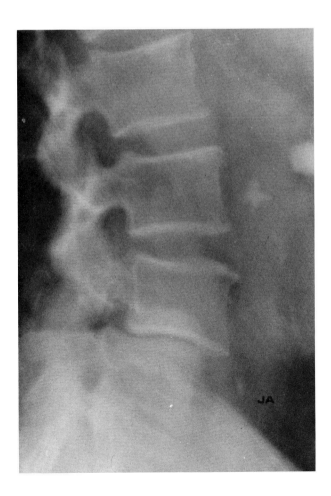

Fig. 40-19. A lateral x-ray film demonstrates a degenerative spondylolisthesis that has slipped almost to its maximal extent of one third the vertebral body. Because of the disk-space collapse and the patient's advanced age, the spine is relatively stable at this level.

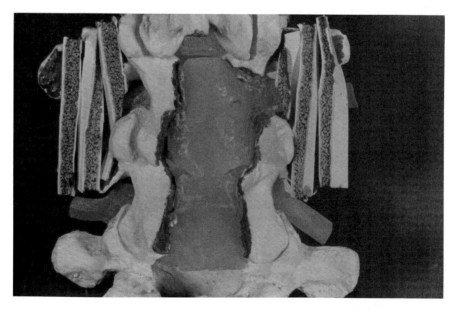

Fig. 40-20. A and **B,** Lateral flexion-extension myelograms demonstrate instability with occlusion of the dye column in extension. In this young and dynamic form of spinal stenosis, fusion would probably be appropriate.

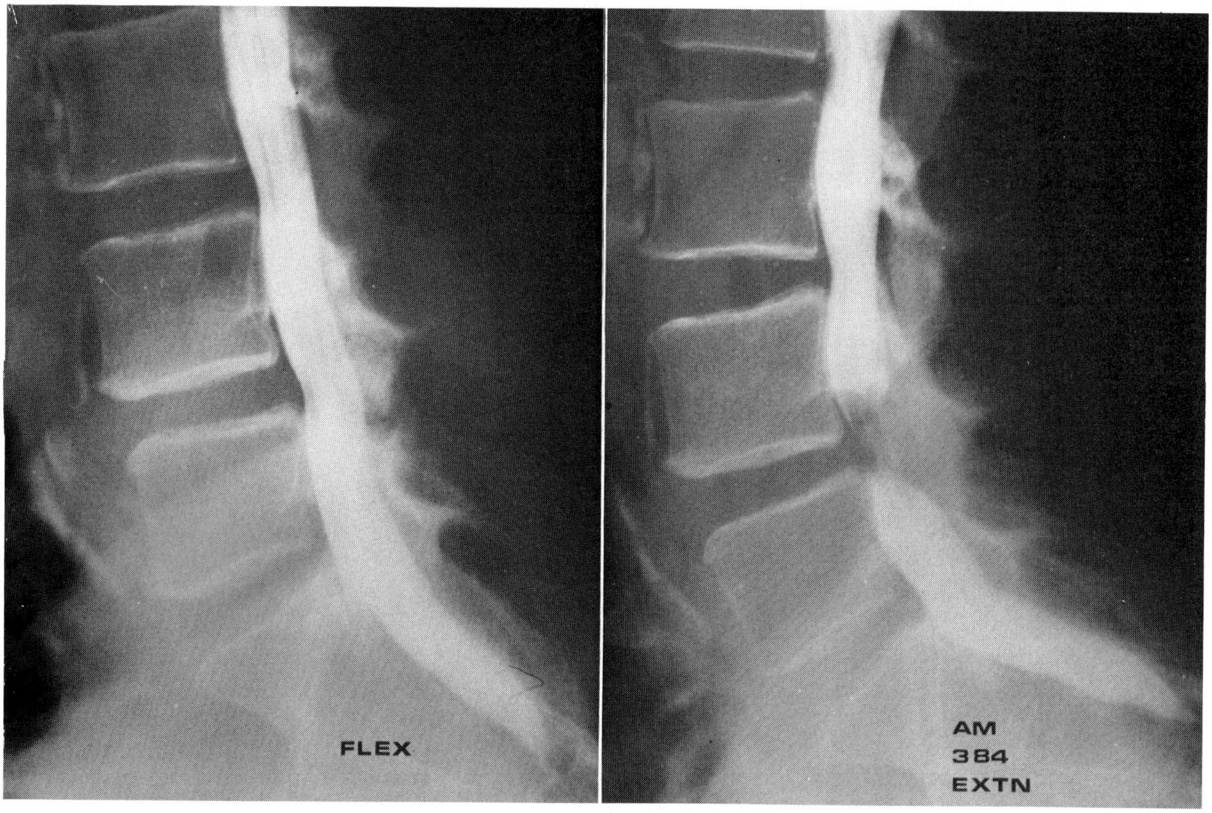

Fig. 40-21. A bilateral lateral fusion has been performed with cortico-cancellous bone strips being applied to the decorticated transverse processes and lateral gutters of the L4 and L5 vertebrae.

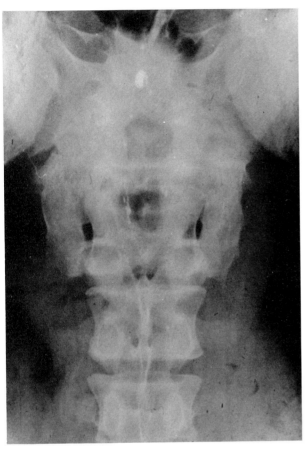

Fig. 40-22. A mature and stable bilateral lateral fusion is seen in this anteroposterior x-ray film of the lumbar spine.

My own indications for lumbar fusion in spinal stenosis include the excision of more than one facet joint at any spinal level, a patient under the age of 50, individuals with a low intercrestal line or a "dynamic spinal stenosis" as seen on flexion extension films. This last syndrome is not seen very commonly, although the lateral flexion-extension myelograms in Fig. 40-20, *A* and *B* show such an individual with a normal myelogram in flexion and complete occlusion of the dye column in extension. These individuals have a dynamic stenosis in every sense of the word, and

the progressive disk collapse after lumbar decompression is likely to produce significant spondylolisthesis and axial symptoms, as well as appendicular symptoms.

Lumbar fusion

When lumbar fusion is to be performed, the preferential approach is a bilateral lateral fusion, after the manner of Wiltse.[7] This usually can be done rather easily through the midline approach (Figs. 40-21 and 40-22). The ablation of the posterior elements in spinal stenosis surgery usually precludes the consideration of a midline fusion in any event, but the bilateral lateral fusion is to be preferred to midline posterior, posterior lumbar interbody, or anterior lumbar interbody fusions. Although supplemental techniques such as autogenous fat grafting, electrical stimulation of fusions, and internal and external supports have been used, the real success of spinal stenosis surgery lies in the control of hemorrhage, the treatment of the proper spinal levels, and the adequacy of decompression and stabilization. If these techniques and principles are kept in mind, the high level of success achieved in simple disk surgery can be approximated, and a happy result will ensue for both the surgeon and the patient.

BIBLIOGRAPHY

1. Burton, C.V.: Successful surgical management of lateral spinal stenosis. In Stouffer, E.S., editor, Instructional course lectures: The American Academy of Orthopaedic Surgeons, vol. 24, St. Louis, 1985, The C.V. Mosby Co.
2. Kirkaldy-Willis, W.H., and McIvor, G.W.D.: Spinal stenosis, Clin. Orthop. **115:**2-144, 1976.
3. Kirkaldy-Willis, W.H., Wedge, J.H., Yong-Hing, K., and Reily, J.: Pathology and pathogenesis of lumbar spondylosis and stenosis, Spine **3:**319-328, 1978.
4. Rothman, R.H., and Simeone, F.A., The spine, vol. 1, Philadelphia, 1982, W.B. Saunders Co.,
5. Tarlov, I.M.: The knee-chest position for lower spine operations, J. Bone Joint Surg. **49A**(6):1193-1194, 1967.
6. Verbiest, H.: A radicular syndrome from developmental narrowing of the lumbar vertebral canal, J. Bone Joint Surg. **36B:**230-237, 1954.
7. Wiltse, L.L.: The paraspinal sacrospinalis-splitting approach to the lumbar spine, Clin. Orthop. **35:**116-122, 1964.

Index